Multidimensional Approach to Quality of Life Issues

Braj Raj Kumar Sinha
Editor

Multidimensional Approach to Quality of Life Issues

A Spatial Analysis

Springer

Editor
Braj Raj Kumar Sinha
Department of Geography
Institute of Science
Banaras Hindu University
Varanasi, Uttar Pradesh, India

ISBN 978-981-13-6957-5 ISBN 978-981-13-6958-2 (eBook)
https://doi.org/10.1007/978-981-13-6958-2

Library of Congress Control Number: 2019934350

This Springer imprint is published by the registered company Springer Nature Singapore Pte Ltd.
The registered company address is: 152 Beach Road, #21-01/04 Gateway East, Singapore 189721, Singapore

Foreword by P. P. Karan

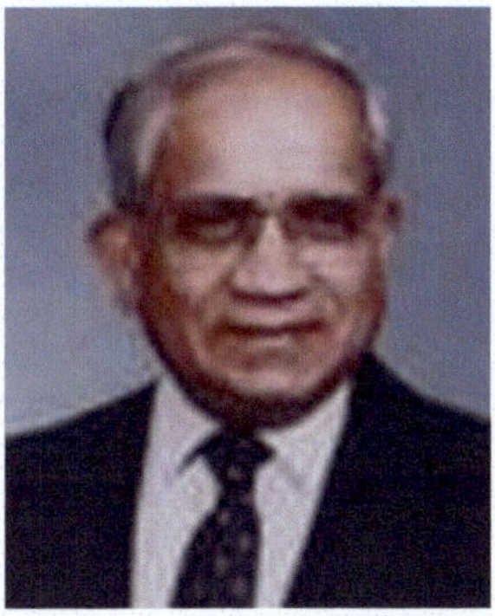

Professor Braj Raj Kumar Sinha's edited volume on the quality of life comes not a moment too soon. The quality of life has stagnated in most countries. In addition to economic, environmental and social evaluations of both positive and negative aspects of life, aspects of culture, values and spirituality are also the key domains of the overall quality of life. This book contributes to the overall assessment of the quality of life in various regions and countries. The contributors brought together in this volume represent some of the most incisive minds working on various aspects of the broader quality of life in various areas of the world. They are experts and researchers. Their individual insights and findings have been drawn together and multiplied through the masterful curation of Prof. Sinha, who has a rich tradition of scholarly research focused on human resources and the quality of life. This book brings insight and ideas on the quality of life from scholars around the world, and their expertise on the topic is deep and broad. Focusing on a range of key issues, the book has captured the scale and complexity of as well as the need for resetting policies at the national and state levels. It is rare to find a group of scholars as accomplished and diverse as those represented in this volume. Their research builds a strong foundation for a real dialogue about the quality of human resources at a time when a generational change in human resources will set the course for decades to come.

This book will promote an international conversation which will help provide a crucible for new ideas and a new commitment to research that could restore the path to a better quality of life. This excellent volume will be a very valuable resource to key policy framers and decision-makers as well as scholars in social sciences interested in the quality of human resources.

Lexington, KY, USA
March 2018

Prof. P. P. Karan
University Research Professor
Department of Geography
College of Arts and Science
University of Kentucky

Foreword by Sudeepta Adhikari

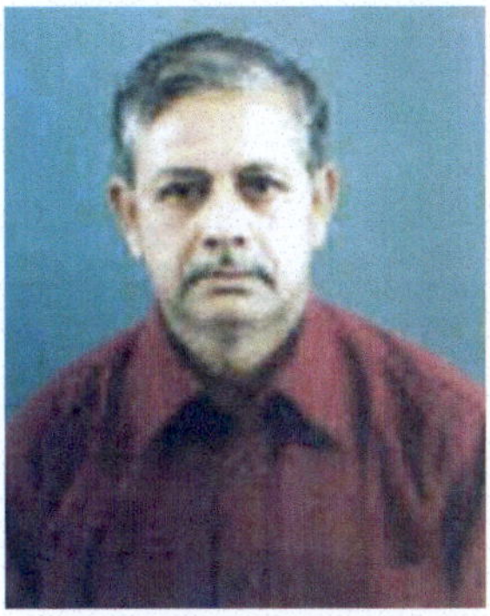

Multidimensional Approach to Quality of Life Issues: A Spatial Analysis is an edited volume by Prof. Braj Raj Kumar Sinha that necessarily comprises chapters on various issues, pertaining to the quality of life. Contributors of the chapters of the book, belonging to the countries of the developed world, developing world and underdeveloped world, or more specifically of the countries of the core economy, peripheral economy and semi-peripheral economy, have attempted to elucidate the meaning of the quality of life in their respective countries through their valued contributions. Contributors of the developed and/or the core economy countries like the USA, the UK and Canada in their respective contributions to the volume have attempted to reveal their conceptualizations of the quality of life, and impending issues, while the contributors of the peripheral countries (vast majority of the countries of the world belong to the category of the peripheral economy, with no role, or stake in the world economy) like Nigeria, Romania, Bangladesh, Nepal, Sri Lanka, etc., in their respective contributions to the volume have spoken of it in different ways, which do not specify clearly the philosophical and methodological stances of the quality of life. The contributors of the semi-peripheral countries like China and India in their respective contributions to the volume have drawn a parallel between the developed and underdeveloped *episteme* of the quality of life and made their deductions over the issues. Conceptually, the concept of the quality of life is multidisciplinary, and as such, it is holistic, because it incorporates every aspect of human's daily life in its fold. It is not exclusively economic; rather, it has cultural, social, political and recreational underpinnings. The volume is well expressive of the varied views of different corners of the world on the quality of life and related issues of it. Most of the contributions to the volume are scientific in nature, but a few contributions reveal a sustained kind of phenomenological underpinnings. The volume is, therefore, characterized by such contributions that tend to make it an *exemplar* that might open up new opportunities for further researches (both applied and fundamental) on the quality of life. The edited volume will be highly useful to academics, bureaucracy and planners, particularly those involved and engaged in both micro-level planning and macro-level planning, pertaining to improving and enhancing the human quality of life.

(Sudeepta Adhikari)

Patna, Bihar
January 2019

Dr. Sudeepta Adhikari
Professor of Geography
Department of Geography
Patna University

Preface

The quality of life is a global challenge for the twenty-first century. It is a multidimensional concept and includes various social, cultural, economic, political, demographic and environmental aspects. These aspects play a foundational role in the life condition of people everywhere. The quality of life is a key element of social planning, the aim of which is to promote and enhance the quality of life of an individual; of a family or inhabitants of a village, town, region, state and nation; and of the world by reducing detrimental conditions or circumstances over a given time. In this direction, the sustainable development and environmental justice approach would positively work in maintaining and promoting the quality of life of people.

Despite these, studies on the quality of life in the field of geography have been scanty as geographers haven't to date paid much attention to this topic. The significance of space, time and society (the main domain of geographers) in the context of QOL has prompted me to collect and compile scholarly contributions from across continents in book form to fill an important gap in the literature on QOL.

This book includes 27 chapters, and these are organized into four parts. **Part I** includes six papers and systematically describes the perspective of theoretical dimension.

'Introduction: An Overview of the Quality of Life' as a first chapter by **the Editor** is of special interest to the readers as it addresses in greater detail the historical perspective, concepts and definition, dimensions, significance, determinants, indicators and method of evaluating the quality of life. Such a comprehensive picture on the quality of life in a holistic form is scarcely available in the existing literature of the subject under study.

The work of **Upuli Perera and Collins Adjei Manesh (UK)** on 'Housing Affordability as a Reflexivity of Quality of Life' is a significant contribution to this book. They address housing as one of the basic necessities of life. According to them, housing enhances the quality of life of individuals in diverse ways. This chapter specifically explores the reflexivity of housing affordability on the quality of life. It starts first by discussing the concept of the quality of life and highlights various elements or attributes of the quality of life. It continues by focusing on the concept of housing and housing affordability to trace the divergent views expressed on these concepts and how these views influence the quality of life. The last section of this chapter treats housing affordability and its reflexivity on the quality of life by discussing how the indicators and measurement of housing affordability have changed over space and time and how such changes have reflected in the present thinking of the quality of life. The chapter makes significant contributions in both theory and practice. It contributes to the existing knowledge on the concept of the quality of life by bringing on board housing affordability and its linkages with the quality of life. It also highlights various elements or indicators that are critical to both housing affordability and the quality of life that policy-makers can dwell on to make informed decisions to enhance the well-being of the general public.

Christopher Cusack (USA) took into consideration the sustainable development and the quality of life as an important global issue and tries to focus on historical evidence and present concerns, connecting sustainability with the quality of life, well-being and human development, well-being and environmental performance as well as on planning for sustainable cities. In his opinion, the quality of life addresses peoples' perceptions of their position in life in relation to their culture, values and expectations, and environmental protection, economic growth and social equity. These are the important aspects of quality of life.

The study of **Vinita Yadav (New Delhi)** on 'Quality of Life: Dimensions and Measurement' is based on theoretical concepts. She said measuring gross national product (GNP) and per capita measures defined the quality of life in the 1970s. The measurement did reflect the economic growth of the country but did little to assess the qualitative aspects of individuals. The sustainability of the economic momentum and its trickle-down effect on the quality of life were questioned. The quality of life assessment at only societal level provides limited solution, so measurement shall be at societal and individual levels to bring differential assessment. With an emphasis on smart cities within region, the emphasis has again been laid in policies on equitable and effective balanced development of the region. In the light of this, the paper tries to resolve the mystery regarding the concepts, definitions and measurement of the quality of life.

Agomoni Tikadar (Kolkata) has thrown light on the social indicators of the quality of life. She considered social indicators as a tool for the observation and analysis of social change. The social change essentially means people living a better life, witnessing the fulfilment of not only economic needs but also social, psychological and other needs. According to her, this aspect of the quality of life can be studied with the help of social indicators in social sciences. Therefore, this chapter deals with the development of the concept of the quality of life. It includes the subjective and objective perspectives, utilitarian and capability approach as well as the welfare approach. The nature of social indicators used in assessing the quality of life has also been discussed from two subjective and objective perspectives.

The study of the quality of life of slum dwellers as carried out by **Brijendra Nath Singh and Braj Raj Kumar Sinha (Varanasi)** is based on the theoretical approach. In their opinion, the quality of life of slum dwellers is generally poor due to the lack of basic facilities and services. Their poor living and economic conditions, the result of inadequate access to safe water, sanitation and other infrastructures, unemployment or low-paid workers, poor housing quality, over-crowding and insecure residential status in combination with other reasons degrade their quality of life. As a result, they remain a vulnerable section of the society. Rapid urbanization is one of the important causes of the growth of slums. This study aims at representing the conceptual background of different aspects of the quality of life of the slum dwellers. In this, the authors have focused on the concepts and definition of the quality of life, selecting criteria/indicators of determining the quality of life, salient characteristics and concepts and methods in studying the quality of life of slum dwellers in space and time.

Part II includes the description and analysis of seven chapters relating to different demographic dimensions.

An assessment and evaluation of Status of Quality of Life and its Distribution in Nepal by **Krishna Prasad Poudel (Nepal)** is of great academic interest. This chapter is based on the ideas of human development and highlights the condition of the quality of life in spatio-temporal context after the restoration of democracy in 1990. Nepal has been practising more liberal and participatory democratic practices in the development process, and as a result, the distribution of the quality of life was expected to be more equitable, justifiable and uniformly distributed over the country. But database information reveals not much difference between 1996 and 2014 even despite the changes in the political system, governance pattern and power nexus after the people's movement and restoration of democracy in the 1990s. The expectation of people towards the change in their quality of life after the restoration of democracy did not match properly. It also has a widening gap between a few accessible core districts and several peripheral inaccessible districts. Therefore, a better corrective measure has to be adopted for the enhancement of the quality of life of the people as a whole.

S. M. Shah Mahmood and Ishrat Islam (Bangladesh) have made a sincere attempt in demonstrating the underlying facts relating to involuntary displacement and its impact on the quality of life in the eastern fringe of Dhaka. Several land development projects in the fringe area of Dhaka City cause the local people for involuntary resettlement. This study examines the quality of life of the relocated people in their present and previous locations from socio-economic perspectives. Their study is based on the data collected from 350 relocated families who had to move from their original residence owing to four land development projects of Dhaka. Approximately 3920 families were identified as relocated from these project areas. Findings show that overall socio-economic condition of the relocated people has degraded from their previous status. The occupation of local people at new location was totally changed. Their housing condition and access to utility facilities were also deteriorated. Social network plays a vital role in enhancing the quality of life of people. Respondents explained that they lost their social network due to move from their original locations. This research would be a guiding source for the policy-makers to deal with the issues as per rules and regulations.

Onipede Wusu (Lagos, Nigeria) highlighted the effects of contraception on the quality of life among ever-married men in Nigeria. He pointed out that contraception is low in Nigeria and over 60% of the population is in the undesirable quality of life. Several factors have been fingered for the pervasive poor quality of life, but little was known about the role of contraception, especially among men. This study analysed the 2013 Nigeria Demographic and Health Survey male data. The analysis involved 8828 ever-married males, aged 15–49. Hierarchical regression technique was used. The results show that national awareness of any contraceptives was 99%, ranging between 94% (modern method = 93%) in north-east and 98% (modern method = 97%) in south-south. The use of any method was highest in south-west (36%; modern methods = 24%) and lowest in north-west (7%; modern method = 2%). The condom was most used in all regions. The R-square change of the hierarchical regression indicates that contraception elevated the explanatory power of the model in all regions. The new R-square ranged between 26% in south-east and 61% in north-west, with an increase ranging between 0.2% in south-west and 0.6% in north-central. After adjusting for selected socio-economic factors, modern contraception and the quality of life's indicators were significantly and positively associated with north-central ($\beta = 0.05, p < 0.01$), north-east ($\beta = 0.04, p < 0.05$), north-west ($\beta = 0.03, p < 0.05$) and south-west ($\beta = 0.05, p < 0.05$). Traditional methods significantly and negatively predicted the quality of life in north-central ($\beta = -0.06, p < 0.01$) but positively in north-east ($\beta = 0.04, p < 0.05$) and north-west ($\beta = 0.06, p < 0.001$). Therefore, modern contraception and traditional contraception are the significant factors in any efforts targeting the elevation of male's quality of life in almost all regions in Nigeria.

According to **Mahmood Aslam and Sushil Dalal (New Delhi)**, the quality of life can be assessed by analysing living conditions such as the standard, the level and the living style of people. It can be inquired objectively by generating a list of information such as economic activities, social conditions and living environment. Displacement and resettlement of human population due to the construction of large dams affect the physical and social conditions of the displaced families. The resultant resettlement process modifies the source of income and changes the expenditure and consumption patterns and the nature of disease at household level. In this paper, they have made their attempt to examine the subjective as well as the objective quality of life in terms of economic activities and social conditions such as health and education through an understanding of living environment among the Bhil and related tribes which have been displaced by the construction of Sardar Sarovar Dam on River Narmada in the western part of India. The socio-economic conditions of this tribe after resettlement have taken a turn towards realignment through redistribution of land and division of labour in both agricultural and non-agricultural sectors of economy. Social and cultural changes have also taken place among the tribal communities after their resettlement.

Fazeeha Azmi (Sri Lanka) highlights the perceptions of the quality of life among the first generation of protracted women IDPs in Mandalakkuda camp in the district of Puttalam, Sri Lanka. The purpose of her study was to explore the perceptions about the quality of life among the first and second generations of protracted internally displaced women who were living in Mandalakkuda camp in the district of Puttalam. The study is based on the 20 qualitative interviews with women from the first and second generations. Collected information and data were analysed under emerging themes in the interviews. Perception of the quality of life was found varying significantly across different generations. Women from the first generation valued mainly the non-material aspect of quality of life, while second-generation women emphasized much on the non-material aspect of the quality of life.

The work of **S. C. Mukhopadhyay (Kolkata)** is on the 'Aspects of the Quality of Life in India and its Macro Region'. He made an attempt to reveal the facts that density of population in India, in general, and north-east macro-region India, in particular, have been increasing (2011 Census) very rapidly since 1991. An analysis of 2011 Census revealed that the higher rate of population growth has increased large number of population in India especially in the east and north-east macro-regions including Andaman–Nicobar Islands. This causes difficulty in maintaining the quality of life in both the rural and urban areas as referred by the sociologists, economists and politicians. Recently, the economists have highlighted an index of the quality of life (2005) with the major eight points like material well-being, health, political stability and security, family life, community life, climate and geography, job security and political freedom. They have also presented an idea of the quality of life in terms of different statistics, regression statistics—tables of some countries score from 1 to 10 (Global 2005) including the so-called developing–undeveloped countries.

Assessment and evaluation of Quality of Life Among the Aged in India: Anthropological Insights as carried out by **Reetinder Kaur and Rohit Kumar (Chandigarh)** are of great academic interest. Their study is an attempt to understand the dimensions of life satisfaction and the quality of life among the rural elderly. Their study is based on the data collected from the 160 elderly living in and around Naggar Village situated in District Kullu of Himachal Pradesh. The results of their study show that the elderly describe their life satisfaction in terms of financial self-sufficiency, social network and social support, religious disposition and satisfaction with their health conditions. They have suggested that a holistic all-inclusive policy must be drafted to address the life satisfaction and the quality of life issues among the elderly in India, especially the elderly women.

Part III combines the description and analysis of seven chapters relating to sociocultural and economic dimension of the quality of life.

Nurul Islam Nazem and Md. Anwar Hossain (Bangladesh) made an assessment and evaluation of Strategic Infrastructure Supporting the Quality of Life in Dhaka. Their paper explores the role of strategic infrastructure in facilitating a good living environment to live a quality life. They have argued that the presence of adequate service infrastructure with good accessibility by the people provides a better quality life. The paper highlights that Dhaka has been suffering from a high infrastructure deficit. The failure of plan for adequate infrastructure, especially for transportation network, housing, drainage, water, sanitation and electricity substantially add to development costs. It is not only the present level of infrastructure but also that Dhaka fails to protect its future infrastructure provisions due to poor planning and management. The study also shows that where infrastructure has been planned and provided, they have been supported required impulses towards the quality living of the people. Besides physical infrastructure, social and economic infrastructures are equally important. Health and education facilities and services which are highly inadequate in the region make Dhaka one of the poorly living city regions in the world.

Spatial analysis of educational facilities and the quality of life in Haveri District of Karnataka as carried out by **Nagaraj H., S. L. Karlawad and L. M. Pujar (Mysore)** provides an empirical example of current research in spatial context in India. They emphasized the adequacy of appropriate educational facilities for the improvement in life quality of modern civilized community. They have used health, education, social, economic and other aspects as suitable criteria in measuring the quality of life. They underlined that these indicators among others reflect the quality of functioning of a social system and efficiency of its economic welfare. They have made an attempt to examine the spatial distribution of educational facilities, identify the different levels of educational facilities in the district and suggest the priorities to reduce spatial disparities in the quality of life. For the fulfilment of these objectives, they have employed a composite Z-score method.

The chapter of **Angshumita Chakraborty and L. N. Satpati (Kolkata)** on 'Vulnerability, Resilience and Quality of Life: A Micro Level Study of Ghoramara Island in the Sundarban Region of West Bengal, India' is also an important chapter to this volume. The study area 'Ghoramara' selected for the present problem is an isolated island of the Sundarban which has already become popular as a vanishing island. Frequent attack of different environmental hazards like cyclone, flood, tidal surge, periodic waterlogging, etc., arising out of extreme climate events affects the quality of life of the islanders. As a result, poor and marginalized people suffer the most, resulting in poor living condition as well as outmigration of the inhabitants in a large number and emergence of environmental refugees. In this context, this paper focuses on different dimensions of resilience like human, financial, social, physical and natural capital of the people of the study area to deal with climatic shocks so that it helps to strengthen the adaptive capacity of the vulnerable community to sustain a decent quality of life of this fragile area.

The study of **Gary Greening and George M. Pomroy (USA)** on parks, recreation and other open space areas is an interesting and useful addition to this volume because these activities generally provide numerous quality of life benefits and typically have positive impacts on property values. For a complete understanding of different dimensions of such benefits and impacts on the quality of life, the authors have taken into consideration the South Middleton Township (a less studied suburban area) for a case study. The authors have employed the regression analysis to see the impact of adjacency and proximity of parks and open space on the quality of life and assessed property values. They stated that the results of the statistical analysis are not conclusive, suggesting a need for further consideration across a wider number of municipalities and open space types.

Industrialization and urbanization being the cultural phenomena contribute a lot to the social, cultural and economic development and life condition of the people of an area. **Aurel Gheorghilaş (Romania)** in his paper has made an attempt to highlight the impact of restructuring of two important Romanian automotive industries (S.C. Aro S.A. Câmpulung Muscel and S.C. Automobile Dacia S.A. Pitesti) on the features of the geographical space and the demographic profile such as age, sex, rural–urban migration, a concentration of population mainly in the urban areas, suburbanization, expansion of the urban network, functional integration of rural settlements in metropolitan regions and quality level of life.

A study on anthropogenic activities and its impact on the social well-being and health condition of people living on wetlands/water bodies conducted by **Ishtiaq A. Mayer, Sheraz A. Lone and Manzoor A. Wani (Srinagar, Kashmir)** is a very informative and important contribution to this book. In this paper, Ishtiaq and his co-authors have thrown light on geographic environment, income status, economic activities, housing pattern, morbidity pattern and its role in projecting inequalities in well-being of a particular section of people (boatmen) in Srinagar City, India. They have also stressed on formulating a holistic policy for the future location/allocation of healthcare facilities in accordance with physical accessibility to duly serve the need for the welfare of population of Srinagar City.

Michael O'Neal Campbell (Canada) has presented another interesting paper and stated that the human quality of life is influenced not only by the societal relations and the physical environment, but also by human–animal relations. This chapter examines the links between QOL and possibilities for big cat—human reintroductions in El Salvador. There is evidence of societal support for big cat reintroductions as supportive of QOL and conservation. However, there may be serious impacts on QOL from such reintroductions, due to the small size of the country, high human population density, the reduction in suitable habitat due to past war, the proximity of such habitat to farmland and urban centres as well as the lowered population of prey animals. Isolated forests, excessive human hunting of prey animals and the devastating effects of the recent civil war also militate against a successful reintroduction.

Part IV comprises seven papers and exhibits the underlying facts or ideas relating to urban- and environment-related dimension of the quality of life.

Keshav Bhattarai and Dalerne Budd (USA) have presented a literature-based study on the quality of life (QoL) and evaluated the environmental, physical, psychological, social, economic and political dimensions concerning the quality of life. In support of this, they have taken into consideration Nepal as a case study where rapidly growing municipalities face sustainability issues due to the lack of resources and essential infrastructure. Their study reveals that rural-to-urban migration and emigration to other countries have contributed to the separation of family members. Similarly, divided families cause various types of serious social disruptions. So in order to improve the QoL, small- and medium-sized cities need investment in infrastructure and basic services, while metropolitan cities require competitive development strategies, efficient policy-making, urban and regional planning and environmental management. The quality of life of rural people is possible through the access to essential services.

The chapter of **Gabriel Simion and Marioara Rusu (Romania)** on 'Land Use Patterns: Key Element of Quality of Life in the Metropolitan Area of Bucharest' is a significant contribution to this part of the book because land use and land cover changes are noticed as an emerging trend of study in the field of quality of life. They have made their attempt to characterize different land use patterns in the BMA and identify the goods and services produced by those different land use patterns. The investigations were completed by field observations, questionnaires and interviews with local stakeholders. Secondary data on population were obtained from the National Institute of Statistics. The result of their study pinpoints that within the Bucharest Metropolitan Area land use pattern has undergone a major change over the last 20 years. Such major change is noticed through the conversion of forests and agricultural land into residential, industrial and commercial uses. Such change is observed supporting the quality of life of its population.

The chapter, 'Links between Human Quality of Life and Gulls in Urban Areas', written by **Michael O'Neal Campbell (Canada)** is quite distinct than other papers as it exclusively discusses the role of floral and faunal species on the human quality of life, of course, with a focus upon aesthetic and conflictual aspects. The author in this chapter has demonstrated both the positive and negative impacts of human–avian (gulls) interactions on the human quality of life in urban areas. The positive impacts of close human–avian association include wildlife observation and conservation values. The negative impacts include predation of valuable animals, noise, building and vehicle damage, food theft, intrusive scavenging of human residences and even attacks on people and companion animals. In terms of QOL, the negative impacts outweighed the positive impacts. The positive impacts were nevertheless important enough for more effective management and further study. This analysis is useful for both QOL and conservation studies.

The contribution of **Mariana Nae and Liliana Dumitrache (Romania)** through their study on 'Post-Socialist Urban Changes and Role Strain in Assessing the Quality of Life: The Case of Bucharest, Romania' is of great importance to this part of the book. It is because of the fact that the trend and pattern of urban transformation in the era of rapid urbanization profoundly affect the human quality of life. Urban transformations such as urban fragmentation, urban land use and urban economic restructuring as emphasized in this study are generally caused by multiple driving factors and the expertise of many actors. The study focuses on the potential role strain in assessing the quality of life in Bucharest City after 28 years of post-socialist urban transformations. The authors have taken help of voluminous data and used binary logistic regression to find out the role strain of personal health status, access to health care, unemployment and low wages, housing conditions and housing affordability as well as environmental risks in the assessment of the quality of life. They have extended appropriate suggestions also for the improvement of the quality of life of the city people.

The work of **Jun-Fan Wu (China)** is similar to that of the above contribution. It is also an interesting and useful addition to this volume. Wu Jun-Fan has also opined that there is a close relation of transformation of urban land use with the quality of life. From this viewpoint, the author has taken the Old Shanghai Town, a city located on the eastern edge of the Yangtze Delta, for a detailed study of the transformation of urban land use from the traditional period to the period of modernization with the perspective of the quality of life. The author has tried to explain the connection between the mode of urban land use and regional environment as well as natural and social factors that affect urban land use and the quality of life of the inhabitants of the Old Shanghai Town.

Management of green spaces in urban areas is currently becoming a worldwide focal theme of study in the field of urban environment from the perspective of the human quality of life. In this context, the study of **Michael O'Neal Campbell (Canada)** on 'Adaptive Management of Green Spaces and Life Quality in Glasgow (Scotland) and Ottawa (Canada)' is very appreciative and adds a new thought to this book. He has rightly stated that the green spaces (greenbelts surrounding urban areas and greenhearts within urban areas) are very vital for urban ecological health and the concept of this encompasses air quality, wildlife presence and habitat development, and the human quality of life. According to him, adaptive management (a broadly sourced evaluative methodology for project appraisal) is eminently suitable for the analysis of the role of green spaces in human life quality. The analysis is based on information derived from interviews with personnel employed in relevant institutions, time series images and maps, and point count surveys of birds and mammals. The main focus of this study is on the utility of an adaptive management perspective applied to two established 'green' cities: Glasgow in Scotland (UK) and Ottawa in Canada. Both cases showed the use of tenets of the AM framework, especially at the project identification design and implementation phases, but with more issues at the monitoring and evaluation phases, and consequent possibilities for policy adjustment. The results call for general management theory and urban planning.

The household-level quality of life study from a small town as carried out by **Mahuya Sen and Braj Raj Kumar Sinha (India)** is another important contribution to this volume. The authors have considered household as the basic residential unit for the study. The objective of this chapter was to evaluate the quality of life of urban inhabitants at the household level. For this, Bolpur (a town for national importance) from Birbhum District, West Bengal, eastern India, was taken into consideration as a study area. The study is based on the primary data collected from 350 households. The quality of life at the household level was found varying across the households of different social groups, different educational achievement, income and occupation categories. The quality of life of medium-sized families was found relatively better than that of larger families. Majority of households belong to lower income category. Only a small number of households fall into the category of higher educational achievement but enjoy a better quality of life. The families belonging to service sector also enjoy a better quality of life.

Varanasi, Uttar Pradesh, India Braj Raj Kumar Sinha

Acknowledgements

I am most grateful to each of the contributors to this edited book for his/her scholarly contribution, tremendous support and patience. I would like to express my deep appreciation to Prof. P. P. Karan, a legendary social and cultural geographer of Indian origin, working in the Department of Geography/Japanese Studies, University of Kentucky, Lexington, USA, for his encouragement and foreword. I also wish to keep on record my deep sense of gratitude to Prof. Ashok K. Dutt, an internationally reputed geographer in the field of urban geography and planning; an ambassador of Indian geography to the USA; presently, Professor Emeritus, Geography and Planning; and Professor Emeritus of Urban Studies, The University of Akron, OH 44325-5005 (USA), for his benevolence, good suggestions and academic encouragement. I remain ever grateful to my wife Mrs. Meera Rani Sinha and my daughters Ekta Sinha and Chaitanya Sinha for their love, constant inspiration, assistance, sacrifice, perseverance and endurance in achieving the goal of this publication. Thanks are also due to Ms. Shinjini Chatterjee, Executive Editor, Human Sciences, Springer Nature, New Delhi, for accepting the manuscript, meticulously handling it and finally publishing this book.

Varanasi, Uttar Pradesh, India

Dr. Braj Raj Kumar Sinha
Professor, Department of Geography
Institute of Science
Banaras Hindu University

About This Book

The book titled *Multidimensional Approach to Quality of Life Issues—A Spatial Analysis* is an attempt at viewing the concept of the *quality of life* in varied approaches, angles and dimensions. Different institutions and scholars of social sciences have viewed it in different perspectives. Each has its own way of approaching the concept. A geographer views the concept from spatial and temporal dimensions in order to demonstrate spatial inequality or areal differentiation in the quality of life.

The book is crafted in a way as to incorporate all the major dimensions of the quality of life, and the papers included in this book are of different disciplinary characterizations and reflect each of the dimensions in a very expressive way, with a necessary focus upon *space, place, time* and *society*. Epistemologically, the concept of the quality of life is a holistic one as it takes into the whole. There are 27 papers, belonging to different dimensions and perspectives, drawn from the scholarly contributors from the USA, Canada, the UK, China, Romania, Sri Lanka, Bangladesh, Nigeria, Nepal and India. All the papers have been categorized into four parts: Part I—Theoretical Dimension; Part II—Demographic Dimension; Part III—Sociocultural and Economic Dimension; and Part IV—Urban- and Environment-Related Dimension.

There are a number of books on the quality of life, each with certain disciplinary limitation and boundary. Geography, being a science of synthesis, sustains disciplinary transcending into the fields of science and social sciences and takes into account the *whole*, and therefore, the book provides a comprehensive outlook to the concept of the quality of life. The papers have been arranged accordingly so as to make the book wide-ranging from philosophical and methodological points of view. The book is, by and large, sustained by statistical and cartographic characterization that distinguishes it from the other books, available on the quality of life. The QOL dimensions have been *spatially* evaluated that show another distinctive feature of the book. The book is illustrated with maps, diagrams and tables which facilitate the discourse on QOL and may help the readers to understand the theme at regional, national and international levels. In fact, this book takes a comprehensive view of different dimensions of the quality of life and provides fresh insights into the thought and a broad understanding of the current issues. The book will add a new facet to the existing literatures on the theme under discussion.

All the papers, included in this book, are socially relevant and time-referent, fit and quite useful to understand the complexities of the contemporary social scenario, plagued by material and relational inequalities. Thus, this book will be a source of indispensable reference and serves the interest of geography students and scholars as well as academicians, researchers, research scholars and students of other allied subjects such as economics, sociology, philosophy, anthropology, social work, technology, science and medical science. It will also help those who are engaged in carrying out further research into the field of the quality of life, regardless of their disciplinary affinities, besides being interested in understanding the complex interconnections of different dimensions and issues of the quality of life concept.

Contents

About the Editor

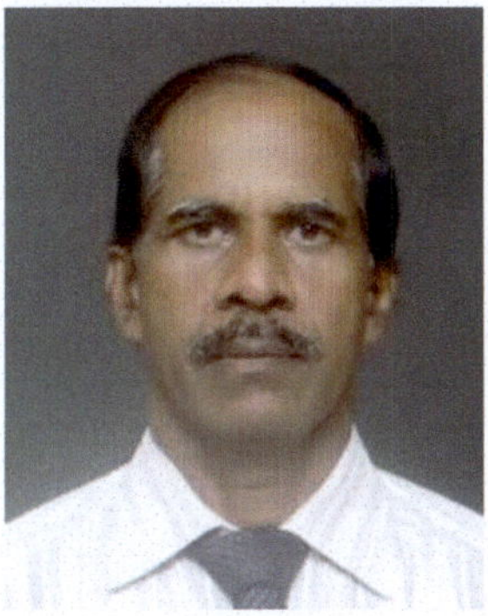

Braj Raj Kumar Sinha is Professor of Geography at Banaras Hindu University, Varanasi, India. He obtained B.A. (Hons.) and M.A. from Patna University, India and Ph.D. from the Maharaja Sayajirao University of Baroda, India. He has previously worked at Visva-Bharati (a Central University), Santiniketan, West Bengal from 1988 to 2007 (last appointment as professor). Professor Sinha's current areas of teaching and research interest are population geography, cartography, resource geography and development studies. He has more than 65 research papers/articles and two books to his credit with national and international publishers. Professor Sinha has been the Vice-President and member of the Executive Council of the National Association of Geographers of India. Dr. Sinha was one of the members of the Editorial Board of the International Journal of Field Studies, UK. He is currently member of the Editorial Board of Human Geographies—Journal of Studies and Research in Human Geography and a member of the International Board of Directors of the Asian Urban Research Association (AURA, Akron, USA). He has visited Czech Republic, South Korea, Romania, UK, USA, Canada, Australia, Thailand and Indonesia for academic purpose.

Part I
Theoretical Dimension

Chapter 1
Introduction: An Overview of the Concept of Quality of Life

Braj Raj Kumar Sinha

Abstract The term '*Quality of Life*' comprises a complex and multidimensional concept, which is rather difficult to define, identify, categorize and analyse. It has vast scope and includes various elements of social, cultural, economic, political and environmental aspects. It is one of the important and challenging social issues of the twenty-first century. Quality of life does not remain the same in the whole life of someone, rather it varies from one stage of lifespan to another and from one type of spatial unit to another because every aspect of life of a person or persons is always influenced by the environment. The study of quality of life of the people of an area can be at any spatial level such as local, regional, national and international level. It can also be studied across social structure such as ethnicity, race, tribes, caste, religion, linguistic culture, gender, age groups, economic and cultural categories, etc. Quality of life of any person or persons of a defined region at a particular point of time is a composite picture of several objective and subjective or quantitative and qualitative variables. This chapter sheds light on the historical perspective, concepts and definition, dimensions, significance, determinants and method of measuring quality of life.

Keywords Multidimensional concept · Environment · Lifespan · Spatial level · Composite picture · Objective and subjective variables

1.1 Epitome

The phrase '*Quality of Life*' comprises a complex and multidimensional concept, which is rather difficult to define, identify, categorize and analyse. It has a very wide scope and includes various elements of social, cultural, economic, political and environmental aspects. This concept has been of great interest to the researchers, academicians, administrators, planners and government officials, because it is a key element of a sincere social planning, the aim of which is to promote and enhance

B. R. K. Sinha (✉)
Department of Geography, Institute of Science, Banaras Hindu University, Varanasi, UP, India
e-mail: sinha_brk@yahoo.co.in

B. R. K. Sinha (ed.), *Multidimensional Approach to Quality of Life Issues*,
https://doi.org/10.1007/978-981-13-6958-2_1

the quality of life of the people by reducing the detrimental conditions of social inequalities or circumstances existing in the society. In fact, it is one of the important and challenging social issues of the twenty-first century. Quality of life does not remain the same in the whole life of someone, rather it varies from one stage of lifespan to another and from one type of spatial unit to another because every aspect of life of a person or persons is always influenced by the environment (the surrounding conditions or situation in which a person or group of persons live and spend time). Such surrounding conditions may be natural/physical, or human, or both together, which is being spoken of as *social milieus*.

In fact, the QOL can be considered as a universal concept which can easily be applied in the context of even a single person or persons or group of persons or people of an area at a given point of time. Therefore, a study of the quality of life of a person or persons or group of persons or people of an area can be at any spatial level such as local, regional, national and international level. For more detail, it can also be studied across social structure such as ethnicity, race, tribes, caste, religion, linguistic culture, gender, age groups; economic and cultural category and so on.

The quality of life is normally interpreted as the condition of life of each person or people of any area which results from the combined effect of a number of factors of ecological, demographic, social, cultural, economic and environmental aspects. The word 'quality' refers to that which makes a particular object what it is! It reflects in identity whereas life is considered as a state of existence of individuals. In view of the fact that quality of life of any person or persons of a society of a defined region at a particular point of time is a composite picture of several variables of objective and subjective categories or of quantitative and qualitative categories. In fact, the quality of life of both the rural and urban people remains as one of the important contemporary social issues in the world. This issue especially for the developing countries remains more crucial and challenging. Therefore, there is a need for an extensive research for more purposeful social planning.

This chapter sheds light on the Historical Perspective, Concepts and Definition, Dimensions, Significance, Determinants and Method of Measuring quality of life.

1.2 Historical Perspective

The following literature in chronological order right from the earlier to the recent period witnesses the development of the concepts of quality of life:

After having gone through the quality of life related literature, it was found that the work of Seth James (1889) was probably the first in the history of development of the concept of quality of life. While discussing the nature of ethical end or standard as social welfare, Seth James (1889, p. 43) stated that 'in order to an ethical theory, we must not regard the mere quantity, but also the quality, of the "life" which forms the moral end'. Seth through this study tried to reflect his premier idea among the scholars that both the 'quantity' and 'quality' of life should be taken into consideration from the point of view of promoting welfare activities to enhance happiness or quality of life of individual members.

Ellwood, C. A. (March 1902, pp. 229–232) carefully went through and intensively studied the earlier works or writings of Aristotle (384–322 B.C.) and tried to reflect ideas or facts and philosophy which Aristotle wrote concerning the individual's 'good life' and 'living well' perceived in the organized 'household', 'village' and 'state' guided by the 'law' or 'science'. In Aristotle's view, the science of the household stands for the 'relations of master and slave, husband and wife, parent and children' and the art of money getting. Such philosophical ideas of him seem to draw attention towards the state or condition of life of an individual or group of individuals residing in the organized household, village, society and state. The art of possessing or getting money should also have a definite limit. The sum of money should be adequate for freedom and a happy life. But it should not be more because the money ends in living well. Everyone has desire to have a desirable life, i.e. a good or happy life and it is possible only by virtue of perfect society or social ethics. For this, a perfect state (the state having virtues of welfare to its people) or in other words, the state which is happy and doing well for 'good and happy life' and 'living well'. Such notions are closer to the concept of quality of life of the people of a particular spatial unit at a given point of time, though the words 'quality of life' was not mentioned in the works of Aristotle.

After integrating the literature concerning the definition and measurement of quality of life **Elyse W. K.** (May 1992, p. 1) found that the concept of quality of life was newer in comparison to the concept of public happiness which was popularly used as a measurable quantity by the political economists in the past. Elyse further pointed out that there is scarce literature about the exact time of the origin of the term 'quality of life'; however, the wider use of quality of life started from 1961, the year during which this term was used in a speech of President Lyndon Johnson. Initially, 'the term was used most often in conjunction with such concerns as environmental pollution or urban deterioration, the context within which it is now used in much broader' scale and received greater attention by the scholars and researchers of different disciplines at global level.

The idea of **Meeberg, G. A.** (1993, pp. 32–38) is almost similar to that of the above. Meeberg also considered quality of life as 'a phrase which was first used shortly after the Second World War and has, since then, been overused and infrequently defined'. Most of the attempts to deal with quality of life occurred in the 1960s.

After consulting relevant literature **Farquhar, M.** (1995, pp. 1439–1440) stated that the term 'quality of life' became more popular after the Second World War. The popularity was increased 'through a range of media from television and magazine advertisements to political speeches and newspaper headlines'. Realizing the importance of this quality of life was given a place 'in the report of President Eisenhower's Commission on National Goals in 1960' with a major focus on objective indicators relating to education, economic growth, health, welfare and the defence of the non-communist world. The late 1960s saw a major shift from the objective indicators to subjective indicators such as 'personal freedom, leisure, emotion, enjoyment, simplicity and personal caring'. The term 'quality of life' was commonly used in speeches and emphasis was given on research in the social and medical science subjects such as sociology, psychology, medical and nursing science, economics, philosophy, history and geography. **Farquhar** also mentioned that from the mid-1970s the term 'clinical interventions' concerning health was also used in the field of medical science along with the increasing importance and use of quality of life in social science. But, in fact, medicine and nursing science focused mainly on quality of life related to health to examine only one domain of quality of life, i.e. physical functioning.

The views of **Roy, I. B.** (1997, p. 229) was similar to that of the above as he also mentioned that prior to the concept of quality of life the term 'life quality' was articulated in the early 1960s and this was first indicated within the 'Report of President Eisenhower's Commission on National Goals', published in 1960 that included concern with individual's views on such issues as health and welfare. Latter in **1964**, **Lyndon B. Johnson** made a speech in which he coined the term quality of life and made clear the distinction between objective and subjective components.

Bowling, A. (1999, p. 10) tried to focus on evaluating and measuring health-related quality of life and while doing so he pointed out that the 'quality of life was introduced by Medline as a heading in 1975, and accepted as a concept by Index Medicus in 1977'. He also mentioned that right from 1970s there had been 'an explosion of interest in the subject, with an increasing number of citations of quality of life in the medical literature'.

Smith, A. (Nov 2000, pp. 2–5) noted that the concept of quality of life was found related to Aristotle's (384–322 B.C.) ideas of 'the good life' and 'living well'. After searching literature, Allison found that 'the first use of the term quality and life was found in an article written by James Seth in 1889 (p. 43)'. Seth believed in morality and put forth the statement that while talking about quality of the 'life' one must consider both the quantity and quality domains of life. Quality of life emerged as an important concept particularly in the second half of the twentieth century. Smith emphasized that the use of the word quality of life in both official and non-official discussions as well as global curiosity of research grew from 1950s. Latter in 1994 several countries such as Denmark, Canada and United Kingdom laid much more emphasis on the study of quality of life and started quality of life research centres, funds were generated and studies carried out for enhancing the quality of life of the people. In addition to such attempts, the World Bank, World Health Organization and the United Nations were also actively engaged in enhancing the quality of life of people of developing and war-affected countries.

After having gone through the literature related to quality of life, **Forward, S.** (Sept 2003, p. 5) stated that the concept of quality of life is not the exclusive result of the twentieth century, it has a link to the historic idea of Aristotle (384–322 BC) referring to the terms 'the good life' and 'living well'. He advocated that the quality of life became very interesting topic of research during the recent period of his work. He studied the work of Smith (2000, p. 4) and quoted that 'the term quality of life was first used in a statement by James Seth in 1889'. Smith himself noted this statement from the article of Seth, J. (1889, p. 43). Forward, Sonja also further tried to make a temporal link with the advancement in the concepts of quality of life through his review of related literature between 1930 and 2002. After reviewing literature related to quality of life, **Massam, B. H.** (2002, p. 144) explained that from 1930s onward different researchers from different areas took an initiative and interest in 'defining, investigating and measuring QOL using different perspectives'. Particularly, 1933 was marked as an important year for William Ogburn (a sociologist from Chicago) who prepared the two-volume report on 'the recent social trends' for the Hoover administration and opened the way to appear the quality of life as one of the developmental items of the then government. Latter in 1960, the students of Ogburn made a significant contribution 'in the emergence of the social indicators' Sharpe, A. (1999, p. 6). Sharpe noted that this effort gave impetus to the blossom of the social indicators movement in the 1970s in dealing with the quality of life concept in social sciences. Similarly, Massam (2002, p. 144) also noted that development in the field of computer science in the 1970s helped increase social indicator and quality of life movement as well as creation of a specialized journal 'the social indicator research' as an important event. Forward, S. (Sept 2003, p. 5) took the idea from a Baltimore journalist and noted that the study of quality of life involves both the objective criteria such as 'income, education, crime rates, housing prices and infant mortality' and the subjective criteria such as 'people's feelings about their neighbourhood and the environment'. Some valuable works carried out before 1960 were also praiseworthy in the field of advancement of the concept of quality of life. The work of Samuel Ordway (1953) and Fairfield Osborn (1954) was also a step forward in the area of quality of life. (**Snoek, F. J.**, 2000, p. 24) stated that 'there is no certainty as to the origin of the term Quality of Life' but favoured the work of Samuel Ordway and Fairfield Osborn as a milestone in the field of quality of life. Further, he gave more emphasis on quality of life than that on the quantity of goods. **Forward, S.** (Sept 2003, p. 5) further noted that the scholars working in the field of quality of life between 1950 and 2000 gave more emphasis on the qualitative attributes of subjective category such as 'health, education, personal freedom, enjoyment and welfare' in defining the concept of happy and well life, rather than the quantitative or material indicators of quality of life. This caused more interest among the scholars to work in the field of quality of life. As a result, Denmark, Canada and United Kingdom established several research centres with a view to study the quality of life of their people. In addition to this, the World Bank, World Health Organization and the United Nations also worked and contributed a lot for the enhancement of quality of life of people globally.

Berlim, M. T. & Fleck, M. P. A. (2003, p. 249) have focused on the relation between the condition of life and health and described that in the earlier period the term 'good life' instead of the term 'quality of life' was commonly used by the experts of different disciplines. They considered that the 'concept of "quality of life" is a fairly new one'. According to them, the QOL became as a catchphrase in 1975 in medical literature but its effective and methodical study began in the early 1980s particularly in oncology and soon it came out into existence as a significant trait of medical examination related to disease and its treatment.

Similarly, **Pennacchini, M., Bertolaso, M., Elvira, M. M., & De Marinis, M. G.** (2011, pp. 99–103) mentioned in the abstract of their paper that the catchword 'quality of life' was popularly used in the literature of medicine and philosophy. Practitioners in medicine and philosophers started using quality of life as an indicator in dealing with health-related matters in the 1960s and 1970s. As a result, scientists working in the field of medicine and philosophy during these periods showed their enthusiasm in preparing and examining the tools or implements to be used in measuring health and quality of life. Nevertheless, such tools or implements were found lacking with some notional and technical difficulties in the use of quality of life in medical science. At the same time, some investigators regarded quality of life as a condition of individual life, whereas in the opinion of some others, it was found useful with a view to treat a patient, and therefore suggestions were made for the improvement in the concept and approach of the subject. Similarly, 1980s and 1990s also witnessed the difference of opinion among the thinkers and philosophers engaged in studying quality of life. Some scholars and philosophers in 1980s believed in the ethical decisions based on the expected outcome or consequences of the action. Such scholars 'used QoL to formulate moral judgment' and were known as the 'consequentialist philosophers'. As against them, the scholars of 1990s believed in 'health and happiness', the result of subjective approach and they were known as 'welfarist philosophers'. Thereafter, conceptual concern of scholars with regard to quality of life declined. But physician's interest in the use of quality of life in medical practices continued.

Fagge, R. (2012) wrote 'the Disillusioning of Mr. Priestely, Chap. 4' in which he stated that in 1953, J. B. Priestley told readers of the New Statesman that the 'The English People should have a good life', a statement that included an element of desperation as he believed that this good life was slipping further from view in the years following 1945. Priestley's wartime doubts about the saliency of the post-war world, and its ability to deliver a decent QOL for the people of Britain, hardened in the years that followed as he became progressively more disillusioned with the rise of mass society, the Cold War and pattern of domestic politics.

The work of **Kladivo, P. & Halás, M.** (2012, pp. 49–50) on quality of life is also important. According to them, the works on quality of life first appeared in the 1960s and the 1970s. The works carried out during these periods were from a psychological or an environmental side. The role of some geographers in studying social indicators of quality of life in spatial context was also important particularly during the 1970s. The work of Smith, D. M. (1973) on the geography of social well-being in the United States: an introduction to territorial social indicators and the work of Knox, P. L. (1975) on social well-being: a spatial perspective was very important.

El Din H. S.; Shalaby, A.; Farouh, H. E., & Elariane, S. A. (2013, p. 87) have tried to trace the history of quality of life concept and said that recently the 'quality of life' as a concept caused much inquisitiveness among the scholars. They advocated that quality of life is formally or practically the result of the study of the scholars of the last century; however, its concept reflects the idea of 'the good life' and 'living well' developed by Aristotle during 384–322 BC. Like Allison Smith, Forward, S. and others, they also mentioned that the idiom 'quality of life' was first developed and used by Seth, James (1889, p. 43). Seth, James also emphasized that in the study of quality of life both the quantitative and qualitative dimensions of quality of life should be given importance.

The chronologically arranged quality of life related studies as carried out by the above scholars show that it was **Seth, James** who formally used first the term 'Quality of Life' and this should be considered as a benchmark in the history of development of the idea of quality of life. However, some other studies from the above provide an idea that the concept of QOL practically and pronouncedly emerged during the 1960s and 1970s. This is also noticed that medical researchers and scientists have taken more interest in the study of quality of life and that is why there is dominance of scholarly literature on quality of life in the field of medical science. They have also used quality of life as an instrument in measuring health, disease and illness. Towards the end of twentieth century, there was greater attention on the status of health rather than simply on quality of life. As a result, many researchers in the field of medical and nursing science gave much more emphasis on 'health-related quality of life' as against the term 'quality of life'. But now in modern time, the study of quality of life has become interdisciplinary and has spread to science, medical science, technology, social science, environmental science, etc. More specifically, the study on quality of life is being carried on in economics, geography, sociology, philosophy, psychology, anthropology, environmental studies, home science, social work, social policy and in different subjects of medical and nursing science.

1.3 Concepts and Definition

Concepts stand for abstract ideas or underlying facts as primary characteristics of a concerned subject. Cognitive psychologists and philosophers assume concepts are the basic constituents of thought and belief. Concepts allow one to sort objects, properties, events and relations into classes on the basis of shared features thereby allowing a person to think about an item in a manner that abstracts from many of the particularities of the specific item. Thus, concepts allow us to create a knowledge base from our past experiences and provide an organizational structure for that knowledge base. Definitions function to fix meaning of a word or phrase in the context of some language thereby eliminating vagueness and/or ambiguity. In other words, definitions function to try to minimize vagueness and ambiguity in argument and discourse (Wallis, C., 2015, pp. 1–28).

The term quality of life has been in practice for a long time as a focal theme of research in several subjects but yet there is no unanimity among the scholars regarding its concrete definition. Quality of life is a complicated and multidimensional frame and needs various approaches from varied viewpoints. Several scholars from different disciplines have made their efforts in defining the word quality of life. Following literature shed light on the concepts of quality of life:

Stanley, M. G. (1973, p. Foreword) took into consideration the notion of quality of life as an expression of well-being of a concerned person. In other words, it is an individual's opinion about his/her well-being (the source of happiness in a given environment) that results from the function of a combination of several quantitative and qualitative attributes. Personal opinion about happiness may not be always the same because a set of things causing one's happiness changes from one point of time to another even at the same place.

According to **Symposium Planning Group** (1973, pp. 1–4), the quality of life refers to the subjective condition of an individual and can only be partially explained by using such terms as trained, happiness, educated, welfare, self-fulfilled, satisfied, reason, purpose, etc. The same holds true of their opposites: discontent, illiterate, frustrated, apathetic, alienated, etc.

Similarly, **Andrews, F. M.** (1974, pp. 280–381) focused on well-being and stated that it is largely perceived to denote the grade of condition of life, the result of the pleasure, happiness, satisfaction, etc. a person gets, enjoys, feels and experiences in the part of life spent. Various miseries in the life of someone also happen and negatively affect the quality of life which the concerned person can refrain. Andrews, Frank M. further considered well-being/quality of life as a result of the interplay of both the objective and subjective criteria/indicators. According to him, the objective indicators consist of 'counts of various types of phenomena' and subjective indicators include 'people's perceptions and feelings'. In broader sense, objective indicators are considered to include the quantitatively measurable criteria 'such as crime rates, population densities and unemployment figures'. Such population components can be directly measured and quantified and can be used while evaluating quality of life of people of a given area at a given point of time. As against this, subjective indicators include those phenomena in measuring well being or quality of life which are based on the statement of individual's 'perceptions, feelings, responses, and the like'.

Kladivo, P. & Halás, M. (2012, pp. 49–60) laid emphasis on the subjective (endogenous) and objective (exogenous) approaches to the study on quality of life. Subjective approach deals with the subjective dimension relating to feelings, perceptions, opinions and such other phenomena of a person(s) and objective approach deals with the objective dimension relating to a wide range of quantitatively countable parameters of quality of life. From this point of view, these two are also called as subjective and objective dimensional approaches to the study of quality of life. In other words, quality of life is a result of the multiple indicators of subjective and objective types relating to demographic, social, cultural, economic, psychological, political and environmental dimensions.

The concept of quality of life as explained by the **World Health Organization** (1976, p. 312) is succinct, clear, meaningful and important and encompasses the broad range of elements determining quality of life. WHO defined quality of life as the state of life that results from the 'combination of the effects of the complete range of factors such as those determining health, happiness (including comforts in the physical environment and a satisfying occupation), education, social and intellectual attainments, freedom of action, justice, freedom of operation'.

Flanagan, J. C. (1978, pp. 138–147) also focused on the objective and subjective indicators of measuring quality of life. According to him, the former includes income, marital status and such other elements, whereas the latter includes happiness, life satisfaction, contentment, pleasure and such other elements forming quality of life concept.

George, L. K. & Bearon, L. B. (1980, pp. 6–7) are also of the same opinion as mentioned above. According to them, there are four important aspects in the concept of quality of life of the people of an area. The two of them belongs to objective and reflects statistically quantifiable aspects and the other two belongs to subjective category and mirrors the personal assessment of the life condition. The four basic aspects according to them are the status of health, socio-economic status, life satisfaction and self-esteem. Although, it cannot be claimed that only these four components would be sufficient to completely evaluate the status of quality of life, these four are from among the unlimited number of components of quality of life.

The study of **Nagpal, R. & Sell, H.** (1985, pp. 1–2) on subjective well-being as a measure of quality of life has been very popular and quoted in the work of several scholars. According to him, the quality of life concept includes several occurrences happening in the part of life spent by someone and cause positive or negative effects in terms of pain and pleasure, happiness and unhappiness, limitations and freedom, mental, physical, social, psychological well-being or ill-being. In fact, the quality of life of a person or persons or people of an area can be judged on the basis of subjective responses concerning varied life aspects determining condition of life of the same person or persons or people. Nagpal and Sell consulted the works of some other scholars such as Andrews, F. M. & Withey, S. B. (1976), Campbell, A. & Converse, P. (1970) and Najman, J. M. & Levine, S. (1981) and stated that the quality of life is 'a composite measure of physical, mental and social well-being as perceived by each individual or by each group of individuals, and of happiness, satisfaction and gratification involving mainly such non-esoteric life concerns as health, marriage, family, work, financial situation, educational opportunities, self-esteem, creativity, belongingness and trust in others'.

Valentei D., Kavasha, A. & Ivanov, S. (1986, pp. 8–9) considered quality of life as a result of the type of vital functions and interpreted it in quite different ways. According to them, it is measured in the form of social stability of health, cultural and occupational skill levels, mobility in the labour sphere and so on.

According to **Lawton, M. P.** (1991, p. 6), quality of life is an outcome of the combined function of various objective and subjective aspects and is considered to involve multi-dimensions. It is normally evaluated on the basis of an assessment of personal perceptions as well as social and economic criteria applicable to the persons under investigation.

Qasim, S. Z. (1993, p. viii) considered 'quality of life' as a holistic one which encompasses not only the physical and economic improvements but also the social, cultural and even perhaps the political ideas of community. He included per capita income, life expectancy, levels of education, communication facilities, transportation, health and hygiene, energy availability, etc. as various aspects of development in measuring condition of life.

The World Health Organization Quality of Life Group (1995, pp. 1405) tried to highlight the three distinctive features such as subjective-concerning individual's opinion regarding self-health functioning or state of health; multifaceted-concerning condition of physical health, psychological condition, social condition and faith in spirituality and religion composing condition of life and positive and negative characteristics of quality of life. In extension of such facts, quality of life is defined as 'individual's perception of their position in life in the context of the culture and value systems in which they live and in relation to their goals, expectations, standards and concerns'. In fact, the concept of quality of life has a very wide scope of combining several complicated domains such as state of physical health, psychological state, extent and degree of freedom, state of relation in the society, faith and acceptance in spiritual and religious activities as well as adaptation to the prevailing environmental condition. In brief, the quality of life, according to WHO Group, is subjective and involves diverse aspects of positive and negative nature, for instance, pleasure and pain, happiness and unhappiness, satisfaction and dissatisfaction, contentment and discontentment, comfort and discomfort, dependence and independence and the like, and is called as multifaceted concept.

The approach of **Farquhar, M.** (1995, p. 1440) about the concept of quality of life is to some extent different from the others. He asserted that the quality of life is defined differently by different experts and noted that it is a complicated notion because varied persons look differently and incorporate dissimilar matters. Likewise, Aristotle's interpretation about the good life describes that every individual considers and evaluates different items differently at different points of time owing to situation in which the concerned person live. In other words, meaning of quality of life varies in terms of its conception. Some researchers consider several general measures and some other particular measures.

Shookner, M. (15 Oct, 1997, p. 5) has made an attempt to define quality of life in his own way. According to him, it can be defined as an outcome of the role of interconnections of sociocultural-, economic-, health- and environment-related situation that influence humans and the process of change in the society.

Nussboum, M. C. & Sen, A. (1999 p. 3) stated that a person's life can be perceived as a result of the amalgamation of 'various doings and beings' (commonly known as functionings) and include basic and complicated elements such as well-fed, disease-free, having self-esteem, maintaining human nobility, participation in community activities, etc. Nussbaum and Sen, however, have not directly used the word 'quality of life' but different basic and complicated elements reflect the idea of quality of life. Brock, Dan (1999, p. 96) has used the 'concept of a "good life" to refer to the quality of life of persons in its broader interpretation', (in Nussboum and Sen 1999).

Smith, A. (Nov 2000, pp. 5–6) noted that there is no universal definition of quality of life which can please every researcher working in this field. This is because of the fact that different scholars/researchers have taken into account different elements or phenomena related to condition of life from different angles while defining quality of life.

The view of **Massam, B. H.** (2002, pp. 143–145) regarding the definition of quality of life is almost similar to that of the above. He stated that there is slight consensus amidst the researchers and other experts with regard to the exact definition/meaning of quality of life. Even despite this, numerous documents mention the quality of life as a consequence of the combined role of sociocultural, economic, environmental and other conditions. It is also considered as the cause or source of an idea or opinion of someone about the quality of life where such notions and views can impact the well-being of people of a place. He further reviewed related literature and noted QOL in terms of pleasure, comfort, contentment in one's life and other characteristics such as needs and desires, aspirations, life styles preferences, existing social and economic activities, climate, equality of cultural institutions, etc. determining condition of good life.

Similarly, **Berlim, M. T. & Fleck, M. P. A.** (2003, pp. 249–252) also stressed that there is no final yardstick for measuring QOL. According to them, there is no any exclusive meaning of the word 'quality of life', especially in the field medical science. Though, it has a very wide notion and includes different dimensions such as physical, psychological and social functioning as well as an understanding of state of health, discomfort, contentment and self-satisfaction concerning condition of life.

From the above literature, it is quite apparent that different institutions, scholars and researchers from science and social science subjects have viewed the concept of quality of life in different perspectives. Each has its own way of approaching the concept. An economist approaches it from a material well-being point of view and a sociologist looks from a social point of view such as differences in social identity. A psychologist has a cognitive way of viewing the quality of life concept, a political scientist looks at the freedom of political choice and participation, whereas a geographer views the concept of QOL from a spatial viewpoint to trace the spatial inequality in it. In fact, quality of life is all about the state of life—whether happiness or despair or satisfaction or dissatisfaction. Life may be full of happiness, if all the needs are fulfilled, it is happiness, and if not, it is despair. It is more of an abstract and subjective rather than an objective reality. The quality of life is, therefore, more a theoretical concept rather than an empirical one. However, it comprises three important dimensions of overall individual need satisfaction: 'having, loving and being' (Erik, A.,1999, pp. 89–94). According to him, *having* refers to the basic needs for survival, i.e. food–nutrition, air, water, resources, amenities and the like; *loving* is more of personal relations such as friendship, affection, love, belongingness and solidarity; and *being* as a dimension lies on the threshold of alienation and self-actualization. Therefore, quality of life is a complicated and multidimensional composition and involves diverse methods from varied conceptual points of view.

In **author's opinion,** the term quality of life stands for the state or condition of life of a person or persons or group of individuals of a particular place at a particular point of time. Generally, it is perceived in a positive sense. However, this is not the fact when one talks in terms of health-related quality of life which has been more popular in the field of medical science and psychology. Quality of Life in positive sense is meant to be free from functional defects or impaired functioning of both the body and mind of an individual. In other words, quality of life in positive sense is dealt with positive health the meaning thereof is a normal functioning of body and mind. Therefore, good quality of life is possible only when both the body and mind work in normal state or when both the body and mind work as naturally designed. But when the body and mind work with functional defects or impaired functioning, the quality of life is perceived in negative sense. This may result due to presence of disease(s) or lack of congenial environment. Thus, good quality of life is the positive residual value or the surplus positive value remained after subtraction of negative composite score value from the positive composite score value of complete range of physical, mental, psychological, social, cultural, economic, political and environmental parameters or variables of both the objective and subjective nature applied for measuring quality of life. The reverse result stands for not good quality of life and shows lack of energy and resilience of the concerned person(s).

1.4 Dimensions of QOL

Dimension stands for the constituent elements or components or aspects or phenomena or any other characteristics of quality of life. Different dimensions and its interactive role determine disparity and variation in the level and state of life of population of a given place and time. Shookner, M. (15 Oct, 1997, p. 6) mentioned several aspects of quality of life which are related to society, economy, environment and a person's physical and mental wellness.

El Din H. S.; Shalaby, A.; Farouh, H. E., & Elariane, S. A. (2013, pp. 89–92) were of the opinion that quality of life involves several different subjects and aspects from the point of view of its study and that is why it is called as having multi-subject and multi-aspect notion. According to them, quality of life encompasses seven dimensions. These are *environmental dimension* that focuses on local or surrounding area's innate characteristics; *physical dimension* stands for facilities, social amenities and social fabrics, utilization of land, basic developmental structure and capital equipments; *mobility dimension* includes approachability, movement of vehicles and other transport-related problems; *social dimension* consists of those parameters which are related to interactive activities with the neighbours and involvement of people in decision-making activities in the community and society; *psychological dimension* relates emotion- and perception-related matters of people in the neighbourhood; *economic dimension* identifies and denotes neighbourhood with a viewpoint of economically gainful pursuits or employment; *political dimension* stands for plans, programmes, schemes of the local bodies and government and its implementation for underpinning the quality of public life. **Massam, B. H.** (2002, p. 145) reviewed several literature related to quality of life and came out with the two major aspects, namely, psychological and environmental. These two dimensions have special bearing on the state of life. In fact, the QOL of an individual depends to a large extent on the external or 'objective' evidence based on information related to material wealth of the same individual and internal or 'subjective' evaluation based on personal understanding or feelings about his/her life. In other words, the psychological dimension stands for individual/personal life quality, self-evaluated state of satisfaction in life and the environmental dimension refers to the quality of life of urban area, a community and a place. While explaining a methodology of measuring human health (**Sinha, B. R. K.**, 2015, pp. 228–232) focuses on different health-related dimensions and the same dimensions may be applicable in case of the study of quality of life.

Therefore, 'quality of life' includes several dimensions such as social, cultural, economic, political, demographic, psychological, environmental, physical and mental, positive and negative, spiritual, emotional, vocational, curative and preventive and other quantitative and qualitative dimensions of objective and subjective nature.

1.5 Determinants/Factors

Qasim, S. Z. (1993, p. x) pointed out that science and technology plays a crucial role in promoting the QOL. Similarly, **Mukherjee, P.** (1993, pp. 1–13) stressed on income, employment, alleviation of poverty, health, education, social amenities and related programmes because these aspects help improve quality of life, and hence there is need for proper planning of these aspects. In the same way, **Bajaj, J. S.** (1993, pp. 15–17) also considered health as an important factor that determines quality of life. He also considered stabilization of population as a prerequisite measure for the enhancement of quality of life. The basic needs such as health, drinking water, food and shelter play important role in improving and maintaining quality of life. **Menon, M. G. K.** (1993, pp. 42–55) took into consideration vocational education and training, employment, population, food and biomass production, water management, energy, transport, shelter and construction, information and telematics, regional holistic development in playing positive role in quality of life. **Sharma, S.** (1993, p. 261); **Naik, C.** (1993, p. 407) have considered the role of mental health and basic education in quality of life.

Shookner, M. (15 Oct, 1997, pp. 6–8) also tried to highlight the factors which normally affect the condition of life of the concerned person(s) and took into consideration the level of income, status in the society, supporting system of the society, job opportunity and working culture and environment, social conditions and natural environment as important determinants of quality of life.

Smith, A. E., Sim, J., Scharf, T. and Phillipson, C. (2004, pp. 794–801) tried to demonstrate the role of determinants in quality of life of persons of 60 and above years. They took into consideration the words variables, attributes, characteristics, factors and determinants as synonymous to each other for signifying the same meaning. To fulfil the objectives of their study, they selected seven factors, namely, 'socio-demographic characteristics, social support, health, material resources, crime, the residential neighbourhood and housing'. These factors/determinants are elaborated in detail in their Table-1(pp. 800–801). Further, they evaluated and explained the quality of life of older people on the basis of potentially more effective social cum demographic variables as well as objective and subjective variables. Social and demographic variables or parameters considered by them were age and sex (biological characteristics of population), marital status (married, unmarried, divorced, widow/widower), social class (profession-based economic activities requiring trained and experienced persons, administrative and bureaucratic personnel, mechanical and vocational persons, specific economic activities in which persons possessing particular skill(s) are gainfully employed), ethnicity, education, physical as well as mental health. Objective criteria based evaluation of condition of life included availability of daily need items, for instance, level of income, availability of adequate food for daily consumption, indemnity for house property and possession of telephone; deprivation (items considered necessary but not available, for example, lack of room warming system, telephone and car service); participation in social activities, time spent in neighbourhood; house-related problems; victim of lawlessness; supporting system from society; illnesses or disabilities that restrict a person's activities in any way. Subjective assessment of quality of life involves opinion about penury; social isolation, which means feeling isolated from society; perception about own health; fear from crime; feeling of loneliness; perception about community integration; satisfaction with accommodation; satisfaction level with neighbourhood and ability to manage financial liabilities. In addition to such purposeful variables, some other relevant variables relating to the above domains may also be considered in measuring life quality of the concerned inhabitants.

Truly speaking, amalgamation of the above variables and their score values in composite form gives the output of overall subjective well-being or subjective quality of life. In other sense, QOL is an outcome or effect of the composite value of several variables or parameters which are related to social and demographic aspects as well as objective and subjective aspects. However, the state and level of life quality can differ from one place to another, from one type of environment to another (in terms of natural and human), from one type of population to another (in terms of social and economic groups/classes). It can also vary on the basis of questions designed or developed and methods adopted for field work, data collection and analysis. That is why, QOL is known as multidimensional.

1.6 QOL: Indicators, Constraints and Measurement

Conceptually, the word 'indicator' is meant to point out a related fact or state or level of something. In other terms, indicator is interchangeably used as an index or measure to unveil or exhibit both the quantitative and/or qualitative characteristics of related aspect(s) under study. This can be used in studying the state or level of given topic, e.g. health, quality of life, human development, human resource development, deprivation and happiness level or the like with reference to a person or group of persons or a place/region/state or a country at a given time (OECD 2008, p. 13). United States Agency International Development (2014, p. Introduction) considered that indicator is a kind of measure that can be directly or indirectly used to show the existing or expected condition or position of a trait or characteristic of a given aspect. Such aspect, e.g. may be related to people, geographical area, social, economic and political aspect, etc. Indicator may be of quantitative or qualitative nature, for instance, fertility ratio, general mortality or infant mortality rate, expectancy of life, etc. Indicator is a kind of sign that shows what something is or what something is likely to be. Actually, this may be anything or any element, e.g. low birth weight as a question in the questionnaire that indicates the state of health. Therefore, an indicator is a general question and a means of information.

Prutkin, J. M. (2002, p. 19) explained some constraints in the way of measuring quality of life. According to him, an assessment or evaluation of quality of life is a tough task on account of involvement of several elements or factors of varied nature and role, importance, selection and applicability of indicators.

Similarly, **Saxena, S.; Chandiramani, K.; Bhargava, R.** (1998, p. 164) also expressed some limitations concerning quality of life measurement. According to them, the idiom 'quality of life' is frequently used as a concept but it is very vague because it involves diverse social, cultural, economic, regional and other aspects and that is why the measurement of quality of life through any designed or arranged schedule of questions in a precise form remains inconclusive. **The World Health Organization Quality of Life Group** (1995, pp. 1406).

The work of **Smith, D. M.** (1977, pp. 33–36) on the quality of life is highly appreciable as he considered different elements relating to improvement of the material quality (housing condition, resources), physical quality (health, reduced violence, preservation of the natural environment), mental quality (education, knowledge, cultural environment) and improvement in the spiritual quality (talents and capabilities, social harmony, moral and ethical stands) of life. Further, he prepared a list of several indicators relating to ecological, demographic, social, cultural, economic, environmental aspects in measuring the status of life quality of the inhabitants of a concerned region.

Jones, E. & John E. (1977, p. 234) also employed some criteria in measuring quality of life. These are per capita and household income, unemployment rate, housing cost, infant mortality, suicide rate, robbery, traffic rate, voting in presidential election, etc.

Ginsberg, E. (1980, pp. 3–4) stated that variation in the pattern of economic growth of an area is by and large a result of variation in qualitative aspects of its inhabitants. It is because of the fact that qualitative attributes of people of an area play a great role in the process of an increase in the level of peace, progress, prosperity and in turn life quality.

Mittal, L. N. (1993, p. 3) and Ghosh, A. K. (1993, p. 11) focused on literacy and education and equitable distribution of resources in raising the quality of life of the people.

Rajesh (1993, pp. 11–12) and Ramaswami, A. and Ram, N. V. R. (1985, pp. 72–73) revealed the importance and role of the quality of human resource (knowledge, skills, attitudes, vigour, attitude, capacity, etc.) and the development of human resources through formal and non-formal education, training, food and nutrition, etc. in maintaining and raising the quality of life of the people. Ramaswami and Ram further added habits, culture, environment, standard of living, number of children, expenditure towards children's education and health awareness, etc. as indicators of destitution and condition of life.

According to **Qasim, S. Z.** (1993, p. 57), GNP or per person income do not truly helps in meeting the basic needs of people. The needs could be many, besides food, clothing, education, health and transport. Maintenance of ecological balance and human rights are as important as the other basic needs. Perceiving various dimensions of the issues of human needs and life quality one gets fully convinced that unless the question of population control is aggressively pursued and some stability is achieved, a real improvement in the quality of life is hard to accomplish. There is utmost urgency for the implementation of two components—literacy and availability of energy from the point of view of improvement in the quality of life.

Singh, N. K. (1993, p. 138) took into account income, employment, health, education, physical environment, human dignity and freedom as quantitative and qualitative indicators in measuring quality of life of the people. **Sarma, E. A. S.; Maggo, J. N. and Sachdeva, A. S.** (1993, p. 107) took into consideration life expectancy at birth, infant mortality rate, crude death rate, literacy rate, per capita income, number of hospitals and dispensaries, telephone exchange, post and telegraph office, per capita availability of food grains, population covered by radio, T.V. as indicator of quality of life.

Hussain Majid (1994, p. 230) has also considered population characteristics such as infant mortality, expectancy of life and literacy as important factors in promoting physical quality of life; however, he added GNP per capita, education and health also in evaluating physical quality of life of the targeted population.

Rajev, A. (2006, p. 143) noted that the spatial variation in the distribution of different urban social groups has been a major area of research among the scholars both in America and in Europe. Such variation not only determines the urban landscape features such as building density and house types but also variation in the quality of life.

Park, K. (2009, p. 16) expressed his opinion that the standard of living and quality of life are not the same rather both are different in its concept. Here, standard of living is basically the result of material-based resources and opportunities (measured by objective indicators), whereas quality of life is the result of a person's subjective assessment about his/her life. In other words, the measurement of quality of life is based solely on the personal opinion and evaluation about satisfaction in his/her life. The most convenient approach of measuring quality of life is to apply the composite index that is calculated on the basis of the sum values of a variety of physical and mental health and other aspect-related indicators. The basic objective of this is to perceive a life of peace, comfort and happiness.

1.7 Variables, Its Composite Measures and Computation of Quality of Life Index

Statistically, the term 'variable' may be a particular thing, element or attribute or a particular characteristic of quantitative or qualitative nature that is used in logical or mathematical calculation to show a variable quantity or quality with reference to a selected or given topic/aspect or task. It varies in situation, space and time. Age, height, eye colour, temperature, rainfall, production, labour input in terms of hours worked, number of hours of television watched in a week or any other such traits are the examples of variables and can be counted or measured and observed. Sometimes it is necessary to make observation of attributes that are not easily observed, such as intelligence or health. These are multidimensional concepts that can be measured using composite variables (https://study.com/academy/lesson/composite-variable-definition-lesson-quiz.html). Composite variable is obtained by merging together the multiple variables (indicators) into a single one. A lone variable or indicator normally does not furnish the needed facts/data or information, but from the combination of two or more one can get meaningful information known as composite value or composite score. In other way, when such composite scores are used in measuring quality of life, it is called composite measures of variables (https://en.wikipedia.org/wiki/Composite_measure).

A 'composite index' is a result of the combination of two or more quantitative and qualitative variables and helps in understanding the status or nature of a subject under study at a certain point of time in an area. This, in other words, according to **United States Agency for International Development** (2014, p. Introduction), combines several particular measures and produces compound result of a complicated, multidimensional and purposeful society-related matters such as penury, rate of progress in mental and physical state, position of supporting capacity, etc. Separate parameter and group of yardsticks can be chosen, systematized and joined to provide subindices exhibiting the major elements or aspects to be examined and studied. For instance, educational subindex may combine measures like literacy, student's enrolment in school, achievement of education. A group of subindices may be combined or summed together to get finally the composite index. Human Development Index (HDI), e.g. includes three aspects of human well-being. These are related to health, education and income.

Composite Scores: After putting assigned positive or negative weight against selected variables of positive or negative nature related to social, cultural, economic, political, demographic, psychological, environmental, physical, mental, spiritual, emotional, vocational, curative and preventive aspects and so on, the total composite scores (an outcome of positive + negative scores) of all variables for each person should be found out.

Thereafter, the percentage of total positive or total negative scores for each person should be worked out. While doing so, the total composite scores (value of total positive and negative scores) should be considered as 100%. Later, Quality of Life Index for the positive and negative performances of each person should be separately calculated dividing the percentage of total positive or negative scores of each person by 100.

Finally, on the basis of variation in the **quality of life index** of the positive and negative performances among the persons under investigation a sequential arrangement of this in certain groups or levels at equal class interval in a convenient manner should be framed for tabulation, cartographic representation and interpretation.

1.8 Meaningful Framework of Positive and Negative Quality of Life Index (QOLI) and Its Level

Following arrangement, for example, can be made to provide a meaningful and acceptable framework for measuring and interpreting level of quality of life of the surveyed persons/individuals or population of an area at any given point of time.

For measuring **Positive Dimension** of Quality of Life, the Index and Level of it can be framed as

i. >0.80 (Very Good), **ii**. 0.61–0.80 (Good), **iii**. 0.41–0.60 (Average), **iv**. 0.21–0.40 (Poor) and **v**. <0.21 (Very Poor).

Similarly, with regard to **Negative Dimension** of quality of life, its level or status and index can be framed as

i. >0.80 (Very High Negative), **ii**. 0.61–0.80 (High Negative), **iii**. 0.41–0.60 (Average Negative), **iv**. 0.21–0.40 (Low Negative) and **v**. <0.21 (Very Low Negative).

Thus, the above approach is considered practically more realistic, appropriate and useful and can be conveniently used in order to fulfil the objective of researchers while working for an evaluation and interpretation of the status and levels of quality of life of the surveyed people/individuals from spatial and temporal perspective point of view. The same approach can also be employed in studying the levels and status of health or human resource development of the concerned person(s), group of persons or population of an area over a specific period of time.

Use: Such sequential arrangement of quality of life Index (QOLI) can be employed to explain the status of quality of life of individuals by age and gender, social class/group, race, ethnicity, religion, educational level, income level and by occupational categories in both the rural and urban areas.

References

Andrews, F. M. (1974). Social indicators or perceived life quality. In *Social indicators research* (Vol. 1). Dordrecht-Holland: D. Reidel Publishing Company.

Andrews, F. M., & Withey, S. B. (1976). *Social indicators of well-being. America's perception of life quality*. New York, USA: Plenum Press.

Bajaj, J. S. (1993). Health as an indicator and determinant of quality of life. In S. Z. Qasim (Ed.), *Science and quality of life*. The Offsetters, Udaichand Marg, Kotla Mubarakpur, New Delhi-110003.

Berlim, M. T., & Fleck, M. P. A. (2003). Quality of life: A brand new concept for research and practice in psychiatry. Revista Brasileira de Psiquiatria (RBP), *25*(4), 249–52, Brazilian Psychiatric Association.

Bowling, A. (1999). Recent interest and developments in measuring health-related quality of life. In *Health-related quality of life: A discussion of the concept, its use and measurement*. http://info.worldbank.org/etools/docs/library/48475/m2s5bowling.pdf.

Brock, D. (1999). Quality of life measures in health care and medical ethics. In *The quality of life* (Nussbaum and Sen, 1999). New Delhi: Oxford University Press.

Campbell, A., & Converse, P. (1970). Monitoring the quality of American life. In *A research proposal to the Russell Sage Foundation*. Survey Research Center, University of Michigan, USA.

El Din, H. S., Shalaby, A., Farouh, H. E., & Elariane, S. A. (April 2013). Principles of urban quality of life for a neighbourhood, housing and building. Nat Res Center (HBRC) J *9*(1).

Ellwood, C. A. (March 1902). Aristotle as a sociologist. In: *Annals of the American academy of political and social science* (Vol. 19). In association with the American Academy of Political and Social Science, UK: Sage Publications, Inc. http://www.ecn.bris.ac.uk/het/aristotle/ellwood.htm.

Elyse, W. K. (May 1992). *Quality of life: Meaning, measurement, and models*. Navy Personnel Research, Arid Development Center, San Diego, California, USA.

Erik, A. (1999). Having, loving, being: an alternative to the Swedish model of welfare research. In M. C. Nussboum & A. Sen (Eds.), *The Quality of Life*. New Delhi: Oxford University Press.

Fagge, R. (2012). *The vision of J. B. Priestley*. Continuum International Publishing Group, The Tower Building, 80 Maiden Lane, Suite 404, New York. https://books.google.co.in/books?isbn=1441163794.

Farquhar, M. (1995). Elderly people's definitions of quality of life. *Social Science and Medicine, 41*(10). Great Britain: Elsevier Science Ltd.

Flanagan J. C. (1978). A research approach to improving our quality of life. *American Psychologist, 33*(2), 138–147. American Psychological Association, Washington, DC, USA.

Forward, S. (Sept 2003). *State of the art report on life quality assessment in the field of transport and mobility*. Sweden: Swedish National Road and Transport Research Institute, Linkoeping. http://www.factum.at/asi/download/ASI_D21_final.pdf.

George, L. K. & Bearon, L. B. (1980). *Quality of life in older persons: Meaning and measurement*. New York (Open Library): Human Sciences Press.

Ghosh, A. K. (1993). Growth of female literacy in India. In *University news*, Monday, November 8, 1993, New Delhi.

Ginsberg, E. (1980). Man and his work. In S. Beach Dale (Ed.), *Managing people at work*. New York: Macmillan Publishing Co., Inc.

Hussain, M. (1994). *Human geography*. Jaipur: Rawat Publications.

Jones, E., & John, E. (1977). *An introduction to social geography*. New York: Oxford University Press.

Kladivo, P., & Halás, M. (May 10, 2012). Quality of life in an urban environment: A typology of urban units of Olomouc. An outcome of a project of the Academy of Sciences of the Czech Republic.

Knox, P. L. (1975). *Social well-being: A spatial perspective*. London: Oxford University Press.

Lawton, M. P. (1991). A multidimensional view of quality of life in frail elders. In J. E. Birren, J. Lubben, J. Rowe, & D. Deutchman (Eds.), *The concept and measurement of quality of life*. New York: Academic Press.

Massam, B. H. (2002). Quality of life: Public planning and private living. In In *Progress in planning* (vol. 58, p. 144), Pergamon: Elsevier Science Limited, U.K.

Meeberg, G. A. (1993). Quality of life: A concept analysis. *Journal of Advanced Nursing, 18*(1), 32–38; PubMed, US National Library of Medicine, National Institutes of Health. http://www.ncbi.nlm.nih.gov/pubmed/8429165.

Menon, M. G. K. (1993). Inputs of science of technology for the improvement of quality of life. In Qasim, S. Z. (ed.) *Science and quality of life*, the Offsetters, Udaichand Marg, Kotla Mubarakpur, New Delhi.

Mittal, L. N. (1993). Women and the educational development processes. In *The university news*, Monday, December 13, 1993, New Delhi.

Mukherjee, P. (1993). Planning for quality of life. In S. Z. Qasim (Ed.), *Science and quality of life*. The Offsetters, Udaichand Marg, Kotla Mubarakpur, New Delhi-110003.

Nagpal, R., & Sell, H. (1985). Subjective wellbeing. Regional Health Paper, No. 7, SEARO (South East Asia Regional Office), WHO, World Health House, Indraprastha, New Delhi.

Naik, C. (1993) Basic education and quality of life. In S. Z. Qasim (Ed.), *Science and quality of life*. The Offsetters, Udaichand Marg, Kotla Mubarakpur, New Delhi.

Najman, J. M. & Levine, S. (1981). Evaluating the impact of medical care and technologies on the quality of life: A review and critique. *Social Sciences & Medicine, Part F: Medical and Social Ethics, 15*(2–3), 107–115. Great Britain: Elsevier Science Ltd.

Nussboum, M. C., & Sen, A. (1999). *The quality of life*. New Delhi: Oxford University Press.

OECD. (2008). *Handbook on constructing composite indicators: Methodology and user guide*. European Commission: JRC.

Park, K. (2009). *Park's text book of preventive and social medicine*. Jabalpur, M.P., India: Banarsidas Bharnot Publishers.

Pennacchini, M., Bertolaso, M., Elvira, M. M., & De Marinis, M. G. (2011). A brief history of the quality of life: Its use in medicine and in philosophy. *La Clinica Teraputica, 162*(3), Societa Editrice Universo, Rome, Itely.

Prutkin, J. M. (2002). *A history of quality of life measurements*. Yale Medicine Thesis Digital Library, Paper 424, Yale University, Yale.

Qasim, S. Z. (1993) *Science and quality of life*. The Offsetters, Udaichand Marg, Kotla Mubarakpur, New Delhi, India.

Rajesh (1993). Population growth, environment and development. In *University news*, Monday, Oct. 25, 1993, New Delhi.

Rajev, A. (2006). *Geography*. Ist Floor, Janakpuri, New Delhi: Spectrum Books Pvt. Ltd.

Ramaswami, A., & Ram, N. V. R. (1985). *Poverty, is it understood?*. New Delhi: Inter India Publications.

Roy, I. B. (1997). *Quality of life for people with disabilities*. Ellenborough House, Wellington Street, Cheltenham, UK: Stanley Thornes (Publishers) Ltd.

Sarma, E. A. S., Maggo, J. N., & Sachdeva, A. S. (1993). Energy, environment and quality of life. In S. Z. Qasim (Ed.), *Science and quality of life*. The Offsetters, Udaichand Marg, Kotla Mubarakpur, New Delhi-110003.

Saxena, S., Chandiramani, K., Bhargava, R. (1998). WHOQOL-Hindi: A questionnaire for assessing quality of life in health care settings in India. *The National Medical Journal of India, 11*(4), AIIMS, New Delhi.

Seth, J. (1889). The evolution of morality. In *Mind* (Vol. 14, No. 53). Oxford University Press on behalf of the Mind Association, UK. http://www.jstor.org/stable/i339152.

Sharma, S. (1993). Mental health and quality of life. In S. Z. Qasim (Ed.), *Science and quality of life*. The Offsetters, Udaichand Marg, Kotla Mubarakpur, New Delhi.

Sharpe, A. (22 July 1999). A survey of indicators of economic and social well-being. In *Paper prepared for Canadian Policy Research Networks*. http://www.csls.ca/reports/paper3a.pdf.

Shookner, M. (15 Oct 1997). *The quality of life in Ontario—1997*. Canada: Ontario Social Development Council & Social Planning Network of Ontario. http://cdcquinte.com/Resources/Quality%20of%20Life-1997.pdf.

Singh, N. K. (1993) An analysis of human development in India in terms of quantitative and qualitative indicators. In S. Z. Qasim (Ed.), *Science and quality of life*. The Offsetters, Udaichand Marg, Kotla Mubarakpur, New Delhi.

Sinha, B. R. K. (2015). A methodology of measuring human health. *Human Geographies—Journal of Studies and Research in Human Geography 9*(2), November 2015, Bucharest, Romania.

Smith, D. M. (1973). *The geography of social well-being in the United States: An introduction to territorial social indicators*. New York: McGraw-Hill.

Smith, D. M. (1977). *Human geography: A welfare approach*. London: Edward Arnold Publishers Ltd.

Smith, A. (Nov 2000). *Researching quality of life of older people: concepts, measures and findings*. Centre for Social Gerontology, School of Social Relations, Keele University, Staffordshire, UK.

Smith, A. E., Sim, J., Scharf, T., & Phillipson, C. (2004). Determinants of quality of life amongst older people in deprived neighbourhoods. *Ageing & Society, 24*. Cambridge University Press, United Kingdom.

Snoek, F. J. (2000). Quality of life: A closer look at measuring patients' well-being. *Diabetes Spectrum 13*(1), 24. American Diabetes Association, USA. http://journal.diabetes.org/diabetesspectrum/00v13n1/.
Stanley, M. G. (March 1973). The quality of life concept: A potential new tool for decision-makers. Research and Monitoring, Environmental Studies Division, The Environmental Protection Agency, United States.
Symposium Planning Group (1973). The quality of life concept: A potential new tool for decision-makers. Research and Monitoring, Environmental Studies Division, The Environmental Protection Agency, United States.
The WHOQOL Group (1995). The World Health Organization Quality of Life Assessment (WHOQOL): Position paper from the World Health Organization. *Social Science Medicine, 41*(10), Great Britain: Elsevier Science Ltd.
United States Agency International Development, from the American People, (2014) African and Latin American Resilience to Climate Change (ARCC), Tetra Tech ARD.
Valentei, D. Kavasha, & Ivanov, S. (1986). *Population and socio-economic development*. Moscow: Progress Publishers.
Wallis, C. (2015). Concepts, meanings, and definitions: Chapter outline. www.csulb.edu/~cwallis/170/text/concepts.pdf.
WHO (1976). WHO Chapter, *30*(8), 312.

Chapter 2
Housing Affordability as a Reflexivity of Quality of Life

Upuli Perera and Collins Adjei Mensah

Abstract This chapter uses housing affordability as a means to understand the dynamic nature of quality of life as a concept. It explores the way in which people utilised housing affordability as a reflexivity of their expectation for quality of life over time and space. Based on the systematic review method, a total of 227 publications that focused on quality of life and housing affordability were reviewed rigorously to retrieve relevant information for the study. The findings of the chapter show that housing affordability is an integral part of the quality of life due to social, economic, and environmental interconnections that exist between them. However, the nature of their interconnections changes over time. Thus, quality of life is a multifaceted concept that varies across different cultures, time, and space as human beings are dynamic agents where the thoughts and needs change frequently. Thus, quality of life is a concept that is subject to construction, negotiation and alteration over time and space. Hence, initiatives or policies towards enhancing quality of life of individuals should take careful attention of such dynamics in order to be more effective.

Keywords Housing affordability · Quality of life · Sustainability

U. Perera (✉)
School of Geography, Earth and Environmental Sciences, Centre for Urban and Regional Studies, University of Birmingham, B15 2TT Birmingham, UK
e-mail: prabudhika@gmail.com; tgup@sjp.ac.lk

Department of Estate Management and Valuation, University of Sri Jayewardenepura, Nugegoda, Sri Lanka

C. A. Mensah
Department of Geography and Regional Planning, University of Cape Coast, Cape Coast, Ghana
e-mail: cmensah@ucc.edu.gh; collinsadjeimensah@gmail.com

B. R. K. Sinha (ed.), *Multidimensional Approach to Quality of Life Issues*,
https://doi.org/10.1007/978-981-13-6958-2_2

2.1 Introduction

Housing is one of the basic necessities of life that enhances the quality of life of individuals in diverse ways. In OECD[1] countries, housing affordability is generally understood as, housing cost that does not take more than 30% of the household expenditure thereby enabling a given household to have sufficient income left for non-housing expenditure (Yuen et al. 2006). Whilst these countries promote housing affordability via tax incentives for rental investment, public subsidies to leverage private investment, and reliance on land use planning system, all such efforts are geared towards improving the quality of life of individuals (Lindstrom 1994). In this regard, housing is recognised to play important role in improving quality of life of individuals because it provides shelter for people to lay their heads, develop their skills, socialise and be educated to engage in different activities of their choice.

Talking about housing affordability and quality of life, more goes into it than just providing residential space to accommodate individuals. This is because there are subjective dimensions of quality of life which vary among individuals and are influenced by time, space and circumstances one finds him or herself in. This makes it important to probe further on how the concept of quality of life has been changing over time as reflective through various housing affordability initiatives pursued in the world since the period of industrialisation to a more contemporary sustainable paradigm era, but available studies have failed to touch on this. It was, therefore, to bridge this knowledge gap that is why this chapter was written. The objective of the chapter is to explore how the understanding of housing affordability can be a reflexive medium of interpreting the changing focus of quality of life of households over the last five decades. This will help to provide a deeper understanding of the relationships between quality of life and housing affordability, and their underpinning variables that have been changing over time and space.

The chapter starts first by discussing the concept of quality of life and highlights its various elements or attributes. It continues by focusing on the concept of housing and housing affordability to trace the divergent views expressed on these concepts and their relationships with quality of life. The last section of this chapter treats housing affordability and its reflexivity on quality of life by discussing how the indicators and measurement of housing affordability have changed over space and time, and how such changes have reflected in the present thinking of quality of life.

2.2 Quality of Life

The concept of quality of life is broad and cut across three major branches of science: Economics, Medicine and the Social Sciences, with each branch offering different views on the conceptualisation of quality of life (Cummins 2005, p. 669). From the

[1]Member countries of Organisation for Economic Co-operation and Development (OECD), all having a democratic system of government and accept the principle of a free economy.

Social Science perspective, quality of life has particularly been conceptualised: (i) as multidimensional that is influenced by personal and environmental factors and their interactions; (ii) to have the same components for all people; (iii) to have both subjective and objective components and (iv) to be enhanced by self-determination, resources, purpose in life, and a sense of belongingness (Cummins 2005). Such conceptualisation has made the quality of life an elusive and diversified concept approached at varying levels of generality from the assessment of societal or community well-being to the specific evaluation of the situation of individuals and groups. This, therefore, makes the quality of life a multidimensional concept that needs to be carefully defined by using different attributes or indicators in which the inclusion and exclusion of indicators should be guided by a given context that quality of life is being used.

There have been the developments of several taxonomies of quality of life. For instance, Ferrans (1996), Felce and Perry (1995, 1996) were in favour of searching suitable indicators to conceptualise the concept. Felce (1997) stressed that quality of life is influenced by six main elements which are material, physical, emotional, social, productive and rights/civic well-being. The World Health Organisation (WHO) on the other hand categorised quality of life into six components: physical well-being, environmental well-being, psychological well-being, social relations, level of independence, and spiritual well-being. In this context, well-being is defined as the state of being happy, healthy and comfortable with life (WHO 1997; Galloway 2006). However, from Social Science point of view, quality of life generally implies the overall satisfaction of one's living. This satisfaction may arise from economic attributes that connect more with material goods, social attributes that are linked to psychological satisfaction and environmental attributes that deal with accessibility to desired natural and physical conditions.

These attributes do possess different dimensions which are either objective or subjective in nature. According to Cummins (2005), the objective dimensions of quality of life are usually the physical attributes that may be in a form of quantities and frequencies of an entity, for example, access to good housing, infrastructure and services, healthy food, etc. On the other hand, the subjective domain of quality of life is within the private consciousness of each individual and it can be verified only through repeated responses provided by the person concerned. These objective and subjective dimensions have further been widely discussed by different scholars such as Felce (1997), Haas (1999), Moons et al. (2006) and Testa and Simonson (1996), Sirgy (1998).

According to Sirgy (1998), the subjective dimension of one's quality of life can arise from either a need-based-expectations (materialist) or cognitive-based-expectations (non-materialist) or both. The need-based-expectation tends to be influenced by social comparisons, like wealth and material possession of family and friends where the cognitive-based-expectations arise via predictive-, past- and ability-based comparisons. With the emergence of postmodernism (the way twenty-first-century people live in; Clapham 2005) thought there has been also a growing concern that quality of life is purely a subjective experience (Haas et al. 2006; Haas 1999) thus it is socially constructed. The other typical view is that quality of life should not be defined 'primarily' in terms of either its objective or subjective components but should rather include both aspects (Cummins 2005) as they both affect the quality of life of an individual. This is particularly true when the quality of life is identified as a measure of collectivises. An example would be assessing the quality of life at a community level, local level or at a regional or national level. For instance, McMahon (2002) in his study of assessing sustainable quality of life in Bristol used five levels of indicators; European common indicators, national and regional headline indicators, stakeholder indicators in Bristol, local-ward and citywide indicators and community group indicators that ranged from waste management, energy, transport, environmental protection, biodiversity, housing and shelter, economy, health and well-being, community safety, social economy, culture, tourism, land use and development, to education and poverty. This implies two things; one is that quality of life should be conceptualised to focus on specific dimensions for a particular purpose such as housing affordability in this case. Second, it needs to be understood that as for many other concepts, quality of life too needs to be assessed relative to the context of time and space.

2.3 Housing

Housing is a term that we are all familiar with. It is a basic need in our lives. However, the meaning associated with housing is not limited to its construction with bricks and mortar or merely a physical element that people choose to live in. It is the engine room of societies as opined by Saunders and Williams (1988, p. 82). Thus, in order to understand the wider meanings given to housing, many social theorists prefer the term home to housing. Saunders and Williams (1988) focusing on Giddens' (1984) structuration theory stressed that home is the routine reproduction of the social world through interaction is accomplished within settings or *locale* which help make such interaction meaningful and to some extent predictable. In this sense, 'home' is a crucial locale which sets the basic form of social relations, interaction and social institutions that are constituted and reproduced. According to Giddens (1984), home is typically a small-scale locale, but can be strongly regionalised internally by modes of activity. Rooms within homes are usually categorised in respect to their characteristic usage in time-space as living rooms, kitchens, bedrooms, etc. Accordingly, a household is the mode of social organisation which is distinctive to home (Saunders and Williams 1988, p. 82). Thus, home, like the nation-state itself may act as an essential constitutive and reproductive element where its meaning can span over a wider scope than the mere dwelling.

Gilman (2002, p. 3) in her book; *The Home; its work and influence* defined home as a human institution which offers rest, peace, quiet, comfort, health and personal expression. It is the place where households accumulate their wealth, assets and social life. Therefore, a home is a locale and the centre in which one's personal satisfaction of life depends on. She further emphasised that home is a governing factor in the formation of character and the direction of life. In the estimation of

Giddens (1984, p. 18), 'a house is grasped as such only if the observer recognises that it is a dwelling with a range of other properties specified by the modes of its utilisation in human activity'. In a study on housing for the hard (homeless sector), Kraus (2001) and Gurstein and Small (2005) explained what home meant to those vulnerable sectors of the society as where one feels safe or one's heaven. To them, housing has been a cornerstone of care. Therefore, creating a home is a wider process of personal self-healing.

All in all, based on the various views discussed above, the housing can be said to be a social establishment where the satisfaction of life mainly depends upon. Furthermore, it inextricably has both social and spatial dimensions. Kemeny (1992, pp. 8–18.) echoed this by indicating that just focusing on home unnecessarily limits the scope of housing research as it does not allow much attention to be given to the various dimensions of housing which are broadly, social and spatial in nature. Thus, a broader overview of housing embraces locational factors and ties housing studies to macro-issues of the nature of the social structure. Therefore, housing needs to be seen as the nuclei of social production and reproduction. It should also be viewed within the integral dimension of markets, environment and society. Therefore, housing is a social institution where quality of life depends on to a great extent.

2.4 Housing Affordability

Whilst housing tends to be the largest investment outlay in a householder's lifetime income, housing affordability is a common way of summarising the nature of difficulty in accessing housing resource (Hulchanski 1995, p. 471). It is the central issue in any housing policy. Many scholarly works often interpret that housing affordability is a phenomenon that is vexed because it means different things to different people (Miles et al. 2000). This makes housing affordability to appear as a term that is ambiguously defined (Linneman and Megbolugbe 1992). This, therefore, raises a number of questions that need to be addressed which are as follows. Why housing affordability seemed to be ambiguous? Why is it being described differently at different times? Similar to the social meaning of housing described earlier, in an economic sense the meaning of housing is different from other commodities. It is considered to be an investment irrespective of whether it is used for personal consumption or as an income generating asset. This is mainly due to its very nature of being highly durable (long life), immovable and the hefty cost that it involves. It is considered as the largest investment (outlay) in a households' lifetime income (Mullins et al. 2006). Thus, home ownership is not only about use value but involves many strands including an appreciation of capital values, and a place of accumulation of wealth by households.

In practice, these social and economic meanings of housing do not operate in a mutually exclusive manner. Michael Stone, a well-known scholar in the field of housing affordability mentions that housing is a principal locus of personal and family life (Stone 1993, p. 10) which means that it is a judgement of socio-economic status of a family. Hence, reflecting on the social meaning of housing mentioned earlier housing can play a role as a catalyst for the accumulation of sociocultural wealth of human societies which could turn it away from economic rationale models. On the other hand, it is also a physical asset base that is build up by a family or a household based on their future expectations and expected circumstances. Mullins et al. (2006, p. 1) state that the housing situation today reflects the patterns of family life need and its investment 60–100 years earlier. Hence, a house is a reflection of private space created or chosen by families based on their perceptual needs and wants which would also fundamentally lead to external changes over the period of time such as economic growth and modernisation of societies.

Clapham (2005, p. 152.) rightly mentioned 'housing' as a means to an end and not an end in itself. Therefore, housing and its affordability are not all about the physical space to prices you pay for that as it appears, but a reflexivity of a rummage around the quality of life within space and time context. Thus, the ultimatum of home ownership or the utility of housing is not merely the consumption of it but it is also the achievement of the overall quality of life in economic, social and physical terms.

The term 'reflexivity' is an ongoing examination of the underlying assumptions and narratives that drive a practice. Generally, it relates to actions and consequences where the cause and effect of such actions can be explained. Harries-Jones (1991, p. 156) explains reflexivity as the 'capacity to act by linking the possibilities of present social action to an alternative epistemology'. Accordingly, this paper uses the term 'reflexivity' to mean the cause and effect relationship between housing affordability and quality of life. Hence, the above-mentioned ambiguity of housing affordability has some relations with the subjective meanings attached to the quality of life that are produced, reproduced, altered and transformed which makes housing affordability ambiguous or vexed. Housing policymakers should explicitly see and accept this intersection between housing affordability and quality of life. Furthermore, the nature of the social order in the society will depend on the ability of people to be able to sustain a particular version of reality as being the objective truth (Clapham 2005, p. 20). As explained in the time and space geography by Hägerstrand (1976), these truths are constantly constructed, negotiated and altered by individuals. Thus, as it is vital to understand the reflexivity of housing affordability and quality of life, it is also important to understand that these subjectivities of quality of life are changing across time and space and do have a reflexive form on housing affordability. Accordingly, the following section throws more light on housing affordability interconnections with quality of life.

2.5 Materials and Methods

The systematic review approach was utilised and this focuses on explicitly searching, appraising and synthesising available literature to satisfy the aim of a topic under study (Victor 2008; Akobeng 2005). The broad nature of the study necessitated this approach which enabled a wider search of the available literature on quality of life and housing affordability to support the study. The systematic review approach helped to avoid bias in the results of the study and also assisted in providing more accurate and reliable conclusions since the approach uses data that have already been tested in other studies. Secondary materials such as books, journals, conference papers and reports related to the topic under study were also taken into consideration. In order to follow a well-organised process or steps to retrieve the required data and provide necessary discussions for the current study different works on systematic review were looked at (Mensah et al. 2016; Uman 2011; Victor 2008; Coren and Fisher 2006; Khan et al. 2003). Below are the processes that were followed to undertake a systematic review of the study.

2.5.1 Formulating a Question to Guide the Review

This was the first process and very important as it provided a scope within which relevant literature was searched. It centred on framing a question to capture the main problem and purpose of the study. It was done to make the review well focused. The broad question posed to guide the review was as follows: *How is housing affordability reflexive of the quality of life of individuals?* Whilst the context of the investigation focused on OECD countries, all publications that were not directly or indirectly related to the above question fell outside the scope of the study.

2.5.2 Identifying Relevant Publications on the Topic Under Study

Necessary efforts were made to assemble relevant publications for the study. Among the major databases that were searched to get publications for the study were Google Scholar, Thomson Reuters, Science Direct, Social Science Research Network, Directory of Open Access Journals (DOAJ), Scopus, JSTOR, Ingenta Connect and Web of Science. In addition to this, Internet engines such as Google, Yahoo, Bing and Ask.com were also searched for further materials. A total of 521 relevant literatures were found at this stage.

2.5.3 Assessing the Quality of Selected Publications

At second stage, total relevant literature arrived were further reduced to 227 publications for final inclusion in the study. This was done in the line with the recommendation of Bowler et al. (2010) who considered six quality assessment criteria for published scholarly works. These criteria were the theoretical basis of the publication, data collection techniques employed, suitability of the target population or unit of analysis, sampling technique adopted, the tools or approach used for analysis and contribution of the publication to the knowledge in the field of study. To enhance the quality of findings of the study, publications which satisfied all or five of the above criteria were included in the study.

2.5.4 Analysis and Synthesis of Evidence

The finally selected publications were subjected to rigorous content analysis to get their main purposes, methods they applied and their major findings and conclusions. These information were collated and analysed to support the discussions of the chapter.

2.6 Housing Affordability and its Reflexivity on Quality of Life

2.6.1 Era of Industrialisation

The preconditions that raised the need to ensure an *affordable decent home* was the nineteenth-century industrial revolution and the accompanying urbanisation in the UK which later extended to the rest of Europe and North America. It generated market responses that packed the newly rural migrant workforce into unsanitary accommodation with inadequate facilities. The pre-industrialised families who were rural, large and self-sustaining were completely changed by modernisation (Mullins et al. 2001) which made families to become urban than rural. During that time when housing was supplied by private landlords and the rents were driven up, the working class could not afford a decent home but to live in a slum while many others sublet their accommodation in order to pay their rents resulting in overcrowded multifamily housing units (Merrett 1979). Urban morphology studies, for example, of Ernest Burgess in 1924, Homer Hoyt in 1939 and Ullman in 1945 (Harvey and Jowsey 2000) clearly reflected this pattern of residential production in the industrial cities, mainly in the West. Such residential production clearly reflected the way households sought their expected quality of life by attempting to gain housing units that they could afford. During that time, the affluent who could afford high earned housing and lived in better environments of inner cities away from industries but had access to many of the services such as schools, hospitals, shopping and clubs. The middle class who too was looking for a better pollution-free environment but could not afford the inner city residential areas settled at downtown residential units. The quality of life of the lower income working class who could not afford and survive with bare minimum needs such as food and shelter was the matter of concern. They could not afford the

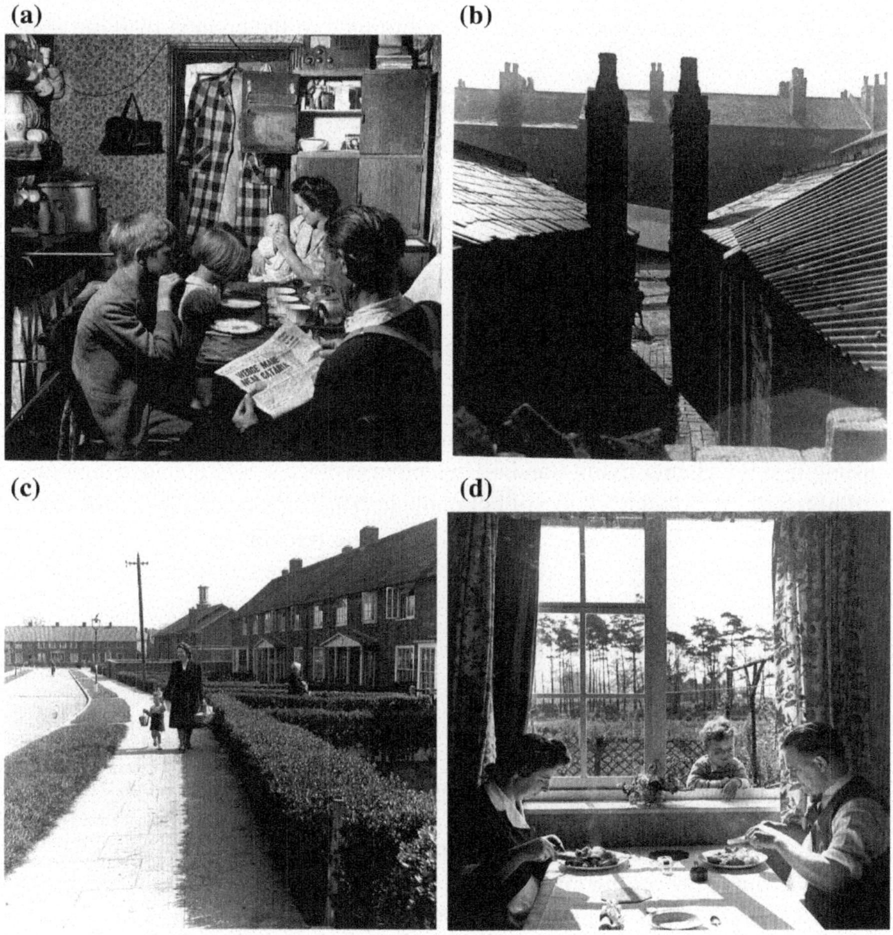

Fig. 2.1 Housing affordability and Quality of Life of working class and middle class in UK during industrialisation. *Source* Brandt et al. (2004, pp. 22, 32, 69, 79)

higher housing prices in the inner city and also the high transportation cost for moving to downtown areas. They had to jeopardise their quality of life by choosing to live in housing units in close proximity to their working places (industries) regardless of exposure to unsanitary conditions and increasing pollutants (see Fig. 2.1).

During that period, the initial knowledge for housing affordability was mainly concerned with the issues of health and amenity that the poor working-class people were facing. Looking into such condition, the Tudor Walters Committee of 1918 (in the context of UK) was appointed to counsel on a decent home for the working class (Swenarton 1981). This attempt was perceived as an idea of reflexivity towards quality of life. The industrial revolution through the post-war period till 1950s and early 1960s played a great role in moving forward the ideas of housing affordability and quality of life; however, such ideas were limited to the context of *basic living standard of the household.*

A and B: *Quality of life of the working class.*
C and D: *Quality of life of the middle class.*

That perception no wonder related to the situation at that time to address extremely poor health and amenity conditions during industrialisation and immediate recovery expectations during the post-war era. The early scientific studies that generally touched on housing affordability by Ernst Engel and Schwabe Herman during 1857 began to probe on how the household budgets of working-class families could be split between the housing and non-housing items to achieve a better standard of life (Reid 1962; Stigler 1954; Winnick 1955). The criteria commonly used was the rule of thumb of 30% (initial guide was 25%). It meant that a working-class household ought to spend 30% of their monthly income on housing and the rest for non-housing consumption for a better living standard, which in essence was to enhance their quality of life. See, for example, works of Feins and Lane (1982), and Lerman and Reeder (1987).

2.6.2 Neo-liberalism and Change of Quality of Life

The social construction of quality of life paradigmatically started changing during 1960s and 1970s. This was largely based on account of the demise of the Keynesian welfare state of the economy and the prominence of neo-liberalism. There was government disinvestment in public housing and the dominance of the production and delivery of housing with the market-driven systems at that time made housing affordability more provoking (Whitehead 1991). For instance, Nelson (1994, p. 401) on the US Congress on housing (1992, p. 8) remarked:

> Since the 1970s there has been a substantial reduction in the number of low rent units in the housing stock and a sharp increase in the number of poor families which resulted in a classic mismatch between supply and demand, leading to higher rents, higher rent burdens, increased overcrowding, increased evictions and increased homelessness.

In Australia, during 1980 and 1990, the profound neo-liberalised housing policies changed the social policy to economic policy which was too apparent in many dimensions of the society (Beer et al. 2007, p. 13). Besides, with the increase of materialism of life the pressure on household budgets started becoming agonising. For instance, a study by Bunting et al. (2004) in Canada showed that a household consumes almost twice as much as housing space during 2003, compared to what they had in 1950, despite the fact that households were much smaller in 2003.

This new economic change led to a collapse of the family supportive wage[2] and brought up a new form of poverty that departs quantitatively and qualitatively

[2]The wage earned by the head of the household that supports all other dependents.

from traditional forms of poverty (Grabb 1996; Bunting et al. 2004). According to Bramley (1994), the reduction of public expenditure on housing in UK coupled with the promotion of home ownership, privatisation, deregulation and the end of approach to housing had typified the post-war period after 1979, and moved the housing market in a different direction. These economic changes and growth patterns resulted in an increase of materialism; and drastic changes in demographic formation centring on nuclei families, lifestyle choices, economic growth patterns and immigration redefined the quality of life beyond the mere standard of living so as the housing affordability.

Thus, the normative frameworks limited housing affordability analysis to housing cost and non-housing cost element needed to be extended in order to accommodate the new changes in lifestyles and quality of life. The residual income approach introduced by Stone (2006a) to measure housing affordability was considered to be a major contribution in the field. The notion of the residual approach suggested that a household could have an affordability problem, if that respective household does not have enough income to meet the minimum standard (essential) of non-housing expenses incurring the housing expenses, regardless of its ratio between housing cost/rent to income ratio. Therefore, a household that spends more than 30%[3] of his or her monthly income but do not have any difficulty in meeting the minimum non-housing cost standard was said to be away from housing affordability issue. This approach rectified the way of liberalism's materialistic lifestyles that brought the quality of life to a different platform and thereby housing affordability. Stone (2006b, p. 151) opined that 'most fundamentally housing affordability is an expression of the social and material experiences of people, constituted as households in relation to their individual housing situations' along with the collapse of the family supportive wage, the middle-class women were expected to demonstrate competence at several tasks. With the changing of family hygiene, dietary habits, the working women and childcare altogether changed the architectural elements of a house which needed more than one attached bathroom, en-suite kitchens compatible with modern energy, servant's rooms and many others.

Furthermore, the quality of life of people started to depend not only on the *quantity* of goods but also on the quality of those goods. In view of this, the privatisation and deregulation of the housing markets led to people appreciating the quality of the housing units they live in. Households were no longer satisfied with houses that were just affordable but they started insisting on their quality. This change of thinking pattern was reflected in works of scholars such as Lerman and Reeder (1987), Thalmann (1999), and Quigley and Raphael (2004) developing indicators of housing affordability by combining the conventional rent income ratio with a quality-based rent income ratio. They started presenting ideas that housing affordability should be viewed beyond the mere housing costs by taking into account the impact of the long-term nature of housing, its quality and other elements.

These new dimensions of quality of life under open market economies, finally influenced the cost and space elements of housing units, thus on housing affordability.

[3]The normative standards given by the ratio approaches.

2.6.3 Sustainability Paradigm

The sustainability concerns emerged in the late 1960s and 70s as a reaction to the degradation of the environment and societies well-being in the post-war. A new economy was intensified during the turn of the twentieth century, as a reaction to the neo-liberalism led consumerism. This informed notable changes in people's lifestyle.

It largely renewed the interest of the ways in which quality of life should be defined. With the eco-centric view of the world, people started realising that quality of life does not merely depend on the material well-being that one would personally acquire but rather started to propel on its longevity and what it acquires as a community at large. People were informed that the unnecessary consumption of resources at present would jeopardise their quality of life in future. Therefore, the conventional presumption that the 'affordable housing should focus on meeting housing needs of the people and not preserving the environment' was challenged (Chiu 2004). There was a growing apprehension that '*environment* has to be safeguarded from deteriorating because such deterioration will diminish the ability of future generations to meet their housing needs' (Chiu 2004, p. 65). Here, the word '*environment'* had a broader perspective beyond the meaning of immediate surroundings. As Saegert et al. (2003, pp. 1472, 1473) mentioned it is the behaviour, the physical and social environment and health that dynamically connect individuals, households, buildings and communities for the liveability of the internal and external living environments. This paradigm shift in the housing need and affordability definitions away from the quality of life concept form pure economic perspective to incorporate environmental and social concerns (Fig. 2.2).

Many of the pre-existing literature that defined and measured housing affordability by merely focusing on 'four walls of the house' based on *house price* (without consideration of liveability, the condition, location and neighbourhood character that a housing unit is associated with) seemed out fashioned (Haas et al. 2006). As a result of this, Salama and Alshuwaikhat (2006) opined that for the purpose of finding a

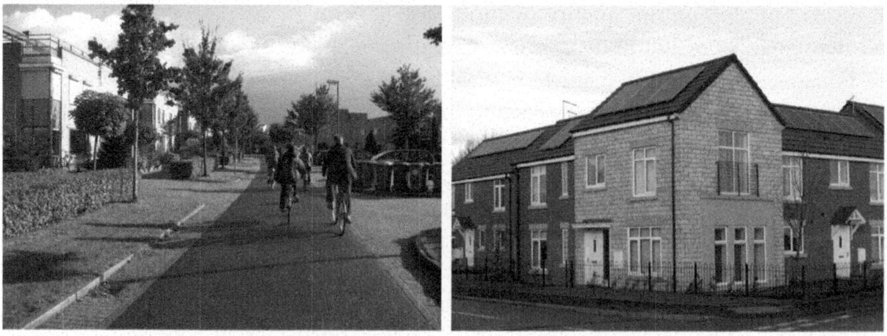

Fig. 2.2 Housing estates designs to incorporate environmental and social-friendly elements such as cycling, roof tops with solar panels. *Source* Falk and Carley (2012), and author

sustainable way to measure housing affordability three dimensions should be looked at. They are the economic dimension which is associated with the financial costs of housing development, the social dimension which includes the sense of belonging and the feeling of togetherness among the inhabitants, and the environmental dimension that encourages water and energy conservation within a building. In the views of Maliene et al. (2008), sustainable housing affordability encompasses 'sufficient in offer, quality (from the technical and provision point of view), economic (greater number of households have opportunities to purchase it and cover the exploitation expenses), ecological (energy saving etc. and comfortless (from the social–psychological point of view)'.

These ideas on housing affordability have now started reflecting in both theory and practice. Many of the contemporary scholarly works on housing affordability highlighted the need for inclusion of ecology as well as the sociocultural sustainability dimensions within the definition and measurement of housing affordability. As such, Chiu (2004) mentioned five elements that the current housing affordability should cover; (a) the social preconditions conducive to the production and consumption of environmentally sustainable housing, (b) equitable distribution and consumption of housing resources and assets, (c) harmonious social relations within the housing system, (d) an acceptable quality of housing conditions and (e) preservation of housing heritage.

Hence, the prior measures of housing affordability were assumed to be in the quantifiable attributes of dwellings and their related cost were viewed within the relationships between the process, the product and the sociocultural aspects of the target population (Salama 2006). In practice, various projects have been built on the broad concept of housing affordability with various aspects of housing affordability such as economic, social and ecology dimensions being key parts of those projects. The end results of those projects have been successes in improving quality of life since they touched on the basic necessities that quality of life depends on. Some notable examples are Sustainable Neighbourhoods in the Netherlands such as Vathorst, Houten and Almere Poort, Affordable Green Neighbourhoods in USA like Essex Crossing—New York, West Grand and Brush—Oakland, Calif and The Sustainable Urban Extensions and New Settlements in UK at areas such as Milton Keynes, Orchard Park, Cambridge, Telford and Dickens Heath in West Midlands, Grand Union Village, London. Furthermore, in establishing the first ever 'quality of life' barometer in the UK, the housing indicator was chosen because housing was a key component of a decent quality of life.

These projects and their reflexivity of quality of life revisited housing affordability as a concept. The examples worthy of attention include the views of the Centre for Neighbourhood Technology (CNT) in the United States. Their suggestion of measuring locational affordability is Housing plus Transport Affordability Index which takes into consideration six neighbourhood variables[4] and three household variables[5] (Haas et al. 2006). The range of the CNTs' method varies from building houses to their connection with jobs and neighbourhoods. Mulliner et al. (2013) proposed the Complex Proportional Assessment (COPRAS) method of Multi-Criteria Decision-making (MCDM) to assess the sustainability of housing affordability, which is capable of taking into consideration numerous decision criteria. They applied this method with a total of 20 weighted criteria[6] including a wider range of economic, environmental and social criteria. Broadening the concept of housing affordability with social and environmental considerations, on the other hand, is reflexive of the shift away of the quality of life concept; from single- or unit-based view (satisfaction of one's personal life or household's life) towards the more pluralist view. It is no longer a thing an individual can attain alone but requires collective efforts and responsibility.

2.7 Conclusions

In sum, quality of life is a multifaceted concept with its scope cutting across many disciplines. This chapter highlighted how it is linked to housing affordability. Housing affordability provides a means to reflect how the quality of life was understood and has changed over different periods of time from industrialisation to the sustainability paradigm. Over the years, its' focus has shifted from mere material gains to encompass broader aspects of human well-being. Through this, the chapter argues, what is perceived to constitute quality of life today may not be necessarily the same in future. Quality of life is conceptually subjected to be constructed, negotiated and altered over time-space.

References

Akobeng, A. K. (2005). Understanding systematic reviews and meta-analysis. *Archives of Disease in Childhood, 90*(6), 845–848.

Beer, A., Kearins, B., & Pieters, H. (2007). Housing affordability and planning in Australia: The challenge of policy under neo-liberalism. *Housing Studies, 22*(1), 11–24.

---

[4]Residential density, job density, average block size in acres, transit connectivity index, job density, average time journey to work, household income, household size, commuters per household.

[5]House price in relation to income, rental costs in relation to incomes, interest rates and mortgage availability, availability of social and private rented accommodation, availability of affordable home ownership products, safety (crime level), access to employment.

[6]Opportunities, access to public transport services, access to good quality schools, access to shops, access to health services, access to child care, access to leisure facilities, access to open green public space, quality of housing, energy efficiency of housing, availability of waste management facilities, desirability of neighbourhood area, deprivation in area, presence of environment problems (e.g. litter, traffic).

Bowler, D. E., Buyung-Ali, L. M., Knight, T. M., & Pullin, A. S. (2010). A systematic review of evidence for the added benefits to health of exposure to natural environments. *BMC Public Health, 10,* 456.

Bramley, G. (1994). An affordability crisis in British housing: Dimensions, causes and policy impact. *Housing Studies, 9*(1), 103.

Brandt, B., James, P., & Sadler, R. (2004). *Homes fit for heroes: Photographs by Bill Brandt, 1939–1943.* UK: Dewi Lewis Publishing.

Bunting, T., Walks, A. R., & Filion, P. (2004). The uneven geography of housing affordability stress in Canadian metropolitan areas. *Housing Studies, 19*(3), 361–393.

Chiu, R. L. (2004). Socio-cultural sustainability of housing: A conceptual exploration. *Housing, Theory and Society, 21*(2), 65–76.

Clapham, D. (2005). *The meaning of housing: A pathways approach.* UK: The Policy Press.

Coren, E., & Fisher, M. (2006). *The conduct of systematic reviews for SCIE knowledge reviews.* London, United Kingdom: Social Care Institute for Excellence.

Cummins, R. A. (2005). Moving from the quality of life concept to a theory. *Journal of Intellectual Disability Research, 49*(10), 699–706.

Falk, N., & Carley, M. (2012). *Sustainable urban neighbourhoods: Building communities that last.* York, UK: Joseph Rowntree Foundation.

Feins, J. D., & Lane, T. S. (1982). *How much for housing?: New perspectives on affordability and risk.* Abt Books.

Felce, D. (1997). Defining and applying the concept of quality of life. *Journal of Intellectual Disability Research, 41,* 126–135.

Felce, D., & Perry, J. (1995). Quality of life: Its definition and measurement. *Research in Developmental Disabilities, 16*(1), 51–74.

Felce, D., & Perry, J. (1996). Adaptive behaviour gains in ordinary housing for people with intellectual disabilities. *Journal of Applied Research in Intellectual Disabilities, 9*(2), 101–114.

Ferrans, C. E. (1996). Development of a conceptual model of quality of life. *Research and Theory for Nursing Practice, 10*(3), 293–304.

Galloway, S. (2006). *Quality of life and well-being: Measuring the benefits of culture and sport: A literature review.* Edinburgh, Scotland: Scottish Executive Social Research.

Giddens, A. (1984). *The constitution of society: Outline of the theory of structuration.* Cambridge: Polity press.

Gilman, C. P. (2002). The home: Its work and influence. Rowman Altamira (reprint of Gilman, C.P. (1903) The Home: Its Work and Influence). New York: McClure, Phillips.

Grabb, E. G. (1996). *Theories of social inequality: Classical and contemporary perspectives.* Toronto, ON: Harcourt Brace and Co.

Gurstein, P., & Small, D. (2005). From housing to home: Reflexive management for those deemed hard to house. *Housing Studies, 20*(5), 717–735.

Haas, B. K. (1999). A multidisciplinary concept analysis of quality of life. *Western Journal of Nursing Research, 21*(6), 728–742.

Haas, P. M., Makarewicz, C., Benedict, A., et al. (2006). *Housing & transportation cost trade-offs and burdens of working households in 28 metros.* Center for Neighborhood Technology, 2.

Hägerstrand, T. (1976). *Innovation as a spatial process.* Chicago, IL: University of Chicago Press.

Harries-Jones, P. (1991). Making knowledge count: Advocacy and social science. McGill-Queen's Press-MQUP.

Harvey, J., & Jowsey, E. (2000) *Urban land economics.* Macmillan.

Hulchanski, J. D. (1995). The concept of housing affordability: Six contemporary uses of the housing expenditure-to-income ratio. *Housing Studies, 10*(4), 471–491.

Kemeny, J. (1992). *Housing and social theory.* London and New York: Routledge.

Khan, K. S., Kunz, R., Kleijnen, J., & Antes, D. (2003). Five steps to conducting a systematic review. *Journal of the Royal Society of Medicine, 96*(3), 118–121.

Kraus, D. (2001). Housing for people with alcohol and drug addictions: An annotated bibliography. City of Vancouver.

Lerman, D. L., & Reeder, W. J. (1987). The affordability of adequate housing. *Real Estate Economics, 15*(4), 389–404.
Lindstrom, B. (1994). *The essence of existence. On the quality of life of children in the Nordic countries—theory and practice in public health.* Doctoral thesis, Nordic School of Public Health, Gothenburg, Sweden.
Linneman, P. D., & Megbolugbe, I. F. (1992). Housing affordability: Myth or reality? *Urban Studies, 29*(3–4), 369–392.
Maliene, V., Howe, J., & Malys, N. (2008). Sustainable communities: affordable housing and socio-economic relations. *Local Economy, 23*(4), 267–276.
McMahon, S. (2002). The development of quality of life indicators—a case study from the City of Bristol, UK. *Ecological Indicators, 2*(1), 177–185.
Mensah, C. A., Andres, L., Perera, U., & Roji, A. (2016). Enhancing quality of life through the lens of green spaces: A systematic review approach. *International Journal of Wellbeing, 6*(1), 142–163.
Merrett, S. (1979). *State housing in Britain*. Routledge & Kegan Paul London.
Miles, M. E., Berens, G., & Weiss, M. A. (2000). *Real estate development: Principles and process*. Urban Land Institute Washington, DC.
Moons, P., Budts, W., & De Geest, S. (2006). Critique on the conceptualisation of quality of life: A review and evaluation of different conceptual approaches. *International Journal of Nursing Studies, 43*(7), 891–901.
Mulliner, E., Smallbone, K., & Maliene, V. (2013). An assessment of sustainable housing affordability using a multiple criteria decision making method. *Omega, 41*(2), 270–279.
Mullins, D., Murie, A., & Leather, P. (2006). *Housing policy in the UK*. Palgrave Macmillan Basingstoke.
Mullins, D., Reid, B., & Walker, R. M. (2001). Modernization and change in social housing: The case for an organizational perspective. *Public Administration, 79*(3), 599–623.
Nelson, K. P. (1994). Whose shortage of affordable housing? *Housing Policy Debate, 5*(4), 401–442.
Quigley, J. M., & Raphael, S. (2004). Is housing unaffordable? Why isn't it more affordable? *The Journal of Economic Perspectives, 18*(1), 191–214.
Reid, M. G. (1962). *Housing and income*. University of Chicago Press Chicago.
Saegert, S. C., Klitzman, S., Freudenberg, N., et al. (2003). Healthy housing: A structured review of published evaluations of US interventions to improve health by modifying housing in the United States, 1990-2001. *American Journal of Public Health, 93*(9), 1471–1477.
Salama, A. (2006). A life style theories approach for affordable housing research in Saudi Arabia. *Emirates Journal for Engineering Research, College of Environmental Design, 11*(1), 67–76.
Salama, A. M., & Alshuwaikhat, H. M. (2006). A trans-disciplinary approach for a comprehensive understanding of sustainable affordable housing. *Global Built Environment Review, 5*(3), 35–50.
Saunders, P., & Williams, P. (1988). The constitution of the home: Towards a research agenda. *Housing studies, 3*(2), 81–93.
Sirgy, M. J. (1998). Materialism and quality of life. *Social Indicators Research, 43*(3), 227–260.
Stigler, G. J. (1954). The early history of empirical studies of consumer behavior. *The Journal of Political Economy*, 95–113.
Stone, M. E. (1993). *Shelter poverty: New ideas on housing affordability.* Philadelphia: Temple University Press.
Stone, M. E. (2006a). A housing affordability standard for the UK. *Housing Studies, 21*(4), 453–476.
Stone, M. E. (2006b). What is housing affordability? The case for the residual income approach. *Housing Policy Debate, 17*(1), 151–184.
Swenarton, M. (1981). *Homes fit for heroes: The politics and architecture of early state housing in Britain.* Heinemann Educational Books.
Testa, M. A., & Simonson, D. C. (1996). Assessment of quality-of-life outcomes. *New England Journal of Medicine, 334*(13), 835–840.
Thalmann, P. (1999). Identifying households which need housing assistance. *Urban Studies, 36*(11), 1933–1947.

Uman, L. S. (2011). Systematic reviews and meta analyses. *Journal of the Canadian Academy of Child and Adolescent Psychiatry, 20*(1), 57–59.
U.S. Congress. Senate. Committee on Banking, Housing and Urban Affairs. (1992). Report to accompany S. 3031, National Affordable Housing Act Amendments of 1992. 102d Cong., 2d sess., Report 102-232. Washington, DC: U.S. Government Printing Office. (Cited in Nelson, K. P. (1994) Whose shortage of affordable housing? *Housing Policy Debate*, *5*(4), 401–442).
Victor, L. (2008). Systematic reviewing. *Social Science Update, 58,* 1–4.
Whitehead, C. M. (1991). From need to affordability: An analysis of UK housing objectives. *Urban Studies*, *28*(6), 871–887.
Winnick, L. (1955). Housing: Has there been a downward shift in consumers' preferences? *The Quarterly Journal of Economics, 69*(1), 85–98.
World Health Organisation (1997). *Measuring quality of life: The World Health Organization quality of life Instruments* (WHO/MSA/MNH/PSF/97.4). Geneva, Switzerland: World Health Organisation.
Yuen, B., Kwee, L. K., & Tu, Y. (2006). Housing affordability in Singapore: Can we move from public to private housing? *Urban Policy and Research, 24*(2), 253–270.

Chapter 3
Sustainable Development and Quality of Life

Christopher Cusack

Abstract Awareness of the need for sustainable development is increasing throughout the world. The goals of sustainable development, oriented around the "three E's"—environmental protection, economic growth, and social equity, also correlate with quality of life considerations. Quality of life addresses peoples' perceptions of their position in life in relation to their culture, values, and expectations. Using measures such as the life satisfaction rating and the human development index, both available from the United Nations Development Programme (UNDP), a positive correlation between self-assessed well-being and overall life satisfaction becomes evident. The UNDP also provides an environmental performance index which likewise correlates with well-being. These correlations appear at both national- and city-specific scales. Achieving progress in quality of life through sustainable development, particularly at the city level, requires careful planning that is both place and culture specific and that involves community and citizen input. Improving quality of life and meeting the needs of the present through sustainable development will help ensure greater likelihood of likewise accommodating the needs of future generations.

Keywords Sustainability · Well-being · City

3.1 Introduction

Improving the quality of life for individuals around the world is an admirable goal. However, the means to achieve such a goal or even accurately measure the concept of quality of life remains largely elusive. Quality of life considerations may be managed at various geographic scales, though at the finest level it is the individual that truly matters. It is of little value for a country or a city or even a neighborhood to be considered as having a relatively high quality of life to an individual who does not share in such well-being. In this situation, a rising tide does not necessarily lift

---

C. Cusack (✉)
Department of Geography, Outdoor Recreation, and Planning, Keene State College, Keene, NH 03435-2001, USA
e-mail: ccusack@keene.edu

B. R. K. Sinha (ed.), *Multidimensional Approach to Quality of Life Issues*,
https://doi.org/10.1007/978-981-13-6958-2_3

all boats. Yet, this does not mean that aspirations toward higher qualities of life at all levels should be disregarded, as proper planning efforts can indeed lead to success. At the neighborhood level, it is noted that residents of those neighborhoods considered "green" are more likely to achieve superior health, happiness, and equity (Gilderbloom 2016). In fact, projects and plans aimed at overall well-being in the neighborhood and beyond are frequently of value for their service toward another valuable objective relating to sustainable development. Indeed, the concepts of quality of life and sustainable development are not at all dissimilar and efforts to improve one may well positively affect the other as well.

An understanding of these concepts reveals the underlying connectivity between the two. With its emphasis on the individual, the World Health Organization Quality of Life (WHOQOL) Group defines quality of life as the perceptions of individuals with regards to their own personal goals and expectations, their standards, and their concerns (Feng and Hsieh 2009). Clearly, it can be expected that individual goals, in many cases, will be the same as it is in case of air and water quality, economic opportunity, and personal safety. Individuals in accordance with these and other issues aim at improving general quality which in turn will also improve the plight of the individual. Yet, inequities remain and individual well-being remains elusive for many. Addressing the issue of inequity, and complementing desires for economic and environmental vitality, is the concept of sustainable development. Brought into popular lexicon via the publication *Our Common Future*, also known as the Brundtland Report, sustainability has been defined as development that meets the needs of the present without comprising the ability of future generations to meet their own needs (World Commission on Environment and Development 1987). More recently, this definition has been explicated as development that generates economic growth, distributes benefits equitably, regenerates the environment, and promotes people (Moşteanu et al. 2014).

Thus, by assimilating individual concerns into a collective conscious, sustainable development seeks not only the environmental protection and economic vitality, but social equity as well. This balance between the three E's of sustainability (Fig. 3.1), as well as between the collective and the individual have made sustainable development one of the great challenges of the twenty-first century. It also reflects the fact that the "quality of life of the world's children in 2050 will depend on our decisions of today" (Göpel 2010, 62). While progress in quality of life and progress in sustainable development are mirroring processes, there are also shared constraints in terms of assessment and achievement. Most notably, concepts of well-being and sustainability are influenced by culture. Relevant literature, therefore, emphasizes the need for greater cultural awareness and heightened intercultural dialog, while noting that different people hold different views of the environment (Gambini 2006; Pellicer 2008). Even prosperity itself has different meanings for different cultures and peoples. As noted by Bijl (2011, 160), the act of building new roads may indicate prosperity and investment in the future or it may be associated with shorter commutes and more leisure time. Still others, however, may consider additional road building to be a detriment to nature and a use of resources that could be better applied toward alternative transportation measures. Both communities and people are unique, and

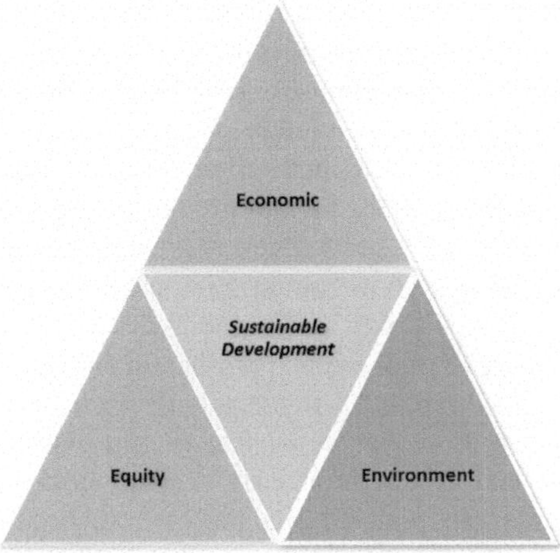

Fig. 3.1 The three E's of sustainable development

their approach to sustainable development and their quality of life considerations vary from one to another, as well as change over time for a single community (Fischer and Adjo 2011, 40).

3.2 Historical Evidence and Present Concerns

The mission of generating new development and retrofitting the existing built environment in a sustainable fashion, while at the same time seeking to improve the quality of life of the populace, may well appear daunting. Efforts to accomplish these tandem tasks, however, must be undertaken in order to ensure that future generations have the same opportunities that are available today. History has shown that cities and even civilizations have waxed and waned as a result of attitudes and actions toward natural resources and the environment. While much has been made of ancient Rome collapsing from within, with environmental degradation being plausibly identified as a contributor, there are numerous additional examples of societal ruin that are far more closely aligned with negative impacts on the environment. The work of Diamond (2005) highlights the collapse of civilizations such as Easter Island, the Anasazi, and Greenland Norse as an outcome of such environmental travails like deforestation, overfishing, and soil degradation. It has similarly been hypothesized that the disappearance of the Mayan cities, so too Angkor Wat, is directly attributable to environmental problems such as the lack of water (Bugliarello 2011).

Parallels between present-day cities and societies and those of past demise are not difficult to perceive. Concerns of rising sea levels are already raising the specter of environmental refugees and the displacement of residents of low-lying islands, such as Tuvalu and the Maldives. Similarly, warming sea temperatures as an instigator of cyclones and ultimate rise in the sea level itself has been explored (Walsh et al.

2012). Nor are concerns limited to Small Island nations of the South Pacific, as coastal nations and cities across the world are faced with similar threats. Yet the environment alone does not comprise sustainable development nor is it the singular quality of life consideration. Economic and social dysfunctionalities have also hastened the demise of earlier societies and can negatively impact both cities and nations today. One needs only to look at the social and economic dysfunction of some of the present-day rustbelt cities in the United States. More dramatic are the continuing horrid living conditions of places such as Harare, Zimbabwe, which according to the *Economic Intelligence Unit* consistently ranks among the worst cities in the world where people live even despite of high crime, poor health care and public transit, and civil unrest.

The principal difference between historical correlation and declining sustainability and societies as well as present-day concerns is essentially a matter of scale. Heretofore, such concerns were city or civilization specific, whereas today such concerns transcend national and even international boundaries to reach levels of global concern. By many accounts, the challenge of this century is to critically examine the economic and environmental realities of the day, and to set aside short-term conveniences for the creation of more sustainable regions characterized by protection of the environment, social justice, and economic vitality (Ziegler 2009). This challenge can be undertaken at all levels of scale. The individual can choose to walk more or take the bus to work. Neighborhood groups can coalesce and reduce crime and improve social cohesion through watch groups and community gardens. Cities can examine their budgets and seek more equitable returns on the allocation of revenue. Nations can collaborate in order to take on pressing global concerns. An appealing quality of life, good governance, sufficient food, water, energy, employment, housing, and education, as well as health care, transportation, aesthetics, and more. These are the characteristics of a truly sustainable society that throughout history have caused societal transcendence or demise (Bugliarello 2011). The pressing question then is whether or not individuals, cities, and nations choose to follow the path of sustainability.

3.3 Connecting Sustainability with Quality of Life

What must be understood is that, despite the best of intentions, if people are not satisfied with their current quality of life they cannot be expected to make sacrifices that may potentially benefit future generations. This necessarily obligates sustainable development programs to address present-day well-being in addition to that of future generations (Morrill in Stoltman 2011, 376–377). In a similar fashion, it is difficult for many to accord higher levels of concern to the needs of future generations than to those in desperate need today. Thus, a truly holistic approach to sustainable development does not address only the environment but also the economic and social concerns, and offers the optimal opportunity for success. Fortunately, as noted, efforts to improve the quality of present populations are frequently those that address the very issues of sustainability. On this point, the literature is clear; quality of life and sustainability are in large part one and the same:

i. "The concept and content of quality of life and sustainability are similar" (Feng and Hsieh 2009, 15).

ii. "At its heart, sustainability is a concept which accords central status to quality of life for present and future generations, at home and abroad" (Bijl 2011, 158).

iii. "Sustainability, then, can be viewed as a state where the key goals of sustainable development are satisfied, a high quality of life is achieved, and the environment is preserved" (Fischer and Adjo 2011, 39).

iv. "Today the indicator of quality of life is widely tied with the concept of sustainable development and is an important part of it" (Lotfi et al. 2011, 232).

deVries and Petersen (2009, 1007) note that literally hundreds of definitions of sustainable development have been proffered over recent decades. Seeking to summarize these definitions and to highlight interdisciplinary nature of sustainability, they themselves define sustainable development as "a quest for developing and sustaining 'qualities of life.'"

By establishing this deep-rooted connection between sustainability and well-being, the very definition of "quality of life" is at some level at one with that of sustainability. Moreover, both sustainable development and the concept of quality of life may be defined and measured in a variety of ways. In fact, Bell and Morse (2008) point out that an entire journal, *Quality of Life Research*, is dedicated to study of the topic. Usage of the term "quality of life" is increasing measurably in relevant literature, with the term "sustainability" likewise becoming increasingly common since 2000 (Barrington-Leigh and Escande 2018). Although somewhat vague in meaning, and certain to vary from person to person and place to place, the existence of similarities among tools measuring these concepts has been noted (Lotfi et al. 2011, 232). This similitude affords some opportunity for comparative analysis, and provides the theoretical basis for study of the concept. While some studies employ the objective approach and statistically analyze variables considered to influence quality of life, other approaches are more subjective in their analysis. The Subjective Well-Being (SWB) approach assesses quality of life by simply asking people how happy/unhappy and content/discontent they are with their life (de Vries and Petersen 2009, 1008). A wide array of literature focuses on the dimensions of quality of life and SWB (Botha 2016). Similarly, the *Human Development Report* put out by the United Nations Development Programme includes an overall life satisfaction rating by country. This ranking is based on self-perceptions of well-being, with the specific survey question being posed as such: Please imagine a ladder, with steps numbered from zero at the bottom to ten at the top. Suppose we say that the top of the ladder represents the best possible life for you and the bottom of the ladder represents the worst possible life for you. On which step of the ladder would you say you personally feel you stand at this time, assuming that the higher the step the better you feel about your life, and

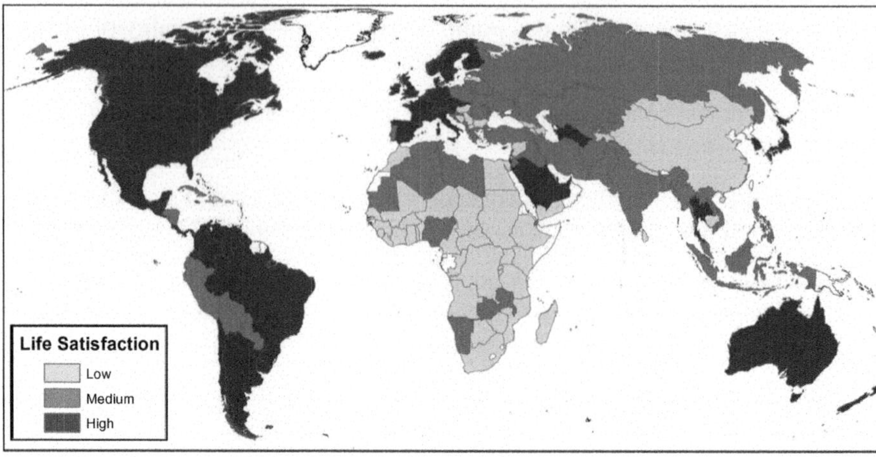

Fig. 3.2 Life satisfaction ratings

the lower the step the worse you feel about it? Which step comes closest to the way you feel? (UNDP 2011, 157).

With the typical survey including at least 1,000 surveys of randomly selected individuals, a viable cross section of a country can be generated. Responses to this quality of life question ranged from a low of 2.8 in Togo to a high of 7.8 in Denmark. The African continent lacks even a single country wherein people self-profess a relatively high quality of life, with a majority of the countries of the continent joining Togo in the lowest category. In contrast, Western Europe and North America are almost exclusively in the highest satisfaction classification. Asia ranges from high to low, with most countries in the middle range of satisfaction (Fig. 3.2).

3.4 Well-Being and Human Development

These results demonstrate that quality of life considerations follow a general economic trend; the countries with the greatest professed life satisfaction and scoring toward the top of the ladder are typically those categorized as having very high human development. Human development, also measured by the UNDP publication, is generated via a composite of three indicators of progress: a country's wealth, as measured by its Gross National Income (GNI); its health, as measured by life expectancy; and its education, measured by years of schooling. The resulting value is placed in a global Human Development Index (HDI). Values range from 0 to 1, with higher values representing higher human development. As with the overall life satisfaction ranking, a Scandinavian country has the highest HDI (Norway at 0.943) and a sub-Saharan African country has the lowest (the Democratic Republic of the Congo at 0.286). From several studies, it is found that almost all countries of

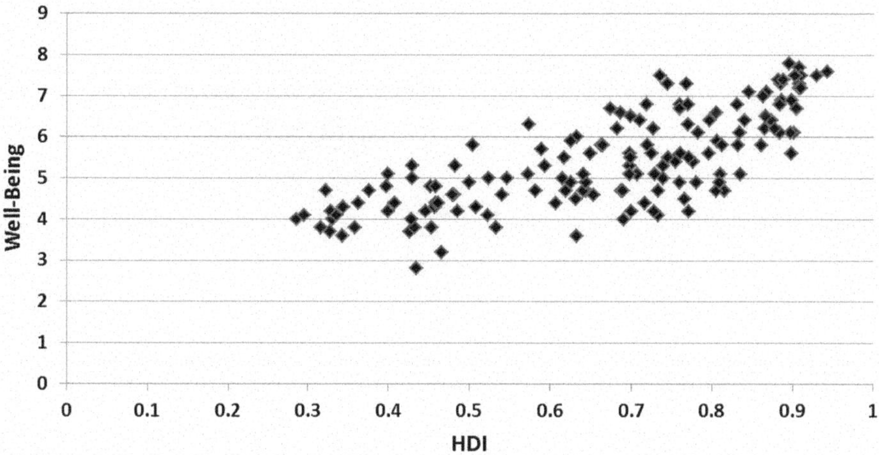

Fig. 3.3 Correlation between well-being and human development index

the world have progressed in their HDI levels over time, with fertility and female schooling being the greatest predictors of such progress (Molina and Purser 2010). Single greatest threat to this progress is the impact of war (Ward 2015). Countries in strife are hard pressed to demonstrate any improvements in HDI or any measurement related to quality of life. Despite an upward trend of progress, geographic disparities continue to remain in the HDI and are reflected in a correlation with overall life satisfaction scores. The correlation between human development index scores and self-assessed well-being scores is perhaps unsurprising (Fig. 3.3).

The coinciding upward trends of both values denote the obvious fact that overall life satisfaction is clearly influenced by such variables as health, wealth, and education. Such coinciding trends are important because the standard of living concept focuses on economic welfare while quality of life includes culture, religious aspects, and the environment (Ioncică and Petrescu 2016). From this correlation, however, the impact of the environment on quality of life considerations remains unclear. In order to determine the extent of this correlation, the well-being variable can be evaluated in light of an environmental performance index. Any association between the two variables would indicate that the quality of the environment has an impact on the quality of life. This, then, reinforces the principles of sustainable development and the need for consideration of the environment in any economic agenda. To ascertain some measures of the impact of environment on human well-being, the environmental performance index is used as a composite measure of sustainability. This index, calculated by the UNDP, comprises 25 performance indicators across ten policy categories and this covers both the environmental public health and ecosystem vitality (UNDP 2011).

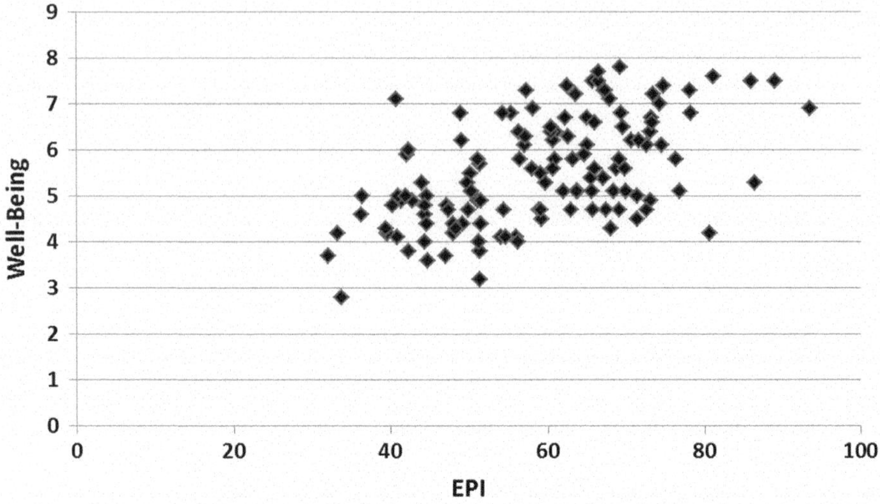

Fig. 3.4 Correlation between well-being and environmental performance index

3.5 Well-Being and Environmental Performance

The environmental performance index ranges from 0 to 100, with the lowest score and highest score, respectively, belonging to yet another sub-Saharan African country (Sierra Leone with a score of 32.1) and Scandinavian country (Iceland with a score of 93.5). The correlation between the EPI and reported well-being may also be readily noted as shown in Fig. 3.4. From this figure, it is clear that the relationship between well-being and HDI is not as pronounced as it appears; however, there is a definite positive trend between well-being and environmental performance index. Countries on the lower end of the EPI spectrum tend to be on the lower rung of the well-being ladder, while countries with higher EPI scores demonstrating correspondingly higher well-being scores. The general linkage between the two variables is apparent, though it may also be noted that every country does not follow positive trend. For instance, the neighboring countries such as Albania and the former Yugoslav Republic of Macedonia (F.Y.R.O.M.) have relatively high score on the EPI, but show only marginal overall life satisfaction. Albania, with a score of 86.4 on the EPI, reveals only a 5.3 on the well-being ladder. Similarly, F.Y.R.O.M. has a score of 80.6 on the EPI but only 4.2 score on overall life satisfaction. Conversely, Costa Rica, with a lower score of 57.3 on the EPI shows a much higher life satisfaction rating of 7.3.

Keeping such anomalies aside, the trend is obvious; countries with higher environmental performance index scores typically demonstrate higher overall life satisfaction scores. The policy implications of these findings are considerable. The overall life satisfaction correlates positively with both the HDI and environmental performance and indicates that in terms of environment and economy one cannot be sacrificed for the other. This is noteworthy in all countries of the world, but perhaps it is most important for the developing countries of the global south. Within these countries, economic progress is generating the rise of a new global middle class. The rise of such a class will undoubtedly be associated with increase in consumption of material goods and energy resources, and hence there is need for development to take on all the trappings of sustainability. Yet increase in income alone has been shown to play only a limited role in happiness, with family, health, environment, freedom, and other variables also critically influencing perceptions of well-being (de Vries and Petersen 2009, 1008). Therefore, awareness of the intrinsic value of nature and of other variables is more difficult to quantify economically. This may help to engender holistic development that considers equity and the environment in tandem with economic growth.

The difference between economic growth and economic prosperity makes a critical distinction. Growth being a more crass term is found frequently associated with money. Prosperity is a broader term that includes the nonmonetary aspects of quality of life. The need for the prosperity to be sustained and inclusive has been similarly acknowledged (Greenwood and Holt 2010, 164). The notion that income or other objective indices of wealth do not necessarily correlate with increased quality of life. This statement can be supported through an example of a swimming pool. As pointed out by Angur et al. (2004, 47), "To one swimming pool owner it may represent prestige and success, making him feel better about himself and his life generally. To another, the pool may represent a burden of time, energy and money. It is not uncommon to find the symbols of affluence accompanied by great dissatisfaction and frustration, or very humble conditions where much happiness prevails." The swimming pool example reveals the subjective nature of quality of life considerations and the difficulty in measuring such a concept with objective indices. It also reveals that perceived quality of life varies from person to person, just as it varies over time and over geographic space.

These difficulties should not mean that improvements in quality of life are not sought; rather they demonstrate the need for place- and culture-specific measures to be enacted. Despite its "multidimensional construct", achieving progress in quality of life through sustainable development planning has been advocated as a necessary objective (Fischer and Adjo 2011, 40). What is not the answer is a one-size-fits-all approach to sustainable development that is more likely than not to be doomed to failure due to the incredible diversity of both the human and natural worlds. The success of sustainable development initiatives is thought to be dependent on how closely they align with and contribute to a sense of place in a given space. The very concept of "place" has emerged as central to sustainability, with stronger emotional ties being associated with greater opportunity for success in sustainable development initiatives (Dale et al. 2008, 279). This would indicate that the instability associated with migration (forced or otherwise) hinders the feelings of belonging so vital to a strong sense of place. A sense of belonging also contributes to overall quality of life. As such, migration must then be accepted as a critical challenge to both QOL and sustainable development initiatives. Moreover, whether the migration is occurring within or between countries, it is typically directed toward cities.

3.6 Sustainable Cities

Highlighted as a seminal moment in the history of human settlement, the year 2007 marked the first time that a majority of the human population lived in urban as opposed to rural areas. Driven by natural increase but even more so by migration, the percentage of urbanites is projected to only increase (Beall and Fox 2007, 4). Rapidly increasing urbanization is now a hallmark of the global south and confirms the pressing need for growth to occur with some semblance of sustainability measures in place. Rapid urbanization brings concomitant escalations in population density, traffic congestion, and pollution. However, with no such concomitant improvements to living conditions guaranteed, the chance for development to occur sustainably will likely suffer alongside overall quality of life (Morrill in Stoltman 2011, 376). The livability of a place has itself been proffered as being synonymous to quality of life, and that the common experiences along with the ability of the city to meet the needs of its populace are directly tied to quality of life (Lotfi et al. 2011, 232). The need to focus on the city is clarified by the introspection advocated by Beall and Fox (2007, 4), "So when we – as students, policy makers, or development practitioners – ask ourselves what kind of world we want to live in 10 or 20 years from now, we must also ask ourselves what kind of *cities* we want to live in." McCarney (2015) echoes this sentiment by noting that cities are taking worldwide center stage not only in sustainable development, but also in the very prosperity of nations.

Currently, many cities exhibit a dual existence with gleaming skyscrapers juxtaposed with dismal slum settlements. An estimated one in three urban denizens, more than one billion people, lives in slums. The conditions in these slums are so dire that the very dignity of the human person is in total neglect (Girard et al. 2003). Basic necessities for life, such as adequate medical care, potable water, and public sanitation all are veritable luxuries in urban slums across the world. In the slum bidonvilles of Nairobi, for example, fecal contamination has even affected piped water and has led to the spread of cholera and hepatitis. The effects of these and other diseases reveal the suffering of the slum populace and are too easily measured by the infant mortality rate which is upward of three times higher in the Nairobi slums than in the city as a whole (Unger and Riley 2007; Davis 2006). For all its problems, Nairobi is only a fraction of the size of such megacities as Lagos, Nigeria, Dhaka, Bangladesh, and Delhi, India. The environmental and economic problems facing these and other megacities are commensurate with their immense sizes and make the need for sustainable development all the more critical.

The plight of the current urban milieu and the impact of current conditions on quality of life and sustainable development in the global south have been recognized. "Nowhere is the commitment of cities to environmental sustainability more vital than in developing countries, where urban demographics are growing rapidly and current total population accounts for 82% of the world population. This underscores the need for growth and prosperity to sustain and fulfill basic needs. Economic growth may be vitally important, but it must be sustainable if any city is to achieve prosperity" (UN Habitat 2012, 79). Yet, living conditions of most of the cities in the developing world are most dire, and the global south by no means holds a monopoly on urban poverty. Even in the most affluent countries, people can be found living on city streets in need of assistance for food and shelter. Many cities of the United States, for example, are experiencing depopulation and simultaneous erosions of tax base and social life. Negative forces at work in the communities of these cities include increasing rates of unemployment and violence. These challenges have reached the public conscience to the point that many believe that the United States is now faced with a diminishing quality of life (Angur et al. 2004, 47).

3.6.1 State of the World's Cities

In an effort to assess the quality of urban life, UN-Habitat produces an ongoing publication series focusing on the state of the world's cities. The 2012–2013 edition focuses on the prosperity of cities and provides an overall prosperity index generated through the interplay of several indices. These indices are particularly valuable in examining the nexus between quality of life and sustainable development in cities. One index measures quality of life while three others measure the three E's of sustainable development; economic productivity, environment, and equity. UN-Habitat (2012, 14) specifically defines the contribution of each index as given below:
i. Quality of life: Enhances the use of public spaces in order to increase community cohesion, civic identity, and guarantees the safety and security of lives and property.
ii. Productivity: Contributes to economic growth and development, generates income, and provides decent jobs and equal opportunities for all by implementing effective economic policies and reforms.
iii. Equity and social inclusion: Ensures the equitable distribution and redistribution of the benefits of a prosperous city, reduces poverty and the incidence of slums, protects the rights of minority and vulnerable groups, enhances gender equality, and ensures civic participation in the social, political, and cultural spheres.
iv. Environmental sustainability: Values the protection of the urban environment and natural assets while ensuring growth, and seeking ways to use energy more efficiently, minimize pressure on surrounding land and natural resources, minimize environmental losses by generating creative solutions to enhance the quality of the environment.

These four individual indices may then be combined to generate an overall composite score of quality of life and sustainable development for each city measured. Results reveal remarkable similitude between cities and the nations within which they reside. Wealthier countries, with higher life satisfaction ratings (refer back to Fig. 3.2), typically contain cities with higher composite scores for quality of life and sustainability. The cities with the highest overall scores are those found in Europe and in developed countries such as the United States, Canada, or Australia (Fig. 3.5). Cities in Asia range from low to high on the composite score, again seemingly dependent on the level of development of each country. Cities in south Asia typically rank in the

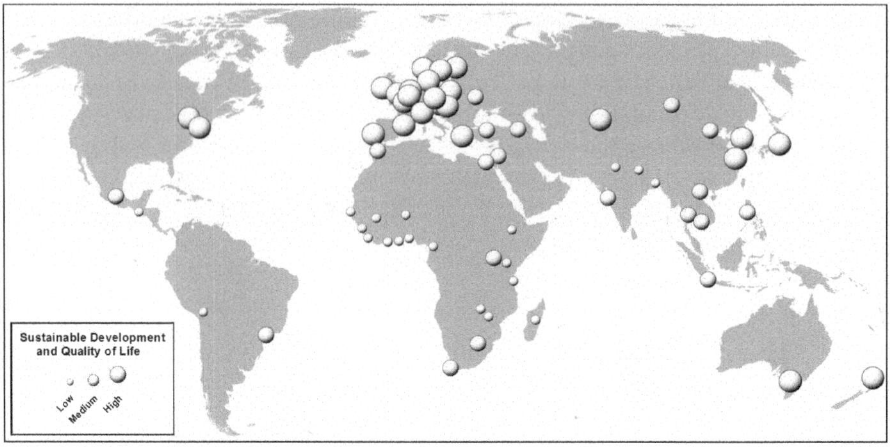

Fig. 3.5 Sustainable development and quality of life

lowest category, in Southeast Asia they fall in the medium category, and in east Asia they rank High. The African continent contains 13 of the 15 lowest ranked cities. Thus, while the scale of measurement may change, these results confirm those at the national level and reinforce the already well-understood need for basic necessities as part of the human condition. Without shelter, food, water, or economic opportunity, conditions of cities and of individual human beings are likely to be coarse and largely bereft of confidence or expectation of progress. In so many cases, to provide basic necessities is to improve quality of life.

3.6.2 Cities and Environmental Advantage

Despite the abject poverty and dreadful living conditions for so many individuals in so many cities, paradoxically cities serve as economic engines and offer perhaps the greatest potential for sustainable development. The correlation between urbanization and economic development has long been noted, with cities nurturing the exchange of commodities, activities, and ideas. Frequently, bastions of democracy and gender equality, which contribute to the quality of life for so many, cities are also sites of production and consumption and are a magnet to millions of migrants in the developing world (Cusack 2011). In terms of demography, urban populations have higher densities and lower birth rates. Resource use in cities tends to be more efficient than in the countryside. As a result, cities demonstrate real opportunities for fostering sustainability. As evidence, in metropolitan areas throughout the United States, per capita emissions are notably lower than the US average. On a yearly basis, residents of Manhattan account for 14,127 fewer pounds of carbon emissions than the typical suburban New Yorker (UNDP 2011, 40). Likewise, the provision of water and sewer lines as well as more formalized education and healthcare systems contribute to life expectancies in megacities of the developing world to be greater than their national averages (Atkinson et al. 2014).

Cities of course remain major sources of pollution and poverty, yet offer the greatest potential for gain in terms of both sustainability and quality of life. As such, the development of new cities and the retrofitting of existing cities may offer the optimal opportunity to attain the goals of sustainable development while at the same time improving the quality of life for untold millions. This understanding of the potential of cities necessitates that they be viewed not solely with a negative lens. For instance, the ecological footprint approach, which measures the amount of land that a city needs to sustain itself, is likely to show that a city's footprint is disproportionately larger than those generated in rural areas. While the ecological footprint provides a useful statistic, it cannot serve as the sole representative of a city and all its potential. Among those advocating a paradigm shift from one that contemplates cities as part of the problem to one that recognizes their potential as part of the solution is Smith (2012). Likewise, Boschmann and Kwan (2008) point out that the urban regions of the United States provide an ideal context for developing socially sustainable agendas oriented around urbanization and transportation.

3.6.3 Sustainable City Planning

These observations parallel calls for quality of life to continue to serve as a focal point of the planning profession. Lotfi et al. (2011, 234), argue that urban quality of life "has always been the central focus of urban planners." This focus, however, must take place at the appropriate scale, as heavy-handed top-down mandates are less likely to succeed. Attitudes toward quality of city life have been found to be influenced by attitudes toward quality of neighborhood life (Angur et al. 2004, 47). Therefore, land use planning necessarily should take place and support development at the human scale (Pinderhughes 2008, 14). Here again, care must be taken so that sustainability planning complements rather than conflicts with quality of life considerations. For instance, reducing air pollution and traffic congestion is an admirable goal of sustainable urban development; however, if the means to achieve these ends by forcing people to sacrifice the freedom and comfort of their personal automobile there may be an attendant reduction in perceived quality of life (Moreno and Ruiz 2008, 161). Rather, sensible approaches that may be emulated from one city to the next offer the optimal opportunity for improvements to quality of life while following the path toward sustainable development.

Among these approaches is to provide more choice in terms of housing, transportation, and other urban elements. The city of Denver, Colorado, has been working on the most extensive multimodal transportation expansion in US history. Other examples include Sustainable Seattle, and the Sustainable City Award in Europe which is bestowed upon cities working to become more sustainable (Bell and Morse 2008, 78). These efforts do not have to be earth-shattering, as simply painting building rooftops white reduces air-conditioning costs by 50% in a one-story building. Green roofs planted with grass or vegetation demonstrates the same effect and can reduce runoff while providing food through hydroponic greenhouses (Smith 2012, 311). An oft-cited example from the developing world is that of Curitiba, Brazil, which is identified as following sustainability principles in managing its growth. China, home to 16 of the world's 20 most polluted cities, has identified 113 key cities for environmental protection. Of these, the city of Rizhao has emerged at the vanguard of sustainability (Kwan 2010, 218). The policies being implemented not only put these 113 cities on the path toward sustainability, they also will result in a higher quality of life for the collective populace in terms of cleaner air and healthier environments.

3.7 Conclusion

The parallels between quality of life and sustainable development are without question. Quality of life addresses peoples' perceptions of their position in life in terms of their culture and values and in relation to their goals and expectations. In these respects, quality of life is at the very heart of sustainability, as many consider the essence of sustainability to be about people's standards and concerns (Beall and Morse 2008, 17). With the world's population continuing to grow, and with so many of the earth's inhabitants only "surviving" as opposed to truly "living", sustainable development offers a means to accommodate future populations while at the same time improving qualities of life. Efforts should, therefore, be made to achieve these tandem goals. Such efforts must be place and culture specific. While successful practices and pioneering efforts may be replicated, there is no one-size-fits-all approach to sustainable development. As noted by Eckersley (2016), what makes a good life, in all its complexity and richness, is difficult to quantify or measure. What works in one country or city may need modification before application in another. Plans should be made at the human scale and with community and citizen input. The will of the people is all too likely requisite for successful sustainable development. Currently, self-assessments demonstrate higher satisfactions with life quality in the more developed cities and countries of the world. However, with virtually all future population growth to be occurring in cities of the developing world, steps must be taken now to provide sustainable living conditions that provide for the human dignity of all.

References

Angur, M. G., Widgery, R., & Angur, S. G. (2004). Congruence among objective and subjective quality-of-life (QOL) indicators. *Alliance Journal of Business Research*, 47–54. http://ajbr.org/index.htm.

Atkinson, G., Dietz, S., Neumayer, E., & Agarwala, M. (2014). *Handbook on sustainable development*. Cheltenham, UK: Elgar Edward Publishing Limited.

Barrington-Leigh, C., & Escande, A. (2018). Measuring progress and well-being: A comparative review of indicators. *Social Indicators Research, 135,* 893–925.
Beall, J., & Fox, S. (2007). *Urban poverty and development in the 21st century: Towards an inclusive and sustainable world.* Oxford: Oxford GB Research Report.
Bell, S., & Morse, S. (2008). *Sustainability indicators: Measuring the immeasurable?.* London: Earthscan.
Bijl, R. (2011). Never waste a good crisis: Towards social sustainable development. *Social Indicators Research, 102,* 157–168.
Boschmann, E. E., & Kwan, M. P. (2008). Toward socially sustainable urban transportation: Progress and potentials. *International Journal of Sustainable Transportation, 2,* 138–157.
Botha, F. (2016). The good African society index. *Social Indicators Research, 126,* 57–77.
Bugliarello, G. (2011). Critical new bio-socio-technological challenges in urban sustainability. *Journal of Urban Technology, 18*(3), 3–23.
Cusack, C. (2011). Sustainable urban development and transportation. In J. P. Stoltman (Ed.), *21st century geography: A reference handbook* (pp. 345–354). Thousand Oaks, California: Sage Publications Inc.
Dale, A., Ling, C., & Newman, L. (2008). Does place matter? Sustainable community development in three Canadian cities. *Ethics, Place and Environment, 11*(3), 267–281.
Davis, M. (2006). *Planet of slums.* London, U.K.: Verso.
deVries, B., & Peterson, A. (2009). Conceptualizing sustainable development: An assessment methodology connecting values, knowledge, worldviews and scenarios. *Ecological Economics, 68,* 106–1019.
Diamond, J. (2005). *Collapse: How societies choose to fail or succeed.* New York City: Viking Press.
Eckersley, R. M. (2016). Is the West really the best? Modernisation and the psychosocial dynamics of human progress and development. *Oxford Development Studies, 44*(3), 349–365.
Feng, C.-M., & Hsieh, C.-H. (2009). Implications of transport diversity for quality of life. *Journal of Urban Planning and Development, 135*(1), 13–18.
Fischer, J. M., & Adjo, A. (2011). Quality of life, sustainable civil Infrastructure, and sustainable development: Strategically expanding choice. *Journal of Urban Planning and Development, 137*(1), 39–48.
Gambini, B. (2006). Cultural assumptions against sustainability: An international survey. *Journal of Geography in Higher Education, 30*(2), 263–279.
Gilderbloom, J. (2016). Ten commandments of urban regeneration: Creating healthy, safe, affordable, sustainable, and just neighborhoods. *Local Environment, 21*(5), 653–660.
Girard, L. F., Forte, B., Cerreta, M., De Toro, P., & Forte, F. (Eds.). (2003). *The human sustainable city: Challenges and perspectives from the habitat agenda.* Aldershot: Ashgate.
Gopel, M. (2010, November–December). Guarding our future: How to protect future generations. *Solutions,* 1.
Greenwood, D. T., & Holt, R. P. F. (2010). *Local economic development in the 21st century: Quality of life and sustainability.* Armonk, New York: M.E. Sharpe Inc.
Ioncică, D.-E., & Petrescu, E.-C. (2016). Slow living and the green economy. *The Journal of Philosophical Economics, IX*(2), 85–104.
Kwan, C. L. (2010). Rizhao: China's green beacon for sustainable Chinese cities. In W. W. Clark III (Ed.), *Sustainable communities* (pp. 215–222). New York: Springer.
Lotfi, S., Faraji, A., Hataminejad, H., & Ahmad, P. (2011). A study of urban quality of life in a developing country. *Journal of Social Sciences, 7*(2), 232–240.
McCarney, P. (2015). The evolution of global city indicators and ISO37120: The first international standard on city indicators. *Statistical Journal of the IAOS, 31,* 103–110.
Molina, G. G., & Purser, M. (2010). *Human development trends since 1970: A social convergence story.* Human Development Research Papers (2009 to present) HDRP-2010-02, Human Development Report Office (HDRO), United Nations Development Programme (UNDP).

Moreno, M., & Ruiz, J. P. (2008). Sustainability of urban transport: Common strategies and individual actions. In L. C. Heberle & S. M. Opp (Eds.), *Local sustainable urban development in a globalized world* (pp. 161–174). Aldershot: Ashgate.
Morrill, R. W. (2011). Geography of well-being. In J. P. Stoltman (Ed.), *21st century geography: A reference handbook* (pp. 367–377). Thousand Oaks, California: Sage Publications Inc.
Moşteanu, D., Mihăilă-Lică, G., Halmahgi, E.-E., & Moşteanu, R. (2014). The sustainable development-human development. *Land Forces Academy Review, 19*(1), 106–113.
Pellicer, G. E. (2008). Educational changes for sustainable cities: Autonomous knowledge. In L. C. Heberle & S. M. Opp (Eds.), *Local sustainable urban development in a globalized world* (pp. 203–210). Aldershot: Ashgate.
Pinderhughes, R. (2008). Alternative urban futures: Designing urban infrastructures that prioritize human needs, are less damaging to the natural resource base, and produce less waste. In L. C. Heberle & S. M. Opp (Eds.), *Local sustainable urban development in a globalized world* (pp. 9–18). Aldershot: Ashgate.
Smith, P. D. (2012). *City: A guidebook for the urban age*. London: Bloomsbury.
Unger, A., & Riley, L. W. (2007). Slum health: From understanding to action. *PLoS Med, 4*(10), 1561–1566.
UN Habitat. (2012). *State of the world's cities report 2012/2013: Prosperity of cities.*
United Nations Development Programme (UNDP). (2011). *Human development report 2011. Sustainability and equity: A better future for all.* New York: UNDP.
Walsh, K., McInnes, K., & McBride, J. L. (2012). Climate change impacts on tropical cyclones and extreme sea levels in the South Pacific—A regional assessment. *Global and Planetary Change, 80–81,* 149–164.
Ward, V. E. (2015). A guide to human rights in the contemporary world. *Perspectives on Global Development and Technology, 14,* 287–297.
World Commission on Environment and Development. (1987). *Our common future: The report of the World Commission on Environment and Development.* New York: Oxford University Press.
Ziegler, E. H. (2009). The case for megapolitan growth management in the 21st century: Regional urban planning and sustainable development in the United States. *The Urban Lawyer, 41*(1), 147–182.

Chapter 4
Quality of Life: Dimensions and Measurement

Vinita Yadav

Abstract Measuring Gross National Product (GNP) and per capita income defined Quality of Life (henceforth QoL) in 1970s. It did reflect the economic growth of the country but contributed little to assess the qualitative aspects of individuals. The sustainability of economic momentum and its trickle-down effect to lesser the divide were questioned to achieve QoL. QoL assessment at only societal level provides limited solution, whereas individual level brings differential assessment. Equitable and effective balanced development of a region needs special attention and proper emphasis on formulating and implementing QoL related plans and policies. The chapter aims to resolve the mystery regarding the definitions and measurement of QoL.

Keywords Quality of life · Well-being · Economic dimension · Human development index

4.1 Introduction

The application of QoL concept is wide and subjective. QoL analyses the standard of living of the society in all domains of life (Chen et al. 2016). QoL has many of the sub-themes, i.e. human development, health care, employment and environment. Social, economic, psychological and spiritual dimensions also measure QoL, both qualitatively and quantitatively (Kullenberg and Nelhans 2015). Each of these dimensions manifests differently in different regions. The QoL is also measured differently for homeless, hierarchical needs' assessment, understand the policy relevance and for sub-national level analysis. QoL is a multifaceted concept used to measure both urban and rural population. It reflects the gap between people's desire and their present way of life. The chapter has two parts: first part deals with meaning

V. Yadav (✉)
Head of the Department, Department of Regional Planning, School of Planning and Architecture, 4 Block - B, Indraprastha Estate, New Delhi 110002, India
e-mail: v.yadav@spa.ac.in

B. R. K. Sinha (ed.), *Multidimensional Approach to Quality of Life Issues*,
https://doi.org/10.1007/978-981-13-6958-2_4

of QoL and second section explains the measurements to assess QoL, use of QoL in special cases as well as summarizes the understanding of QoL.

4.2 Quality of Life (QoL): Meaning and Determinants

For developing an understanding of QoL, it is important to bring clarity about the concept. Smith (1973) was the first geographer who used services availability, consumption and expenditure pattern indicators to understand QoL. Since then, QoL is defined in the context of health care, work and politics on one hand and people's involvement in achieving valuable goals on the other. QoL encompasses the concepts of well-being and happiness rather than only wealth (Green and Haines 2008).

Planning takes into account various economic aspects such as land, ownership of assets, etc. with or without focus on life's quality. The development's measurement only in terms of Gross Domestic Product (GDP) and physical expansion serves a limited purpose as it is closely linked with QoL of citizens. According to Azad et al. (2015), QoL concept should not be merely based upon the economic aspect of standard of living but also upon the physical health, education, research, social belonging, recreation and environment to understand the regional disparities in the region. Hence, individual's voice needs to be considered for improving QoL (OECD 2011).

The inclusion of parameters governing QoL in the planning process will help to develop regions. In planning domain, focus on QoL aims at holistic welfare of societies in terms of economic, social and environment aspects. Planners use QoL with respect to the service and amenities delivery in order to identify the optimal solution for upliftment of the backward region. In QoL, substantial parameters of economic development with focused domestic production are taken into consideration. It is different from the concept of standard of living as the former deals with overall well-being including wealth, health, employment and education, whereas the latter deals with income (Dhar 2011). The higher production capacity of an individual results in more production which, in turn, brings an improvement in standard of living indicating social, health, cultural and economic well-being (Turkoglu 2015).

Al (2008) discusses issue related to defining, measuring and scaling the QoL. QoL is a broad concept and mostly measured with the help of Gross Development Product (GDP), whereas it is only one of the measures to assess economic well-being. There is a radical shift from per capita income to Human Development Index (HDI). HDI includes life expectancy and literacy. Social inclusion and gender sensitivity lead to emergence of concepts such as HDI, Gender Inequality Index and Multi Dimensional Poverty Index to gauge QoL (UNDP 2010).

McCall (1975) describes QoL as a measure to comprehend the people's 'happiness requirements'. QoL is individual's perception of their position in relation to their goals, expectations, standards and concern. The culture and value systems impact the achievement of life's goals. Person's personal beliefs and state of mind affect

QoL (Bowling 2001). It has not only been a recent basis for policy formulation, but its use is extensive in healthcare and commercial sector.

According to Bajaj (1993), key determinants of QoL are availability of essential services and goods to the weaker section. The services include health care including immunization, safe drinking water and nutrition. Additionally, social well-being and esthetic values also need to be added as criteria.

Annual Human Development Report, UNDP (1997) examines health by life expectancy, educational achievement, secondary and tertiary enrolment and wealth by taking indicator of per capita GDP based on Purchasing Power Parity (PPP) to assess the standard of living.

World Bank (2006) focuses on generating employment opportunities to reduce the poverty levels of 2.8 billion people living below US$ 2 per day and 1.2 billion people earning less than US$ 1 a day to improve their QoL.

Nordenfelt (1993) approaches the QoL concept from two perspectives: happiness and health aspects. It includes theories on happiness, human welfare, concept of subjective health and measurement of QoL in healthcare. Galloway et al. (2006) gave various definitions of QoL related to sport and culture.

In urban areas, QoL is affected by factors such as crime levels, effectiveness of law enforcement, internal stability and relations with neighbouring countries. The physical spaces with smart infrastructure, access to medical facilities, educational opportunities, use of technologies and investment in public services rank higher in QoL assessment. Pollock and Barry (2003) emphasize that neighbourhood planning improves the QoL of residents. Linkage between physical and programme planning helps to incorporate social programme into plans. The people's vision gets translated into the goals and achievable objectives of projects.

Sun (2005) assesses the QoL at neighbourhood level to measure livability of residential areas. Drawing from numerous subjects, QoL is a multi-scale concept measuring human needs with well-being. Such objective and subjective elements are also called approaches. It measures the well-being of an individual in terms of happy years, i.e. length of happily lived life (Veenhoven 2007).

Mercer (2017) analyses the data on Quality of Living of worker's well-being in 231 countries. In 2017, cities located in Western Europe are on the top, whereas war-torn cities are at the bottom. Vienna topped the list followed by Zurich and Auckland, whereas Bengui located in Central African Republic and Baghdad, Iraq are at bottom of the list.

Science does provide solution for improving QoL but still certain phenomenon is beyond the understanding of science. An individual's contentment was also considered as an important contributor to QoL (Findlay et al. 1988) but one has to be first satisfied in terms of provision of basic services and infrastructure (Costanza 2008).

4.3 Measurement of Quality of Life

QoL differs significantly between urban and rural areas, males and females, and organized and unorganized sectors (Mukherjee 1993). QoL is multi dimensional and categorized into five dimensions. Out of five dimensions, physical well-being and social well-being are widely used, whereas material well-being, emotional well-being and development and activity are some other dimensions (Felce and Perry 1995). A few other dimensions are psychological, cognitive, spiritual and environmental. The subjective approach describes feelings, perceptions and mental state, whereas objective approach considers measurable indicators to analyse QoL (Ira 2003). The study of QoL also helps to deal with issues faced by new towns across the regions (Sarag et al. 2013).

Nussbaum and Sen (1993) highlight the measurement and assessment of QoL. Gross National Product (GNP) is widely used indicator to measure the QoL but it is also measured as utility to assess happiness. Bajaj (1993) considers per capita income, rate of economic growth, Physical Quality of Life Index (PQLI), satisfaction of minimum needs and holistic approach combining satisfaction of a variety of physical as well as socio-cultural needs to assess QoL.

Khalil (2012) assesses QoL with the help of social life, access to transport networks, urban economy, residential quality, environment quality and access to urban service-related indicators. Becker et al. (1995) used questionnaires for measurements of multi dimensional QoL. It gives the domains of indicators and conceptual framework for different sets of QoL studies.

WHO (1997) gives the scoring, strengths of instruments and its usage in different fields for measuring QoL. It further gives the domains and facets within the domains, which uses QoL measurements.

According to Cobb (2000), usual methods applied in measuring QoL are generalized and overly simplified. The indicators based on non-utilitarian premises, such as Sen's capabilities approach, have reached the conceptual stage and future research is required to concretize in this direction.

The study of Veenhoven (2000) focuses on the definition and classification of QoL. The author considers long and happy life as one of the important indicators. The livability, life-ability, external utility and inner appreciation are varied types of QoL.

Becker et al. (2003) study the impact of longevity on the evaluation of welfare. The evaluation of differences in welfare is done through comparison of about 49 countries by giving monetary values to the longevity gains between 1965 and 1995. Life expectancy gains evolve as an important component of improvements in welfare.

Stiglitz et al. (2009) argue that income, consumption and wealth are relevant measures to assess the well-being of citizens than domestic production. The production is an indicator to assess the level of employment. The quality of product matters more than quantity.

Findlay et al. (1988) asked people about methods, indicators and importance of different criteria in contributing to a high QoL. The aim was to find out common factors to compare the cities in terms of measuring QoL.

Haq et al. (2010) analyse empirically intra-district variations in quartiles classes as good, fair, medium and poor QoL in Punjab at Tehsil level. Kahneman and Deaton (2010) distinguishes between emotional well-being and life evaluation. The health and aloneness are forecaster of emotions, whereas income and education impact the life. The latter's satisfaction is directly linked with income.

According to Diener and Suh (1997), there are several alternatives indices, i.e. social, subjective well-being and economic to measure QoL. WHO (1997) demonstrates details of various instruments used to measure QoL. It provides the instruments and indicators used in each of the domains, stages in development of instruments and their strengths.

Narayana (2009) brought out the issue of non-comparability of variables used in education index of HDI.

Health definition incorporates well-being (WHO 1948). According to Hennessy et al. (1994), health-related QoL involves both objective and subjective assessments. They are particularly useful for evaluating efforts in the prevention of disabling chronic diseases. Such data can inform health policy, planning and practice. Michalos (2004) believes in cohesion between social indicators and health-related QoL. The earlier studies point out that how abstract the social indicators are. Since then, health-related QoL is understood as a multi dimensional concept (Calman 1987) and includes both objectives and subjective perspectives (Testa and Simonson 1996).

Lambiri et al. (2007) reveal that there is a positive correlation between decision taken to locate house and business vis-à-vis QoL. The concept is multi dimensional and hence, it requires the quantitative indicators for assessment.

Lazim and Osman (2009) used mathematical modelling based on fuzzy sets theory. Lagory et al. (2001) examined the QoL among the homeless. Amongst life chances and life choices factors, former is more pertinent in influencing QoL.

4.4 Quality of Life: International Assessment

The Economist (2005) has developed a new QoL index for 111 countries where at the scale of four, people's satisfaction level is categorized as very, fairly, not very or not at all satisfied. The average scores (on a scale of one to ten) from comparable life satisfaction surveys were assembled for 2000 for 74 countries. The multivariate regression is used to assess various factors associated with life satisfaction. The factors such as material well-being, health, life expectancy at birth have been chosen. Beta-coefficients regression analysis is used to categorise the indicators into most and least important. However, its simplified implementation has more people answering the query despite it is not being able to capture their feeling.

The difference exists between male and female with respect to the socio-economic characteristics. Eckermann (2000) paper studies the gender perspective but study is restricted to Australia. It concludes that women's QoL is worse than men. The author points out that the gap is not just evident in developing countries but also in developed countries. It also identifies number of suicides among men, which require special attention.

Foster (1977) used industrial samples from North America to study economic well-being. The workers were given questionnaires that dealt with questions regarding QoL and economic variable. The questionnaires included questions such as whether the employees would relocate if the industry relocates? It concludes that both economic and QoL considerations are important in the location decision-making process. Urban relocations were preferred to rural relocations.

Requena (2003) empirically analyses relationship between social capital, contentment and QoL in the workplaces. Social capital involves trust, loyalty, and communiqué.

Di Tella et al. (2003) conclude that happiness depends upon the macroeconomic variables such as Gross Domestic Product (GDP). The welfare state pays off the people for unemployment.

Liu (1977) assesses quantitatively the urban economic and non-economic QoL in large U.S. metropolitan areas with population greater than 500,000 in 1970. Individual economic well-being represented by both flow and stock variables such as income and wealth, and community economic health considerations such as industrial productivity, economic diversity and income distribution were included to assess economic quality. Non-economic QoL was assessed through various social, political and environmental factors such as various types of trade-offs and feedback impacts. Data were collected both from primary and secondary sources to fit a social accounts model to generate economic and non-economic indicators. The large metropolitan areas were classified in accordance with the index values of the indicators. The trade-offs between economic growth and changes in non-economic conditions among the urban areas were studied, and policy implications were deduced and recommended.

Moller (2007) gave the trends of QoL for South Africa over the years from 1983 to 2004. The domains of study include urbanism, housing backlog, poverty, policy changes, changes in governments and its effect on QoL of the people.

Rossouw and Naude (2008) stated that investigators used subjective pointers to determine people's perception of non-economic QoL. Though income is important for QoL, yet non-income element could make an important difference.

4.5 Conclusion

There are different definitions and measurements, which exist to assess the QoL. It is measured not only in terms of well-being but also a contrast is visible in studying it quantitatively or qualitatively. There is a positive correlation between the indicators of QoL and level of their success in planning (Ebrahimzadeh et al. 2016). In order to take help of QoL studies in decision-making, Gastil (1970) encourages taking more specific and quantitative social indicators rather than highly abstract and broad aspects. According to Milbrath (1979), objective indicators are imperfect for deducing QoL. Hence, subjective indicators must supplement it. Different regions have varied QoL. Hence, region-specific analysis can provide a viable strategy for bringing improvement in overall well-being. Smart Region's study can be effective only if societal and individual's QoL will be improved.

Acknowledgements I am thankful to students i.e. Aman Singh Rajput, Mehak Chhabra, Sadhana Manthapuri and Toshi Yadav for their help in literature review.

References

Al, R. C. E. (2008). An integrative approach to quality of life measurement, research, and policy. *Surveys and Perspectives Integrating Environment and Society (SAPI ENS)*, 1.1.

Azad, A. F., Bostoni, M. K., & Anvari, M. R. (2015). Assessment of the life quality of urban areas residents (The case study of the city of Fahraj). *IOSR Journal of Engineering, 05*(07), 31–36.

Bajaj, J. S. (1993). Health as an indicator and a determinant of quality of life. In S. Z. Qasim (Ed.), *Science and quality of life* (pp. 15–32). New Delhi: The Offsetters.

Becker, G. S., Philipson, T. J., & Soares, R. R. (2003). The quantity and quality of life and the evolution of world inequality. *The national bureau of economic research (NBER)*. Working paper no. 9765. Retrieved from http://www.nber.org/papers/w9765.

Becker, M., Shaw, B., & Reib, L. (1995). *Quality of life assessment manual*. Madison: University of Wisconsin.

Bowling, A. (2001). *Measuring disease: A review of disease-specific quality of life measurement scales*. Buckingham: Open University Press.

Calman, K. (1987). Definitions and dimensions of quality of life. In N. Aaronson, J. Beckman, J. Bernheim, & R. Zittoun (Eds.), *The quality of life of cancer patients* (pp. 81–97). New York: Raven.

Chen, S., Cerin, E., Stimson, R., & Lai, P. C. (2016). An objective measure to assessing urban quality of life based on land use characteristics. *ELSEVIR Science Direct: Procedia—Environmental Sciences, 36*, 50–53.

Cobb, C. W. (2000). *Measurement tools and the quality of life*. San Francisco: Redefining Progress.

Costanza et al. (2008). An integrative approach to quality of life measurement, research, and policy. *Surveys and Perspectives Integrating Environment and Society (SAPIENS), 1.1*, 1 (1). Retrieved from http://journals.openedition.org/sapiens/169.

Dhar, U. (2011). Positivism and its impact at workplace. In A. K. Chauhan, & S. S. Nathawat (Eds.), *New facets of positivism*. New Delhi: Macmillan.

Di Tella, R., Macculloch, R. J., & Oswald, A. J. (2003). The macroeconomics of happiness. *Review of Economics and Statistics, 85*, 809–827.

Diener, E., & Suh, E. (1997). Measuring quality of life: economic, social, and subjective indicators. *Social Indicators Research, 40*, 189–216.

Ebrahimzadeh, I., Aziz Shahraki, A., Akbar Shahnaz, A. & Myandoab, A. M. (2016). Progressing urban development and life quality simultaneously. *City, Culture and Society, 7*, 186–193. Retrieved from http://dx.doi.org/10.1016/j.ccs.2016.03.001.

Eckermann, L. (2000). Gendering indicators of health and well-being: Is quality of life gender neutral? *Social Indicators Research, 52*, 29–54.

Felce, D., & Perry, J. (1995). Quality of life: Its definition and measurement. *Research in Developmental Disabilities, 16*(1), January–February, 51–74.

Findlay, A., Morris, A., & Rogerson, R. (1988). Where to live in Britain in 1988: Quality of life in British cities. *Cities, 5*(3), 268–276.

Foster, R. (1977). Economic and quality of life factors in industrial location decisions. *Social Indicators Research*, *4*, 247–265.

Galloway, S., Bell, D., Hamilton, C., & Scullion, A. (2006). Well-being and quality of life: Measuring the benefits of culture and sport-a literature review and thinkpiece. *Scottish Government*.

Gastil, R. D. (1970). Social indicators and quality of life. *Public Administration Review*, *30*, 596–601.

Green, G. P., & Haines, A. (2008). *Asset building and community development* (2nd ed.). Los Angeles: Sage Publications.

Haq, R., Ahmed, A., Shafique, S., & Malik, A. (2010). Variation in the quality of life within Punjab: Evidence from MICS, 2007–08 (with Comments). *The Pakistan Development Review*, *49*, 863–879.

Hennessy, C. H., Moriarty, D. G., Zack, M. M., Scherr, P. A., & Brackbill, R. (1994). Measuring health-related quality of life for public health surveillance. *Public Health Reports*, *109*, 665–672.

Ira, V. (2003). *Two dimensions of the quality of life as perceived by rural and urban populations* (pp. 6–13). Institute of Geonics, Academy of Sciences.

Kahneman, D., & Deaton, A. (2010). High income improves evaluation of life but not emotional well-being. *Proceedings of the National Academy of Sciences*, *107*, 16489–16493.

Khalil, H. A. E. E. (2012). Enhancing quality of life through strategic urban planning. *Sustainable Cities and Society*, *5*(1), 77–86. https://doi.org/10.1016/j.scs.2012.06.002.

Kullenberg, C., & Nelhans, G. (2015). The happiness turn? Mapping the emergence of "happiness studies" using cited references. *Scientometrics*, *103*(2), 615–630. https://doi.org/10.1007/s11192-015-1536-3.

Lagory, M., Fitzpatrick, K., & Ritchey, F. (2001). Life chances and choices: assessing quality of life among the homeless. *The Sociological Quarterly*, *42*, 633–651.

Lambiri, D., Biagi, B., & Royuela, V. (2007). Quality of life in the economic and urban economic literature. *Social Indicators Research*, *84*, 1–25.

Lazim, M. A., & Osman, M. T. A. (2009). A new Malaysian quality of life index based on fuzzy sets and hierarchical needs. *Social Indicators Research*, *94*, 499–508.

Liu, B. C. (1977). Economic and non-economic quality of life: empirical indicators and policy implications for large standard metropolitan areas. *American Journal of Economics and Sociology*, *36*, 225–240.

McCall, S. (1975). Quality of life. *Social Indicators Research*, *2*, 229–248.

Mercer. (2017). *2017 City Rankings*. Retrieved from https://mobilityexchange.mercer.com/Portals/0/Content/Rankings/rankings/qol2017e784512/index.html.

Michalos, A. C. (2004). Social indicators research and health-related quality of life research. *Social Indicators Research*, *65*, 27–72.

Milbrath, L. W. (1979). Policy relevant quality of life research. *The Annals of the American Academy of Political and Social Science*, *444*, 32–45.

Moller, V. (2007). Quality of life in South Africa—The first ten years of democracy. *Social Indicators Research*, *81*, 181–201.

Mukherjee, P. (1993). Planning for quality of life. In S. Z. Qasim (Ed.), *Science and quality of life* (pp. 1–13), New Delhi: The Offsetters.

Narayana, M. R. (2009). Education, human development and quality of life: measurement issues and implications for India. *Social Indicators Research*, *90*, 279–293.

Nordenfelt, L. (1993). *Quality of life, health and happiness*. England: Avebury.

Nussbaum, S., & Sen, A. (1993). *The quality of life*. New York: Oxford University Press.

Organization for Economic Cooperation and Development (OECD). (2011). *OECD better life initiative-executive summary*. Retrieved from https://gnse.files.wordpress.com/2011/09/executive-summary_your-better-life-index.pdf.

Pollock, L., & Barry, P. (2003). *Planning handbook*. Chicago: Local Initiatives Support Corporation.

Requena, F. (2003). Social capital, satisfaction and quality of life in the workplace. *Social Indicators Research*, *61*, 331–360.

Rossouw, S., & Naudé, W. (2008). The non-economic quality of life on a sub-national level in South Africa. *Social Indicators Research, 86*, 433–452.
Sarag, H. E. D., Shalaby, A., Farouh, H. E., & Elariane, S. A. (2013). Principles of urban quality of life for a neighborhood. *HBRC Journal, 9*(1), 86–92.
Smith, D. M. (1973). *Geography and social justice: Social justice in a changing world*. Hoboken: Wiley Blackwell.
Stiglitz, J. E., Sen, A., & Fitoussi, J. P. (2009). Report by the *Commission on the measurement of economic performance and social progress*. Retrieved from http://ec.europa.eu/eurostat/documents/118025/118123/Fitoussi+Commission+report.
Sun, Y. (2005). *Development of neighbourhood quality of life indicators*. University of Saskatchewan: Community-University Institute for Social Research.
Testa, M. A., & Simonson, D. C. (1996). Assessment of quality-of-life outcomes. *The New England Journal of Medicine, 334*(13), 835–840.
The Economist. (2005). *The economist intelligence unit's quality-of-life index, the world in* 2005. Retrieved from https://www.economist.com/media/pdf/QUALITY_OF_LIFE.pdf. February 1, 2017.
Turkoglu, H. (2015). Sustainable development and quality of urban life. *ELSEVIR Procedia—Social and Behavioural Sciences, 202*, 10–14.
UNDP. (1997). *Human development report* 1997. *United Nations Development Programme (UNDP)*. New York: Oxford University Press.
UNDP. (2010). Human development report 2010–20th anniversary edition. *The real wealth of nations: pathways to human development*. New York: UNDP.
Veenhoven, R. (2000). The four qualities of life. *Journal of Happiness Studies, 1*, 1–39.
Veenhoven, R. (2007). Subjective measures of well-being. In McGillivray (Ed.), '*Human well-being: concept and measurement* (pp. 214–239). New Hampshire: McMillan, Chapter 9.
World Bank. (2006). World bank group working for a world free of poverty. Washington, DC: World Bank Group. Retrieved from https://siteresources.worldbank.org/EXTABOUTUS/Resources/wbgroupbrochure-en.pdf.
World Health Organisation (WHO). (1948). *The constitution of the World Health Organisation*. Washington, DC: WHO.
World Health Organisation (WHO). (1997). *WHOQOL: Measuring quality of life*. Geneva: Division of Mental Health and Prevention of Substance Abuse.

Chapter 5
Concept of Social Indicators and Quality of Life in Social Sciences

Agomoni Tikadar

Abstract The social indicators are regarded as a tool for the observation and analysis of social change. The social change essentially means people living a better life, witnessing fulfilment of not only economic needs but also social, psychological and other needs. This aspect of a quality life can be studied with the help of social indicators in social sciences. Therefore, the present paper deals with the development of the concept of quality of life. It includes the subjective and objective perspective, utilitarian and capability approach and welfare approach. The nature of social indicators used in assessing quality of life has also been discussed from two subjective and objective perspectives.

Keywords Subjective approach · Objective approach · Utilitarian approach · Capability approach · Quality of life · Welfare approach · Social indicator

5.1 Development of Social Indicators in Social Sciences

The concept of social indicator is a new perspective to human living and strongly disagrees to the earlier view of economic indicators as the basis of human development. The development of social indicators can be traced back to the 1960s in the form of social indicators movement which marked a new way of measuring well-being of people in our society. It was Raymond Bauer (1966) at an early stage, who invented the term and basic concept of social indicators. In his definition, social indicators were 'statistics, statistical series, and all other forms of evidence that enable us to assess where we stand and are going with respect to our values and goals'.[1] Duncan (1969) wrote extensively about the existence of 'social indicators movement'. This

[1] Noll, H. H. (2002): 'Social Indicator and Quality of Life Research: Background, Achievement and Current Trends' pp. 7, published in Genov, Nicolai Ed. (2002) *Advances in Sociological Knowledge over Half a Century*. Paris: International Social Science Council.

A. Tikadar (✉)
Deshbandhu College for Girls, University of Calcutta, Kolkata, India
e-mail: agomoni@gmail.com

B. R. K. Sinha (ed.), *Multidimensional Approach to Quality of Life Issues*,
https://doi.org/10.1007/978-981-13-6958-2_5

was followed by a wide acceptance of social indicators in America. Many American scholars such as Sheldon and Moore, Ferriss, Campbell and Converse, Caplan and Barton had put forward their views on such development.[2]

It was then Drewnowski (1980) who said social indicators were essentially a measuring tool. They were not only a tool but also an integral part of the social sciences. They have a theoretical basis that can find solution to the construction of relevant social indicators. According to Noll (2002), it was Alfredo Niceforo who shaped an approach of comprehensive welfare and quality of life measurement. Thus, the concept of social indicator research spread from the United States to Europe and other countries and international organisations. This kind of research was undertaken with a sense of mission and was known as 'Social indicators movement'.[3]

In the late 1960s and early 1970s, due to political factors, the movement took a backseat. It was also the growing dissatisfaction among policymakers with the economic indicator like Gross National Product (GNP) per capita due to which the social indicators gained importance again. It was also getting clear that growth-oriented strategies were failing to take care of social welfare. Thus, the concept of human well-being started getting more emphasis, and there was a shift from an economic approach to that of a welfare approach. Social indicators have gained importance in analysing social change. The social change means people living a better life, development of not only economic needs but also social, psychological and other needs. This aspect of a quality life can be studied with the help of social indicators in social sciences. Therefore, the present article shall deal with the development of the concept of quality of life.

5.2 Determining Quality of Life

The study of social change and development with the help of quality of life starts with the basic question that what human wants to lead a quality life. Different scholars have given different perspectives on human needs. Dalkey and Rourke (1973) tried to identify group value judgement with respect to the determinants of quality of life. The components, which were essential for a good quality of life included life, care, affection, self-respect, peace of mind, emotional stability and sex. They have explored the subjective, psychological, individualistic, emotional aspect of quality of life. According to Koelle (1974), the quality of life is determined by four primary goals, i.e. material, physical, mental and spiritual goals. He had observed that when these goals are compared with other preferences, material goals are viewed as more important in the developing nations than in the developed nations. Morris (1980)

---

[2]Kenneth C. L. and Alex C. M. (2018) Fifty Years after the Social Indicators Movement: Has the Promise Been Fulfilled? An Assessment and an Agenda for the Future, *Social Indicators Research*, 135(3), 835–868.

[3]Noll, H. H. (2002): 'Social Indicator and Quality of Life Research: Background, Achievement and Current Trends' pp. 7, published in Genov, Nicolai Ed. (2002) *Advances in Sociological Knowledge over Half a Century*. Paris: International Social Science Council.

did not give an all-round definition or idea of QOL, but assumed that people would desire low infant mortality, high life expectancy at age one and would also like to be basically literate. Hence, he gave the idea of a Physical Quality of life based on these indicators without measuring freedom, justice, security or other intangible goods.

More recently, Lane has defined ‘quality of life not only as a state, but as a process which includes subjective and objective elements. In his approach, he particularly emphasises the active role of personal experience and the capacity of individuals—in his terms the quality of persons—as a constitutive element of life quality: Quality of life is properly defined by the relation between two subjective or person-based elements and a set of objective circumstances’.[4]

5.3 Utilitarian and Capability Approaches to Quality of Life

The Utilitarian view treats ‘preferences, choices, or tastes as private, individual, unconditioned, and arbitrary. Even abstract preferences, such as the desire for security or freedom, are considered to be formed inside each individual. According to utilitarian theory, QOL involves the satisfaction of the desires of individuals, and the good society is defined as one that provides the maximum satisfaction or positive experiences for its citizens’.[5]

The utilitarian and non-utilitarian views about values and quality of life dispute over the nature of being human. The utilitarian thinks that people have individuality and that it is not wise to study their private desires or internal feelings. Therefore, we see that economists and utilitarians are opposed to value judgement of individuals.

According to Sen (2003), Quality of Life is determined by human capabilities, which is the characteristic of a person to function in this world and lead a full life. He said that instead of depending on a utilitarian view, human capabilities to achieve certain basic functions are more logical. The basic functioning like to live a healthy life, education, etc. are valued everywhere but there are other components like happiness, security, etc. which are equally important but the weightage of these vary person to person, culture to culture and region to region.

According to Cobb (2000), the Gross Domestic Production (GDP), the Measure of Economic Welfare (MEW), the Index of Sustainable Economic Welfare (ISEW) and the Genuine Progress Indicator (GPI), all have a utilitarian influence, with social or environmental meaning in it. He has acknowledged an alternative way of thinking about quality of life in the work of nobel laureate Amartya Sen in his capability approach.

---

[4]Noll, H. H. (2002): ‘Social Indicator and Quality of Life Research: Background, Achievement and Current Trends’ pp. 10, published in Genov, Nicolai Ed. (2002) *Advances in Sociological Knowledge over Half a Century*. Paris: International Social Science Council.

[5]Cobb, C. W. (2000): ‘Measurement tools and the quality of life’. *Redefining Progress*, 7–9.

5.4 Welfare Approach and Quality of Life

Human beings mostly consider their well-being, based on the satisfaction of their 'perceived needs and wants'.[6] Different scholars have given different perspectives of human needs. Lasswell and Kaplan (1950) have observed welfare values and deference values as human needs. Welfare values include the well-being of individual in terms of health, safety, wealth, skill and enlightenment (knowledge, etc.), deference values include the respect, rectitude and affection derived from relationships with people. Dahl and Lindblom suggested survival, psychological gratification (through food, sex, sleep and comfort), love and affection, respect, self-respect, power and control, skill, enlightenment, aesthetic satisfaction, excitement and novelty as human needs.[7] Maslow has suggested a hierarchical arrangement; he proposed that 'higher' needs emerge successively as lower ones are satisfied. Well-being is composed of a variety of objects—health, happiness, association, rights and freedom.[8]

5.5 Objective and Subjective Approach

There are two distinctive concepts of indicators used in quality of life—first the objective approach and second the subjective approach. In recent years, another trend has emerged that tries to combine both these approaches; the objective approach in one end deals with the component of available resources (health, education, amenities, justice, income, etc.) and capacities to meet needs with these resources. The subjective approach deals with the psychological state or a person's perception of his life. This can include his state of mental peace, happiness and sadness. Thus, the emerging recent concept of Quality of Life is more holistic and comprehensive that creates a perfect balance between the material and non-material needs.

The objective approach is based mainly on the studies conducted by the Scandinavian welfare researchers following the tradition set by Jan Drewnowski and Richard Titmus. As per this approach, welfare is thought as the 'individuals command over or under given determinants, mobilizable resources, with the help of which he/she can control and consciously direct his/her living conditions'.[9] The Scandinavian approach focuses almost exclusively on resources and objective living conditions. Sen (1993)[10] has put forward a concept about welfare and quality of life in his 'capability approach'. He has said that the capability approach considers quality of life to

[6]Smith David (1977): *Human Geography: A Welfare Approach*, Edward Arnold (Publishers).

[7]Smith David (1977): *Human Geography: A Welfare Approach*, Edward Arnold (Publishers).

[8]Drewnowski (1974): *On Measuring and Planning Quality of Life*, Mounton, The Hague.

[9]Noll, H. H. (2002): 'Social Indicator and Quality of Life Research: Background, Achievement and Current Trends' pp. 7, published in Genov, Nicolai Ed. (2002) *Advances in Sociological Knowledge over Half a Century*. Paris: International Social Science Council.

[10]Sen, Amartya (1993): 'Capability and Well-Being' published in M.C. Nussbaum, A. Sen. Eds. *The Quality of Life*, Oxford: Clarendon Press, pp. 30–53.

be conceived and measured directly in terms of functionings and capabilities instead of resources or utility. The core of well-being is the ability to achieve valuable functionings, e.g. A school has toilets, kitchen and drinking water for students; it is not the resources that decide a good quality of life, the capability of the user is in question, can they use it? If no, may be due to lack of water in the toilets or lack of clean water in tube well or leaking roof of the kitchen, hence, it is understood that overcoming the problem might not be possible and hence the capability of the students to use these resources is poor; hence, the living condition is also poor.

The subjective approach has been adopted by the American researchers based on subjective indicators which focus on the outcomes of conditions and processes. 'The American school is strongly influenced by social psychology and mental health research, which emphasise subjective experience. Hedonic well-being is the principal benchmark against which state actions and societal development are to be measured. This school uses subjective indicators such as happiness or life satisfaction to measure QOL'.[11] The followers of this approach have emphasised on welfare and quality of life which has to be subjectively perceived and experienced by the individual, e.g. the ground reality of access to resources in school is found to be poor which impacts to anxiety, illness, psychological issues, unhappiness and exclusion from education. Thus, subjective well-being of an individual citizen is the primary objective of social development and is important in measuring the quality of life. However, Diener and Suh (1997) also said 'subjective well-being is not a state of simply being merry without having any deeper concerns. The central elements of well-being, a sense of satisfaction with one's life and positive effective experiences, are derived from the context of one's most important values and goals…if objective and subjective indicators converge, the researcher can make more definitive conclusions about quality of life. Social indicators and subjective well-being measures are complementary. Not just ingredients alone, but also how they are cooked determines the taste of the final meal'.[12]

5.6 Conclusion

The quality of life has been conceptualised and measured by two traditions in social sciences: social indicators research and quality of life outcomes in health and social policy research. The quality of life studies has done extensive social reporting and specific age group studies, e.g. on women, immigrants, children and elderly people who have helped in raising several socio-economic issues of present society. It has given a new direction to the concept of human well-being and human development.

[11]Grünberger Sigrid & Omann Ines (2011): 'Quality of life and sustainability links between sustainable behaviour, social capital and well-being' presented at the *9th Biennial Conference of the European Society for Ecological Economics (ESEE)*: 'Advancing Sustainability in a Time of Crisis', Istanbul, Turkey, pp. 2.

[12]Diener, E & Suh, E (1997): 'Measuring quality of life: Economic, social, and subjective indicators', *Social Indicators Research*, 40(1–2), pp. 189–216.

It has also brought forth comparative analysis on living condition of people in our society both at national and international levels. It has helped us in building theoretical models, empirical analysis, causes and changes of human well-being. However, the rise of objective and subjective indicators which was a debating issue earlier has been replaced by Amartya Sen's Capability approach. Nowadays, new concepts are emerging based on his approach which is being studied and quality of life measurement is getting further refined in terms of selection of new indicators. Thus, human development studies based on quality of life needs to incorporate new debates and ideas to completely capture the notion of human well-being in our society.

References

Bauer, R. A. (1966). Social indicators and sample surveys. *Public Opinion Quarterly, 30*(3), 339–352.

Cobb, C. W. (2000). *Measurement tools and the quality of life*. San Francisco: Redefining Progress. http://citeseerx.ist.psu.edu/viewdoc/download?doi=10.1.1.201.9685&rep=rep1&type=pdf.

Dalkey, N. C., & Rourke, D. L. (1973). The Delphi procedure and rating quality of life factors. In *The quality of life concept* (pp. 209–221).

Diener, E., & Suh, E. (1997). Measuring quality of life: Economic, social, and subjective indicators. *Social Indicators Research, 40*(1–2), 189–216. http://web.yonsei.ac.kr/suh/file/Measuring%20quality%20of%20life_Economic%2C%20social%2C%20and%20subjective%20indicators.pdf.

Drewnowski, J. (1974). *On measuring and planning quality of life*. Mounton: The Hague.

Drewnowski, J. (1980). Social indicators, quality of life and economic theory a suggestion for establishing a theoretical basis for social indicators and quality of life research. *Philosophica, 25*(1), 15–32. http://www.philosophica.ugent.be/fulltexts/25-3.pdf.

Duncan, O. D. (1969). *Toward social reporting: Next steps* (p. 41). New York: Russell Sage.

Grünberger, S., & Omann, I. (2011). *Quality of life and sustainability links between sustainable behaviour, social capital and well-being*. Presented at the 9th Biennial Conference of the European Society for Ecological Economics (ESEE): Advancing Sustainability in a Time of Crisis, Istanbul, Turkey.

Koelle, H. H. (1974). An experimental study on the determination of a definition for the quality of life. *Regional Studies*.

Lasswell, H. D., & Kaplan, A. (1950). *Power and society: A framework for political inquiry*. New Haven, CT: Yale University Press.

Morris, M. D. (1980). The physical quality of life index (PQLI). *Development Digest, 18*(1), 95.

Noll, H. H. (2002). Social indicator and quality of life research: Background, achievement and current trends. In N. Genov (Ed.), *Advances in sociological knowledge over half a century*. Paris: International Social Science Council. http://www.gesis.org/fileadmin/upload/institut/wiss_arbeitsbereiche/soz_indikatoren/Publikationen/isscnoll.pdf. Accessed on 25 June 2017.

Sen, A. (1993). Capability and well-being. In M. C. Nussbaum & A. Sen. (Eds.), *The quality of life* (pp. 30–53). Oxford: Clarendon Press.

Sen, A. (2003). Capability and well being. *Oxford scholarship online*. http://existencia.org/files/alt-eco/quality.pdf.

Smith, D. (1977). *Human geography: A welfare approach*. Edward Arnold (Publishers).

Chapter 6
Quality of Life of Slum Dwellers: A Theoretical Approach

Brijendra Nath Singh and Braj Raj Kumar Sinha

Abstract Quality of life (QoL) of people living in slums has been a matter of great concern to the scholars of different disciplines. The life condition of slum people is pathetic due to lack of basic facilities of their day-to-day life. They are socio-economically and politically deprived and poor section of urban society. They suffer from hazardous environmental conditions, and as a result they are called as vulnerable population or at risk population. Most of the slum dwellers live a low standard and uncomfortable life. Rural-to-urban migration, particularly in the developing countries, is one of the most important causes of slum growth. This paper aims at developing the conceptual and theoretical ideas concerning the life quality of slum dwellers and focuses on the concept and definition, indicators, classification, slum population characteristics, methods of measurement, and concluding remarks for the improvement in quality of life (QoL) of slum dwellers.

Keywords Quality of life (QoL) · Slum dwellers · Vulnerable · Urbanization · Population characteristics

6.1 Introduction

Quality of life (QoL) of slum dwellers has been an interesting topic of research in the field of population and urban geography. Rapid urbanization lead migration is one of the important causes of slum growth in cities. Living condition of most of the slum dwellers is not good owing to insufficient availability of potable water, lack of cleanliness, basic infrastructure and other services. Unsatisfactory housing quality, congestion and poor residential condition also affect condition of life of slum dwellers. Several studies supported that the life quality of people living in slums is

B. N. Singh (✉)
Department of Geography, Banaras Hindu University, Varanasi, UP, India
e-mail: bsingh422@gmail.com

B. R. K. Sinha
Department of Geography, Institute of Science, Banaras Hindu University, Varanasi, UP, India
e-mail: Sinha_brk@yahoo.co.in

B. R. K. Sinha (ed.), *Multidimensional Approach to Quality of Life Issues*,
https://doi.org/10.1007/978-981-13-6958-2_6

hazardous and poor due to above-mentioned problems as well as due to their physical location along the road, railway line, sewerage drains, low river embankment, canal, on low lands and on other high-risk physical locations.

Insecure residence, substandard housing, overcrowding, inadequate infrastructure and services, lack of proper healthcare facilities, improper health care delivery system, and other problems affect health and quality of life related to health. So, the overall condition in slums needs to be improved. From this viewpoint, governmental and non- governmental organizations work for the rehabilitation of slum dwellers in urban areas especially of the big cities. Vale (2007, p. 8) said that the nineteenth and early twentieth centuries witnessed first the growth of slums as a common feature in the USA and Europe. However, in recent period, the trend of faster growth of slums is predominantly noticed in urban regions of the developing and undeveloped countries. Health being a precious wealth is considered as an important sign of human well-being. It is based on the different norms of health. Health of inhabitants depends on the number of doctors, hospitals, fresh drinking water, unpolluted environment and other health-related problems. Pollution in environment badly affects the condition of human health in several ways and causes several diseases among the slum dwellers. In this context, it is imperative to note that there is need to pay proper attention to the quality of life (QoL) of persons residing in slums with a viewpoint of maintaining sustainable development both in more and less income countries. Integration of quality of life (QoL) in development policies and programmes for long-term perspectives should be included in the study of slum dwellers, Vale (2007, p. 8).

6.2 Concepts and Definitions of Quality of Life (QoL)

Quality of life (QoL) is an ambiguous and multidimensional concept and conceptually includes every aspect of a person's life. Quality of life (QoL) has also been defined as a result of different components of the physical and religious aspects of life to which a person accomplishes life goals. Broadly speaking, the quality of life (QoL) is categorized into two major parts—objective and subjective quality of life. Barcaccia (2013, p. 1) has defined QoL as 'the general well-being of persons and societies, outlining negative and positive features of life'. It also includes satisfaction of life that comes out from status of health, family condition, educational attainment, employment status, property/income, religion-related beliefs and the environment. Quality of life (QoL) has both the national- and international-level developmental activities and polity.

Diener et al. (1999, pp. 276–302) have defined the 'quality of life (QoL) as a condition of life. It broadly encompasses how an individual measures the "goodness" of multiple aspects of their life'. It also includes emotion concerning events occurred in life of someone, personal nature, satisfaction in working activities, individual relation and need-based satisfaction in life.

In simple words, we can say that quality of life (QoL) is broader than living standard and status of material possession in one's life. Quality of life (QoL) is normally the result of the combination of working situation or atmosphere, relation of society and politics, health status and cleanliness, educational background, condition of economy and other quality of life-\related elements.

Andelman et al. (1998, p. 3) discussed the quality of life (QoL) and said that, 'quality of life aggregates the seven domains like 1. Wellbeing, 2. Health, 3. Productivity, 4. Intimacy, 5. Safety, 6. Community and 7. Emotional well-being of persons'. They also focused on other aspects related to both the objective and subjective dimensions of a person's life (Fig. 6.1).

While thinking about quality of life Bowling (1999, p. 2) presented a model in which he laid emphasis on innate capacity of someone, an attempt made by the family of someone and society. The connotation of the notion of quality of life is determined by the way a reader uses the term and creates an image about it as well as the status and items of him/her in the structure of society and politics. Therefore, meaning of the quality of life is not constant rather varies from person to person as per his/her idea or concept (Fig. 6.2).

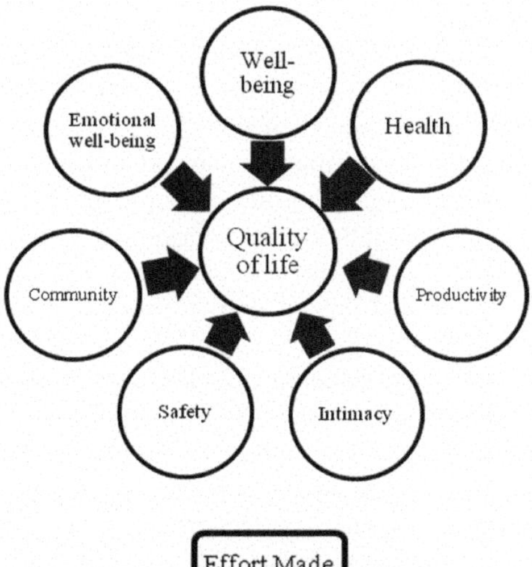

Fig. 6.1 Quality of life (QoL) dimensions. *Source* Prepared by Authors (2016)

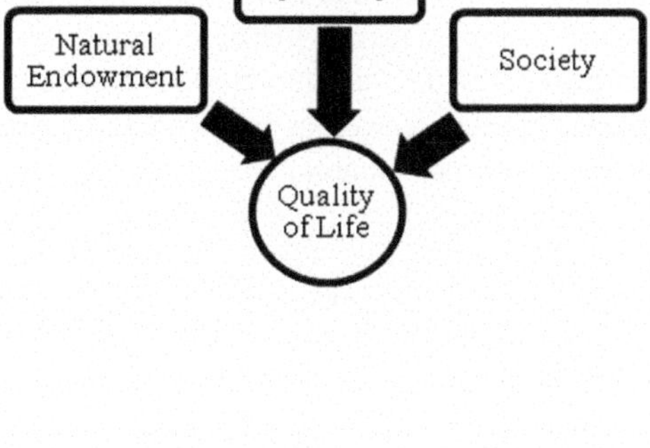

Fig. 6.2 Quality of life (QoL) as a natural endowment. *Source* Prepared by Authors (2016)

Vicente Royuela et al. (2007, pp. 4–5) have said that in recent times the quality of life (QoL) study has emerged very usual, interesting and interdisciplinary and scholars from different disciplines have taken much interest.

Rogerson (1999, pp. 969–985) tried to emphasize the competitive role of cities in determining the status of quality of life (QoL). While emphasizing, he said that life quality is more significant than job opportunities, costs of living and tie in family. According to him, cities are the centre of concentration of economic, political, trade-cum-commercial and several other activities and these in turn directly and indirectly affect the quality of life urban citizens.

Different scholars have given different definitions of quality of life (QoL); however, there is an agreement with regard to the determinants that are related to the natural surroundings, condition of houses, atmosphere, contamination, educational and health aspects. It has been argued that the perceptions and experiences of an individual about his/her life are important from the perspective of evaluation of life conditions in space and time. Quality of life is generally measured differently in different ways; however, the subjective and objective evaluation is more appropriate and acceptable approach.

Jacksonville Community Council (2000, p. 1) considered quality of life as a feeling of happiness, contentment or satisfaction that results from surrounding conditions in which the person lives.

Glaeser et al. (2001, pp. 27–50) have accepted the same meaning of quality of life that was given by a group of academicians of the International Society. This society had defined quality of life as the extent to which the life of an individual remains desirable versus undesirable and subjective versus objective.

Chesire and Magrini (2006, pp. 23–37) noted that majority of scholars from economics generally do not believe in a definite definition of quality of life, rather they lay more emphasis on indicators or variables that determine quality of life.

Helburn (1982, pp. 445–456) stated that the emphasis of current researches are on the notion of quality of life, place and its characteristic features and environmental conditions in which people live and spend time.

According to Sen (2009, pp. 2–4) quality of life is considered as an extent of well-being of a person or group of persons. It is an intangible concept, and hence the direct measurement of this is difficult. Not only this, it also involves physical and psychological dimensions where the former combines food and nutrition, health, health and safety and prevention from pain and infirmity and the later relates tension, anxiety, happiness and other emotion-related conditions. It is in fact not possible to speculate the quality of life of a certain person because the characteristics of a person are different from the characteristics of another person. However, higher average level of diet, shelter, as well as freedom and rights can grossly help increase quality of life of population of an area.

In reality, the concept of quality of life is broader and explains that how well society supports happiness and satisfaction in life of its residents. Perceptions of safety and low crime rates are assumed to be important ingredient of positive quality of life.

6.3 Indicators or Parameters for Measuring Quality of Life

Measurement of quality of life of population of an area depends on several parameters. Different scholars have used different indicators in measuring life quality. Andelman et al. (1998, p. 3) have identified seven indicators such as material well-being, health, stability in the politics and security, life of family, life of community, equality in gender, as well as political liberty for calculating the quality of life index.

Mercer (2011) added two more indicators such as Climate and Geography, and Job Security to that of the seven indicators as proposed by Andelman et al. (1998, p. 3) and calculated the quality of life index.

Andrulis et al. (2004) took into consideration that different avenues and choice of its selection help the person(s) in determining quality of life as developed by Amarty Sen. Recently, attempts have been made towards technical and scientific ways in measuring quality of life.

Stiglitz et al. (2009) laid emphasis on the concepts of subjective well-being and welfare approach in measuring quality of life. The World Values Survey developed the most inclusive subjective approach based on personal beliefs and values in measuring quality of life. In addition to this, objective approach has also been taken into consideration. European Environment Agency (2009) studied several areas of a person's life such as economic condition, housing condition, employment and work–life balance, health, subjective well-being and perceived quality of life and applied in 25 European Union member states.

Subasinghe (2015, pp. 36–65) was of the opinion that quality of life can be divided into objective and subjective categories. Objective and subjective are also considered as important dimensions, indicators, measures and approaches in studying quality of life and can be applied both at the individual and societal levels. Objective measure includes quantifiable indicators like per head income, rate of literacy, employment, labour force and its participation rate and the like, whereas subjective measure includes feelings of happiness, satisfaction, contentment, etc.

Campbell et al. (1976) have also studied quality of life at the individual level in which he observed the role of characteristics and views of individuals in determining the level of quality of life. In this sense, quality of life is the degree of happiness or unhappiness, satisfaction or dissatisfaction in the life of concerned person or persons.

6.3.1 Indicators in Context of Spatial Location

Royuela et al. (2007, pp. 2–3) stated that different spatial locations differ in terms of its environment in which people live and spend life. For example, the environment of metropolitan cities is quite different from the environment of places located away from it. The different environmental conditions differently affect the quality of life of different spatial locations.

Similarly, Florida (2002, pp. 743–775) also stated that the quality of goods or services pulls quality of labour. That is why, the places having better quality of goods and services pull better quality of labour in the cities of United States. Further, he highlighted the significance of human resources in leading to growth of economy. In this way, he underlined the significance of quality of life parameters as the driving forces behind the selection of location of the highly skilled labour power. In other words, the places having highly skilled labour seem to have better quality of life.

Berger et al. (1987, pp. 761–778) and Stover and Leven (1992, pp. 737–754) have suggested that the evaluation of quality of life should include those necessary conditions which can increase personal satisfaction and happiness. Their studies focused on the locations of the places and their characteristics in order to enhance the quality of life of the concerned places.

Türksever and Atalik (2001, pp. 163–187) tried to focus on the aspects related to objective and subjective category of quality of life in the context space and time. They have also taken into consideration status of health, climatic condition, gathering of people, sport-related aspects, condition of houses, journey to workplace and pollution of environment as important determinants of quality of life.

(Diener 2006, p. 4) selected several indicators relating to society, culture, economy and natural environment in measuring quality of life of municipality in which people live.

6.4 Classification of Quality of Life Indicators

In general terms, indicator stands for a thing that indicates the state or level of something. Indicator may be of positive or negative nature. Indicators show the actual aspects of life and its condition. With the help of the selected indicators, one can measure quality of life of the people. Indicators indicate overall scenario and information about the aspect of study. For example, social indicators indicate the social status of the concerned fields of the study. Different scholars defined the social indicators in different ways.

Greg Bognar (2005, pp. 561–562) took into consideration that social indicators and data related to them work as proxy measure for welfare. Social indicators are normally employed in the assessment of condition of someone's life in the society. Social indicators can suitably be applied in the welfare study of common members of society as well as in the study of welfare of particular group of population in particular locations and societies. In fact, the combined effect of both the social and economic indicators provides detailed and broader idea of welfare and life condition of an individual. The research works in the field of social indicators received more attention during the period of 1970s.

Indicators of quality of life are also known as variables or measures and are classified into the category of subjective and objective measures or indicators. The subjective and objective measures are also known as subjective and objective approaches and after assessment quality of life is called as subjective and objective quality of life. Subjective QOL is based on personal assessment about feeling of satisfaction or happiness and other positive or negative sense or attitude in life, whereas objective quality of life is based on the calculation of quantitative data such as per person income or property, number of persons employed, percentage of literacy, participation of labour force in economic activities, etc.

6.5 Methods and Concept of Measuring Quality of Life

The measurement and geographical analysis of quality of life involves various types of statistical methods and cartographic techniques. Different statistical methods help the researchers in making assessment of quality of life of targeted population, may be general or slum population. The chi-square $(X)^2$ test can also be used to get the significance level of the result. Sinha et al. (2016, pp. 402–410) have studied the social amenities of slums in India. In this study, the 'Z' score method has been used for the calculation of social amenities index. In the calculation of 'Z' score value, the score of both the quantitative and qualitative indicators of positive and negative characteristic relating to social amenities of slum dwellers was taken into consideration. After the calculation of index, the choropleth map of India was prepared to show the actual status of the slum dwellers.

With the help of Ginni's coefficient method, deprivation index can also be calculated for the slum dwellers and results can be shown with the help of choropleth maps which can be prepared in Arc Map software. Broadly, the quality of life index can be calculated using the following three methods.

1. 'Z' Score method,
2. Chi-square $(X)^2$ test method and
3. Ginni's coefficient method.

Thus, the final results can be displayed with the help of choropleth map. The comparison of age and sex structure between the slum dwellers and general population can be shown with the help of age–sex pyramidal diagrams and histogram. Thus, it is clear that there are several ways to calculate the quality of life index and the cartographic representations can be made with the help of different cartographic techniques to show the spatial and temporal patterns.

Royuela et al. (2003, pp. 51–74) in their study have calculated the composite quality of life index in tabular form in detail. They have classified all the indicators in three broader categories. These are individual opportunity for progress, index of social equilibrium, and community conditions of life. Further, they made subheadings of them.

On the basis of the above table, one can easily calculate the quality of life index for both the general and the slum population.

6.6 Slum Population: Characteristics and Quality of Life

National Family Health Survey-3 (2005–06, p. 5) has estimated that the India's total urban population by 2030 will exceed 550 million. In the present time, the ratio of slum population in most of the urban centres is substantially high. The general living and health condition of such population is poor and this is a matter of great concern to the government, administration, academicians. Slum population is also taken into consideration as an indicator of poverty. Slums are very thickly populated locations of poors. The environmental condition also remains unsatisfactory.

It would be imperative to understand the meaning of slums. There are several indicators which help us in defining slums. UN-Habitat (2002) has demonstrated the characteristics, indicators and definition of slums in greater details. One can define the slums on the basis of different characteristics or indicators like accessibility of water, accessibility of sanitation, housing quality, presence of more population, tenure security, etc. Such indicators directly reflect the living conditions and can be used in evaluating the level of quality of life of slum population of an urban area.

Characteristics of slum population provide an idea about the living conditions of slum dwellers. Characteristics of slum dwellers play a significant role in explaining the level of quality of life. Particular characteristic has particular reflection on overall condition of a given population. Characteristics concerning personal opportunity for development, equilibrium in the society, conditions of community life as mentioned by Royuela et al. (2003, pp. 51–74) as well as the characteristics as mentioned by UN-Habitat (2002) characterize the life conditions of the slum dwellers of an area.

Jha and Tripathi (2014, pp. 171–183) has also studied the quality of life of slum population in Varanasi city. They have also used different types of parameters for defining quality of life of the slum population. These were source of lightening; fuel used for cooking, source of drinking water, housing condition, sewerage disposal facility, place of waste dumping, medical facility, literacy, female literacy and types of ration cards. Their study shows that the level of quality of life of slum dwellers in Varanasi city is of low and very low category. Housing condition, literacy and medical facilities are poor. Inadequate supply of piped water in the slum areas is a major problem. Similarly, the lack of proper waste disposal facility and poor sewage system lead to pollution- and health-related problems and in turn negatively impact life condition of slum population.

Depending upon such characteristics, one can say that the quality of life of slum population generally differs because living conditions and lifestyle of the slum dwellers are quite different from that of the general population. That is why the study of different population characteristics becomes essential. Following are the major characteristics of slum population with regard to quality of life.

6.6.1 *Demographic Characteristics*

Demographic characteristics are important in the study of life condition of slum population. The demographic as well as socio economic conditions of slum residents are different from that of the non-slum residents. The composition of age and sex shows the predominance of young age population in slums as against that of the general population of non-slum urban areas. Migration, being a dynamic cultural phenomenon, greatly affects the age–sex composition and growth of population especially in large cities. Most of the cities show agglomeration of economic activities and working-age group people caused by age-selective in-migration. Normally, the sex ratio among the slum population is found lower than that non-slum population. Census of India 2011 shows that the percentage of younger age group population in slums is higher than that of non-slum population. Slums are characterized by the presence of more number of children and lesser number of older people. All these characteristics directly or indirectly affect the level of quality of life of the residents of slums.

6.6.2 *Economic Characteristics*

Economic characteristics are also related to overall life condition of population in general and of slum population in particular. In general terms, slum dwellers are mostly found engaged in the informal sector of economy, whereas the general populations are found engaged in formal sector of economy. The employment opportunity for the general population is greater than that of the slum dwellers. The earnings of general population are found much higher than the earning of slum dwellers. So, the slum dwellers enjoy less income opportunity than the general population. All these may be owing to higher education and skills among the general population than that of the slum population. Such prevailing conditions affect to a large extent the quality of life of slum dwellers.

6.6.3 *Poverty Related to Slum Resident*

Poverty is one of the important characteristics of slum population and negatively affects the quality of life of slum dwellers. Poverty is one of the economic characteristics and the incidence of this in slums is very high in comparison to that of the non-slum areas. A comparison between slum households and households of general population reveals that the life conditions of slum population are far below the condition of general population because the level of poverty is much higher in the slum areas compared to that of the general population.

6.6.4 Household Amenities

Housing amenities are considered as social amenities. Such amenities denote the infrastructure or facility availability within the premises. Household condition of general population is much better than that of the slum dwellers. Slums have much poorer housing conditions in comparison to that of the non-slum dwellers. Housing conditions are measured by the materials of construction, over number of residents, housing ventilation, whereas social amenities are measured by the availability of the lighting, cooking, latrine, drinking water, sewerage and other essential facilities. Most of the people are poor and their housing conditions also remain poor because in most cases houses are very congested and overall quality of houses is poor. Such houses lack minimum basic services, for instance, potable water, facilities of functional toilets, improved cooking system and proper cooking. Lack of all these basic services causes several infectious diseases and other problems which the slum dwellers have to always face. The overall living conditions of slum dwellers of the developing countries are more pathetic alarming compared to that of the developed countries. All the problems related to housing directly or indirectly harm the general health conditions and in turn affect overall quality of life of slum population.

6.7 Challenges Related to Quality of Life of Slum Dwellers

Challenge stands for a kind of situation or condition in which someone has to make an attempt in planned way to tackle successfully the fixed task. Here, challenges are related to the problems of slum dwellers. As mentioned above, slum dwellers face several problems in their daily life that are connected to the society, culture, economy, polity and environment. Slum people need social, cultural, economic, political and environmental facilities from the point of view of their welfare. Overall condition of life of the slum dwellers is poor owing to scarcity of required resources and services. In other word, slum dwellers have to face the challenges of limited employment opportunities and income. They also face the problems of insufficient housing space, scanty and poorly developed infrastructure, unhygienic environmental condition, lack of social security, inadequate health and educational opportunities and facilities. They need proper education, skill, proper social support system and other opportunities of their livelihood.

Slum dwellers basically reside in the poor building structures made of low quality of materials like plastics, wood, grass, mud and other materials. UN-Habitat (2014, pp. 1–9) describes slum household as a living unit in which several persons live together in any way and lacks either potable water or facilities related to hygienic environment, adequate living space, durable housing and ownership security. Lack of these conditions adversely affects quality of life of slum people.

Poor housing is a vital problem which the slum dwellers have to face. Structural quality, housing durability, construction of temporary houses are important problems in slums. Normally, slum dwellers make their houses temporarily for certain time and they migrated from one place to another place. It is not good for the social security purpose. The houses of slum dwellers are kuccha in nature. The structural quality of houses is generally not good as houses are basically built by the low-grade materials like wood, mud, soil, grass, asbestos and other material. All these are not suitable for health and adversely affect life condition of slum population.

Slum households are normally characterized by overcrowding, lack of adequate space, public areas, and these are big problems. It is found due to lack of adequate and proper spaces in slum areas. Slums are usually the location of dense settlements. In general, housing density in the slum areas is found with 6–9 persons per room which is a matter of great concern.

Accessibility of improved or pure water to the slum dwellers is another major problem. Impure water generates several kinds of water-borne diseases which harm the general health condition of slum dwellers. Open sewer drain lines and its overflow in front of houses, unplanned water pipeline are also major causes of the several diseases.

Sanitation facility is very essential for the healthy life. A healthy life increases the working efficiency of the people and changes the life condition. Slum dwellers generally face sanitation problems and as a result most of the slum dwellers are affected by several kinds of health-related problems. Thus, one can say that lack of sanitation facility adversely affects the quality of life of people living in slum areas.

Security tenure is also an important aspect of slums. Security is very essential for the general people as well as slum dwellers. Most of the slum dwellers do not have any kind of permanent ownership of houses. They also suffer from some other house-related problems. All of the above problems and conditions are the causes of poor quality of life of the people living in slums. They enjoy less social amenities as against the general people of the society.

Health of slum dwellers is another challenging issue. Quality of life and health are very interlinked to each other. Normally, slum dwellers have below average level health which is caused by the lack of several essential amenities. General health condition, infant and general mortality rates remain higher in slum areas as against non-slum areas. According to W.H.O. (2010), the expectancy of life at birth of poor slum population is lower than that of the propertied urban population. Slums people also suffer from several chronic diseases.

In terms of education, slum dwellers are far away from the educational facilities and they generally do not have accessibility of good quality education provided by governmental and non-governmental organizations. Most of the children of the slums areas do not attend school. The percentage of literate and educated people in slum areas is quite lower than that of the general population of the society. Education for All Global Monitoring Report of the UNESCO (2012) pointed out that the level of education of the poor slum population remains even less than the average educational levels of the rural areas. This is also a challenging issue of study in the field of slum population.

Employment and job opportunity help increase quality of life. It is observed that there is predominance of general population in formal sector activities while on the other side slum dwellers basically get work in informal sector of economy. Mostly, slum dwellers work in menial economic activities.

6.8 Concluding Remarks

From the above, it is observed that quality of life of slum population is nowadays a matter of great concern to the governments, administrators, planners as well as academicians because increasing slum population causes major threats to health and quality of life. Slum population acts as a barrier in the way of sustainable urban development. Over the period of few decades, the percentage share of slum population has substantially increased. As a result, slum population creates problems relating to housing, drinking water, sanitation, health, education, employment, electricity, transport and environment in urban areas. These are the major challenges for the urban sustainability and quality of life. Therefore, there is a need to ensure the required facilities in the slum areas to help promote the quality of life. Governmental as well as non-governmental organization's efforts in this regard would be a positive step to change the socio-cultural life of the slum dwellers. Following suggestions or strategies would be a positive approach in solving slum problems and in enhancing quality of life.

Slum population should be made educated and trained to enable them to get work in both the formal and non-formal economic activities. Urban slum population should be mobilized and empowered in terms of certain capacities for enhancing their life conditions. Skill enhancement programmes should be launched and implemented for capacity building of the slum population. There should be arrangement of the affordable housing and other social amenities for the slum dwellers. Government should make arrangement of the potable drinking water in the slum areas and drainage facilities, and sanitation system should also be improved to function properly to reduce water-borne diseases. Government should also ensure adequate educational and health facilities in common with the electricity and cooking fuel like LPG gas in the slum-dwelling areas. Regular health camps may be arranged by the local governments for improving health conditions and quality of life of the slum dwellers. All these can be linked to the process of upgrading slums.

References

Andelman, R. et al. (1998). Quality of life: Definitions and terminology. In A. C. Robert (Ed.), *A discussion document from the international society of quality of life studies*, International Society of Quality of Life Studies, Vol. 3.

Andrulis, D. P., Reid, H. M., & Duchon, L. M. (2004). *Quality of life in the nation's 100 largest cities and their suburbs: New and continuing challenges for improving health and well-being*. The Social and Health Landscape of Urban and Suburban America Report Series, USA.

Barcaccia, B. (2013). Quality of life: Everyone wants it, but what is it?. *Forbes/Education*. Retrieved on 25 Aug 2016.

Berger, M. C., Blomquist, G. C., & Wladner, W. (1987). A revealed-preference ranking of quality of life for metropolitan areas. *Social Science Quarterly, 68,* 761–778.

Bognar, G. (2005). The concept of quality of life. *Social Theory and Practice, 31*(4), 561–562.

Bowling, A. (1999). Health-related quality of life: A discussion of the concept, its use and measurement background. In *Presented at the Adapting to Change Core Course*, September 2, 1999.

Campbell, A., Converse, P. E., & Rodgers, W. L. (1976). *The quality of American life: Perceptions, evaluations, and satisfactions*. New York: Russell Sage Foundation.

Chesire, P., & Magrini, S. (2006). Population growth in European cities: Weather matters—But only nationally. *Regional Studies, 40*(1), 23–37.

Diener, E. (2006). Guidelines for national indicators of subjective well-being and ill-being. *Journal of Happiness Studies, 7*(4), 397–404.

Diener, E., Suh, E. M., Lucas, R. E., & Smith, H. L. (1999). Subjective well-being: Three decades of progress. *Psychological Bulletin, 125*(2), 276–302.

European Environment Agency. (2009). *Ensuring quality of life in Europe's cities and towns: Tackling the environmental challenges driven by European and global change*. EEA Report 5/2009, Office for Official Publications of the European Communities, Luxembourg.

Florida, R. (2002). The economic geography of talent. *Annals of the Association of American Geographers, 92*(4), 743–775.

Glaeser, E. L., Kolko, J., & Saiz, A. (2001). Consumer city. *Journal of Economic Geography, 1,* 27–50.

Helburn, N. (1982). Geography and the quality of life. *Annals of the Association of American Geographers, 72,* 445–456.

Jacksonville Community Council. (2000). Quality of life in Jacksonville: Indicators for progress. Jacksonville, Florida (p. 1), Available on - https://www.sustainable.org/creating-community/inventories-and-indicators/150-jacksonville-community-council-inc.

Jha, D. K., & Tripathi, V. K. (2014). Quality of life in slums of Varanasi city: A comparative study. *Transactions, 36*(2), 171–183.

Mercer. (2011). Quality of living survey report. Retrieved on 14 Aug 2016 from http://www.mercer.com/articles/quality-of-living-survey-report-2011 & http://www.economist.com/media/pdf/quality_of_life.pdf.

National Family Health Survey-3. (2005–06). Health and living conditions in eight Indian cities, Ministry of Health and Family Welfare Government of India, International Institute for Population Sciences Deonar, Mumbai, Vol. 5.

Rogerson, R. J. (1999). Quality of life and city competitiveness. *Urban Studies, 36*(5–6), 969–985.

Royuela, V., Suriñach, J. Y., & Reyes, M. (2003). Measuring quality of life in small areas over different periods of time. Analysis of the province of Barcelona. *Social Indicators Research, 64*(1), 51–74.

Royuela, V., Moreno, R., & Vayá, E. (2007). Is the influence of quality of life on urban growth non-stationary in space? A case study of Barcelona, Institut de Recerca en Economia Aplicada, Documents de Treball (pp. 4–5).

Sen, M. (2009). *Comparison of rural and urban quality of life of Bholpur P. S., Birbhum, W. B.*, Ph.D. Thesis, Department of Geography, Visva-Bharti Santiniketan, pp. 2–4.

Sinha, B. R. K., Singh, B. N., & Nishad, P. (2016). Characteristics of slum population in India. In R. Rachamawati (Ed.) *The 13th international Asian urbanization conference rapid urbanization and sustainable development in Asia* (pp. 402–410). Badan Penerbit Fakultas Geografi (BPFG), Universitas Gadjah Mada, Yogyakarta, Indonesia. ISBN 978-979-8786-58-7.

Stiglitz, J. E., Sen, A., & Fitoussi, J.-P. (2009). *Report by the commission on the measurement of economic performance and social progress*, The Commission, Paris. Retrieved on 26 Aug 2016 from http://www.stiglitz-sen-fitoussi.fr/en/index.htm.

Stover, M. E., & Leven, C. L. (1992). Methodological issues in the determination of the quality of life in urban areas. *Urban Studies, 29*(5), 737–754.

Subasinghe, W. (2015). Quality of life study on slum dwellers with special reference to Sri Lanka. *International Journal of Scientific Research and Innovative Technology, 2*(3), 36–65.

Türksever, N. E., & Atalik, G. (2001). Possibilities and limitations for the measurement of the quality of life in urban areas. *Social Indicators Research, 53,* 163–187.

UNESCO. (2012). *Education for all global monitoring report*. Retrieved on August 27, 2016, from UNESCO website.

UN-Habitat. (2002). Retrieved on August 24, 2016, www.unhabitat.org/whd.

Un-Habitat. (2014). World Habitat Day, Vices from slums, United Nation Health Settlement Programme (pp. 1–9). Retrieved on August 27, 2016, from www.unhabitat.org/whd.

Vale, L. (2007). *From the Puritans to the projects: Public housing and public neighbors*. Cambridge: Harvard University Press.

W.H.O. (2010). Urban heart, www.who.org.

Part II
Demographic Dimension

Chapter 7
Status of Quality of Life and Its Distribution in Nepal

Krishna Prasad Poudel

Abstract After the restoration of democracy in 1990, Nepal has been practicing more liberal and participatory democratic practices in development process. Therefore, it was hypothesized that the distribution of quality of life has been speculated more equitable, justifiable, and uniformly distributed over the country. Data for the analysis were mainly taken from the Human Development Index (HDI) of two successive Human Development Reports jointly prepared and published by the Government of Nepal and United Nations Development Programme (UNDP) Nepal in 1998 and 2014. Both the reports were prepared by the independent Nepalese scholars and the index was computed by the "goal posts" suggested by the UNDP. Since the changes in political system, governance pattern, and power nexus after the people's movement and restoration of democracy in 1990s, there is a progress in mean index value but the distribution pattern of HDI in 1996 and 2014 does not show much difference. Even some accessible and better scored Tarai districts in 1996 showed a downward trend on quality of life. The expectation of people toward the change in their quality of life after the restoration of democracy did not match properly. It has also widening the gap between a few accessible core districts and several peripheral inaccessible districts. Therefore, a better corrective measure has to be adopted for the enhancement of the quality of life of the people as a whole.

Keywords Democracy · Human development index · Quality of life · Spatial distribution · Development

7.1 Introduction

The present land mass of Nepal was fragmented into several small political kingdoms and states in the long historical past. Only after two and a half century ago, small states were unified by the then King of Gorkha, Prithivi Narayan Shah, who ruled his dynasty. After him, the dynasty was ruled by 13 kings. But, in between that time

K. P. Poudel (✉)
Central Department of Education, Tribhuvan University, Kathmandu, Nepal
e-mail: kpoudel.pokhara@gmail.com

B. R. K. Sinha (ed.), *Multidimensional Approach to Quality of Life Issues*,
https://doi.org/10.1007/978-981-13-6958-2_7

period, in 1847, the Ranas took over power from the King and remained the de facto rulers for 104 years. The people along with the Shah King Tribhuwan (grandfather of last King, Gyanendra Shah) revolted against the Rana oligarchy, and in 1951, the Rana regime gave way to democracy. However, the ushering of democracy was not completely free of political turmoil. Nepal had followed different governance practices over the years as of the Hindu tradition, culture, and religion even after the 1951 revolution. After the long period of political instability and practices of interim constitution between 1951 and 1957, Nepali Congress formed a government through election under the multiparty government system for the first time in the history of Nepal. But that could not continue and in 1959 then King Mahendra took over rules and dissolved all constitution and government system. He then introduced the partyless Panchayat system. After almost 30 years of Panchayat system, in 1990, democratic governance system was reinstated by the people's movement, and then, the first democratic constitution of Nepal was promulgated in 1991. According to that constitution, Nepal was declared as the Hindu Kingdom, and King was the supreme ruler and the multiparty democracy was in the practice.

Less than 6 years after the restoration of the multiparty system, the Communist Party of Nepal-Maoist started an armed insurgency in 1996 claiming that the people had not yet received justice. In the decade long armed conflict more than fifteen thousand Nepalese lost their lives, thousands were displaced and hundreds disappeared. Terror, instability and infrastructure damage took its toll in the nation. In the meantime, the entire family of King Birendra was wiped out in the infamous Royal Palace Massacre. But after the decade long Maoist insurgency in the country between the late 1990s and early 2010s, new shifts on socioeconomic thinking and participation on governing systems have been introduced. The Comprehensive Peace Agreement (CPA) between the government, the then seven party alliance and Maoist signed on November 22, 2006, which drove the country toward the new political changes.

The interim constitution of Nepal 2007 was promulgated by incorporating the new political directives and mandate mentioned in the CPA. Kingship was overthrown, republicanism has been institutionalized, secularism was enshrined in the constitution, and the political principle of federalism was introduced. However, the debate over the governance system is still continuing even after the two elections of Constituent Assembly (CA) which had not yet been successful to draft the new constitution. Within these political ups and downs, the atmosphere of politico-economic-development of the country remained highly instable. The quality of life of the people is directly interconnected with the dynamics of the sociopolitical situation.

The census of 1991, the first after the restoration of democracy, collected information on caste and ethnicity (CBS 2014). There have been several changes over social, economic, and development indicators which exert direct impacts on the determinants of quality of life (QOL) of people of the nation after the 1990s political changes. It has been hypothesized that the quality of life after the restoration of democracy has been enhanced and there has been a reduction in development gaps among the accessible and peripheral districts. More participatory, more equitable and power devolution system in the development process has been perceived by the people and those enhance the quality of life in total. By taking these presumptions, this paper tries to find out the status and distribution of quality of life of people based on the available data, information, and documents.

7.2 Concepts, Indicators, and Measurement of Quality of Life (QOL)

Quality of life (QOL) refers to the relative standard of an individual person or a group of people living in a certain geographic area. In the formal texts, QOL is defined differently as per the need, situation and is also varied in the scale of determinants. The dictionary meaning of QOL is "the general well-being of a person or society, defined in terms of health and happiness, rather than wealth".[1] However, it is hard to measure the well-being of a person or society which is explicitly determined by several factors of a person or an individual life which are interconnected at the local community or society as well as national and international scales. The category of quality expresses a given stage in man's cognition objective reality…cognition proceeds from quality to quantity and thence to their unity measures, and any object represents a unity of quality and quantity.[2] From these dictionary meanings, it is clear that the quality is a relative standard of an individual or a group of people living in a certain geographic area measured with the help of certain variables. QOL is widely used in the health science and basically measured through the health indicators of an individual (Burckhardt and Anderson 2003). In social science, the level of well-being or indicators of happiness are new practices. Bhutan is the first champion of using gross national happiness (GNH) indicator in spite of gross domestic products (GDP) to measure the economic standard of the country as usually adapted by other countries in the world. Since 1971, Bhutan has rejected GDP as the only way to measure progress. In its place, Bhutan has practiced to measure prosperity through formal principles of gross national happiness (GNH) and the spiritual, physical, social, and environmental health of its citizens and natural environment (Kelly 2012). The logic behind the happiness measurement is that economic output is a crude measure of national success. It accounts for negative transactions (like sales of handguns) as much as positive things (like education spending). Rich people do tend to be happier. But the same is not true for countries: the U.S., for example, has become richer without improving well-being overall.[3]

Following different practices on measuring the well-being of the people, some macroscale determinants of the quality of Life (QOL) in Nepal have been compiled from different sources of information. In the meantime, some micro-level indicators have also been compiled to measure the QOL for the period of 20 years after the restoration of democratic governance system in Nepal since 1991. Hence, the macro-

[1] http://www.collinsdictionary.com/dictionary/english/quality-of-life. Accessed on 15 August 2016.

[2] http://encyclopedia2.thefreedictionary.com/quality+of+life, Accessed on 20 September 2016.

[3] http://www.fastcoexist.com/3017037/the-10-happiest-countries-in-the-world-and-why-were-not-one-of-them. Accessed on 20 September 2016.

level indicators have been used to compare the condition of life with the regional and global perspective, the micro-indicators have been used for the overview the adopted governance systems in the current geographic-politico-economic context of the country. Finally, the conclusions have been drawn with a view to obtain the actual result after the analysis of required data.

7.3 Methodology and Data Sources

Mahbul Ul Haq (1998: 2) wrote in his book that for the last several decades, human development remained in the shadow of economic development. Economic development alone cannot give the justifiable result in the overall development. Rich countries having a good income, high gross domestic products (GDP) and high gross national income (GNI) also suffer from several social issues like income distribution gap between rich and poor, unemployment, prostitution, social crimes, and so on. His long essay "Reflections on Human Development" has defined human well-being which is closely interlinked with the quality of life. He clearly connoted that "people are both means and the end users of economic development." He has addressed certain indicators to measure human well-being of nations or certain geographical area through objective terms. Such objective indices can be used to compare different geographical regions or nations to get an idea to move forward as well as to make the comparison within the states or regions to put the targeted improvement in the given time.

In the 1990s, United Nation Development Programme (UNDP) initiated Human Development Report (HDR) at global as well as at the national level. In Nepal, UNDP Nepal Office had given this responsibility to an independent organization (Nepal South Asia Center) to prepare the Nepal Human Development Report 1998 as a benchmark of the initiation to measure the human dimension of the development (NESAC 1998). Since then almost every year the HDR of the country has been prepared by the independent researchers. Following the same pattern, the issue of HDR 2014 was published (UNDP 2014). Both of these issues are highly important because the first issue contains the data and information of the initial years of the restoration of democracy in the country in 1990s, and second, the latest issue, has been prepared after almost two decades of democratic exercise in the development process. Within this time interval, the Millennium Development Goals (MDG) for several activities has also been completed. Therefore, in preparing this article, the data on QOL have been extracted from these two publications. Analysis of data has given a clear impression of national progress from the new practice of development after a long autocratic development practice in the country. In this study, attempts have been made to see variation in the pattern of spatial distribution of change in HDI that took place over the years. For the spatial distribution of changing QOL over time, district level human development index (HDI) from the abovementioned two reports has been taken here. The HDI is used to measures three important attainments, i.e., health, education, and income in a relative term of certain spatial territory (Haq 1998;

NESAC 1998; NPC and UNDP 2014). These reports state that HDI reflects average achievements in three respects: A long and healthy life, measured by life expectancy at birth; knowledge, measured by adult literacy and mean years of schooling; and a decent standard of living, measured by GNI per capita in purchasing power parity (PPP$) (NPC and UNDP 2014).

Keeping in mind the above concepts the HDI score of each district given in two reports, i.e., Nepal Human Development Report 1998 and 2014, jointly published by UNDP Nepal and National Planning Commission of Government of Nepal has been analyzed. Other required information were collected from the records of Central Bureau of Statistics (CBS) of Government of Nepal, Nepal Rastra Bank, Ministry of Finance of Government of Nepal and also from some different open sources. For the analysis of variation in the spatial pattern of distribution of HDI scores, preparing maps and scatter diagram Geographic Information System (GIS) and Statistical Package of Software for Social Sciences (SPSS) have been used as the convenient tools and techniques.

7.4 Geographical Characteristics of Nepal

Nepal is a sovereign landlocked country of Asia. It is situated in the central part of the Himalayas between 26° 22′ and 30° 27′ N latitudes and 80° 04′ and 88° 12′ E longitudes, and covers an area of 147,181 km^2 with diverse geographical conditions. The country is landlocked by India on three sides with 1880 km boundary and by the Tibet Autonomous Region of the Peoples' Republic of China in the north. The elevation ranges from around 60 m above sea level in the southeastern alluvial plains to 8,848 m at the peak of the Mount Everest.

Nepal's physiography ranges from alluvial plains in the tropical lowlands to very rugged and snow and ice covered Himalayan Mountains. The range includes five major physiographic zones elongated from west to the east, including the High Himalaya, High Mountains, Middle Mountains (or Middle Hills), *Siwalik* (or *Chure*), and *Tarai* (LRMP 1986). These zones are composite form of three ecological belts, i.e., Mountain (2700–8848 m)[4], Hill (between 600 m and 2700 m) and Tarai (between 60 m and 600 m in approximation), whereas for the purpose of development, country was divided into five regions, i.e., eastern, central, western, mid-western, and far-western. Following these regionalization schemes, most of the socioeconomic data are aggregated into 15 subregions (3 ecological zones × 5 Development Regions). Despite these regional practices and also with the database organized over the years a few international organizations are putting their own regionalization schemes (NPC and UNDP 2014; CBS and The World Bank 2013).

[4]Above the mean sea level (msl).

7.5 Demographic Characteristics of Nepal

The total population of the country was 18.5 million in 1991, 22.7 million in 2001 and 26.5 million in 2011. The trend of population growth during inter-census period was 2.10% between 1981 and 1991 (CBS 1995: 2) and 2.25% between 1991 and 2001 (CBS 1992), whereas the growth rate was sharply declined to 1.35% between 2001 and 2011 (CBS 2014: a). As of the 2011 census report, the country has 130 ethnic groups, 124 different mother tongue/dialects and 10 different religious/cultural groups of the people. The current crude birth rate and crude death per 1000 population are 24.3 and 8.3, respectively. Total fertility rate remains 2.6%; infant mortality rate was 4.6 in 1000 live birth. Currently, life expectancy at birth is 68.4 years (CBS 2012).

7.6 Indicators of Economic Growth

The economic survey of Nepal (MoF 2014) cited the World Economic Outlook published by IMF in April 2014, revealed that Nepal has not been able to make substantial progress on economic growth front. Except only in 2008, the rest years after the 2007–2012 have the change within 3.4–4.8% and the projection for the year 2013 and 2014 is also almost the same (Table 7.1).

Global production that increased by 3.2% in 2012 grew by just 3.0% in 2013. The economy of developed countries that expanded by 1.4% in 2012 grew by 1.3% in 2013. Likewise, the growth rate of the economies of emerging and developing countries remained at 4.7% in 2013 as compared to 5.0% growth recorded in 2012. IMF has also projected the global growth of 3.6% in 2014. While comparing the world output growth among the neighboring countries of Nepal, i.e., India and China; Nepal is far behind (NRB 2013). However, looking into the consumer price over the same period, it has not much changed among the neighboring countries as well as in the advanced countries (Table 7.2). This is quite clear that Nepal has a similar trend of consumer price as the neighboring courtiers are following despite its economic growth trend.

Table 7.1 World output growth (annual percent change)

Year	2007	2008	2009	2010	2011	2012	2013p	2014p
World	5.4	2.8	−0.6	5.3	3.9	3.1	3.1	3.8
China	14.2	9.6	9.2	10.4	9.3	7.8	7.8	7.7
India	10	6.2	9.6	10.8	6.3	3.2	5.6	6.3
Nepal	3.4	6.1	4.5	4.8	3.9	4.6	3	4

p = projection
Source World Economic Outlook (WEO), April 2013 and update July 2013

Table 7.2 Consumer price in selected geographical region (annual percent change)

Year	2007	2008	2009	2010	2011	2012	2013p	2014p
Advanced economies	2.2	3.4	0.1	1.5	2.7	2.0	1.5	1.9
China	4.8	5.9	4.8	−0.7	3.3	5.4	2.6	3.0
India	6.4	8.3	10.9	12.0	8.6	9.3	10.8	10.7
Nepal	6.2	6.7	12.6	9.5	9.6	8.3	9.6	8.3

p = projection
Source World Economic Outlook (WEO), April 2013 and update July 2013, cited in Nepal Rastra Bank, 2013

The first HDR of Nepal prepared by the independent experts in 1998 reported that the HDI of the country was 0.325. For the calculation of HDI, the data of 1996 were used. In that year life expectancy at birth was 55 years, per capita purchasing power parity (PPP) income was U.S. $ 1186; adult literacy rate was 36.72 and mean year of schooling was 2.254 years. However, the HDR 2014 prepared was based on data of 2011 census, life expectancy at birth was 68.90; adult literacy rate was 59.57 and the mean schooling year was 3.90; the per capita purchasing power parity (PPP) income was US $ 1160. The calculated arithmetic mean HDI was 0.541 and the geometric mean was 0.490 (NPC and UNDP 2014: 90). These reports had certain "goal posts" for calculating the HDI as designated by UNDP. However, in the course of time, there have been several changes and updates in the basic calculation. The changes on calculation do not show exact comparison over changes; hence, the figures provide certain spatial distribution pattern and easy to compare the visualization across the country. From this point, analysis of HDI and its pattern of distribution across the ecological belts, development regions and districts have been made for the visualization of development after the changes on governance system in the country since 1991.

7.7 Distribution of the HDI and Its Changes Between 1998 and 2014

In 1998, it was reviewed that Nepal had made very slow but gradual improvement in human development in all years between 1960 and 1996, except 1993. The indices indicated that deprivation in access to income was much higher than deprivation in health and knowledge which meant more egalitarian distribution of health and education than of income (NESAC 1998: 39). The Nepal HDR 2014 summarizes the indicators of HDR, since the first HDR was published in 1998; it revealed both inequalities in human development across geographical regions and social groups, and the extent and direction of progress. The status of human development can then be appreciated in the context of economic, social, and political policies pursued by the State (NPC and UNDP 2014: 11). The disparity of HDI was clearly visible in spatial

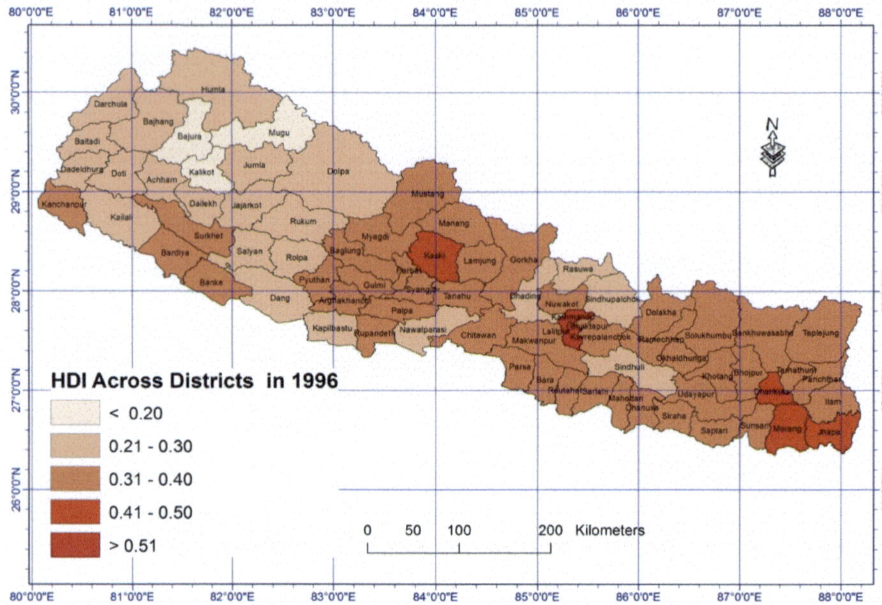

Fig. 7.1 HDI across districts 1996

distribution pattern across districts, ecological belts, and the development regions. In 1998, the clear distinction was visible on rural and urban nature of human settlement distribution. Mostly the private investments were highly concentrated in the urban areas and welfare measures have long shown a high level of disparity between urban and rural areas (NESAC 1998: 40). Because of these reasons, the HDI value tended to be higher close to the urban settlements. Similarly, the southern plain area has the high potentiality of agricultural production and better concentration of infrastructure (Poudel 2013). The spatial distribution of HDI on two points of time (i.e., 1996 and 2014) shows the pattern of distribution more clearly (Figs. 7.1 and 7.2). In 1996, the high concentration was visualized in the Kathmandu and Lalitpur districts and then the second highest concentration was in Jhapa, Morang Dhankuta, and Kaski districts. In 1996, all the districts of Eastern Development Region and the western development region have more or less the uniform HDI; however, large disparity appeared in Central Development Region and Mid-Western Development Region. According to the HDI of 2014, the spatial distribution pattern has an increasing trend in disparity.

The HDI value in Central Tarai is relatively lower than that of many other districts. The scatter plot (scatter diagrams) of the 2 years HDI show that the concentration of many Tarai districts was on the lower part of the 2014 HDI (Fig. 7.3).

It is quite interesting that in 1996, most of the Tarai districts were in good position of development. The HDI was better in comparison to that of almost all the Mountain districts and some of the Hill districts. After the restoration of democracy in 1990 the

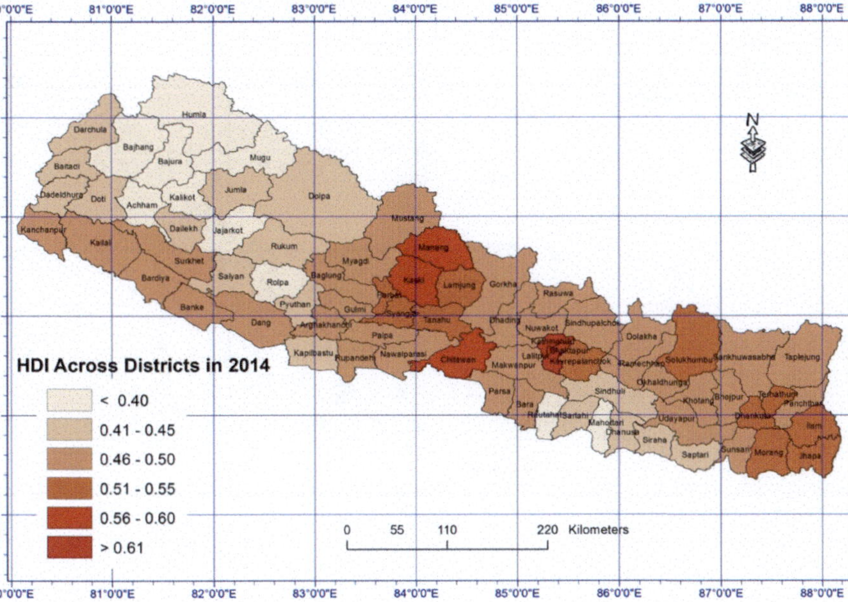

Fig. 7.2 HDI across districts 2014

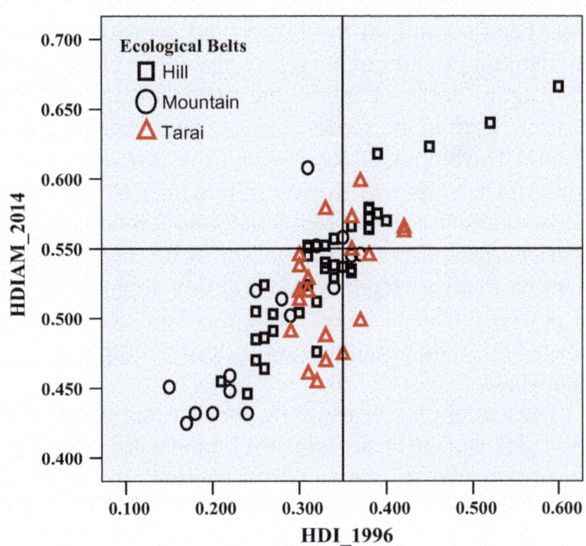

Fig. 7.3 Scatter plots of HDI 1996 and arithmetic mean (AM) HDI of 2014 across ecological belts

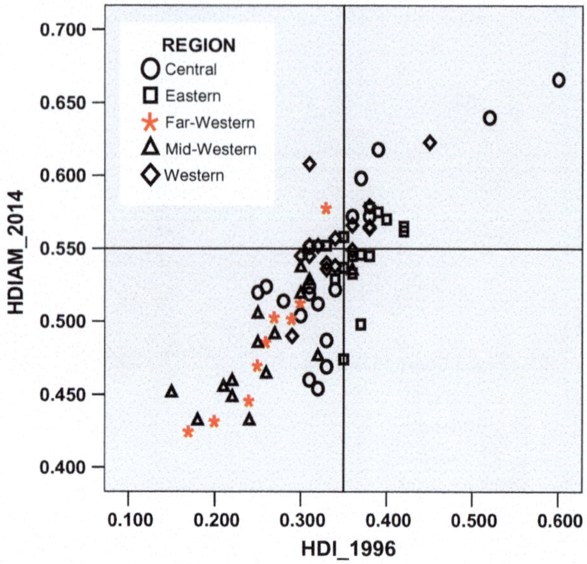

Fig. 7.4 Scatter plots of HDI 1996 and arithmetic mean (AM) HDI of 2014 across Development Regions

political participation of the Tarai was better, and democratic exercise on resource distribution has been better implemented. Several local and regional political parties have been coming in the power and decision-making process was claimed more equitable and participatory. Despite these changes over the last two decades the HDI figure does not follow the same direction. In 1996 only five out of 20 Tarai districts were in the second lowest order. Among them, two districts were from the Central Development Region and the rest three were from mid-western and far-western Development Region. While in 2014, the scenario was changed drastically. Three districts, Sarlahi, Mahottari, and Rautahat came into the lowest level and two districts, Dhanusa and Kapilbastu in the second lowest level of HDI. Except for Kapilbastu all are from the Central Development Region and also the large majority of powerful leaders representing the Tarai community are from these districts. The nexus of decision-making power does not replicate the quality of life of the people as a whole.

The scatter plot clearly show the distribution of HDI of 1996 and arithmetic mean (AM) HDI of 2014 across Development Regions (Fig. 7.4). The concentration of progress between 1996 and 2014 was high in the districts of Kathmandu Valley and some Hill districts. A large number of districts of far-western region were not in good position.

7.8 Conclusion

From the analysis of the status of quality of life and its distribution, it is found that all the indicators of quality of life showed a good progress over the period of last two decades. In general, the mean life expectancy year of the people also increased from 55 year to 69 year, average literacy rate increased from 37% to 60%, and mean schooling years increased from 2.25 to 3.90. On the other hand, the per capita purchasing power parity (PPP) did not show any progress. It was U.S. $ 1186 in the previous year, and in 2014, it was U.S. $ 1160. Despite the slow economic growth, the social indicators showed a better position. However, in the last two decades, the distribution across the districts shows some unevenness and changes in the previous trend. Mostly, the better figures were confined in few accessible districts and the large numbers of remote districts had no sign of progress. Even after the political change from centralized Panchayat system to more participatory multiparty democratic systems after 1990s, some districts represented a good number of representation of people in decision-making power, yet such districts showed declining scores of indicators. This result shows some unhealthy practices in overall progress in quality of life of the people. Therefore, there is a need for developing some corrective measures, plans, and policies and its timely implementation to enhance the quality of life of the people with due consideration of spatial distribution and regional variation in overall developmental resources.

Annex

Appendix 7.1 Distribution of HDI value across districts, development region, and ecological belts 1996

Ecological belt	Development region	<0.20	0.21–0.30	0.31–0.40	0.41–0.50	>0.51
Mountain	Eastern			Sankhuwasabha, Taplejung, Solukhumbu		
	Central		Rasuwa, Sindhu-palchok	Dolakha,		
	Western			Mustang, Manang		
	Mid-western	Mugu, Kalikot	Dolpa, Jumla, Humla			
	Far-western	Bajura, Bajhang	Darchula			

(continued)

(continued)

Ecological belt	Development region	<0.20	0.21–0.30	0.31–0.40	0.41–0.50	>0.51
Hill	Eastern			Khotang, Panchthar, Okhaldhunga, Bhojpur, Udayapur, Ilam, Terhathum, Dhankuta		
	Central		Dhading, Sindhuli	Makwanpur, Nuwakot, Ramechhap, Kavrepalan-chok, Bhaktapur		Lalitpur, Kath-mandu
	Western			Gorkha, Myagdi, Gulmi, Arghakhanchi, Baglung, Palpa, Parbat, Lamjung, Syangja, Tanahu	Kaski	
	Mid-western		Jajarkot, Dailekh, Salyan, Rolpa, Rukum	Pyuthan, Surkhet		
	Far-western		Achham, Doti, Baitadi, Dadeld-hura			
Tarai	Eastern			Siraha, Saptari, Sunsari	Jhapa, Morang	
	Central			Dhanusa, Rautahat, Bara, Mahot-tari,Sarlahi, Parsa, Chitawan		
	Western		Kapilbastu, Nawal-parasi	Rupandehi		
	Mid-western		Dang, Bardiya	Banke		
	Far-western		Kailali	Kanchanpur		
Total		4	22	44	3	2

Appendix 7.2 Distribution of HDI value across districts, development region, and ecological belts 2014

Ecological belt	Development region	<0.4	0.41–0.45	0.46–0.50	0.51–0.55	0.56–0.60	>0.61
Mountain	Eastern			Solukhumbu, Taplejung, Sankhuwasabha			
	Central			Rasuwa, Dolakha, Sindhupalchok			
	Western			Mustang		Manang	
	Mid-western	Dolpa, Mugu, Humla, Kalikot	Jumla				
	Far-western	Bajhang, Bajura	Darchula				
Hill	Eastern			Khotang, Panchthar, Bhojpur, Udayapur, Okhaldhunga	Terhathum, Ilam, Dhankuta		
	Central		Sindhuli	Makwanpur, Ramechhap, Nuwakot, Dhading	Kavrepalanchok	Bhaktapur	Lalitpur, Kath-mandu
	Western		Rukum, Dailekh,	Palpa, Myagdi, Arghakhanchi, Gorkha, Baglung, Gulmi	Syangja, Parbat, Lamjung, Tanahu	Kaski	
	Mid-western	Rolpa, Jajarkot	Dadeldhura, Pyuthan,	Surkhet,			
	Far-western	Achham	Salyan, Baitadi, Doti				
Tarai	Eastern		Saptari, Siraha,	Sunsari	Jhapa, Morang		
	Central	Sarlahi, Mahot-tari, Rautahat,	Dhanusa	Parsa, Bara	Chitawan		
	Western		Kapilbastu	Rupandehi, Nawalparasi			
	Mid-western			Dang, Banke, Bardiya			
	Far-western			Kanchanpur, Kailali			
		12	14	33	11	3	2

References

Burckhardt, C. S. & Anderson, K. L. (2003). The quality of life scale (QOLS): Reliability, validity, and utilization. *Health and Quality of Life Outcomes 1*, 60. https://doi.org/10.1186/1477-7525-1-60, http://www.hqlo.com/content/1/1/60.

CBS and The World Bank. (2013). *Nepal: small area estimation of poverty 2011 (summary and findings)*. Kathmandu: Central Bureau of Statistics and The World Bank, Nepal.

CBS. (1992). *National population and housing census 1991 (National Report)*. Kathmandu: Central Bureau of Statistics.

CBS. (1995). *Population monograph of Nepal*. Kathmandu: Central Bureau of Statistics.

CBS. (2012). *National population and housing census 2011 (National Report)*. Kathmandu: Central Bureau of Statistics.

CBS. (2014). *Population monograph of Nepal (volume I population dynamics)*. Kathmandu: Central Bureau of Statistics.

Haq, M. U. (1998). *Reflection on human development*. Delhi: Oxford University Press.

Kelly, A. (2012). The observer, Thimphu, Bhutan, Saturday 1 December. http://www.theguardian.com/world/2012/dec/01/bhutan-wealth-happiness-counts.

LRMP. (1986). Land utilization report. Land resources mapping project (LRMP), kenting earth sciences limited, Government of Nepal and Government of Canada.

MoF. (2014). *Economic survey, fiscal year 2013/14*. Kathmandu: Ministry of Finance, Government of Nepal.

NRB. (2013). *Macroeconomic indicators of Nepal*. Kathmandu: Nepal Rastra Bank.

NESAC. (1998). *Nepal human development report 1998*. Kathmandu: Nepal South Asia Center.

NPC and UNDP. (2014). *Nepal human development report 2014: Beyond geography unlocking human potential*. Kathmandu: National Planning Commission Government of Nepal and United Nation Development Programme, Nepal.

Poudel, K. P. (2013). *National development plan and urbanization in Nepal (conference paper), presented at the 12th international Asian urbanization conference on 'urban dynamics, environment and health: Challenges for the twenty first century, organized by the department of geography, Banaras Hindu University, India, December 28–30, 2013*.

Chapter 8
Impact of Involuntary Resettlement on Quality of Life of Relocated People in the Eastern Fringe of Dhaka City, Bangladesh

SM Shah Mahmood and Ishrat Islam

Abstract Involuntary resettlement and quality of life are one of the important themes of research. Real estate is considered as one of the most lucrative sectors of business, and land market is extensively controlled by influential groups of private real estate developers. Because of high land price in central city areas of Dhaka, the majority of the land developers are attracted in the fringe areas of this city where vast tracts of wetland and agricultural land are available at lower price. In many cases, local people are exploited by the developers and forced to sell their land. The relocation of these local people in different areas of the country can be identified as involuntary resettlement of people. The objective of this study is to explore the quality of life of the relocated people in their present and previous locations from socioeconomic perspectives. This study is based on the information collected from relocated families who had to move from their original residence because of four land development projects of Dhaka. Approximately, 3,920 families were identified as relocated families from these project areas. About 350 relocated household heads were surveyed by a prestructured questionnaire. This research used snowball sampling for the questionnaire survey. A set of indicators were studied to assess and compare the present and past status of the socioeconomic condition of relocated families. Data were collected on housing condition, services, social network, occupation, income and expenditure, landownership, etc., for fulfilling research objective. It was found from the research findings that over all socioeconomic condition of the relocated people have been degraded from their previous status. At present, about 67.7% of the local people who were the owner of land in previous locations do not own any land at present. Similarly, local peoples' occupation structure was changed significantly at their current location. Their housing condition and access to utility facilities are also deteriorated. Social network plays a vital role to enhance the quality of life of people. According to the respondents, they had lost their social network as they moved out from their original location.

SM Shah Mahmood · I. Islam (✉)
Department of Urban and Regional Planning, Bangladesh University of Engineering and Technology (BUET), Dhaka, Bangladesh
e-mail: ishratislam.buet@gmail.com

SM Shah Mahmood
New York City Department of Environmental Protection Police, New York City, USA

B. R. K. Sinha (ed.), *Multidimensional Approach to Quality of Life Issues*,
https://doi.org/10.1007/978-981-13-6958-2_8

Keywords Dhaka · Involuntary relocation · Land development project · Socioeconomic condition · Quality of life

8.1 Introduction

Dhaka is the administrative and economic heart of Bangladesh and one of the fastest growing megacities in the world. According to Bangladesh Bureau of Statistics (2012), Dhaka alone has the highest concentration with 44.39% of the total urban population and 8.5% of the national population. Dhaka's population has increased between 17.88 and 25.09% since 1951 (Islam 2009). There is limited availability of land for housing and the costs of lands are gradually increasing. Therefore, nearly two-thirds of the urban population is facing difficulties getting land within a convenient distance from their place of work (Islam 1993). There has been rapid growth and thorough land use conversion in the Dhaka city. It ranges from rural agriculture to urban residential, industrial, and institutional uses (Fatema 2003). Urban fringe areas are dynamic in nature, which go through changes over time. It has been noted by Clark (2009) that low-cost land availability in fringe areas attracts developers with speculative motive, and this act is supported due to the lack of comprehensive planning, rules, and regulations. With the growing demand for housing, the private land development companies have a leading role in the land market and a major influence on land development and planning in Dhaka (Roy 2007). According to Haque (2012), the city of Dhaka and its fringe areas are experiencing continuous land development by unprincipled real estate companies. Logan and Molotch (1987) observed that land is considered a product and is controlled by a specific class of landowners. But in case of poor and marginal farmers, this scenario is not applicable because they face immense difficulties to keep a hold over their own land in the city of Dhaka, especially in its fringe areas. A loss of occupation, social network, and physical dislocation can result when fringe people are dislocated from their own land. On the other hand, to buy a small piece of land to build a house, a middle or lower middle-class individual in the urban fringe has invested his whole life's savings. It is understandable that a middle and working class family cannot effort to buy a land within the city. As a result, they become land less and drove away from the main city (Jamuna Multipurpose Bridge Authority 1993). To ensure the reasonable sharing of cost and benefit of development projects among the residents it is necessary to study the consequences of involuntary resettlement in the life and livelihood of the affected people. The decision to shift one's residence is voluntary and involuntary (in Lobo and Kumar 2009). In case of voluntary shift, people move away for reasons ranging from better economic opportunities to a safe social or natural environment. The major factor here is the free will of the person to move. According to Adesina (2007), multiple factors such as disasters, ethnic, religious or political conflicts, and development projects are responsible for involuntary dislocation. Development projects both by government and private sector left people with no option but to accept involuntary resettlement and redesign their life and livelihood in a new place leaving all their memories and social ties behind.

It is understood that development projects will bring benefit to people of all sections of society and their quality of life would be improved eventually. Nowadays, in economics and political science, the quality of life of a population is a significant factor, and it is linked with a planning and decision making process. It is determined by a variety of social and economic influences (in Young 2008). The factors connected with quality of life (QOL) are covers a wide range. For example, health situations, recreational facilities, social communication, education opportunity, cultural ethics, work atmosphere, safety, housing condition, and more.

Dhaka as the capital city is experiencing high rate of urbanization and private sector is significantly involved in land and housing sector development. About seventy seven (77) private land developer companies are registered with RAJUK (The Capital Improvement Authority of Dhaka) according to Private Residential Land Project Regulation, 2004. These companies have land development projects within the jurisdiction of RAJUK area. This research focused on people who are displaced from their local area due to private land development projects. The research tried to compare the quality of life of these displaced people before and after relocation. Selected indicators of "Quality of Life" has been addressed in this research which includes landownership, housing condition, occupational status, income and expenditure, access to utility, facilities, and social network. Again safety, freedom of expression, compensation, and living environment are also considered as indicators of quality of life. The displacement of local people took place through a complex process. A detail investigation was conducted on the issue of safety, freedom of expression, compensation, and living environment during the displacement process faced by the local residents of the study areas who were mostly involuntarily displaced by the private land developers. In this backdrop, the research aimed to study the process and nature of relocation of local people due to land development projects. It also compared the quality of life of relocated people before and after relocation.

8.2 Selection of Study Area and Data Collection Approach

About seventy seven (77) private land developer companies are registered with RAJUK to operate their business. This research included 5% of private land developers who have land projects in Dhaka. Four land development project areas were considered as study area to survey the people displaced due to these development projects. Selection criterion for study area is based on the size of the projects from the year 2000–2010. Only those land projects were considered which had development approval by RAJUK. Four land projects selected for the study are Green Model Town (Project area: 200 ha) of Amin Mohammad Foundation Ltd, United City (Project area: 73.33 ha) of Neptune Development & Holding Ltd, Pink City (Project area: 120 ha) of Xenovally, and Ashiyan City (Project area: 466.67 ha) of

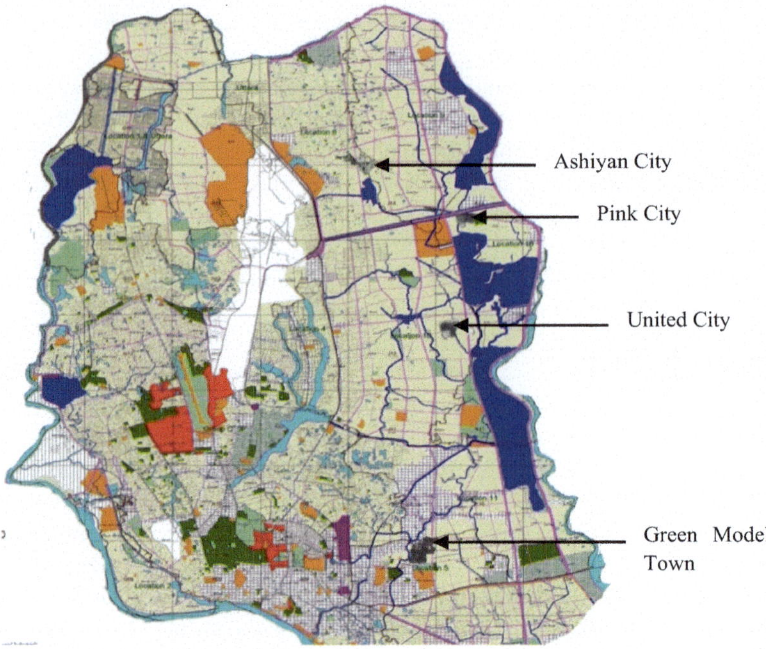

Fig. 8.1 Area of land development projects (study areas) in the fringe area of Dhaka. *Source* Field survey, 2011

Ashiyan Land Development Ltd. Location of these land development projects at the eastern fringe of Dhaka is shown in Fig. 8.1.

Data was collected from both primary and secondary sources to fulfill the research objectives. This research required a substantial amount of primary data because there was no previous study conducted on relocation of local people due to private housing projects. A semi-structured questionnaire survey was conducted to collect data from the relocated people. To assess the present and past status of socioeconomic condition of relocated families a set of indicators were studied. There was no authentic information and specific number of relocated families in any government offices. It was a challenging task to find out the information of relocated families. Though original local residents sold their land and moved to different places, some of local people were still living in the areas adjacent to the study areas, and they had information about the displaced families. At first, survey team collected information from these local residents. Again, local primary school teachers, local religious leaders (*Imam*), local NGOs workers and clubs provided information about present address of the displaced people. Focus group discussion and interviews of local key informants played a vital role to explore the number of displaced families and their present area of residence. Based on the information from the abovementioned sources, approximately 3,920 families were identified as displaced families who had landownership in project areas (study area). About 350 displaced household heads were surveyed. This research used snowball sampling for questionnaire survey. Snowball sampling also called network or chain sampling. Residents of adjacent land development projects were the main introducing section for snowball sampling and data were collected from the people who had left their original area and settled in different locations of Dhaka and outside Dhaka. Face to face interview was conducted with the sample population. In addition, information on housing projects was collected from various secondary sources like RAJUK (Capital Improvement Authority of Dhaka), Real Estate and Housing Association of Bangladesh (REHAB), offices of land developers, and advertisements published in media and website. Secondary data was also collected from various government, nongovernment, and international organizations.

8.3 Displacement and Relocation Process of Local People

Dislocation of people can happen due to civil encounters, natural and man-made disasters, and development projects including large and small scale (in Lobo and Kumar 2009). According to Lobo and Kumar (2009), development projects have an impact on people's lives in different ways. Some are forced to leave their homes and relocate in different places. They are known as displaced persons. Households are affected by the projects, and then, there are changes in the use of natural resources. As a consequence of the development, affected people are losing physical and non-physical belongings, for example, house, land, social networks, and so on (Asian Development Bank 1998).

The Oxford dictionary (1995) defines resettlement as settle in new or previous location, while the same dictionary defines relocation as move to a new location. Both relocation and resettlement terminology are used by the majority of social scientists who have studied the movement of people in new locations (Yan and Qian 2003; Yuefang and Steil 2003). Lobo and Kumar (2009) noted that the decision to shift one's residence may be voluntary or involuntary. In case of voluntary shift, people move away for reason ranging from better economic opportunities to a safe social or natural environment. The major factor here is the free will of the person to move. On the other hand, a variety of factors such as disasters, ethnic, religious, and political encounters and development projects have caused involuntary displacement. According to Asian Development Bank (1998) development projects result in involuntary resettlement and affected people have to rebuild their lives, incomes, and asset bases in new locations. Turton (2006) defines forced relocation as when persons are forced to leave their homes or land for whatever reason. He does not find any difference between the ideas of forced resettlement and the development of convinced resettlement. Turton's definition of forced relocation involves the use of power within parties.

The relocation process of local people due to private housing projects in the four study areas is a complex process. To get information about the relocation process, a number of indicators were studied such as original place of settlement, duration of living in original settlement, influential actors, factors that influenced relocation process, selling of the land in original settlement, satisfaction of the owner regarding selling price, nature of pressure faced by the local residents in land transfer process, area of relocation, etc.

8.4 Actors Involved in Land Transaction Process

It is evident from this study that a number of actors played significant role to displace people from their place of origin. Primarily four actors played a vital role; they are land developers, middleman/musclemen, local officials, and local people.

Land development sector is considered as one of the most lucrative business field. Land developers of the four study areas engage middle man/land broker, local young political party leaders to buy land from local people using various tricks. Amin Mohammad Group established the Green Model Town project and Neptune land developer implemented the United City project. Both the developers have engaged the middlemen to acquire land from local people. The owner of the Pink City is a politician. At first, the authority of the Pink City started their journey to set up the land development project on the owner's own land and later started to acquire the surrounding land with the help of local musclemen.

Middlemen/musclemen are the person who creates connection between land developers and local people. From field investigation, it was found that usually middlemen/musclemen are the local residents who have good knowledge about over all local conditions. It was informed by local people that in most of the cases middlemen/musclemen were involved with ruling political party to get the political favor. In most of the cases, middlemen get a percentage from land developers after he negotiates a deal between the developer and the landowner. In some cases, land developers engaged with the local musclemen to threat and pressurize the local people for selling their land. They also maintain strong connection with political leaders, local administrative body and officials, land officers, social influential persons, and young mobsters for continuing their activities without any interruption.

From focus group discussion and field experience, it is understood that the local administrative body is always in favor of developers. As a result, most of the respondents were reluctant about taking support from local administrative officials. The officials of the land offices also play a vital role to provide support to the activities of the land developer.

From the field investigation it was found that the main occupation of local people in their original area was agricultural. Most of the respondent got their land through inheritance (81.4%). They were permanent residents of the study areas for more than 20 years. It is evident from the field investigation that the displaced people with limited access to power structure were easily exploited by the developers and their associates.

8.5 Factors Related with Displacement and Relocation of Local People

From field investigation, it was apprehended that sell of land was made both in voluntary and involuntary manner. Respondents in the sample survey expressed their view regarding causes for land selling. Voluntary causes of land selling included issues like "good land price" (16%) and "commitment from developers to get a job" (26%). Again, involuntary causes mentioned by the respondents are "family security" (30%), "false land documents of disputed piece of land parcel" (15%), and "uninhabitable condition created by the developers" (13%) (Fig. 8.2).

"Family security" refers to the mental and physical pressure on the people from both developers and the local musclemen. From field investigation, it was found that the musclemen made various types of social pressure and panic to acquire the land from the local people such as eve-teasing, threats, throwing stone at houses in midnight, and so on. From field survey, it was found that 30% respondent indicated issue of family security for selling their land. In case of Pink City, the local people primarily mentioned about "family security" as the causes of land selling. It was found that a significant number of people from Hindu religion were relocated from the study area due to family insecurity. The people who did not want to sell their land to the developers took few steps against the developers' activities, but their protest was not successful due to the political pressure.

Good land price (16%) was another issue for relocation of the local people from their original homestead. Majority of the local people do not have enough education and are not well aware of future consequence. Most of the relocated people inherited their land. As a result, they were easily motivated by the developers for selling their land with a handsome financial offer. Though land price per *katha* (local unit of measurement which is equivalent to 720 sq.ft.) was 5–10 lakh in study areas but in some cases, land developers offered up to 15 lakh per *katha* to the local people.

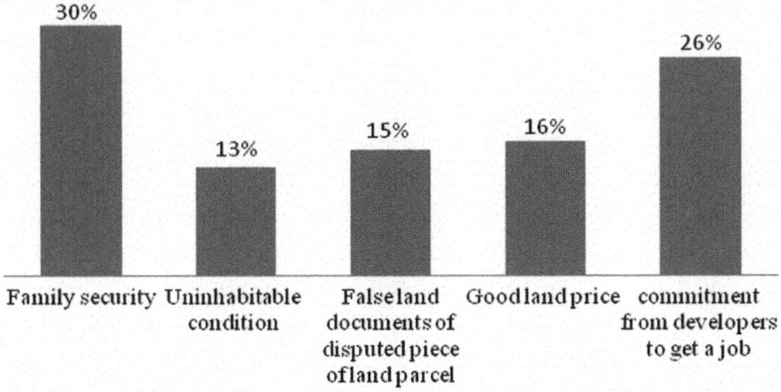

Fig. 8.2 The reasons for land selling by the local people. *Source* Field survey, 2011

Commitment from developers to get a job (26%) was another reason for selling the land by the local people. This criterion was common for Green Model Town and United City projects. The land developers gave the assurance to the local people that if they sell their land, their relatives may get a job in the company. But from field experience, it was found that local people never got a job in the land developer's office after they sold their land.

From the field survey, it was found that all the developers tried to identify the disputed parcels of land in their project areas. It is easier for the developers to get hold of such properties where there were dispute about ownership of land among the successors. In this process, middlemen acted as a data collectors from field level and arrange false documents of disputed parcel of lands. During field survey 15% relocated households indicated about the false land document produced by land developers and this was the prime cause of their relocation. Islam (2009) described that in most of the cases land developers, at the beginning of the projects buy small parcels of low land in a scattered manner. In course of filling these low lands, they intentionally spread out sand on surrounding plots and make all the adjacent plots unproductive for paddy cultivation. As a consequence, owners of those plots are compelled to sell their land to the developer and the process continues with the expansion of the project. It can be noted here that low lying wetlands and agricultural land are very common in the study areas. Here, the developers recognized that most of the people were engaged in agriculture. So, if agricultural land is filled with the sand, local people will be bound to sell their homestead at low price. In case of Ashiyan City project, the water and gas lines of the households were cut off to compel the residents to sell their land.

Local owners are also threatened by the developers to sell their land (in Haque 2004). From field investigation, it was found that 13% relocated household indicated that "uninhabitable condition" was created by the developers which forced them to relocate. Developers often occupy lands of absentee owners and government owned (*Khas*) land. During the field investigation, a number of residents were found who are still living in the area under severe threat of eviction.

Based on field survey, it can be said that major portion of the respondents of the survey did not try to protest the process of forcible (involuntary) relocation by any form of social or legal assistance (66.3%). Only 33.7% of the respondents tried to protect their land by social or legal assistance. Here occupational and social status of the local people played imperative role regarding their initiatives to protect their lands from developer.

In most of the cases, it was evident that the bargaining power of landowner was very low, as local musclemen who acted as middle man favored the land developers by fixing land at a low price. From the field investigation, it was found that land price varies with some criteria. For example, the price of homestead was different from the price of agricultural land. Developer had to pay more money to get the homestead land than that of agricultural land, as it was the business policy to get the whole land easily. The developers believed that, it would be easier for them to get the agricultural land if they buy homestead land at the beginning. Likewise, social and political power of local people also determined the selling price of land. Those who had strong political linkage got extra benefit than common local people.

8.6 Money Transfer Procedure and Satisfaction About Land Price

From the four study areas, some common scenarios have been found regarding money transfer procedures between the local people and developers. The field survey reflected that most of the respondents did not get their whole money at a time. It was found that about 28% of people got the money by one cheque but 72% people did not receive the whole amount of money at a time. In most of the cases, middlemen are engaged in money transfer process between land developers and local people. Middlemen also took percentage of the land selling money from both local people and developers. The role of the Middleman varied from place to place and developer to developer. In some cases, the middlemen gave threat to the local people that they will not receive any money if they take any step against the activities of the Middleman. As middlemen had the political support, they exercised the power to deprive the local people of their rights. From the field survey of four land projects, it was found that there were no project offices in projects areas. Thus, the people cannot make any communication with the office of the land developer. They had the only option to negotiate with the middlemen for land selling money. Most of the respondents in the sample survey were not satisfied (79.4%) with their land price.

Though both voluntary and involuntary procedures were used for relocation, this research outcome clearly shows that maximum local people were displaced from their original location through the involuntary procedure. During the displacement process, the basic right of the people to protect their property was violated. The safety and security of local residents were severely threatened by the developers and their associates. It indicates ruthless deterioration of the quality of life of local people during the displacement process.

8.7 Places of Relocation

It was found from field survey that most of the respondents were interested to live nearby their previous location. But in reality, job opportunity placed prime consideration for choosing a new place (Fig. 8.3).

The first priority of the displaced people was to search for a new job or new land for living in adjacent areas. It is obvious from Fig. 8.3 that 44.6% household were relocated to the areas ranging between 1 and 5 km away from the previous location. From the survey, it was found that only 4.6% household moved beyond 15 km from

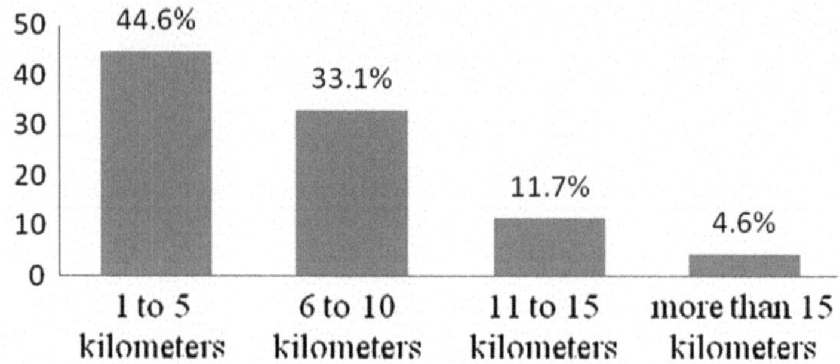

Fig. 8.3 Distance between existing and original place. *Source* Field survey, 2011

the original location. Less than 20% relocated in districts outside Dhaka city such as in Comilla, Khulna, Noakhali, and Gazipur.

8.8 Quality of Life After Relocation

During dislocation, people lose natural, man-made, social, and human capital (in Ahsan 2007). Displacement of local people from their foundation and poverty are connected together by many social researchers. There have been a number of researches where the Model of Cernea (1999) has been used as a structure. For example, Mahapatra (1999) uses the model to assess India's relocation from 1947 to 1997. Displacement of local people from their own land has many negative social effects (Yuefang and Steil 2003). Similarly, Pokharel (1995) mentioned that once people lose their own land, income, other assets and move to new environments, they are powerless to use their traditional abilities. The efficiency of their land drops, as does their food security. Resettlement has many negative impacts on communities, social organizations, and it disrupts informal networks and so on. To compare the quality of life of the respondents before and after relocation, a set of indicators have been studied such as landownership, housing conditions, access to utilities and services, occupation, income and expenditure, social network, and more.

*8.8.1 Land*ownership

Due to relocation, landownership has been changed drastically. From the field survey, it was found that the people without lands in previous locations were hardly found. But at present, most of the people (67.7%) have no land. Previously, 43.1% of people had land between 10 and 20 *katha* but now, it is decreasing to remain 6.9%. People whose land was more than 20 *katha* but now they no land (Table 8.1). Though some

Table 8.1 Present and previous landownership

Land size (One *Katha* = 720 sq.ft.)	Previous landownership (%)	Present landownership (%)
Above 20 katha	3.4	0
10–20 katha	43.1	6.9
5–9 katha	28.0	0.9
1–4 katha	25.4	24.6
No land	0	67.7
Total	100	100.0

Source Field Survey, 2011

people got the money at a time from the developers by selling their lands, most of them could not afford to buy a new parcel of land at any other place due to high price.

8.8.2 *Occupational* Status

It is learned from the field survey that at present, local people's occupational structure is totally changed from previous locations. For example, the percentage of respondents previously engaged in agriculture and labor sector were dramatically changed. The percentage of people involved in agriculture was reduced to 16.6% from 42.3% as they changed their locations of residence. Similarly, the percentage of respondents engaged in labor force was increased from 22.9% to 56.6%. At the same time, small business and large business percentage are reduced from previous to present. One interesting point was that private and government service holders have shown no change between previous and present occupation (Fig. 8.4).

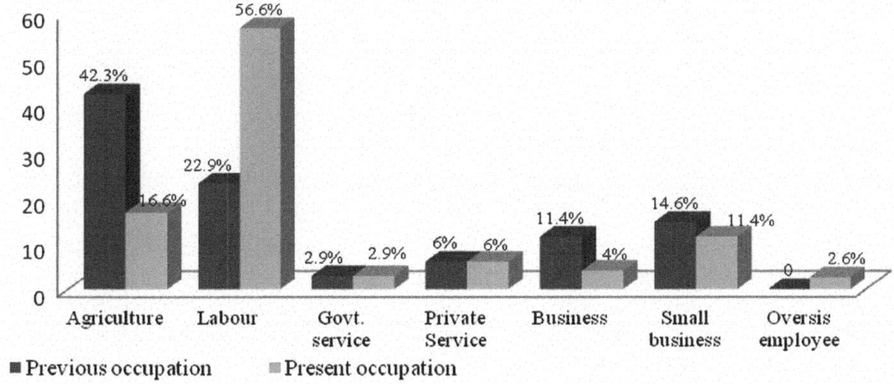

Fig. 8.4 Previous and present occupation. *Source* Field survey, 2011

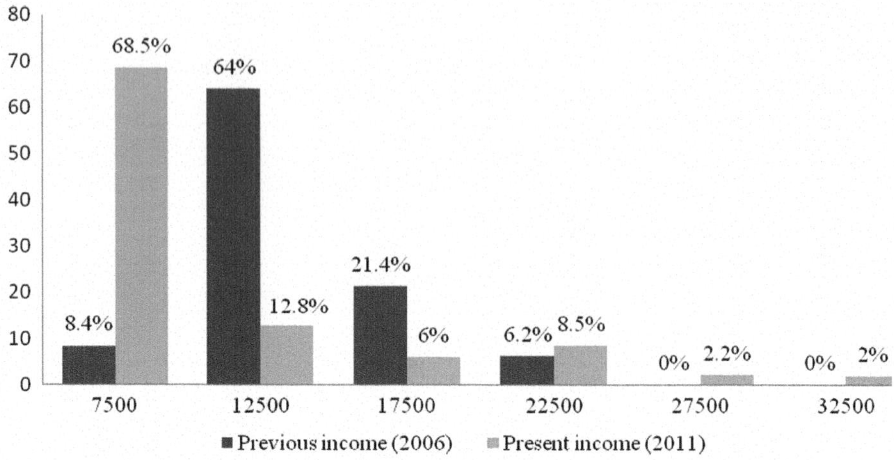

Fig. 8.5 Present and previous income and expenditure. *Source* Field survey, 2011

8.8.3 Income and Expenditure

From the field survey, it can be said that the overall income range is reduced from previous to present. The average inflation rate of Bangladesh is 8.28, and it has been considered while calculating the income for the years 2006 and 2011. This is to note that 100 BDT of 2011 is equal to the 67.182 BDT in 2006 (BDT 80 = 1 US dollar). After the valuation of money, it can be said that in previous locations, most of the people had an income between 15,000 BDT and 20,000 BDT but at present, it ranges from 5,000 BDT to 10,000 BDT (Fig. 8.5) So it can be said that local people's actual income was reduced at present than previous locations.

8.8.4 Housing Condition

Most of the respondents in the sample survey live in rented houses at present locations (67.7%); only 32.3% lived in their own home. On the other hand, in previous locations, 100% of respondents lived in their own home.

It was found from the field survey that at present, 33.7% of households belonged to kutcha house whereas previously it was only 7.7%. Such houses were built with a temporary structure constructed with bamboo, thatch, mud, corrugated tin sheet, etc. Similarly at present semi-pucca (semipermanent structure) house types reduced to 9.5% from previous locations. Likewise, 27.7% household belonged to Pucca (permanent structure) house in previous locations which came down to 11.1% in the present locations (Fig. 8.6).

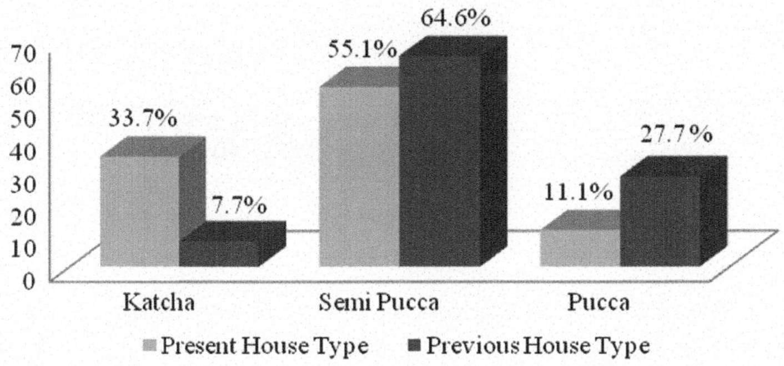

Fig. 8.6 Present and previous house type. *Source* Field survey, 2011

8.8.5 Utility Facilities

From the field survey, it was found that in previous locations, most of the households (92.9%) had electricity connection but at present, 37.1% of households did not have access to electrical connection. It was found from the field survey that in previous locations, 74.9% of households were under gas supply whereas this percentage was only 25.1% at present locations. It was found from the field survey that most of the households had water availability in their house in previous locations (91.4%). Only 8.6% did not have their own supply, they mainly collected from their neighbors. On the other hand, 68.9% household had water availability and 31.1% did not have water connection in their house at present locations. As a result, a huge percentage collected their water from the surroundings.

8.8.6 Social Network

The socioeconomic study of Dhaka city demonstrates that 60–70% of families of Dhaka city have their close relatives living in the same region (Siddique 1991). Similarly, friendship grows between relatively similar natures of people (Brown 1973). In the present study, the primary social network was described by relatives and friendship networks within the neighborhood area. Similarly, the secondary social network in the neighborhood was described by the level of participation of the respondents in the activities of the neighborhood-based organizations.

It was understood from the field survey that maximum local people lived adjacent to their relatives, friends in their previous locations (70.6%). This percentage has significantly dropped to 35.7% in present locations (Fig. 8.7).

It is important to identify the involvement of people with neighborhood organization for measuring social network. The ultimate nature of bonding with the neighborhood can be understood by the concerns of the residents toward problems of neighborhood and initiatives taken by them for solving these problems and for upgrading

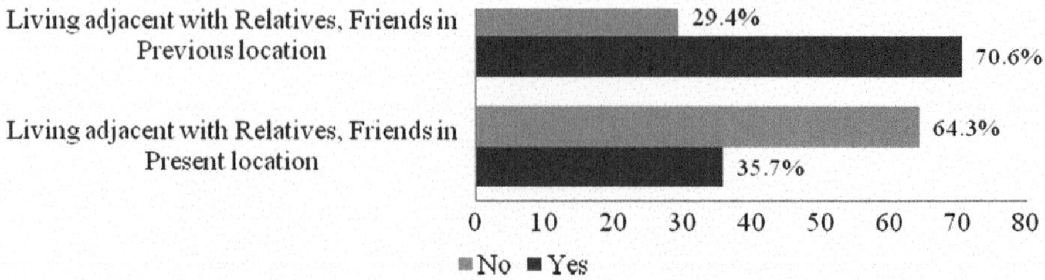

Fig. 8.7 Relatives, friends living in adjacent to each other in present and previous locations. *Source* Field survey, 2011

the overall socioeconomic environmental condition of the neighborhood. Residents of a neighborhood usually do these actions by forming a neighborhood-based association (in Coulthard et al. 2002). Such neighborhood-based club or organization may be a cultural club, neighborhood development club, sports club, religious club, and so on. From the survey, it was found that only 36.9% are involved with neighborhood organization in present locations. But this percentage was 73.1% in their previous location. For example, Jubo Somity (Sports club) was established by Holan Nama Para's resident in Dakkin Khan Union, Dhaka. Similarly, residents of adjacent areas of Pink City established so many clubs like "Dumni Somaj Unnayan" (neighborhood development club). In present locations most of the respondents are tenants. This played a vital role for involvement with neighborhood organizations and in turn affected their quality of life. As tenant families, they do not have the provision of membership or have no chance to control a club. As a result, they feel alienated in the neighborhood and have no voice regarding various social issues. This is not a healthy sign of from the point of view of their quality of life.

8.9 Consequences of Relocation

Many development projects ultimately increase poverty by dislocating large numbers of local people. According to World Bank, unsuitable new sites can lead to loss of livelihoods and social capital, and may increase cultural isolation, poverty, and people may return to their original community leaving the new sites. Risk of impoverishment is inherent in the process of relocation of local people from their original places through a number of sources. Findings of this research supported social researchers' judgement about the consequence of relocation. According to Michael Cernea's (2000), impoverishment risks management and reconstruction model (IRR model) for resettling displaced population, eight risks are identified that resettled people have to cope with in order to successfully protect their lives from impoverishment. Table 8.2 shows the analysis of study findings according to the eight risk indicators of "Cernea Model".

Table 8.2 Analysis of study findings according to "Cernea Model"

Eight risks after relocation	Before relocation	After relocation	Findings from study area
Landlessness	0% respondents were landless	67.7% landless	In previous location, maximum people had land between 10 and 20 katha
Joblessness	42.3% involved with agriculture	56.6% people are day labor	Day labor had no fixed income and had no job security
Homelessness	100% people had own home	32.3% have own home	Maximum local people turned as landless people
Marginalization	Most of the people's income ranges between BDT 10,000 and 15,000	Most of the people's income ranges between BDT 5,000 and 10,000	Evaluate income range between two locations based on the inflation rate
Food insecurity	Most of the people's income ranges between BDT 10,000 and 15,000	Most of the people's income ranges between BDT 5,000 and 10,000	Relocated people in the vulnerable condition
Increased morbidity and mortality	–	–	Not considered in this study
Loss of access to common property resources	–	–	Not considered in this study
Social disarticulation	• 70.6% people lived beside relatives and friends • 73.1% people had involvement with neighborhood organization	• 35.7% people lived beside relatives and friends • 36.9% people have involvement with neighborhood organization	Primary social network described by relatives and friendship networks, secondary social network described by the level of participation in the neighborhood organizations

Source Field Survey, 2011

8.10 Conclusion

The current land laws and regulations, including the Acquisition and Requisition of Immovable Property Ordinance II (1982), have failed to adequately address the needs of those affected and displaced people. Land Acquisition Ordinance (LA Ordinance) of Bangladesh does not have any provision for resettlement/rehabilitation but only the monetary compensation to the property loser. In most of the cases, this money cannot compensate for 25% of tile losses (in Khatun 2005). For the calculation of compensation, the land acquisition officials at the district have to depend on records of rights and records of transfer of property. But to avoid taxes, general people show a lower value of the land.

According to the "Private Residential Land Development Rules 2004", entrepreneur of a private residential project must own precisely the complete land area (100%) without any shares, if the entrepreneur fails to own maximum 10% of the total land locally for any reason from any land or house owner (in special case maximum 15% of the total land with the permission of the committee formed by the government), can be proposed for land acquisition through the law and in such circumstance the entrepreneur must appeal for land acquisition with proper reason supporting his proposal. Under the Sub Act (1) and the Acquisition and Reacquisition of Immovable Property Ordinance, 1982 (Ordinance No. II of 1982), owners of the acquired land or house must be paid an extra 50% value for the property. This Act also mentioned that owners of the acquired land or house must be provided a Rehabilitation Plot in the project area with 50% discount from the present rate of the developed plot as their land or house has been acquired for the project. All the acquired landowners must be rehabilitated and such indigenous dwellers must be provided with Rehabilitation Plot where accurately their previous houses/infrastructures were and Layout Plan must be produced accordingly. In this Sub Act, indigenous means such person who has been dwelling in that house or land since 1971 or before, or has been inherited the land or house according to the CS Record.

It is clearly evident from the research outcome that maximum local people were displaced from their original location through the involuntary procedure. Serious deterioration of the quality of life particularly disruption of life and livelihood and the safety issue of family members were the major concern which forced them to sell their land. Masum also noted that the development of urban fringe land follows in informal ways without proper rules and regulations in most developing countries. The research also demonstrations that overall quality of life of relocated people in their new place have been declined significantly matched to that of their previous area of residence, which eventually supported the opinion of social scientists regarding adverse effect of relocation (Cernea 1999).

It is alarming to note that urban fringe is mainly used in the capital city of Bangladesh for asset gathering of influential actors at the price of relocating local individuals and declining their quality of life. Access to the legal and administrative structure is very limited for the general people in Bangladesh. Existing rules and regulation required to be revised for protecting local people's right. The proposed National Policy on Resettlement and Rehabilitation (NPRR) should be implemented as soon as possible. It has to be kept in mind that the fruit of economic improvement will be of no use if the oppression of people continued and social justice is denied in the name of development.

Acknowledgements The researchers like to express their gratitude to Department of Urban and Regional Planning, Bangladesh University of Engineering and Technology (BUET) for proving all sorts of support to conduct this research work.

References

Adesina, A. (2007). *Socio-spatial transformations and the urban fringe landscape in developing countries*. United Nation University Institute For Environment And Human Security (UNU-UHS) Summer Academy On Social Vulnerability And Resilience Building In Mega city, Germany.

Ahsan, M. (2007). *Involuntary resettlement in jamuna bridge project: Impoverishment risks and reconstruction measures (MDS Thesis)*. Dhaka, Bangladesh: Development Studies Program, BRAC University.

Jamuna Multipurpose Bridge Authority. (1993). *Revised resettlement action plan*. Dhaka: Report of Jamuna Multipurpose Bridge Authority.

Asian Development Bank. (1998). *Handbook on resettlement: A guide to good practice*. Manila: Asian Development Bank.

BBS. (2012). *Population and housing census 2011 socio-economic and demographic report*. Bangladesh Bureau of Statistics, Statistics and Informatics Division (SID), Ministry of Planning, Government Republic of Bangladesh, Dhaka.

Brown, H. (1973). *Man and his environment: A psychological introduction, in city as a social system* (pp. 13–43). Bletehley: Urban Development Unit, Open University Press.

Coulthard, M., Walker, A., & Morgan, A. (2002). *People's perceptions of their neighbourhood and community involvement*. London: National Statistics Publication.

Clark, D. A. L. (2009). *Environmental challenges to urban planning: Fringe areas, ecological footprints and climate change. Key challenges in the process of urbanization in Ho Chi Minh City*. Vietnam: Governance, Socio-Economic, and Environmental Issues.

Cernea, M. M. (2000). *Impoverishment risks, risk management, and reconstruction: A model of population displacement and resettlement*. Paper was presented to the UN symposium on hydropower and sustainable development. Retrieved from http://communitymining.org/attachments/254_population_resettlement_IRR_MODEL_cernea.pdf.

Cernea, M. M. (1999). *The need for economic analysis of resettlement: A sociologist's view*. Washington DC: The World Bank.

Fatema, R. (2003). *Analysis of land suitability for urban development in the Easter fringe area of Dhaka city: An application of multicriteria evaluation technique* (MURP Thesis). Department of Urban & Regional Planning, Bangladesh University of Engineering and Technology (BUET), Dhaka, Bangladesh.

Haque, M. J. (2004). Impact of private land development on the environment of the eastern fringe area of Dhaka (Phd Thesis). Department of Urban & Regional Planning, Bangladesh University of Engineering and Technology (BUET), Dhaka, Bangladesh.

Haque, K. N. H. (2012). *The political economy of urban space: Land and real estate in Dhaka City*. Bangladesh: Institute of Governance Studies, BRAC University.

Islam, I. (2009). *Wetlands of Dhaka metro area: A study from social, Economic & Institutional perspectives*. Bangladesh: A H Development Publishing House, Dhaka.

Islam, N. (1993). The Bangladesh situation in urban management capacity CUS bulletin on urbanization and development, No. 24 and 25. Center for Urban Studies, Dhaka, Bangladesh.

Khatun, H. (2005). Development induced displacement and rehabilitation in Bangladesh: Challenges and perspectives. *Oriental Geographer, 49*(2).

Lobo, L., & Kumar, S. (2009). *Land acquisition, displacement and resettlement in Gujrat: 1947–2004*. Delhi, India: SAGE Publication.

Logan, J., & Molotch, H. (1987). *Urban fortunes: The political economy of place*. Berkley: University of California Press.

Mahapatra, L. K. (1999). Testing the risks and reconstruction model on India's resettlement experience. In M. Cernea (Ed.), *The economics of involuntary resettlement: Questions and challenges*. The World Bank: Washington DC.

Oxford Dictionary. (1995). *Oxford* (9th ed.). Oxford: Oxford University Press.

Pokharel, J. C. (1995). *Population displacement and compensation planning in Kulekhani hydro-electric project, Nepal* (pp. 139–150). in Hari Mohan Mathur (ed). op. cit.

Roy, S. (2007). *A study on private residential land development activities in Dhaka and their compatibility with DMDP structure plan (1995–2015)* (*MURP Thesis*). Department of Urban & Regional Planning, Bangladesh University of Engineering and Technology (BUET), Dhaka, Bangladesh.

Siddique, K. (1991). *Social formation of Dhaka City- A study in third world urban society.* Dhaka University Press Limited.

Turton, D. (2006). Who is a forced migrant? In C. J. De Wet (Ed.), *Development-induced displacement: Problems, policies and people*. Oxford: Berghahn Books.

Yan, T., & Qian, W. (2003). Rural resettlement and land compensation in flooded areas: The case of three gorges project, China. *Asia Pacific Viewpoint, 44*(1), 35–50.

Young, R. D (2008). *Quality of life indicator systems–definitions, methodologies, uses, and public policy decision making South Carolina indicators project publications*. Retrieved February 27, 2015, from http://www.ipspr.sc.edu/scip/documents.asp.

Yuefang, D., & Steil, S. (2003). Three gorges project resettlement: Policy, planning and implementation. *Journal of Refugee Studies, 16,* 422–443.

Chapter 9
Regional Analysis of Effects of Contraception on Quality of Life Among Ever Married Men in Nigeria

Onipede Wusu

Abstract Use of contraception positively affects quality of life of people of a society. The quality of life of Nigerian people is not satisfactory due to several factors including contraception. This study analyses the 2013 Nigeria Demographic and Health Survey data concerning males. The analysis involved 8,828 ever married males from 15 to 49-year age group. Hierarchical regression technique was used in the analysis. Results of the study show that national awareness about any contraceptive was 99%, ranging between 94% in North East and 98% in South-South. Use of any method was highest in the South West (36%; modern methods = 24%) and lowest in North West (7%; modern method = 2%). The condom was most used in all regions. The R square change of the hierarchical regression indicates that contraception elevated the explanatory power of the model in all regions. The new R square ranges between 26% in South East and 61% in North West. After adjusting the selected socio-economic factors, modern contraception and quality of life's indicators were significantly and positively associated in North Central ($\beta = 0.05$, $p < 0.01$), North East ($\beta = 0.04$, $p < 0.05$), North West ($\beta = 0.03$, $p < 0.05$) and South West ($\beta = 0.05$, $p < 0.05$). Traditional methods significantly and negatively influence the quality of life in North Central ($\beta = -0.06$, $p < 0.01$) but positively in North East ($\beta = 0.04$, $p < 0.05$) and North West ($\beta = 0.0$, $p < 0.001$). Therefore, both the modern and traditional contraception are considered as significant factors in enhancing male's quality of life in almost all the regions of Nigeria.

9.1 Introduction

The Quality of Life (QoL) is a complex concept, it is related to health status, physical functioning, psychological adjustment, well-being, life satisfaction and happiness (Rathnayake and Siop 2015). The World Health Organisation (WHO) conceptualisation indicates that QoL is the way people perceive of their position in life in the context of culture and values system in which they live as well as touching on their

O. Wusu (✉)
Department of Sociology, Lagos State University, Ojo Lagos, Nigeria
e-mail: onipedewusu@yahoo.com

B. R. K. Sinha (ed.), *Multidimensional Approach to Quality of Life Issues*,
https://doi.org/10.1007/978-981-13-6958-2_9

pursuits, hopes, standard and desires (Aduloju et al. 2015). In the light of such notion, the study of quality of life becomes important from the point of view of planning for welfare, well-being and happiness of the Nigerian people. The quality of life (QoL) of people in Nigeria is, in fact, poor, unsatisfactory and most challenging. Over a decade, the quality of life of the average Nigerian citizen has suddenly declined and this has been mainly caused by the extreme poverty, which is still pervasive in Nigeria. The majority of population of Nigeria lives with so low income that they can not cover minimum standards of food, water, shelter, medical care and schooling. Zosa-Feranil et al. (2009) rightly stated that the unacceptable QoL is connected to hunger, lack of shelter, sickness, inability to see a doctor, inability of having accessibility to school and lack of knowledge of writing and reading, joblessness, fear for the future, living one day at a time, losing a child to illness caused by unclean water, powerlessness, lack of representation and freedom. As a result the incidence and severity of low QoL in the country is ranked amongst the highest in the world (Anger 2010). Over 60% of the total population (presently >74 million) of the country live under $2 per day poverty line (World Bank 2014). This is an indicative of prevalence of impaired QoL in Nigeria.

Therefore, eradication of extreme poverty will certainly enhance the adequacy of material well-being and personal satisfaction, thereby improve QoL (Fatiregun et al. 2009). Millennium Development Goals and Sustainable Development Goals epitomise the world agenda that targets the enhancement of QoL (Anger 2010; Sachs 2012).

Widespread low QoL in Nigeria has been explained as a function of various factors. The studies have highlighted structural defects, inadequate economic growth, almost total dependence on petroleum and total neglect of other promising sectors, growing unemployment, laziness, poor educational system, poor governance and organised conflict (Ebong and Ogwumike 2013; Olowa 2012; Ucha 2010; Yunusa 2008). The population growth question in improving QoL is still largely controversial. Scholars appear more comfortable with the hypothesis that improving QoL paves way for slow population growth than the other that high population growth promotes low QoL (Lee 2009; Merrick 2002; Sinding 2009; Wusu and Amoo 2015). There is no agreement over the role of population growth in the QoL the world over. While some studies report that population is a significant factor in QoL, others indicate that it is not an important determinant (Ukpong et al. 2013).

In spite of the disagreement, three relatively recent in-depth analyses of the QoL situation in sub-Saharan Africa unanimously suggested that the population question in improving QoL cannot be completely obliterated. The first study asserts that although institutional restructuring and policy are critical in the drive to elevate QoL, the growth rate of the population also matters (Gupta et al. 2011). The other two studies' candid advice was that sub-Saharan African countries would do better in their efforts towards enhancing QoL if a deliberate effort to reduce high fertility rate is incorporated (Cho and Tien 2014; Sinding 2009). The two arguments are summarised in the opening remarks of an article in Peru that government is unlikely to improve QoL if poor families continue to have seven children on the average (Boesten 2007).

Low contraceptive prevalence in sub-Saharan Africa is considered as a crucial barrier to addressing the high fertility situation, fuelling rapid population growth in the region (Campbell et al. 2006). Fertility in Nigeria is still one of the highest in the world in spite of substantial investment in contraceptives over the years while poor QoL is not abating (Anger 2010). National contraceptive use is still as low as 15% (Natioal Population Commission & ICF 2014). What is the importance of contraceptive use in improving the QoL? In the first instance, the identification of the original indicators of the MDGs, which excluded family planning may indicate that world leaders did not consider it important in the battle against poor QoL (Zosa-Feranil et al. 2009). Thus, suggesting no association between family planning and low QoL, although family planning was later given recognition in this regard.

The world leaders that crafted the MDGs' original indicators were not alone in the neglect of the benefits of family planning. A recent study in rural Kenya suggested that in spite of high knowledge of contraceptives, high level ignorance of the benefits exists (Mutombo et al. 2014). However, reports of a few previous studies on the subject suggest that family planning possesses great benefits for QoL (Allen 2007; Bongaarts et al. 2012; Sonfield et al. 2013; Wusu 2011). These studies that analysed the role of family planning in good QoL alluded to the linkages between improving sexual and reproductive health through the use of reliable contraceptive methods and progress in the concomitants of good QoL such as access to better education, improved nutrition and health.

Although a few studies have reported that family planning is key to improving QoL, empirical studies establishing linkages between the two variables are scanty. In fact, in the contexts whereby the population question in QoL is still in doubt, studies on the question are expectedly limited. Thus, the question of the role of population in QoL remains largely unanswered. Most of the ideas on the role of family planning in improving the QoL in Nigeria are speculative, and weak in the empirical foundation. In addition, involving men in the study of family planning in Nigeria is a recent development (Duze and Mohammed 2006). Therefore, we know little about male contraception. In particular, there is poor knowledge about the influence of male contraception on their QoL or that of their households. The critical role men play in almost all aspects of family decision-making in sub-Saharan Africa and in most developing countries underscores the need for studies aiming at considering male contraception and QoL (Mishra et al. 2014; Wusu and Isiugo-Abanihe 2003). This study is about the first to employ nationally representative data in the empirical analysis of the association between male contraception and a demographic indicator of QoL in Nigeria. In addition, this study is important because the regional analysis of the association between contraception and a population related QoL among men has been rarely studied. It is, therefore, a study with the potential of expanding the frontier of knowledge on the impact of male contraception on their QoL.

The question underpinning this study centres on what role contraceptive use plays in QoL in Nigeria. What is the association between male contraceptive adoption and QoL in Nigeria? In the light of these questions, the key objective of this study is to elucidate existing linkages between male contraception and QoL in the geopolitical regions of the country. Therefore, the hypothesis tested in this study is that there is a statistically significant positive association between contraception and indicator of QoL among ever married men in Nigeria.

9.2 Conceptual Framework

Figure 9.1 highlights the conceptual framework hypothesising interaction between the independent (contraceptive use) and dependent variables (QoL) of this study. The study has the assumption that the listed confounding factors (region, age, age at first sex, age at marriage, residence, education, religion, number of wives and number of living children) are likely to influence the association between contraceptive use and QoL independently (Mumah et al. 2015; Wusu 2015). The arrows linking the confounding factors box with those of contraceptive use and QoL represent this association.

The first hypothesis is that contraceptive use is likely to influence QoL directly, hence the first arrow painted pink, a colour different from the confounding factors box. However, it is highly probable that the interaction between the two variables is influenced by the confounding variables (Mumah et al. 2015; Wusu 2015; Wusu and Amoo 2015). Hence, the second arrow connecting contraceptive use and QoL boxes through the confounding factors' box painted blue (the colour of the box). As a result, the analysis controlled for the effect of the last eight confounding factors

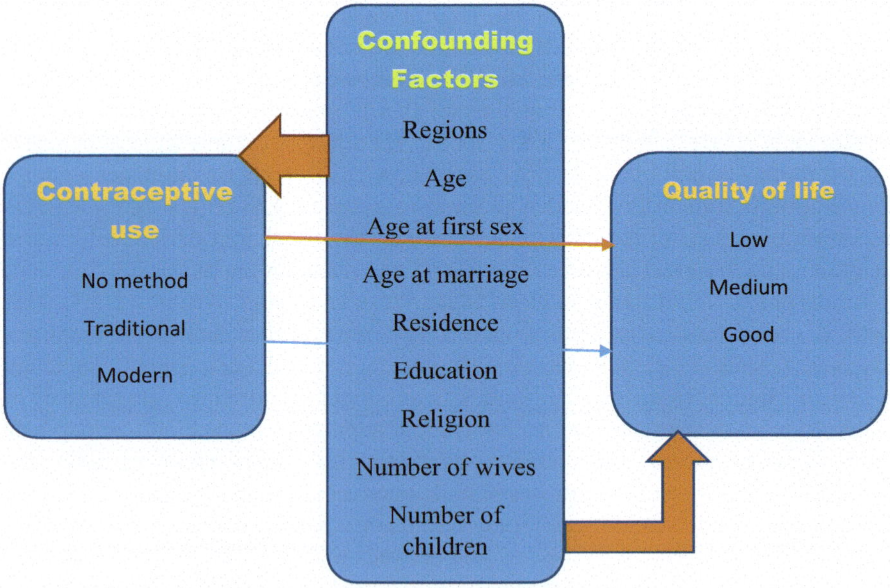

Fig. 9.1 Conceptual framework

while testing the significance of the association between contraceptive use and QoL's indicator in each of the six geopolitical regions in Nigeria.

9.3 Data and Methods

This study analysed the 2013 Nigeria Demographic and Health Survey (NDHS) male data, which is the latest. The analysis involved 8,828 ever married men, aged 15–49, extracted from the male recode data file of the MeasureDHS. The data set is freely available at MeasureDHS.com. Wealth index factor score (3 decimals) variable was used as the indicator of QoL, representing the dependent variable. The adoption of wealth status as an indicator of QoL is based on the assumption that improved wealth status is synonymous with good QoL while poor wealth status should reflect poor QoL. Furthermore, in the QoL indicators itemised by the WHO as well as the adapted definition in this study context, financial situation, housing and accessibility that are crucial to life satisfaction are also used by Measure DHS in deriving the wealth index score (Fatiregun et al. 2009; National Population Commission [Nigeria] and ICF International 2014).

Wealth index factor score is a ratio scale variable, which necessitated the use of the hierarchical regression technique in multivariate analysis. The categorical version of the variable consists of four categories, namely poorest, poorer, middle, richer and richest. Thus, it is a variable Measure DHS constructed from the household living condition or wealth situation to represent proportion poor or not as well as proportion rich or not (representing good or low QoL) in the population. I reclassified the variable into poor, middle and rich (indicating poor, medium and good QoL) at the univariate and bivariate levels of analyses to demonstrate the proportion of the study population in various QoL categories.

Independent variable used in the analysis was MV 313 titled current contraceptive use. It has five categories: no method, folkloric method, traditional method, modern method and don't know. Don't know was declared missing prior to the analysis while folkloric and traditional were classified into traditional. Three categories emerged from the reclassification.

These include using no method, traditional method and modern method. These three categories were used directly in bivariate analysis while they were converted to dummy in the multivariate analysis. Based on the literature, nine confounding variables were selected for multivariate analysis. On the one hand, five ratio variables include age, age at marriage, age at first sex, number of wives and number of living children. On the other hand, education, employment, religion and residence were four categorical variables. For the purpose of description, at univariate level of analysis, the ratio variables were reclassified into categorical version as age (24 or less, 25–29, 30–34, 35–39 and 40+), age at marriage (15–19, 20–24 and 25+), age at first sex (14 or less, 15–19, 20–24 and 25+), number of living children (1–2, 3–4 and 5+) and number of wives (1 and 2+). In contrast, at the multivariate level of analysis, ratio variables were used in their original forms. With the exception of education, the four categorical variables, the original categories were used at univariate and multivariate levels of analysis. Education was reclassified from four categories (no education, primary, secondary and higher) into three (no education, primary and secondary and above). Employment was measured as working and not working, religion as Catholics, other Christians, Islam and Traditionalist (Others declared as missing because of placement difficulty), and residence as urban and rural. But all categorical variables were recorded dummy at the multivariate level of analysis.

The study conducted three levels of analyses. At the univariate level of analysis, percentage distribution of the respondents by all the variables (dependent, independent and confounding) across the six geopolitical regions (North Central, North East, North West, South East, South-South and South West) was done. The bivariate analysis involved the test of association between the dependent variable (categorical version of wealth index, the indicator of QoL) and the independent variable (contraception) by the geopolitical regions. Chi-square test of association between contraceptive use and QoL indicator was carried out. Cramer's V tested the strength or the effect size of the association. Given that the bivariate table has three rows and columns, the decision rule was 0.07–0.21 (means small effect); 0.22–0.34 (means medium effect) and 0.35 and above (means large effect) (Pallant 2007). Multivariate level of analysis constructed hierarchical regression model testing association between the indicator of QoL and contraceptive use while controlling for the confounding variables. All analysis was carried out using Statistical Package for Social Science (SPSS) 20.0.

9.4 Results

9.4.1 Socio-demographic Characteristics of Sample

Table 9.1 shows the distribution of the respondents by socio-demographic characteristics, the independent, dependent and confounding variables involved in the analysis by region. The age distribution indicates that majority of the ever married men interviewed were 30 years and above in the six regions. In particular, a sizeable proportion of the respondents were in the age bracket of 40 years and higher (minimum of 33%). With the exception of South East and South West, a minimum of two-third of the respondents were resident in rural areas in all the regions. Two-third of South East sample and 72% of their counterparts in South West were of urban residence. The residential pattern reinforces the fact that the South West followed by South East remains the most urbanised parts of Nigeria. The religious affiliation shows that Muslims dominate the three regions in the north while Christianity (Catholic and other Christians) was most popular in the south. The educational background of the sampled men shows that most of those from North East and North West reported no schooling while the majority of their counterparts in South East, South-South and South West reported secondary or higher education.

Table 9.1 Percentage distribution of ever married men by selected socio-economic and demographic characteristics by regions in Nigeria, NDHS 2013

Characteristics	Percent					
	North Central N = 1591	North East N = 1603	North West N = 2343	South East N = 650	South-South N = 1316	South West N = 1325
Age						
24 or less	5.2(83)	7.3(117)	5.8(137)	2.9(19)	2.1(28)	3.1(41)
25–29	16.5(263)	18.0(289)	15.3(358)	8.3(54)	12.3(162)	10.0(132)
30–34	20.2(322)	20.6(330)	19.5(457)	17.5(114)	19.4(255)	20.2(268)
35–39	21.9(348)	21.1(339)	21.8(510)	21.8(142)	22.4(295)	24.9(330)
40+	36.1(373)	32.9(528	37.6(881)	49.4(321)	43.8(576)	41.8(554)
Place of residence						
Urban	34.1(542)	20.5(328)	21.9(5120	64.8(421)	31.8(419)	71.5(947)
Rural	65.9(1049)	79.5(1275)	78.1(1831)	35.2(229)	68.2(897)	28.5(378)
Religion						
Catholics	16.7(264)	2.1(33)	2.6(60)	43.4(281)	8.5(111)	4.1(54)
Other Christians	33.8(535)	18.7(299)	4.7(110)	51.3(332)	88.4(1148)	60.3
Muslims	47.6(752)	78.6(1259)	91.7(2128)	1.1(7)	2.1(27)	34.5(457)
Traditionalists	1.9(30)	0.6(10)	1.0(23)	4.2(27)	1.0(13)	1.1(15)
Education						
No schooling	16.5(263)	48.3(774)	52.2(1222)	2.8(18)	1.7(23)	6.6(87)
Primary	19.9(317)	18.4(295)	20.2(474)	36.6(238)	26.7(351)	22.6(299)
Secondary+	63.5(1011)	33.3(534)	27.6(647)	60.6(394)	71.6(942)	70.9(939)
Wealth status						
Poor	26.1(416)	68.5(1098)	67.6(1584)	14.2(92)	8.5(112)	8.6(114)
Middle	28.4(452)	15.7(251)	15.5(364)	19.4(126)	23.5(309)	11.9(158)
Rich	45.4(723)	15.8(254)	16.9(395)	66.5(432)	68.0(895)	79.5(1053)
Contraceptive use						
No method	77.1(1227)	94.8(1519)	92.7(2173)	82.0(533)	80.0(1053)	644.2(851)
Traditional	6.0(96)	0.9(15)	5.0(116)	5.2(34)	6.8(89)	11.4(151)
Modern	16.8(268)	4.3(69)	2.3(54)	12.8(83)	13.2(174)	24.4(323)
Number of living children						
1–2	35.0(501)	32.5(461)	31.3(644)	39.6(231)	37.1(449)	39.3(491)
3–4	32.3(462)	28.7(407)	27.6(567)	33.4(195)	30.9(373)	38.7(483)
5+	32.8(469)	38.9(552)	41.1(845)	26.9(157)	32.0(387)	22.0(274)
Age at first sex						
14 or less	3.1(50)	1.2(20)	0.3(7)	4.0(26)	7.4(97)	4.2(56)
15–19	29.4(467)	15.4(247)	4.6(108)	40.0(260)	58.1(764)	45.9(608)
20–24	22.3(355)	15.2(243)	5.2(122)	35.3(231)	24.3(320)	34.6(458)

(continued)

Table 9.1 (continued)

Characteristics	Percent					
	North Central N = 1591	North East N = 1603	North West N = 2343	South East N = 650	South-South N = 1316	South West N = 1325
25+	45.2(719)	68.2(1093)	89.9(2106)	20.5(133)	10.3(135)	15.3(203)
Age at marriage						
15–19	16.5(262)	21.8(350)	19.2(451)	6.6(43)	13.9(183)	9.6(127)
20–24	33.8(538)	37.9(607)	39.1(916)	17.2(112)	30.1(396)	27.8(369)
25+	49.7(791)	40.3(646)	41.7(976)	76.2(495)	56.0(737)	62.6(829)
Working						
No	1.6(25)	7.9(127)	7.3(172)	2.0(13)	2.3(30)	1.3(17)
yes	98.4(1566)	92.1(1476)	92.7(2171)	98.0(637)	97.7(1286)	98.7(1308)
Number of wives						
One	84.3(1297)	78.7(1226)	73.8(1697)	95.4(595)	90.5(1136)	90.7(1162)
Two+	15.7(242)	21.3(331)	26.2(604)	4.6(29)	9.5(119)	9.3(119)

In a similar vein, the highest proportion in the poor category (indicating poor QoL) were reported in North East and North West while the highest proportion of the rich (indicating good QoL) was in the South West, South-South and South East. Modern contraceptive use was low all over the six regions, but South West followed by North Central, South-South and South East respondents reported relatively higher prevalence. The lowest levels were reported in the North East and North West. Table 9.1 shows that age at first sex was markedly higher in the north, especially in North East and North West, than what obtained in all the southern regions. However, age at marriage was highest in the southern regions with South West having 80% of the men reporting getting married at age 25 or higher. A vast majority reported working. Most of the sampled men indicated monogamous marriage.

Figure 9.2 presents the percentage distribution of ever married men in Nigeria by contraceptive knowledge and region. The figure shows that knowledge of modern contraceptive was almost universal in all regions of Nigeria. National awareness of any contraceptives was 99%, ranging between 94% (modern method = 93%) in North East and 98% (modern method = 97%) in South-South. Use of any methods was highest in South West (36%; modern methods = 24%) and lowest in North West (7%; modern method = 2%). In contrast, most of the sampled men were not using any methods (see Fig. 9.3). Use of any methods was highest in South West (36%; modern methods = 24%) and lowest in North West (7%; modern method = 2%). The condom was the most popular method used in all regions. The pill and injection were the other modern methods of contraception reported by the respondents.

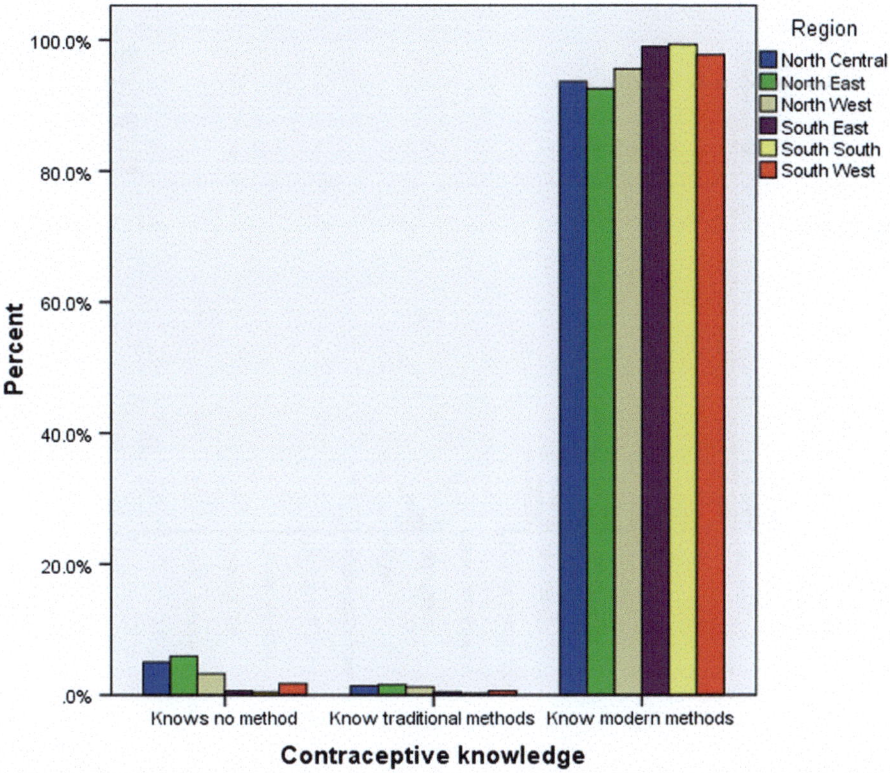

Fig. 9.2 Percentage distribution of ever married men by contraceptive knowledge by regions in Nigeria, NDHS 2013

9.4.2 Association Between Contraception and Quality of Life

Table 9.2 presents bivariate association between contraceptive use and the QoL indicator (wealth status). The association was statistically significant in all regions except in South-South. In North Central, South East and South West, a higher proportion of the respondents using traditional or modern contraceptives indicated middle or rich wealth status (indicating medium or good QoL) compared to those who reported non-use of any methods. It is also striking to note that, with the exception of North East, the highest proportion of ever married men who reported using modern contraceptives indicated rich wealth category (good QoL) in all regions relative to those using traditional methods and not using any methods. In the North East and North West, though the association was statistically significant, the proportions did not exhibit a clear pattern.

Surprisingly, Cramer's V test of effect size or the strength of the association between contraception and QoL indicator was small in North Central, North East,

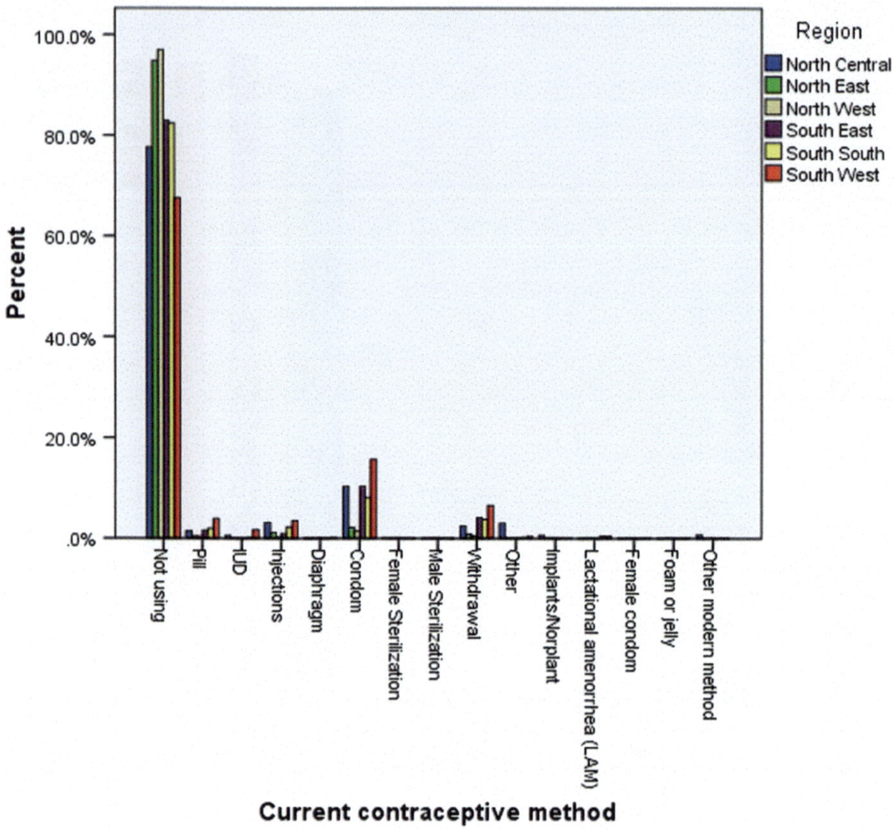

Fig. 9.3 Percentage distribution of ever married men by contraceptive use by regions in Nigeria, NDHS 2013

South East and South West but medium only in North West where there was no clear pattern among the proportions (see Table 9.2).

The beta coefficients of the multivariate hierarchical regression analysis of the association between contraceptive use and indicator of QoL are presented in Table 9.3. To start with, the introduction of contraceptive use elevated the explanatory powers of the models in all regions as evident in the R square change. The R square change indicates the difference between the proportion of change in the indicator of QoL attributable to contraceptive use and the R square which represents the explanatory power of the model prior the introduction of contraceptive use. The change in R square ranged between 0.003 in South West, South-South and North East and 0.005 in North Central, though the change was not significant in South East and South-South as evident in the *p* values (0.159 and 0.056, respectively). Although the change was small across the regions, it is important to note that the change was a

Table 9.2 Percentage distribution of ever married men by contraception and QoL (wealth index) by regions in Nigeria, NDHS 2013

Characteristics	QoL (Wealth Index)					
Contraception	Poor	Middle	Rich	Poor	Middle	Rich
	North Central ($N = 1591$)			*North East* ($N = 1603$)		
No method	29.4(361)	29.7(364)	40.9(502)	70.2(1067)	15.0(228)	14.7(224)
Traditional	16.7(16)	30.2(29)	53.1(51)	40.0(6)	13.3(2)	46.7(7)
Modern	14.6(39)	22.0(59)	63.4(170)	36.2(25)	30.4(21)	33.3(23)
Chi-square	52.63***			46.49***		
Cramer's V	0.18***			0.17***		
	North West ($N = 2343$)			*South East* ($N = 650$)		
No method	70.1(1524)	14.9(324)	15.0(325)	16.3(87)	19.9(106)	63.8(637)
Traditional	37.9(44)	26.6(31)	35.3(41)	2.9(1)	23.5(8)	73.5(25)
Modern	29.6(16)	16.7(9)	53.7(29)	4.8(4)	14.5(12)	80.7(67)
Chi-square	110.28***			14.68**		
Cramer's V	0.22***			0.15**		
	South-South ($N = 1316$)			*South West* ($N = 1325$)		
No method	8.9(94)	24.5(258)	66.6(701)	11.9(101)	12.8(109)	75.3(641)
Traditional	11.2(10)	21.5(258)	66.6(701)	4.6(7)	12.6(19)	82.8(125)
Modern	4.6(8)	18.4(32)	77.0(134)	1.9(6)	9.3(30)	88.9(287)
Chi-square	9.08			38.52***		
Cramer's V	0.08			0.17***		

*significant at $p < 0.05$; **significant at $p < 0.01$; ***significant at $p < 0.001$

reflection of the significant role contraception played in QoL among men in the six regions of Nigeria.

The beta coefficients in North Central region suggest the existence of a statistically significant association between contraceptive use and QoL indicator. The relationship between traditional methods and the QoL indicator was negative. Conversely, modern contraception was positively and significantly associated with QoL in the region. The beta coefficient suggests that a unit increase in modern contraception in the study population resulted in 0.04 improvement in the QoL among men ($p < 0.05$). The coefficients for traditional and modern methods in North East and North West suggest that they were significantly associated with QoL indicator. The associations were positive in both regions. On the one hand, a unit increase in traditional contraceptive use steered 0.04 ($p < 0.01$) and 0.06 ($p < 0.001$) elevation in QoL among men in North East and North West, respectively. On the other hand, a unit increase in modern contraception resulted to 0.04, $p < 0.01$ (North East) and 0.03, $p < 0.05$ (North West) improvement in QoL.

In South East, both contraceptive methods did not significantly predict the indicator of QoL. In contrast, while traditional methods were not significantly associated,

Table 9.3 Coefficients of hierarchical regression on the association between contraception and QoL (wealth index) among ever married men by regions in Nigeria, NDHS 2013

Independent variables	Confounding variables	β coefficients					
		North Central	North East	North West	South East	South-South	South West
Contraception							
No method(r)		–	–	–	–	–	–
Traditional		−0.06**	0.04**	0.06***	0.02	−0.03	0.03
Modern		0.04*	0.04**	0.03*	0.07	0.05*	0.05**
	Age	0.13*** 0.13**	0.03 0.03	−0.05* −0.05*	0.18** 0.18**	0.15*** 0.15***	0.10*** 0.10***
	Age at marriage	0.08*** 0.08***	0.13*** 0.13***	0.12*** 0.12***	0.04 0.03	0.04 0.04	0.11*** 0.11***
	Age at first sex	−0.01 −0.01	−0.05** −0.05**	−0.01 −0.01	−0.02 −0.02	−0.01 −0.01	0.01 0.00
	Place of residence						
	Rural(r)	–	–	–	–	–	–
	Urban	0.52*** 0.53***	0.49*** 0.48***	0.50*** 0.50***	0.10** 0.10**	0.41*** 0.40***	0.54*** 0.54***
	Religion						
	Catholic Christians(r)	–	–	–	–	–	–
	Other Christians	0.19 0.19	0.11 0.09	0.22*** 0.20***	−0.04 −0.05	0.03 0.04	0.41 0.40
	Muslims	0.25* 0.25*	0.18 0.18	0.08* 0.08*	0.04 0.04	0.06 0.05	0.35 0.34
	Traditionalists	0.01 0.01	0.01 0.01	0.04* 0.04*	−0.16 −0.17	−0.04 −0.03	0.08 0.08
	Working						
	No(r)	–	–	–	–	–	–
	Yes	−0.01 −0.01	0.04* 0.03*	0.03* 0.03*	0.01 0.02	−0.03 −0.03	−0.02 −0.02
	Number of wives	−0.02 −0.02	0.06** 0.06***	0.02 0.01	−0.05 −0.05	0.04 0.05	0.03 0.04
	Education						
	None(r)	–	–	–	–	–	–
	Primary	0.09*** 0.10***	0.13*** 0.12***	0.06*** 0.06***	0.39*** 0.38***	0.12 0.11	0.20*** 0.19***
	Secondary+	0.36*** 0.35***	0.45*** 0.45***	0.33*** 0.33***	0.70*** 0.68***	0.36*** 0.35***	0.40*** 0.39***
	Number of living children	– 0.15*** – 0.15***	−0.05* −0.06*	0.02 0.02	−0.20*** −0.20***	−0.16*** −0.15***	−0.11*** −0.11***

(continued)

Table 9.3 (continued)

Independent variables	Confounding variables	β coefficients					
		North Central	North East	North West	South East	South-South	South West
F statistic		161.6*** 141.3***	184.0*** 159.6***	300.6*** 261.7***	17.5*** 15.3***	46.9*** 40.7***	129.5*** 112.0***
F change		9.20***	6.16**	11.57***	1.84	2.88	3.77*
R		0.75 0.75	0.77 0.77	0.78 0.79	0.51 0.51	0.56 0.56	0.74 0.74
R square		0.560	0.589	0.614	0.256	0.313	0.551
R square change		0.565	0.592	0.617	0.261	0.316	0.554
R square difference		0.005	0.003	0.004	0.004	0.003	0.003

Note In each of the cells for confounding variables and R, the upper coefficients represent before contraception was introduced into the model while the lower ones are when contraception was introduced
*significant at $p < 0.05$; **significant at $p < 0.01$; ***significant at $p < 0.001$

modern contraception was significantly and positively associated with the indicator of QoL in South-South and South West. A unit increase in modern contraceptive use amongst men in the two regions would bring about a 0.05 improvement in their QoL.

9.5 Discussion

This study has demonstrated the association between contraceptive use and QoL indicator among ever married men in Nigeria. To start with, the bivariate analysis has shown that contraception and QoL were significantly associated in almost all the regions. Although a higher proportion of traditional contraceptive users indicated medium and good QoL, a staggering proportion of ever married men who used modern contraceptives reported membership of the good QoL category in all regions. In the first instance, the higher proportions of traditional and modern contraceptive users reporting medium and good QoL support the hypothesis that contraception is likely to improve QoL among ever married men in Nigeria. Besides supporting the hypothesis, it is vivid that a higher proportion of men who used modern contraception reported good QoL. In addition, although the effect size or the strength of the bivariate association was small in the majority of the regions, the strength was statistically significant in all regions except in South-South. Thus, this study supports the findings of previous studies that contraception plays a critical role in improving QoL in developing countries (Gupta et al. 2011; Sinding 2009; Wusu 2011).

The multivariate hierarchical regression lends further support to the hypothesis that there is a statistically significant and positive association between contraception and the QoL indicator in the study. First, the beta coefficients testified to the statistically significant positive association between the independent and dependent variables in virtually all the regions. Second, contraception remained statistically significant even when critical confounding factors were controlled for in the model. Third, the increase in R square, though marginal, after contraception was added to the regression models was an indication that contraceptive use elevated the explanatory power of the models on QoL indicator. Thus, this study provides support for the hypothesis that contraceptive use is a crucial determinant of QoL among ever married men in Nigeria.

This study suggests that when population growth is rapid as a result of high fertility owing to low contraceptive prevalence, poor QoL becomes inevitable and if contraception rises, population growth declines and consequently QoL improves (Merrick 2002). If effective contraception is widespread among ever married men, fertility will take a corresponding course leading to sustainable decline and ultimately lowers population growth (Bongaarts 2006). At a national level, low population growth lowers expenditure on consumption and provision of social infrastructures. Resources are therefore freed for investment in capital projects that can prepare the ground for sustainable socio-economic development (Ashraf et al. 2013; Mcnally 2013; Sinding 2009). At the individual level, a man with a manageable family size because he uses reliable contraception to space children and stops childbearing, is likely to have sufficient resources to support the education of the children and improve the QoL of the family (Allen 2007; Anyanwu 2014). In addition, such individuals who plan their family size are likely to make contributions to national domestic savings that are needed to improve national investment and employment, which are important forerunners of improvement in the QoL of citizens (Bloom and Williamson 1998).Therefore, it is critical to address issues related to family planning in Nigeria as a step towards improving the QoL in the country.

As suggested in the findings of earlier studies, men are aware of various contraceptives they can take advantage of and plan their families (Duze and Mohammed 2006; Oni and Mccarthy 1997). The problem family planning programmes have to contend with is the very low prevalence of modern more effective methods in all regions of the country, though the North East and North West reported the lowest prevalence (Avong 2012; Izugbara et al. 2010).There is a need for family planning programmes to address the barriers to contraception in Nigeria that have been identified in previous studies (Srikanthan and Reid 2008; Wusu 2015; Wusu and Isiugo-Abanihe 2007). Addressing those barriers is imperative in order to promote modern contraception among men and women in the country. The condom enjoyed relatively high patronage across the regions, suggesting that family planning programmes may single out the method for promotion, adopting reliable strategies that may increase its prevalence in all regions in the country.

Before concluding it is important to highlight a few limitations of the study. In the first instance, the data set analysed is cross-sectional, as such the results are not amenable to cause–effect interpretation. Also, a few of the bivariate cells in some regions recorded very few frequencies; such small frequencies may have influenced the statistical analysis conducted. There was no way to eliminate such frequencies because they were due to low contraceptive use reported by respondents in the reclassified categories of the indicator of QoL. However, the multivariate analysis could not have been influenced because the continuous version of the indicator was used.

9.6 Conclusion

Nevertheless, the findings present insightful information on the association between contraception and QoL. The study concludes that although the contribution of contraception to the model explaining QoL was small, there is a statistically significant positive association between contraception and QoL even after confounding variables were controlled for, among ever married men in Nigeria. The analysis has shown that levels of contraception and the QoL were low in North East and North West. Nevertheless, the association between modern contraception and QoL was positive and statistically significant in North East and North West and in all other regions except South East. As a result, this study suggests the need for a holistic policy on improving QoL that incorporates family planning with an emphasis on promoting condom use among ever married men in all regions in Nigeria, giving special attention to North East and North West.

References

Aduloju, O. P., Akintayo, A. A., Olofinbiyi, B. A., Awoleke, J. O., Ade-Ojo, I. P., & Dada, M. U. (2015). Predictors of quality of life among infertile women in a South-Western Nigerian teaching hospital. *International Journal of Tropical Medicine and Public Health, 5*(1), 8–12.

Allen, R. H. (2007). The role of family planning in poverty reduction. *Obstetrics Gynecology, 110*(5), 999–1002. https://doi.org/10.1097/01.aog.0000287063.32.

Anger, B. (2010). Poverty eradication, millennium developmant goals and sustainable development in Nigeria. *Journal of Sustainable Development, 3*(4), 138–144.

Anyanwu, C. J. (2014). Marital status, household size and poverty in Nigeria: Evidence from the 2009/2010 survey data. *African Development Review, 26*(1), 118–137. https://doi.org/10.1111/1467-8268.12069.

Ashraf, H. Q., Weil, N. D., & Wilde, J. (2013). The effect of fertility reduction on economic growth. *Population and Development Review, 39*(1), 97–130.

Avong, N. H. (2012). Relationship between religion and use of modern contraceptives among the Atyap in Kaduna State, Nigeria. *Research on Humanities and Social Sciences, 2*(8), 82–89.

Bloom, D., & Williamson, J. G. (1998). Demographic transitions and economic miracles in emerging Asia. *World Bank Economic Review, 12*(3), 419–455.

Boesten, J. (2007). Free choice or poverty alleviation? Population politics in Peru under Alberto Fujimori. *European Review of Latin American and Caribbean Studies, 82*, 3–20.

Bongaarts, J. (2006). The causes of stalling fertility transitions. *Studies in Family Planning, 37*(1), 1–16.

Bongaarts, J., Cleland, J., Townsend, W. J., Besrtrand, T. J., & Gupta, M. D. (2012). *Family planning programmes for the 21st century: Rationale and design*. New York: Population Council.

Campbell, M., Sahin-Hodoglugil, N. N., & Potts, M. (2006). Barriers to fertility regulation: A review of the literature. *Studies in Family Planning, 37*(2), 87–98.

Cho, Y., & Tien, B. N. (2014). *Sub-Saharan Africa's recent growth spurt: An analysis of the sources of growth.* Policy Research Working Paper 6862, Retrieved December 22, 2016, from http://econ.worldbank.org.

Duze, M. C., & Mohammed, I. Z. (2006). Male knowledge, attitudes, and family planning practices in northern Nigeria. *African Reproductive Health, 10*(3), 53–65.

Ebong, S. F., & Ogwumike, O. F. (2013). Economic growth and poverty reduction in Nigeria: An empirical investigation. *Journal of Economics and Sustainable Development, 4*(7), 117–130.

Fatiregun, A. A., Mofolorunsho, K. C., & Osagbemi, K. G. (2009). Quality of life of people living with HIV/AIDS in Kogo State, Nigeria. *Benin Journal of Postgraduate Medicine, 11*(1), 21–27.

Gupta, M. D., Bongaarts, J., & Cleland, J. (2011). Population, poverty and sustainable development: A review of evidence. *Policy research working paper.* Washington DC: Development Research Group, The World Bank.

Izugbara, O. C., Ibisomi, L., Ezeh, C. A., & Mandara, M. (2010). Gendered interests and poor spousal contraceptive communication in islamic northern Nigeria. *Journal of Family Planning and Reproductive Health Care, 36*(4), 219–224.

Lee, R. (2009). *New perspectives on population growth and economic development* Paper presented at the IUSSP 2009 Marrakech.

Mcnally, S. (2013). Global population explosion: Economic and health meltdown. *Journal of the Royal Society of Medicine, 106,* 38–39.

Merrick, W. T. (2002). Population and poverty: New views on an old controversy. *International Family Planning Perspectives, 28*(1), 41–46.

Mishra, A., Nanda, P., Speizer, I. S., Calhoun, L. M., Zimmerman, A., & Bhardwaj, R. (2014). Men's attitudes on gender equality and their contraceptive use in Uttar Pradesh. *Reproductive Health Open Access, 11*(41), 1–13.

Mumah, J. C., Machiyama, K., Mutua, M., Kabiru, C. W., & Cleland, J. (2015). Contraceptive adoption, discontinuation, and switching among postpartum women in Nairobi's urban slums. *Studies in Family Planning, 46*(4), 369–386.

Mutombo, N., Bakibinga, P., Mukiira, C., & Kamande, E. (2014). Benefits of family planning: An assessment of women's knowledge in rural western Kenya. *British Medical Journal Open, 4*(4), e004643. https://doi.org/10.1136/bmjopen-2013-004643.

Natioal Population Commission, & ICF, M. (2014). *Nigeria demographic and health survey 2013.* Abuja, Nigeria, and Rockville, Maryland. USA: NPC and ICF International.

Olowa, O. W. (2012). Concept, measurement and causes of poverty: Nigeria in perspective. *American Journal of Economics, 2*(1), 25–36. https://doi.org/10.5923/j.economics.20120201.04.

Oni, G. A., & Mccarthy, J. (1997). Family planning knowledge, attitudes and practices of males in Ilorin, Nigeria. *International Family Planning Perspectives, 17*(2), 50–54, 64.

Pallant, J. (2007). *Spss survival manual* (3rd ed.). England and New York: Open University Press and McGaw-Hill Education.

Rathnayake, S., & Siop, S. (2015). Quality of life and its determinants among older people living in the rural community in Sri Lanka. *Indian Journal of Genrontology, 29*(2), 131–153.

Sachs, J. D. (2012). From millennium development goals to sustainable development goals. *Lancet, 379,* 2206–2211.

Sinding, W. S. (2009). Population, poverty and economic development. *Philosophical Transactions of the Royal Society, 364,* 3023–3030. https://doi.org/10.1098/rstb.2009.0145.

Sonfield, A., Hasstedt, K., Kavanaugh, M. L., & Anderson, R. (2013). *The social and economic benefits of women's ability to determine whether and when to have children.* Retrieved December 22, 2016, from www.guttmacher.org/pubs/social-economic-benefits.pdf.

Srikanthan, A., & Reid, R. L. (2008). Religous and cultural influences on contraceptives on contraception. *Journal of Obstetrics Gynaeocology Cancer, 30*(1), 129–137.

Ucha, C. (2010). Poverty in Nigeria: Some dimensions and contributing factors. *Global Majority E-Journal, 1*(1), 46–56.

Ukpong, G. I., Ekpebu, D. I., & Ofem, I. N. (2013). Cointegration inferences on issues of poverty and population growth in Nigeria. *Journal of Development and Agricultural Economics, 5*(7), 277–283.

World Bank. (2014). *Nigeria economic report.* Washington, DC.: World Bank.

Wusu, O. (2011). *Contraceptive use and poverty reduction among women in seven West African countries.* Paper presented at the 6th Union for African Population Conference, Burkina Faso.

Wusu, O. (2015). Religious influence on non-use of modern contraceptives among women in Nigeria: Comparative analysis of 1990 and 2008 ndhs. *Journal of Biosocial Science, 45*(5), 593–612.
Wusu, O., & Amoo, E. O. (2015). Feritility behaviour and wealth situation in Nigeria: Evidence from 2013 demographic and health survey. *Social Indicators Research*. https://doi.org/10.1007/s11205-015-1016-4.
Wusu, O., & Isiugo-Abanihe, C. U. (2003). Family structure and reproductive health decision-making among the Ogu of South-Western Nigeria: A qualitative study. *African Population Studies, 18*(2), 27–45.
Wusu, O., & Isiugo-Abanihe, C. U. (2007). Gap in knowledge and use of contraceptives in South-Western Nigeria: A study of *Ogu*. *UNILAG Sociological Review, 8*, 83–106.
Yunusa, M. H. (2008). Incidence of poverty in Nigeria: Causes and consequences. *Journal of International Development, 6*(1), 22–32.
Zosa-Feranil, I., Green, C., & Cucuzza, L. (2009). *Engaging the poor on family planning as a poverty reduction strategy* Vol. Task Order 1.

Chapter 10
Resettlement and Quality of Life of the Bhil Tribe in Sardar Sarovar Dam Area, India

Aslam Mahmood and Sushil Dalal

Abstract Displacement and resettlement of the human population due to the construction of large dams affect the physical and social conditions of the displaced families. The resultant resettlement process modifies the occupational patterns and the nature of health-related problems and, in turn, quality of life at the household level. Post-independence era in India has been earmarked for over all development through the construction of large dams to meet multiple purposes, however, such project has sometimes been opposed by several quarters on various grounds. One of the important criticisms against big dams is its effect on the quality of life of the displaced population. The present paper examines the quality of life among the Bhil and related tribes, which have been displaced by the construction of Sardar Sarovar Dam on River Narmada in the western part of India. The socio-economic conditions of this tribe after resettlement have taken a turn towards realignment through redistribution of land and division of labour. As the size of land holding given to the displaced tribal population has decreased, there is a shift in their occupation from cultivation to agricultural labour. Animal rearing as a source of livelihood has declined drastically except in poultry farming and people have also adopted diverse occupations in non-agricultural fields for their survival. The consumption of food among the resettled families has decreased after resettlement leading to poor health conditions as a result of which occurrence of diseases has increased in spite of increased availability of modern health facilities. Attitude towards health-seeking behaviour has also undergone a significant change, wherein the tribal families which earlier believed in black magic/witchcraft/necromancy and herbal medicine have shifted to treatment through allopathic medicines.

Keywords Bhil · Living environment · Resettlement · Sardar Sarovar Dam

---

A. Mahmood
CSRD, SSS, Jawaharlal Nehru University, New Delhi, India
e-mail: aslammahmood@gmail.com

S. Dalal (✉)
Pt. Neki Ram Sharma Government College, Rohtak, Haryana, India
e-mail: sushil_dalal@yahoo.com

B. R. K. Sinha (ed.), *Multidimensional Approach to Quality of Life Issues*,
https://doi.org/10.1007/978-981-13-6958-2_10

10.1 Introduction

In recent years, considerable stress has been laid on 'The Quality of Life' as a human development index in understanding the impact of socio-economic welfare schemes undertaken by Governments for people. The quality of life can be assessed by analysing living conditions of the people such as the standard of living, the level of their living, and the living style of the people. It can be inquired objectively by generating a list of information containing economic activities, social conditions and living environment of the people. United Nations defines quality of life in terms of human well-being, which is determined by factors such as socio-economic conditions of the population and their healthcare practices, etc. Post-independence era in India has seen over all development in nearly every walk of life. Massive projects have been initiated to develop agriculture, industry, road network, education, health care, urban planning, science and technology, etc. Construction of large dams on several major rivers of India has been found to be necessary for multi-purpose projects of development covering irrigation and generation of hydroelectricity (GOI 1985). Some of such important projects are creation of 'Damodar Valley Corporation' to manage the course of river Damodar, construction of 'Bhakra Dam' on Sutlej river in Himachal Pradesh, mainly for hydroelectricity, Sardar Sarovar Dam over river 'Narmada' in Gujarat, etc. Constructions of big dams, however, are opposed by several quarters on various grounds. It is argued that the main beneficiaries from the construction of these big dams are the big industrialists and farmers and not much attention is paid to the loss of the displaced tribal population which is already marginalized and is not able to take its case to the authorities in any convincing way. One of the important criticisms against these big dams is its effect on the quality of life of the displaced population (Amte 1989; Cernea 1985, 1994; Mathur and Cernea 1995; Mathur and Marsden 1998; Paranjpye 1990; Ramaiah 1998). Shah (2003) has examined the impact of resettlement on the quality of life of second-generation. The present paper examines the effect of the construction of Sardar Sarovar Dam in the western part of India on the quality of life among Bhils and related tribes, which have been displaced by the construction in terms of economic activities and social conditions such as health and food habits.

The research on quality of life has recently acquired momentum, especially after the development of the UN Human Development Index (HDI). While critical attention was paid to it only during 1970s, soon it became the main focus of welfare of human beings globally (Mukherjee 1989). Quality of life is determined by a combination of several social and economic characteristics related to the life of the people of the area (Morse and Berger 1992; NBA; Sangvai 2002; Alagh 1995). A good health enables an individual to lead socially and economically more productive and active life (Karve 1956). The state of good health and well-being of individuals is not a static phenomenon but undergoes a change through a continuing process that depends upon various causative factors such as socio-economic status, nutritional and food intake, educational level, community environment, technology and so on (Naik 1969).

There is no doubt that environment is one of the most important factors which controls the health of an individual or a community (Akhtar and Learmonth 1985). An amalgamation of both environmental and socio-economic factors (Asian Development Bank 1998; Dash 2009; Lobo and Kumar 2009; Singh 1990; Sharma 1986; CSS 1999; Goyal 1996; NCA 1995; Parasuraman 1998; TISS 1993) works as a catalyst for the health of an individual. For example, it is argued that both the physical and social health problems of individuals are rooted in poverty and development (Baviskar 1997; Roy 1999, 2000; Independent Review Team 1997; Thukral 1992; ICLD 1988). However, some of the health problems do not simply arise out of poverty. The developmental levels of the community are also instrumental in having manifold repercussions on the health of people (Colledge 1982).

Quality of life, related to health, measures the capacity of an individual to fight diseases (Good 1996) and enables physical and social conditions favourable to eat, drink and take care of personal hygiene (Eyles and Wood 1982). The World Health Organization (WHO) defines 'health' as a state of complete physical, mental and social well-being. Here, well-being is mapped on the basis of level of health care. The status and level of health care relates to the assessment of treatment and expenditure on curing the diseases of the patient. Hence, the present chapter discusses the quality of life of the displaced tribal people using the socio-economic variables including occupation, living conditions in terms of healthcare practices and food consumption.

10.2 Research Problem

The main objective is to discuss the impact of resettlement on quality of life of the affected tribal communities. The resettlement process has affected the quality of life in general and the levels of living of the tribal population in particular. Therefore, the quality of life in terms of socio-economic conditions and living environment including healthcare measures is needed to be analysed among the tribal population in the state of Gujarat. The state of Gujarat was selected for the case study as a larger part of Gujarat was submerged due to the construction of the Sardar Sarovar Dam on river Narmada as a result of which it has the largest number of resettlement sites.

10.3 The Study Area

Due to the construction of Sardar Sarovar Dam, the resettlement sites are developed in various geographical regions of Gujarat. The Government of Gujarat provided an option to the affected families of Madhya Pradesh and Maharashtra to resettle in Gujarat. The Sardar Sarovar Punarvasahat Agency (SSPA) eventually developed 235 sites in Gujarat to resettle the affected families opting to resettle in Gujarat from all three riparian states. Out of these, ten sites representing different physiographic features have been selected for the present study. Four sites are resettled by the displaced tribal people from the states of Madhya Pradesh and Gujarat and the remaining two sites are resettled by the affected families from Maharashtra.

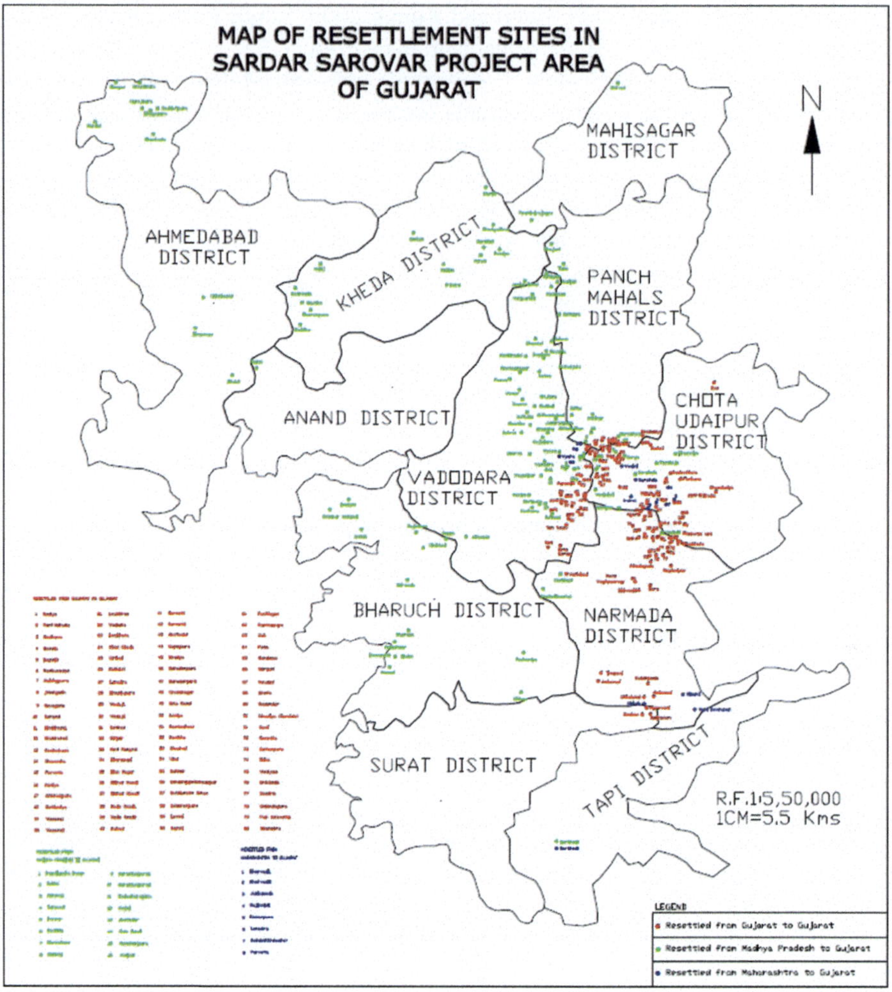

10.4 Methods and Materials

The construction of 'Sardar Sarovar Dam' in the area was an ambitious project of the government which covered three riparian states viz. Madhya Pradesh, Maharashtra and Gujarat. It was considered that as Gujarat has the maximum share in the project, so it has the major responsibility to resettle and rehabilitate the maximum number of affected families in the state. As a result, the Gujarat government developed resettlement sites which are spread over seventeen physiographic divisions in seven districts in the state. On the basis of the physical setting of the region in Gujarat, four sites, i.e. Junarampura, Vyara-1, Vyara-2 and Pansoli from Vadodara Plain, three sites, i.e. Golagamdi, Parveta (MH) and Parveta (Guj) from Orsang-Heran Plain and Vejpur, Gora and Dhefa belonging to Mahi Plain, Narmada Gorge and Lower Narmada Valley have been selected. Using a stratified random sampling technique, the required information through structured questionnaire has been collected to examine the relevant dimensions of the study. A total of 330 households of Bhil tribe have been surveyed from the sample villages.

10.5 Results and Analysis

The economic condition of a family reflects their quality of living. It is controlled by the occupational pattern of the family. The section is broadly analysed into two parts, i.e. occupation and health in terms of dietary habits and diseases.

10.5.1 Occupational Patterns

Occupation is an important parameter to study the quality of life and economic potential of the subject. The displaced families in their original villages were living in close proximity to natural surroundings. Their economic activities were determined by ecological conditions which were integrated and self-sufficient for livelihood. These people were engaged in primary economic activities such as primitive farming, cattle rearing, fishing and hunting-gathering for subsistence. The agricultural labour in the form of *parji* (exchange of labour) system during peak seasons was common in the region. But after displacement, the percentage share of the tribal population engaged in performing these economic activities was affected by social ecology of the recipient areas and has been forced to do work beyond their customary occupations. Hence, it is important to understand changes in the work structure of the affected tribal population.

Depending upon the time devoted to each type of work, the main occupation of the tribal families has been carried out in the survey. Main occupation here refers to the economic activity in which a person works for the major part of the year. The occupation has been divided into six categories, i.e. cultivation, cattle rearing, agricultural labour, wage labour, service and others. The first three categories relate to cultivation and related activities whereas the last three belong to non-agricultural pursuits. The fishing, hunting, gathering and small business have been classified into 'others' category.

A majority of the tribal people are engaged in cultivation and related work. More than 80% of the families are engaged in cultivation in their native villages (Table 10.1). However, the size of the land holdings varies substantially among them.

Table 10.1 Percentage share of occupational structure of the tribal families

Occupation	Before resettlement	After resettlement
Cultivation	83.33	63.33
Cattle rearing	12.74	0.00
Agricultural labour	1.21	21.21
Wage labour	0.00	8.49
Service	1.51	5.45
Others	1.21	1.52
Total	100.00	100.00

Source Compiled from survey data

In the primitive tribal culture, the cultivation is characterized as a traditional system and is labour intensive. Nature plays a dominant role in determining the economic pursuits. Although the percentage share of population in this occupation has declined after resettlement, yet it still attracts more than 60% of the tribal households. This decline does not mean that cultivation is losing its popularity but can be explained in terms of a huge decrease in the land holdings. While the average land holding was more than fifteen acres (including *Jangal khata* land) per household at their native villages, the landholding has now been reduced to more than three times at resettlement sites. However, the number of households having agricultural land has increased due to the provisions made by Narmada Water Dispute Tribunal (NWDT) award. Another important transformation which has been noticed is that the cost of livelihood has increased significantly. So, the people are forced to engage in other occupations to meet out the increased expenditure.

Animal rearing was the second most popular occupation and source of livelihood at the native villages because people could manage to collect fodder for animals from the nearby forest and *Gochar* land. But at resettlement sites, they have lesser number of animals. Here, none of the resettlers has opted for animal rearing as main economic activity. Interestingly, the nature of domestication of animals has changed at resettlement sites. Here, poultry has become more popular whereas in the old villages goat-rearing was more prevalent.

The resettled families do not have an interest in cattle rearing because due to the reduced availability of common property resources, people have started nurturing poultry in the house courtyard. The number of bullocks, too, has fallen to a great extent because their use in agricultural fields has been reduced due to lack of terrain and now they have started using tractors for cultivation and transportation. The agricultural labour as a main occupation was not admired by the resettlers at their native places and less than 1% families opted for it as a main occupation. It was because of the prevalence of *parji* system in which labour was exchanged instead of hiring it. A drastic change in this category at the new sites can be observed and it has become the most important main occupation after cultivation.

Wage labour was not prevalent among the resettled families at their old villages. They were shy to go for other works except for agricultural labour because, in their minds, they were not too educated, trained or skilled to perform non-agricultural work. But at resettlement sites, the growing demand for money to meet out the household expenses has compelled them to go out for wage labour in nearby semi urban and urban areas. As a result, it has become the main occupation of 8% households. The population has mostly adopted works such as house construction (*Kadiyakam*), stone cutting, cotton ginning mill, etc. Some of them have started to drive tractors on rent to cultivate the land as well as use it for earth filling and transporting of stone, etc.

Though the economic gains in the activities like collection and selling of firewood from the forest were negligible in the submerged villages, it played an important role in providing employment to the tribal community. Hunting and fishing had been the basic and ancient occupations of the tribes. Due to their proximity to forests, they had access to the forest produce and river resources. In the modern times when cultivation and domestication of animals have been adopted by the tribal society, they have reduced their dependency on forest and river as a source of food and employment. Gathering was also one of the important forest-based activities, though it was not considered as the main occupation, yet a section of the resettled population still maintains this activity as their traditional occupation. In the old villages, people used to collect forest produce from the nearby areas. They did not carry out these activities at a commercial level and used them for fulfilling their daily requirements like collecting the firewood. Every household consumed a minimum of 5–8 kg of fuel wood per day.

During the lean agricultural period, the people often went out in the forests for gathering of woods, leaves, roots, fruits, etc. In this way, the forests provided a wide range of food items and adequate fuel and firewood. But the situation has radically changed at resettlement sites and this activity is no more popular due to the non-availability of forest land in the nearby areas. Some families are now engaged in household manufacturing works such as basket making, pottery making and have become artisans, ironsmiths, tailors, shopkeepers, vegetable vendors, ice cream vendors, etc. These activities have increased to about 0.9% at resettlement sites. A few of the households had been part of the service sector (in public or private sector) at their old villages, which has increased to more than 5% at new sites.

Thus, the above description of the economic activities of the tribal people indicates a high degree of self-reliance in the submerged villages under the largely non-monetized economy. Although there was no monetary savings by them, the existence of these complementary production sources effectively prevented the emergence of unemployment in their community. But after resettlement, resettled families have become more dependent on employment in the agricultural sector, as well as in the service sector to earn money for their livelihood.

10.5.2 Health and Quality of Life

The problem of health may affect the body in two ways—at mental as well as at physical level. Though both types of health care are important, physical health is more important as it may lead to the mental problems if the physical health of a person is not good. It is observed that the different types of mental disturbances are faced by the tribal people. Most of the households suffer from demoralization followed by stress and anger.

Resettlement in the fragile environment consists of settling on the land that has been already extensively used or is not fit for cultivation and exerts immense mental and physical hardship on the tribal. Besides, people face financial difficulties as well and suffer from the availability of poor information system. After resettlement, the self-sustained system of food intake in the tribal world has been disrupted due to the loss of ancestral agricultural land, and as a result, they have to purchase food items from the market. The expenditure pattern indicates that it has increased after resettlement. It is observed that the tribals who shifted from Gujarat part of Narmada Valley spend more money on managing food as compared to the expenditure done by families of the other two states.

10.6 Change in the Dietary Habits

To see the change in the dietary habits, the frequency of taking meals in a day by the resettled families has been studied. It is interesting to note that more than 45% of the resettled families take meals thrice a day which has decreased at a rate of around 55% at their native villages. Thus, it can be concluded that the condition of resettlers has declined in terms of number of meals consumed in a day. About the quality of food, resettlers also seem to have compromised. The resettled people have reported that they have no choice other than to consume cheaper, poor quality food because the good crops are to be sold in the market. But, before resettlement, the situation was better. They used to adopt the rotation of various crops, and as a result, they had a choice of a wide variety of food.

The quality of food intake has also been greatly influenced in terms of the consumption of non-vegetarian food. Table 10.2 shows that the proportion of families consuming non-vegetarian food among the resettled families has decreased from 43% to 38% after resettlement.

In terms of the frequency of consumption of non-vegetarian food, the maximum number of families consumes non-vegetarian food once in a month followed by once in a week, i.e. 59% and 33% families respectively. However, a large number of the resettlers prepare meat and eggs at home by keeping fowls in house courtyards, whereas fish is bought from the market. It is important to note that the meat and fish, prominent sources of proteins are on the decline from the diet of resettled people. This is mainly because of the non-availability of these food items at affordable prices.

10.6.1 Disease and Health

Food consumption and status of health are two sides of the same coin of the health care. Hence, the status of health of the resettled population at resettlement sites has been studied. In the submerged areas of the tribal tract in Sardar Sarovar Project, the tribals used herbal medicine and traditional methods of magic, etc. But after resettlement, the Government and NGOs have provided modern healthcare facilities at the resettlement sites for their use. Centre for Social Studies (CSS) has pointed out that there are better levels of medical care in or near resettlement sites as compared to the submerged villages. However, Whitehead (1999) found that the government has taken little care in informing the resettlers about the local health problems and they are often served poorly.

The prevalence of different diseases among the resettled population has been given in Table 10.3. It is very surprising to note that the occurrence of different diseases per 10,000 population is found to be higher in case of fever, headache, kamdo (pain in limbs), malaria and stomach pain at resettlement site. However, the diseases such as cold, cough, skin etching and TB have decreased drastically. A large number of the people replied about their stomach problem due to indigestion of food. They used to consume coarse grains such as Bajra, Maize, Kodra, Bhadi and so on in their old villages. The course flour was prepared by grinding with Gharganti (rotary quern). But at resettlement sites, they have started consuming fine flour of wheat which is grinded by flour mills that causes indigestion problems.

Some people also face obesity problem due to declining physical work as a result of the change in the geographical area. Skin diseases have also been reported at their present sites, but it is on a drastic decline after migration. It has been reported that the incidences of fever and malaria are found higher at resettlement sites. It has been observed that vulnerability to illness has increased at resettlement sites.

In the present study, an enquiry about the sources of medical treatment of the sample families was made and results are given in Table 10.4. This table reveals that a number of families used different sources of medical treatment. In their old villages, resettled people took recourse to herbal treatment whereas at resettlement sites government has provided modern medical treatment facilities. The majority of the resettled families take treatment from private or charitable dispensaries and General Hospitals. It is important to note that among the resettled families the tradition of

Table 10.2 Frequency of families consume non-vegetarian meals

	Responses	Before resettlement	After resettlement
1	Yes	43.20	38.17
2	No	33.73	55.03
3	Not responded	23.08	6.80
	Total families	100.00	100.00

Source Compiled from survey data

Table 10.3 Common diseases per ten thousand population

	Name of diseases	Before resettlement	After resettlement
1	Asthma	0.00	3.96
2	Cancer	0.00	3.96
3	Chickengunia	0.00	0.00
4	Cold and vomiting	2318.55	545.89
5	Cough	403.23	110.76
6	Dengue	0.00	0.00
7	Diarrhoea	0.00	15.82
8	Fever	435.48	890.03
9	Headache	66.45	75.16
10	Kamdo	62.26	75.16
11	Leprosy/Paralysis	0.00	0.00
12	Malaria	225.81	383.70
13	Skin disease	342.74	7.91
14	Stomach pain	24.19	134.49
15	T.B.	60.48	43.51
16	Typhoid	20.16	19.78

Source Compiled from survey data

Table 10.4 Sources of medical treatment

	Sources of medical treatment	Percentage of resettled families	
		Before resettlement	After resettlement
1	Medical store	0.36	2.24
2	Private/charitable	31.57	49.91
3	PHC	3.10	5.85
4	CHC	0.73	0.17
5	General hospital	24.09	21.17
6	Badwa/Bhuaa (Quacks)	22.81	14.29
7	Baghat	12.77	5.34
8	Others	4.56	1.03
	Total	100.00	100.00

Source Compiled from survey data

going to Badwa Badwa/Bhuaa (Quacks) has declined from 22.81% to only 14.29%. It is also interesting to note that most of them are not willing to go to Primary Health Centre and Community Health Centre due to non-availability of doctors there at the time of emergency. During the pre-resettlement period, most of the people of the resettled families used to take local or traditional medicines extracted from the forest produce. The '*Bhuaas*' extracted these local medicines from leaves, woods, roots and barks of trees. After resettlement, this facility ceased to exist for them, while allopathic facilities have not been adequately extended to many of them even in the case of a serious illness. The study indicates that a decline in the use of traditional and home-based remedies is mainly because of social disruption, as a result of which most traditional medicine users have dispersed to other geographical regions. The governing reasons for it are non-availability of medicinal plants in the resettled villages and belief of the resettled people that the traditional medicine could not cure modern diseases along with changes in (age structure of the heads of the households) the role of decision-making process in the households which have affected most of the decisions regarding the type and place of treatment. Although the change was found to be positive in favour of modern methods of allopathic treatment, some families continue to resist the use of modern health facilities.

An investigation on the causes of resistance to modern health facilities was also carried out among the affected families. Table 10.5 demonstrates the responses of surveyed families about the causes for their lack of interest. There is a medical cell in SSPA at Vadodara that visits the resettlement sites on a regular basis accompanied by an MBBS doctor.

The findings suggest that the resettled population has yet to learn to make better use of healthcare facilities available in the area and biological adjustment to the changing environment will also take some time.

Table 10.5 Problems faced in receiving medical treatment by affected families

	Problems	Percentage response of resettled families (%)	
		Yes	No
1	Medical facilities not provided by government	48.22	51.78
2	Do not believe in allopathic treatment	8.88	91.12
3	Traditional (herbal) medicine not available	69.23	30.77
4	Poor economic condition	60.95	39.05
5	No transport facilities available to go to health centre	18.34	81.66
6	Non-availability of private medical facilities	33.43	66.57
7	Referral services unaffordable	31.07	68.93
8	No doctor available in health centre	43.49	56.51

Source Compiled from survey data collected

10.7 Conclusion

Construction of Sardar Sarovar dam on river Narmada in Gujarat has displaced large number of people in Gujarat, Maharashtra and Madhya Pradesh due to submerging of their villages. These displaced people have been given resettlement sites and governmental assistance to move to new places leaving their land, economy, history, culture and age-old memoires of their forefathers. This large scale displacement has created several social, economic and cultural problems. The resettlement plays a vital role in assessing the quality of life in terms of standard of living that has been calculated by taking into account variables such as expenditure on food and diseases, dietary change and change in occurrences of diseases at a new area.

The economic conditions have also been analysed by taking occupational patterns. A change in work force may occur after a sudden influx of population on land and availability of resources at resettlement sites. So, it is also important to find out the occupational structure. The results indicate that the self-sufficiency/dependency in terms of economic activities has lessened after resettlement. Although there was no saving at old villages, the existence of complementary production sources prevented the emergence of unemployment.

The results show that a majority of the resettled families before migration were engaged in agriculture and related activities (cultivation, cattle rearing and agriculture labour) and a few families were engaged in non-agricultural activities such as fishing, hunting, wage labour, service and small business. The dependence on cultivation has lessened after resettlement which was the most preferred main occupation among the resettled families. As the main occupation, the proportion of families engaged as agricultural labourers has increased and it has become the second most important economic activity at the resettlement sites. But a decreasing trend has also been observed in cultivation and cattle rearing, fishing and hunting, gathering from the forest and other common areas. The tribals did not find any favourable conditions at the resettlement sites to pursue these activities. Wage labour, too, became vital for sustenance and the percentage share engaged in service and small business has also increased. However, it is still very low at their resettlement sites. In the light of above one can say that instead of self-sufficiency, resettled families have shown more dependency on employment in the agricultural sector as well as in the service sector.

Cattle rearing was the most preferred professions supplementing agriculture by providing subsidiary benefits such as organic manure to the displaced at their native villages. This has been replaced by agricultural labour after resettlement. However, some of the resettled families have started poultry farming at new sites as it was found to be easier. Cattle rearing is on the decline due to the low level of availability of resources and CPR at resettlement sites.

In brief, the tribal population was engaged in several types of occupations in their natural habitat. The majority of families are engaged in cultivation before as well as after resettlement. However, the dependence on cultivation decreased after resettlement and the families started depending more on agricultural labour and wage labour. In wage labour, they are engaged in activities like masonry (Kadiayakam), digging of well, construction at roadsides and so on.

It has been observed from the study area that the resettled people face considerable psychological disturbances at the time of shifting to new sites and as a result, a large number of families suffered from demoralization followed by stress and anger. One of the direct impacts of the transition was seen on their health behaviour. Their expenditure on food, dietary habits, incidence of different diseases, attitude towards traditional and modern methods of medical treatment, all have undergone drastic changes. These changes are of a mixed type—some are on the bright side while others are discouraging.

It was observed that the highest number of resettled families used to take meals three times a day in their old villages. A good percentage of families also consumed food twice a day. But after resettlement, the percentage of families consuming food twice in a day has increased. Majority of the households consumed non-vegetarian food before migration, but the number of families consuming non-vegetarian food has declined after migration. In brief, it can be said that the consumption of food has decreased after resettlement with a further decline in consumption of non-vegetarian food.

The occurrence of diseases such as malaria, pain in limbs, and stomach pain (due to indigestion of food) among the tribals has increased after resettlement. It is pertinent to note that the prevalence of diseases like Asthma, Cancer and Diarrhoea was found in the resettlement area but was not reported from the submerged villages. Although the distance of health centre decreased as compared to pre-resettlement period, the incidents of occurrence of diseases have increased. Some people faced obesity problem due to decline in physical work as a result of change in the geographical area. Although skin diseases declined at their present sites, the incidences of fever, malaria and headache increased at resettlement sites which were low in the old villages.

In the old villages, tribals mostly used herbal treatment. It has been informed that although the government provides medicines to the resettled people, about half of the tribal families responded that the medical facilities are not extended to them. Some of these people, who believed in allopathic medicine, took medicines from private or charitable hospitals as well as general hospitals, while others go for Badwa, Bhuaa (Quacks) and Bhagat. The village-wise expenditure on medical treatment exhibits that while higher expenditure on health in some villages has been incurred due to their proneness to health hazards; in the others, the families spend more money on health due to economic prosperity. The incidence of occurrence of some of the diseases has become high and as a result, the quality of life in terms of food consumption and occurrences of diseases has deteriorated among the resettlers.

In nutshell, it can be concluded that due to change in factors such as the size of landholding, animal rearing practices, loss of traditional medicinal system, etc. the settlers have shown a considerable decline in terms of quality of life. It is visible in a decrease in intake of food as well as a change in the pattern and frequency of diseases. Due to the loss of their natural habitat to which the tribals were habituated and had an organic communication with it in terms of livelihood, pattern of life as well as physical conditioning, the downward trend in terms of health and happiness is quite visible in the resettled community. The material compensation in terms of an alien ecosystem which effectively uproots them from their moorings without any sustaining cultural and ecological ambience plays havoc with a native community which sustains itself on shared belief and natural system. Hence, the study reveals a change in quality of life among resettled people, with a pronounced propensity towards a decline in terms of food, health and satisfaction.

References

Akhtar, R., & Learmonth, A. T. A. (1985). *Geographical aspects of health and diseases in India*. Concept Publishing, New Delhi.

Alagh, Y. K. (1995). *Economic dimensions of the Sardar Sarovar project*. New Delhi: Har-Anand Publications.

Asian Development Bank. (1998). *Handbook on resettlement: a guide to good practice*. Manila: Philippines.

Amte, B. (1989). *Cry the beloved Narmada*. Anandwan: Maharogi Sewa Smiti.

Baviskar, A. (1997). *In the Belly of the river: tribal conflict over development in the Narmada Valley*. New Delhi: Oxford university Press.

Centre for Social Studies. (1999). Monitoring and evaluation of resettlement and rehabilitation programme for Sardar Sarovar Narmada Project: Composite M & E Reports 15 through 24, Surat.

Cernea, M. M. (1985). Involuntary resettlement: social research, policy and planning. In M. M. Cernea (Ed.), *Putting people first: Sociological variables in rural development*. Berkeley: Oxford University Press.

Cernea, M. M. (1994). *Involuntary resettlement in development projects: policy guidelines in World Bank-Financed projects* (Technical Paper no. 80): Word Bank.

Colledge, M. (1982). Economic cycles and health: Towards a sociological understanding of the impact of the recession on health and illness. *Social Science Medicine, 16*, 1919–1927.

Dash, N. R. (2009). Sardar Sarovar Dam: A case study of oustees in Gujarat, India. In Huhua Cao (Ed.), *Ethnic minorities and regional development in Asia: realities and challenges*. Amsterdam: Amsterdam University Press.

Eyles, J., & Woods (1982). The social geography of medicine and health. London: Croom Helm.

Good, B. J. (1996). Mental health consequences of displacement. *Economic and Political Weekly, 31*(24), 1504–1508.

Government of India. (1985). *Report on the committee on rehabilitation of displaced Tribals due to development projects*. New Delhi: Ministry of Home Affairs.

Goyal, S. (1996). Economic perspectives on resettlement and rehabilitation. *Economic and Political Weekly, 31*(24), 1461–1467.

Independent Review Team. (1997). Displacement and rehabilitation in Madhya Pradesh. In J. Drèze et al. (Eds.), *The dams and the nation*, New Delhi: Oxford University Press.

International Commission on Large Dams. (1988). World register on Dams, Paris.

Karve, I. (1956). *The Bhils of West Khandesh: A social and economic survey*. Poona: Deccan College.

Lobo, L., & Kumar, S. (2009). *Land acquisition, displacement and resettlement in Gujarat: 1947–2004*. New Delhi: Sage Publications.

Mathur, H. M., & Cernea, M. M. (1995). *Development, displacement and resettlement: focus on Asian experiences*. New Delhi: Vikas Publishing House.

Mathur, H. M., & Marsden, D. (Eds.). (1998). *Development projects and impoverishment risk-resettling projects affected people in India*. New Delhi: Oxford University Press.

Morse, B., & Berger, T. R. (1992). *Sardar Sarovar project: independent review*. World Bank: Washington D. C, USA.

Mukherjee, R. K. (1989). *The quality of life: valuation in social research*. New Delhi: Sage Publication.
Naik, T. B. (1969). *Impact of education on the Bhils*. New Delhi: Research Programmes Committee Planning Commission.
Narmada Bachao Andolan. (undated). *Narmada: The struggle for life, against destruction*. Chittaroopa Palit for Narmada Bachao Andolan, Baroda.
Narmada Control Authority. (1995). *Master Plan for R & R*, Indore.
Paranjpye, V. (1990). *High Dams on the Narmada: A holistic analysis of the Valley projects*. Delhi: INTACH.
Parasuraman, S. (1998). Socio-economic conditions of people displaced by Durgarpur steel plant. *Man & Development, 20*(2).
Ramaiah, S. (1998). Impact of involuntary resettlement on levels of living. In H. M. Mathur & D. Marsden (Eds.), *Development projects and impoverishment risk- resettling projects affected people in India*. New Delhi: Oxford University Press.
Roy, A. (1999). The greater common good. *Outlook, 5*(19), 54–72.
Roy, A. (2000). The cost of living. *Frontline, 17*(3).
Shah, D. C. (2003). *Involuntary migration: evidence from Sardar Sarovar project*. Jaipur: Rawat Publications.
Sangvai, S. (2002). Narmada displacement: continuing outrage. *Economic and Political Weekly, 37*(22), 2132–2134.
Sardar Sarovar Narmada Nigam Ltd. (undated). Sardar Sarovar project on river Narmada: meeting the challenges of development. Government of Gujarat, Gandhinagar.
Sharma, N. K. (1986). Large Dams-a necessary developmental choice. *Bhagirath, 33,* 55–64.
Singh, S. (1990). Evaluating large Dams in India. *Economic and Political Weekly, 25*(11), 561–574.
Thukral, E. G. (Ed.). (1992). *Big Dams, displaced people: rivers of sorrow rivers of change*. New Delhi: Sage Publications.
Tata Institute of Social Sciences. (1993). Sardar Sarovar project: review of resettlement and rehabilitation in Maharashtra. *Economic and Political Weekly, 28*(33), 1705–1714.
Whitehead, J. (1999). Statistical concoctions and everyday lives: Queries from Gujarat resettlement sites. *Economic and Political Weekly, 34*(28), 1940–1947.

Chapter 11
Perceptions of Quality of Life Among Two Different Generations of Women IDPs in Protracted Displacement in Mandalakkuda Camp in Puttalam District, Sri Lanka

Fazeeha Azmi

Abstract The purpose of this study is to explore the perceptions of quality of life (QOL) among the first and second generations of internally displaced women, who are living in Mandalakkuda camp in the district of Puttalam in protracted displacement for nearly a quarter century. I conducted 20 interviews with women from first and second generations to understand how they perceive QOL. Collected information and data were analysed under emerging themes observed from the interview transcripts. The study showed that the perception of QOL varied significantly across different generations. While women from the first generation valued mainly the non-material aspects of QOL, the second-generation women emphasized much on the material aspects of QOL. It was also possible to note some common dimensions identified by both groups. The study concludes that generation and protracted nature of displacement have implications for how these two groups of women perceive QOL. However, these concerns are hardly acknowledged by solutions proposed by the government to address the issues of Internally Displaced People (IDPs). It is argued that considering the length of time the IDPs are living in displacement, it is important to recognize the generational differences in understanding QOL, in any government-initiated solutions, which seriously influence the decision to return, reintegrate or resettle.

Keywords QOL · IDPs · Protracted displacement · Generation · Women · Resettle

11.1 Introduction

The three-decades-long war between the government of Sri Lanka and the Liberation Tigers of Tamil Eelam (LTTE) ended on 17 May 2009 with a huge human cost. Although the government's military victory brought relief to many people, still a

F. Azmi (✉)
Department of Geography, University of Peradeniya, Peradeniya, Sri Lanka
e-mail: fazeehaazmi@gmail.com

B. R. K. Sinha (ed.), *Multidimensional Approach to Quality of Life Issues*,
https://doi.org/10.1007/978-981-13-6958-2_11

large number of people are living in displacement[1] with unsolved problem caused by the war. The 30-year war displaced a large number of people from all three communities of the country. Among the displaced people, the plight of Muslims who were forcefully evicted by the LTTE in 1990 remains problematic. If one traces the history, 1990 marks a milestone in the displacement history of Sri Lanka. In October 1990, almost all Muslims in the northern districts of Jaffna, Mannar, Vavuniya, Kilinochchi and Mullaitivu were forced to leave by the LTTE rebels with a very short notice, leaving all their belongings behind. The expelled Muslims not only lost their homes, possessions, livelihoods and lands but also their personal identities, history, culture and communities within a single day. The expulsion, which received wider attention at the onset of the event, also resulted in altering the ethno-demographic landscape of the Northern Province. Within a couple of days, a mono-ethnic North was created.

Muslims who were forced to leave made their way mainly towards the government-controlled areas in Vavuniya, Anuradhapura and Puttalam district in the north-western coast (Brun 2000, 2008; Hasbullah 2001; Fazeeha 2012). The Internally Displaced People (IDPs) , who arrived in groups to Puttalam were allocated to various welfare centers. Most of them continued to live in Puttalam since their arrival. Statistics are not available regarding the exact number of IDPs at present due to various complicated problems. According to interviews conducted by Internal Displacement Monitoring Center (IDMC) in 2012, although 75,000 IDPs have registered as returned to their villages, only 21,500 were living permanently in the areas where they have returned to (IDMC 2014). Those who were living in Puttalam, over the course of two decades, have continued to live in temporary camps and while some were able to build houses in Puttalam. Few IDPs are settled in other areas of the country as well. Majority of the IDPs who are living in temporary shelters are neglected by the government and international humanitarian organizations as they are labelled as low priority cases (OCHA 2010; Haniffa 2015).

With the defeat of the LTTE in May 2009, the government of Sri Lanka initiated programmes to solve the issue of protracted displacement. The solutions focussed on return, local reintegration or resettlement without a comprehensive plan or long-term vision. Although the government initiated the above three options, under the large-scale post-war reconstruction agenda, it prioritized and motivated the IDPs to return to their former villages. In breach of the UN guiding principles on internal displacement, return for many displaced persons, especially women, have not been safe, dignified or in some cases not voluntary. According to informal discussions, I had with few elderly IDPs, the IDPs who were returning to their villages in Mannar have not been provided even with basic facilities for a decent return. The government also lacked a proper plan for IDP resettlement until recently.[2] The policy introduced in 2016, addresses the issues related to conflict-affected displacement within the

[1]More than 93,000 people are estimated to be displaced as of late December 2012 (Government statistics as compiled by UNHCR, 31 December 2012).

[2]The Ministry of Prison Reforms, Rehabilitation, Resettlement and Hindu Religious Affairs, released the National Policy on Durable Solutions for Conflict-Affected Displacement in 2016.

framework of international guidelines and right based approach. It also pays attention to conflict-affected protracted displacement (IDMC 2016). However, it lacks clear implementation strategies. Without a clear implementation strategy, the objectives of the policy could not be achieved. Resettlement is not about simple physical relocation of people. It should include a human dimension and produce spaces for permanent settlement and sustained communities (Muggah 2008). Solutions related to return, resettlement and reintegration are very complex as such decisions largely depend on the decision of individuals who are affected. During the time this research was conducted, the Sri Lankan government did not have a resettlement policy for IDPs. However, the government had initiated solutions focused on return, reintegration or resettlement without a clear vision or goal.

Within this uncertain and unclear institutional context among the IDPs, the solutions proposed by the government created a tension. While some of the IDP families accepted the government proposed solutions, many could not do so. It is also important to note that when the northern Muslims were displaced in 1990, the total number of families displaced was 30,000, which during the time of this research has reached nearly 70,000. Therefore, taking a decision on return, reintegration or resettlement had a generational dimension too. Some children were born after forced migration while others who were children during the time of migration has lived a larger part of their youth in Puttalam. Among this group, most young people prefer to live in Puttalam. Among the old, the majority of the IDPs prefer to go back to their former villages if safe return is guaranteed. During the informal discussions held with women from different generations for a project on "Internal displacement and place attachment" in the same camp, it also became evident, that decision related to resettlement, return or reintegration was also linked to how women from two different generations perceive QOL. Influenced by such informal discussions this research tries to explore QOL from a generational perspective. Therefore, the objective of this chapter is to focus on how women from two different generations of IDPs view QOL and its implications for government proposed solution. Although one could imagine a deteriorated quality of life among IDPs generally, it is also important to understand how different the two generations view QOL in the context of return, reintegration and resettlement.

11.2 QOL in the Context of Protracted Displacement

Defining what 'quality of life' is a very difficult task. The concept has been used in many disciplines from a variety of perspectives (Group 1994). It had been equated with the concepts of 'good life', 'well-being', 'happy life' and many other words reflecting the meaning of a satisfactory life. QOL has been approached from quantitative and qualitative perspectives depending on the researchers' philosophical understanding of knowledge (Liu 1975). The differences in knowledge positions have influenced methodologies to study QOL and the research outcomes too. The quantitative approaches to understand QOL included measurable dimensions such as income, housing and level of education. These are a predetermined set of indicators. The need for going beyond quantitative approaches in understanding QOL was raised by many researchers (Binswanger 2006; Rapley 2003; Renwick and Brown 1996). Hence, the current research on QOL acknowledges the importance of considering the multidimensionality of the concept and provides rich literature on the subject.

Since the beginning of this century, research focusing on the subjective qualitative dimensions of QOL showed a rapid increase in addressing its multidimensionality. Among them, the QOL dimensions introduced by the Quality of Life Unit, University of Toronto has received wider attention.[3] The qualitative dimensions of QOL it identifies are based on important domains (Rapley 2003). It identifies three main domains: Being, Belonging and Becoming. Within each domain subcategories are identified, and each subcategory is further divided to include different dimensions of QOL depending on the context. The main domains, which are connected with each other, are very important to understand the subjective QOL, which cannot simply be caught by quantitative measures of QOL. Being is referred to as one's own physical, psychological and spiritual status. Belonging is referred to as the perception of the sense of belonging to the community, which includes physical and social belonging, while Becoming relates to how people connect to the society through volunteering, work and going to school.

Another contribution that influenced my theoretical assumption comes from a geographic perspective. Mikkelson and Nucci (2015) discuss the contribution of geographical methodologies to the study of QOL, influenced by the epistemological and ontological basis of the discipline from positivist and humanist philosophies. They point out the influence of humanistic turn in geography, which provided the space to accommodate a multidimensional perspective to the study of QOL since the late 1970, making changes in the theoretical and methodological approaches to study QOL. Tonon defines QOL as 'degree that determines a person's life to be desirable or undesirable in individual cases. Domains of satisfaction with life are to be understood as the people's judgment, when assessing different areas of their lives' (2015, p. 5). Tonon calls for a more subjective understanding of QOL from the point of an individual and argues QOL should be understood as individual satisfaction related to what they identify as material needs and what they prioritize as subjective and symbolic needs. Hence, it is important to understand, QOL is not only decided by individual needs, but also by the social, cultural, political and geographical spaces which people are living in. Therefore, it is important to understand that the concept of QOL is inherently multidimensional and move beyond a simple set of material aspects, to subjective well-being achievements and agency of people (Nussbaum and Sen 1993).

Understanding QOL in an internal displacement context and particularly in protracted displacement context is complicated and challenging. My position as a qualitative geographer influenced the research methods I chose to study QOL among two generations of IDP women. The study theoretically and methodologically benefits

[3]University of Toronto, Quality of Life Research Unit. http://sites.utoronto.ca/qol/qol_model.htm. Accessed 15.12.2017.

from the works of Quality of Life Unit, University of Toronto and Mikkelson and Nucci (2015). I understand QOL include material as well as subjective dimensions and it is influenced by social, cultural, political and geographical spaces.

11.3 Overview of Study Site: Mandalakkuda and Methodology

Mandalakkuda *Grama Niladari* (GN) division[4] of Kalpitiya is located in the district of Puttalam. The study was undertaken between September 2011 and December 2012. In the Puttalam district, Kalpitiya consists of large number of Muslim IDPs compared to other areas in the district. About 75% of the displaced Northern Muslims are living in this area. At the time of the study, there were nine IDP camps in Mandalakkuda GN division. For this particular research, I selected the Al-Manar U camp in Mandalakkuda. The IDPs in the camp are from villages in Mannar. The total population of this camp was 1,224 that belong to 332 families in 2011. I selected women from 20 families for this study representing two different generations. When I selected women I focused mainly on their ages, as the objective of this research focuses on QOL from a generational perspective. Researching IDPs about QOL from a generational perspective needs a careful methodology. The idea behind the concept of 'generations' in the paper is that 'people born at about the same time grow up sharing a historical period that shapes their views' (Kertzer 1983: 128). Hence, the pre- and post-displacement historical and social contexts are important factors that could have an impact on how women from different generations view QOL. The first generation refers to women who were forced to move as adults (or young adults), and the second generation refers to the children who were below the age of 10 or who were born after the forced migration. I conducted qualitative interviews with 10 women from each, first and second generations. First-generation women were above the age of 55 and second-generation women were below the age of 30. Each interview lasted from 45 min to one hour. Interviews were recorded and transcribed. During the analysis when major themes emerged related to QOL they were identified and used for discussion.

11.4 QOL: First- and Second-Generation Views

The following section sheds light on different dimensions of QOL defined by two groups of IDP women from Mandalakkuda. Their perceptions were framed by previous experiences, present life or anxiety for the future depending on their varying experience in living in displacement. Discussions in the analysis are arranged according to themes. The researcher attempted to remain as descriptive as possible

[4]Lowest administration division in Sri Lanka.

and utilized sections of participants' narratives to verify the themes and highlight QOL in the view of participants.

11.5 Voices from First Generation

This section captures how the first-generation women view QOL. Most of them are married and living with their children or grandchildren. Majority of them are involved in informal income earning activities through which they support their families and themselves. Their level of education is very low and the majority of them have not gone to schools. They have also married at very early ages and are influenced by their cultural practices in their former villages.

11.5.1 Reduced Physical Functioning Health

I met Fathima at her son's home. She was 64 years old at the time of the interview. Since she had become ill due to diabetes, she was confined to home, as she could not move around due to her poor eyesight. When I asked her about what is QOL for her she described:

I have seven children. All were born in Mannar and the youngest one was one year when we moved here. They are all married now and have their own children. When I was in Mannar, while looking after all my children, I worked in our farm also. I did all the household works from cooking to washing. I did not have a domestic maid to help me. I did everything alone. We had all the things we want. Now I cannot walk or help my children. I have become a burden to them. For me what is good quality of life now is to have a good health to support my family. I am worried that day by day I am becoming weak.

Fathima's story indicates how reduced capabilities through declining health contribute to the understanding of QOL, which is related to physical well-being. She still believes she could have supported her children's families had she been in good health. She had been working hard since she left her village in Mannar. Good health is a very important dimension of QOL to elderly people as it enables them to continue working and functioning independently. In the camp context, many older women had experienced health problems related to hard work. Like Fathima, the needs of the elderly population in the settlement are diverse and complex due to growing health concerns in the older years, which is a threat to QOL at old age. Further, the camps they are living have undergone dramatic changes in the demographic and social composition in the past two decades, contributing negatively to the health-related QOL.

Health is also an important indicator of human capabilities which is essential for a good QOL (Sen 1985). In general, in the camp, the old people are suffering from various health problems and particularly women are affected. After years of living in shock, trauma and performing hard physical labour to make a living, most of the IDPs have entered old age with chronic ill health.

Kulsoom who is 58 years old also described the difficulties she encountered when she could not fulfill her obligations towards her family due to poor health. When I asked her about how she views QOL, her reply was:

> Since we moved from Mannar, we had a hard life. All my daughters are married and they face lot of difficulties in living a good life. I was working as labourer in an onion garden. I was supporting my daughters also. I have a problem in my spinal code and I can't work anymore to support them. Good quality of life depends on how healthy you are. You feel it especially when you are old.

Among the first-generation women, their age and poor health, which have reduced their capability to undertake paid or unpaid work, has also put an extra pressure on their remaining years of life. Some of the elderly people continue to work despite poor health, partly for their own needs and partly to meet the needs of their family. With ageing, along with reduced capabilities, mainly resulting from deteriorating health due to physical labour, women who were engaged in agriculture after their displacement are now gradually excluded from such opportunities. Considering the status of health among first generation women, continuous stress caused by an uncertain future related to their livelihood put pressure on their physical and psychological health.

11.5.2 Loss of Social Network

Unlike men in Sri Lankan rural society, women highly depend upon social and familial networks for various purposes in their everyday life. In the camp, first-generation women still experience a feeling of loss in terms of proper social network that they had before they were displaced. When asked about what QOL means to her, Zainabu 66 described:

> Today, generally people have become more selfish. Back in our village, we were almost like one family and that is a good strength. Good quality of life is not about having lot of money. I think if you have family and friends around that is much more worth than money. I feel these are very much absent here in the camps compared to my past life in the village.

Zainabu's story reflects the domain of Belonging in terms of QOL. Belonging is not only about being located physically in a community. To enjoy the QOL, one also needs belonging to the society and community in which they are living. This is about acceptance and access to resources as well. Zainabu does not feel she is socially belonging to the place where she currently lives. Her account also reveals the loss of social network she had before displacement, which she still values as important for QOL rather than money. Beebi who is 70 years old also feels the loss of her former neighbours from her village:

> Here although your neighbour is from the same village, if you are not close with them, they will also be an outsider for us. You can earn money to have a good quality of life. What is

> more important in defining good quality of life is earning good people whom you can trust and who will help each other. Even within family, sometimes I feel, I am alone.

Beebi was worried about not having access to the social relationship and network she had in her village before migration. Few other women from the first generation were also worried about the rapid socio-economic changes taking place in the camp and different types of alienation they have to face not only in the wider society but also within their families. Their stories contribute to another level of belonging which should be looked at from the household level.

11.5.3 Old Age Insecurity

As a consequence of various pressures and problems, the second generation is gradually moving away from agricultural activities and making their livelihoods from other sources. The living arrangements of elderly persons in the camp are gradually changing. In some IDP families, family members are separated due to choosing different options related to the solutions proposed by the government for their problems related to displacement. I met Kareema aged 75 at her home. She was alone. After some initial inquiry about living in displacement, I asked what QOL is for her. She stated:

> I have enough money. All my children give me money. However, they rarely come and see me. For me good quality of life is not money at this age but security. I am living alone. I have three sons. One has moved back to our former village. I am too old to go back to my village though I like to go. My son told he got a land to build a house, which is far away from hospital. Further public transport is not available there. I have to consider this, as I am old. Other two sons are living in Colombo with their families. They are living in a very small room. I did not want to live there, though I like to be with them. It is so sad that we need children around us when we are old. It is not only we depend on them but we feel secure and happy if they are with us.

Women interviewed from the first generation mentioned the issue related to reaching old age as an IDP. The current situation in the settlement shows that the issues the second generation prioritizes in their pursuit of QOL have not only had a direct impact on them, but also they had an indirect impact on their depending family members. Since the arrival of IDPs, economic opportunities in the study area have become extremely competitive. As a result, there has been intense competition between the locals and IDPs for resources and livelihoods (Brun 2003). At present, a few IDPs have returned permanently while others have opted for trans-local life basically due to economic hardships. Some have decided to move out of the camp area like Kareema's sons. Their decision negatively affects the QOL of whom they left behind.

In the Sri Lankan society, the responsibility of looking after elderly parents still depends on the hands of children. Although care facilities are available for elders, generally in the Sri Lankan context, it is not socially accepted for elderly parents to be sent to live in special homes for the elders. Besides, such facilities are not available in the study area. Therefore, any negligence by children will place their elderly parents in a miserable situation and essentially have an impact on their parents' QOL. Kareema is in a similar situation where her children's decision has affected her expectations regarding her future QOL as Tonon (2015) identifies as peoples' judgment related to their satisfaction.

11.5.4 Deterioration of Culture, Tradition, Religion, Unity and Moral Values

In Sri Lankan society, the elderly expect that family and society should listen to their voices too as they are experienced citizens. In traditional Sri Lankan societies, mostly at village level, elderly people generally gain the power to influence family and society through their participation in certain kinds of social and religious institutions. However, this trend, which existed in former villages of IDPs, has slowly being altered by various forces. For Aneesa 55, deterioration of culture, religion and tradition are important aspects in terms of how she views QOL:

> When we talk about quality of life, what I value most is culture, religion and traditions we had once. After arriving in Kalpitiya as IDPS, we lost many things and among them our culture, religion and traditions are important. The younger people are going behind money and they think about the life, which is suitable only for this world. We will die one day and we will not take these things with us. For me quality of life is about living in good culture, following your religion and protecting your tradition.

The first-generation women in the study explained that external social and economic changes have gradually filtered into the camps and former traditions and culture are being replaced by modern ways of life. This trend shows the spiritual dimension of being has been challenged for some IDPs.

11.5.5 Extra Burdens: Struggle, Fear and Desperation

Ayesha 57, lived in a small hut together with her two daughters who are not yet married. After she came to Kalpitiya, she managed to build three houses for her three daughters as dowry, through her hard work. However, she is worried about her inability to build two more houses for unmarried daughters. She was in despair, with no other children to support her. Ayesha's story was a story of struggle, fear, desperation and frustration. When I asked what QOL is for her, she said:

> If I can live my life without fear, struggle and desperation, that will ensure good quality of life. How can I think about such satisfactory life, as I could not still build houses or buy a piece of land for my younger daughters. I am worried about their marriages. If that is settled, I can rest.

Others view Ayesha as a successful woman in the camp, as she was able to build three houses for her daughters' dowry. However, Ayesha is worried whether she would be able to do the same for her two daughters who are not yet married. Ayesha's account shows how she had worked hard for bringing a good QOL for her daughters. For her what QOL means is not directly related to her personal QOL, but it is related to her daughters' well-being. At the same time it is important to note that by devoting herself for the QOL for her children, she is partly satisfied with her "spiritual being".

11.5.6 Without a Future Here or There

First-generation IDP women were worried about their belonging in the host communities as well as back in their former villages. Although the government provided 'return' as one of the solutions to their problems, it failed to provide adequate facilities for a safe return, which many women identified as important for their QOL back in their villages. When asked about QOL, Latheefa a widow who is 70 years reflected her view on QOL as follows:

> Finally, the war is over and we thought we would be able to return happily to our villages and stand on our own feel after almost 25 years and put a full stop to dependent and humiliated life. We thought we would be able to live a good life in our villages with a freedom in our breath. However, people who went to Mannar are very much worried about the situation there. It is not the same Mannar we left. I am worried that I will not be able to live the good life I am dreaming before my death.

Poor living conditions, traumatic memories, an uncertain future and financial worries impose psychological strains on IDPs. Although many first generation women want to go back, they are reluctant due to the lack of resources to start their lives in Mannar. These women mentioned that they would never be peaceful in their homeland. They mentioned those who have already returned to former villages face difficulties in accessing necessities such as food, water, shelter and sanitation in rebuilding their lives back in their villages. They also raised considerable concerns about return, especially since they have lost most of their productive and healthy years in living in temporary shelters. Because in their former villages, they were engaged in agriculture, provided support in post-harvest fisheries and some of them have also helped their families in trade. These livelihoods have become inaccessible in their former villagers for many IDPs due to their protracted displacement. They are very uncertain about the future and this was reflected in their personal view on QOL.

11.5.7 Unemployment of Males

Although living in a completely different socio-economic environment than their villages, after displacement, first-generation women have a widespread social expectation that men should be the primary breadwinner and males' employment defines a family's quality of living. Subaida aged 73 expressed:

> Most of our men here are unemployed and underemployed. If men can have, good jobs and women can take care of the household and children that will be the basis for a good quality of life. Our women now migrate to Middle Eastern countries and men stay at home. This is not good to see.

She was a rich woman before the eviction. She has not studied beyond grade five. She had a very negative image of women who work. She insisted on the importance of maintaining the traditional gender roles to run a peaceful family life. She finds a male's employment as a marker of respect and recognition of a family's QOL. This related to the being and becoming domains of QOL.

11.5.8 Access to Land

Fareeda 58 is from a family who had large agricultural land before their migration. When asked about the meaning of QOL, Fareeda sums it up:

> If you have land to do agriculture, it shows your wealth and status and especially the quality of your life. We have never bought rice from shops. Our family did not have the experience of working in other's land until we came here. For people who did agriculture, land is the main thing that influences the quality of life.

Land was the main source of capital for many IDPs before they were evicted. Land in agricultural societies not only provides means for livelihood but also social prestige. Before the forced eviction, landowners were rich and had comparatively a good QOL. Further, land was commonly used as dowry; house being the other among the IDPs before migration (Brun 2008). Therefore, loss of land is not only a problem related to access to livelihood and QOL but also a problem related to wedding practices.

The narratives above reflect how first-generation women IDPs view QOL. Their views encompassed many dimensions of subjective QOL and what they judge as important in their lives. Their perceptions of QOL were related mainly to reduced physical capacity; loss of social network; declining old age security; deterioration of culture, religion, unity and moral values; extra burdens, struggle and fear; uncertain future; unemployment of males and access to land. From the themes emerged in the narratives of first-generation women IDPs, it is clear that their conceptualizations of QOL is related mainly to social or community and family aspects than individual aspirations. Further, the identified dimensions related to QOL were greatly influenced by pre- and post-migration lives, within the context of protracted displacement and uncertain future.

11.6 Quality of Life: What Does the Second Generation Tell?

The following accounts represent the views on QOL held by the second-generation IDPs in the camp. The second-generation women were below the age of 10 during the time of displacement or born in the camps after displacement. Majority of them have not even seen their parents' villages. They were brought up in a totally different environment compared to their parents. Their level of education is higher.

11.6.1 Employment

Generally, girls who were interviewed from the second generation had forward-looking ideas about QOL compared to the first generation. Unlike their mothers' generation, these young girls did not expect a man (father, brother or husband) should provide for them financially for the rest of their lives in order to have a good QOL. This could be related to the fact that compared to their mothers' generation; there is a tremendous increase in young girls entering education. I met Salma (26) who has just completed her degree in law. When I asked her about QOL she said:

> Our parents did coolie work and we cannot do same type of work. Having a proper job is important to have a good quality of life. I will not accept any job until I find a good one. I have a degree and I want to do a job that matches my qualification and that can help me to live a satisfactory life. For me quality of life depends on your job. I think in order to have a good quality of life it is important that girls should come forward and do jobs.

The main cause of poor quality of life among IDPs is unemployment, or in some cases what can be called as underemployment. Many IDPs continuously struggle to secure a livelihood because job opportunities are scarce in the depressed economic environments of the study area and the country in general. They also face additional difficulties compared with the host population as they lack social capital to overcome administrative obstacles. With the increasing population and a youth population with good educational qualifications, unlike in the past, unemployment and underemployment have become serious issues in the study area. Young girls identified lack of employment and underemployment as an important obstacle to achieve the QOL they want. For them, QOL largely depends on employment. Some young IDPs believed that they had been deprived of their fair chance of employment opportunities in the government sector as their poverty prevents them to access to higher education, technical and vocational educational opportunities in the country which makes them more qualified to a job.

11.6.2 Education

The importance of education in all aspects of life, especially in a camp setting, cannot be overemphasized in understanding QOL. Farsana who is just 19 years expressed her view on QOL:

> I think good quality education is important for a good quality of life. The school in our area is not having many facilities. For example, we do not have teachers for important subjects like English, Math and Science. How can we compete with other students? For me education is essential for good quality of life.

Jaseel, 23 also reflected on the importance of education for QOL

> Without education, we cannot do anything here. We do not have any resources for our future except education. This is important for our quality of life.

QOL in the study areas was linked to education. The importance of education was particularly recognized as an important aspect of QOL. It was felt that good educational opportunities had been lost through forced migration. While IDP youth have equal access to higher education and are eligible to attend state universities free of charge if they pass the entrance examinations, their limited access to good quality secondary education prevents them from getting admission to state universities.

Despite education being provided free of charge in Sri Lanka, the accompanying costs are not affordable for the IDPs. In addition, in some poor families, children who attend school are also burdened with domestic work, especially due to the absence of their parents who work as casual labourers. In such families, girls look after their younger siblings and do household work. Some of them have stopped attending school completely while others do not go to school regularly. Many young women raised many issues in terms of the poor quality of education being responsible for their present situation in terms of QOL. Many families could not afford to send their children to the town schools.

11.6.3 Good Quality Housing

Housing was put forward as a dimension of QOL by many second-generation women. This dimension was identified and discussed primarily in terms of quality of house. Safeena who is 27 years told me her perception on QOL:

> Unlike our parents, we are living in this camp since we were kids. I think for me quality of life is not only about having enough food to eat; it is also about having a good house to live in. Unlike earlier, we are connected with the outer world. Our friends from schools or from our work place visit us. They will judge us by our home. In many occasions I have felt uncomfortable when friends visit me especially if they are originally from Kalpitiya.

Safeena's account not only shows the material dimension of QOL, but also her psychological being. When I visited the houses of my informants, I observed and I was told especially by the young girls that they lack privacy and space in their homes. Like Safeena, others also were worried about their poor housing conditions and they are often too ashamed to invite other friends to visit them in their homes.

11.6.4 Identity

Those who were born after displacement inherit the IDP label from their parents only. They were caught up in a dilemma related to identity within the family and community, as they do not officially qualify to be labelled as IDPs. However, they are grossly categorized as IDPs in official documents and everyday discourses. These young women do not want to return to a place, which they do not know. Their relation to their parents' villages is created through a relational way. Shiyana 20 years put it this way when asked about QOL:

> My parents are teachers. Although my parents were able to support our education and give us a good life unlike many others, our quality of life here is decided by our IDP status. Although my parents want to return, my siblings or I do not want to return. We all were born and brought up here. We will not return. Which also means the IDP label will be with us forever and I personally view even if you have billions you will not have a mentally satisfied good quality of life if you are an IDP. But I do not want to go back to my parents' village, which is known to me only by stories they tell about their villages.

The importance of identity as essential for QOL was put forward by the first generation of IDP women. For the second-generation women too, it was identified as an important dimension of QOL. However, for those who were born after displacement, importance of identity takes a different form though they are not the direct victims of displacement.

11.7 Concluding Reflections

This paper explored the QOL between two different groups of women IDPs. The QOL narratives presented by both first and second generations emphasized different dimensions of QOL. Their perceptions about QOL are embedded within pre- and protracted post-displacement contexts. The IDP women's perceptions of QOL varied according to generations, especially in the way they prioritized the dimensions. While the first generation women prioritized more psychological, social, community and spiritual dimensions of QOL, the majority of the second-generation women prioritized the material dimensions of QOL. Second-generation women prioritized individual aspects related to QOL rather than the community or social aspects. Both generations identified identity as an important marker of QOL. An important finding of this research is that the IDP women's perceptions of QOL, regardless of which generation they belong to are undoubtedly linked to the changing perceptions of QOL, which in turn are influenced, by increasing links with the outside world at local, national and global levels. Their perceptions are shaped by the protracted nature of displacement too.

When expressing their views on QOL, first generation women could not disconnect from their past lives in their original villages. Different ways they conceptualize QOL covered many non-material dimensions. When second-generation women described what they mean by QOL they did not share collective views, rather they focused on personal views which affect them. Unlike the first generation women, they do not have socio-cultural memories of their parents' places of origin. For the second-generation women who were not born in the camp, this may be also due to the fact that some of them hardly remember anything about their places of origin. Besides, the young informants are socially, historically and geographically detached from their places of origin for a long time. The psychological aspects of living in displacement was identified both by first and second-generation women when defining QOL. Experiencing poverty, feeling inferior, humiliated, shame and insecure were captured in their definitions.

When first-generation women talked about their pre-displacement life, they linked the aspects of QOL mainly with material things. However, when I asked what do they perceive as QOL now, I understood their concerns were moving beyond material aspects. It is pertinent to note that QOL for the elderly in the study seems to be not very good as reflected by their narratives. Their narratives reflected a victimhood which led them to relate QOL with negative dimensions. The dimensions articulated by the second-generation women revealed many different aspects of QOL than the first generation. To conclude, it could be argued that perceptions of QOL are changing among different generations of IDP women and this has implications for future decisions on resettlement, return and integration. It is also important to note, that the generational perspective of QOL in a protracted displacement context shed light on important dimensions of QOL which should be recognized in any solutions related to protracted IDP issues.

Ethical Statement 'This chapter is based on the research project "**2012–2014** A No Where Generation: Exploring the sense of place among Internally Displaced Women in the Mandalakkuda welfare camp in Puttalam in the context of resettlement and return. University of Peradeniya, Sri Lanka, Research Grant: Project-No RG/2011/14/A". I thank the University of Peradeniya, Sri Lanka for the financial assistance provided and the anonymous referees, who evaluated the project proposal and report, which this chapter is based on. I also thank the research participants (whose names are anonymized) for their support in providing required and interesting information.'

Participants who participated in providing information to this study were informed about possible dissemination plans for the research presentations, research findings and publications. None of the participants was without any formal school education.

References

Binswanger, M. (2006). Why does income growth fail to make us happier?: Searching for the treadmills behind the paradox of happiness. *The Journal of Socio-Economics, 35*(2), 366–381.

Brun, C. (2000). Spatial practices of integration and segregation among internally displaced persons and their hosts in Sri Lanka. *Norsk Geografisk Tidsskrift, 54*(3), 96–101.

Brun, C. (2003). Local citizens or internally displaced persons? Dilemmas of long term displacement in SriLanka. *Journal of refugee studies, 16*(4), 376–397.

Brun, C. (2008). *Finding a place: local integration and protracted displacement in Sri Lanka.* Colombo: Social Scientists' Association.

Fazeeha, A. (2012). To go or not to go: Struggle for belonging among second generation Muslim IDPs in Kalpitiya in Puttalam district in the context of post war resettlement. In D. Herath (ed), *Healing the wounds of war. ICES* (pp. 167–192). Sri Lanka.

Group, W. H. O. Q. O. L. (1994). Development of the WHOQOL: Rationale and current status. *International Journal of Mental Health, 23*(3), 24–56.

Haniffa, F. (2015). Competing for victim status: Northern Muslims and the ironies of Sri Lanka's post-war transition. *Stability: International Journal of Security and Development, 4*(1).

Hasbullah, S. H. (2001). *Muslim refugees: the forgotten people in Sri Lanka's ethnic conflict.* Nuraicholai: Research and Action Forum For Social Development.

IDMC (2016). New policy on durable solutions in Sri Lanka: The challenge of implementation. Retrieved on 10 Jan 2018 from http://www.internal-displacement.org/library/expert-opinion/2016/new-policy-on-durable-solutions-in-sri-lanka-the-challenge-of-implementation/.

Kertzer, D. I. (1983). Generation as a sociological problem. *Annual Review of Sociology, 9*(1), 125–149.

Mikkelsen C., & Di Nucci, J. (2015). Qualitative methodologies in geography, contributions to the study of quality of life. In: G. Tonon (ed) *Qualitative studies in quality of life.* Social indicators research series (Vol. 55, pp. 63–95). Cham: Springer.

Liu, B. C. (1975). Quality of life: Concept, measure and results. *American Journal of Economics and Sociology, 34*(1), 1–14.

Muggah, R. (2008). *Relocation failures in Sri Lanka: A short history of internal displacement and resettlement.* Macmillan.

Nussbaum, M., & Sen, A. (1993). *The quality of life.* Oxford: Clarendon Press.

Rapley, M. (2003). *Quality of life research: A critical introduction.* Sage.

Renwick, R. E., Brown, I. E., & Nagler, M. E. (1996). *Quality of life in health promotion and rehabilitation: Conceptual approaches, issues, and applications.* Sage Publications, Inc.

Sen, A. (1985). *Commodities and capabilities.* Oxford: Oxford University Press.

Tonon, G. (2015). Relevance of the use of qualitative methods in the study of quality of life. In: G. Tonon (ed) *Qualitative studies in quality of life.* Social indicators research series (Vol. 55, pp. 3–21). Cham: Springer.

United Nations Office for the Coordination of Humanitarian Affairs (OCHA) (2010). Sri Lanka, Common Humanitarian Action Plan, Mid-Year Review.

Chapter 12
Aspects of the Quality of Life in India and Its Macro Region

S. C. Mukhopadhyay

Abstract The density of population in India, in general, and Northeast Macro Region India, in particular, has been increasing (2011 Census) very rapidly since 1991. An analysis of 2011 Census revealed that the higher rate of population growth has increased large number of population in India especially in the east and north-east macro-regions including Andaman–Nicobar Islands. This causes difficulty in maintaining the quality of life in both the rural and urban areas as referred by the sociologists, economists and politicians. Recently, the economists have highlighted an index of quality of life (2005) with the eight major points like material well-being, health, political stability and security, family life, community life, climate and geography, job security and political freedom. They have also presented an idea of quality of life in terms of different statistics, regression statistics—Tables of some countries' score from 1 to 10 (Global 2005) including so-called developing–undeveloped countries.

Keywords Density of population · Urban and Rural areas · Well-being · Social life

12.1 Introduction

The present paper is concerned with a study on aspects of the quality of life in India and its macro region. It relates to some aspects of quality development in terms of a number of dimensions—social, cultural, political as well as economic quality development. It refers to certain characteristics of social life such as free participation and fairness in the distribution of benefits, i.e. to certain moral types of a society such as justice, equity, peace and liberty: UN definition clearly brings back the focus on human endeavour for the process of change which is seen as good. Development is also inclusive of certain other concepts such as liberty, self-

S. C. Mukhopadhyay (✉)
Calcutta University, Kolkata 700019, India
e-mail: satpati.ln@hotmail.com

National Association of Geographers, New Delhi, India

B. R. K. Sinha (ed.), *Multidimensional Approach to Quality of Life Issues*,
https://doi.org/10.1007/978-981-13-6958-2_12

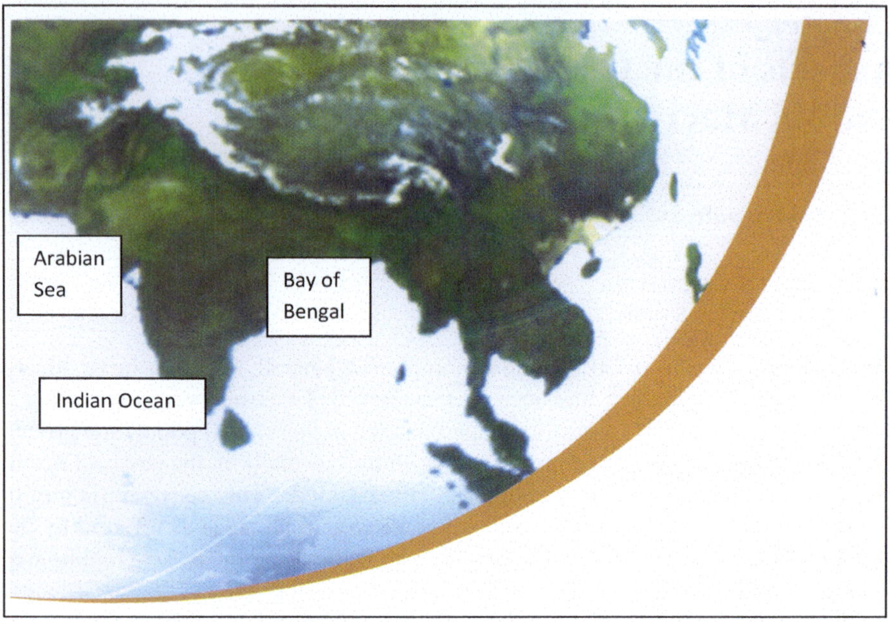

Fig. 12.1 Physical map of India with special reference to its NE Macro Region including the Andaman and Nicobar Islands, a Union Territory (UT) in the eastern part and surroundings, scale 1.50 Million

determination, autonomy, participation and empowerment (Figs. 12.1, 12.2, 12.3, 12.4 and 12.5) (Mukhopadhyay 1997, 1998, 2009, 2011, 2013; Bhattacharyya 1997; Ghosh 2009).

The author has banked upon the modern methodology—the use of Remote Sensing, GIS, Internet, software, etc. including the works of the predecessor and the like. We should agree that development is essentially economic growth and the way to achieve economic growth is through modernization of and increases in industrialization, advanced technology, modern bureaucratic and economic mechanisms. But during the later years of the 1990s and in the beginning of the new millennium, it was found that a large section of the population in the African, Asian and Latin American countries remained poor, undernourished, underfed, underemployed and deprived of the even most basic social and cultural need including our country (India). This led the social scientists to explore the possible causes of such an object of poverty and deprivation existing among the people of the developing nations to come up with alternative theories. These have included particularly those related to the distribution of the wealth mainly in terms of money and the like. This author has tried to establish some aspects of Quality life of India considering North–Eastern Macro Region Andaman and Nicobar Islands too.

Development of a nation is the interplay of politico-eco-cultural phenomena. Based on the active participation of the entire population in hierarchical stages of

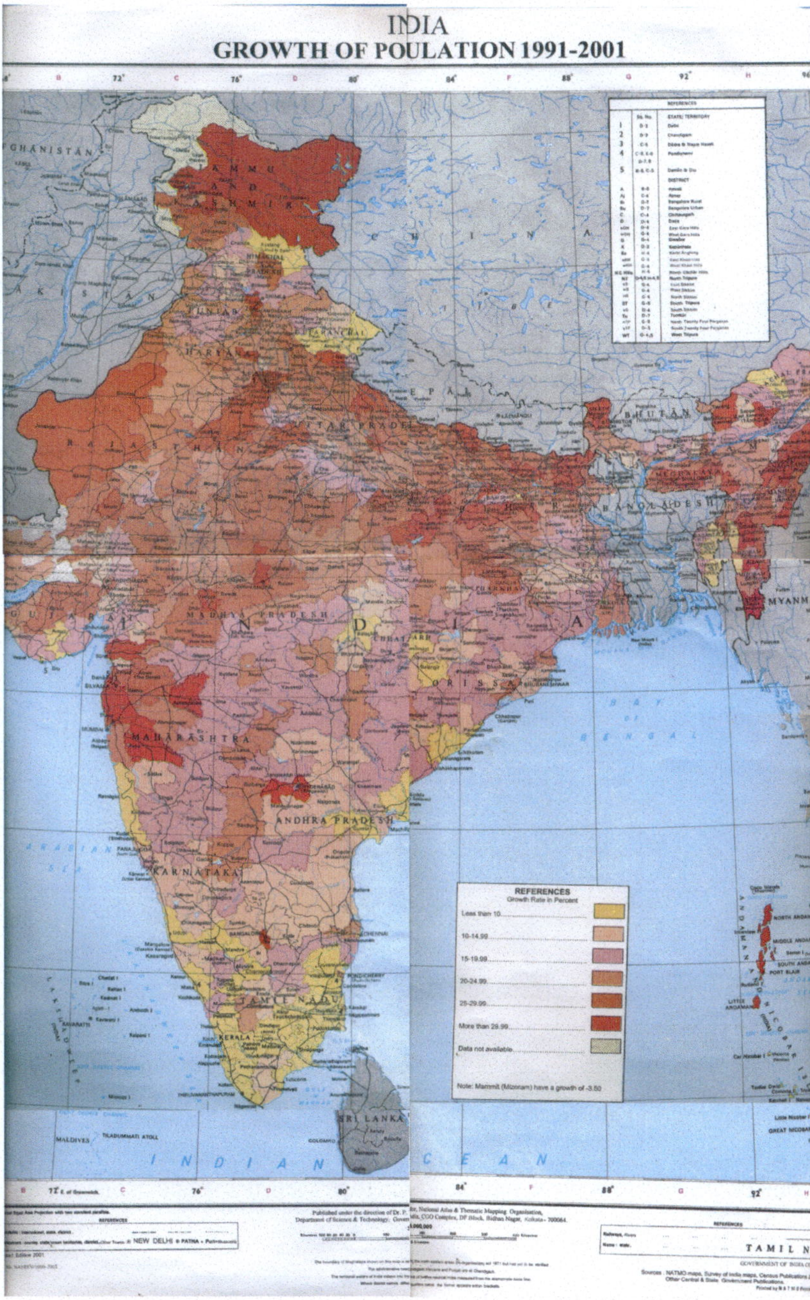

Fig. 12.2 Map of India showing the growth of population on 1991–2001, NATMO (Govt. of India under P. Nag)

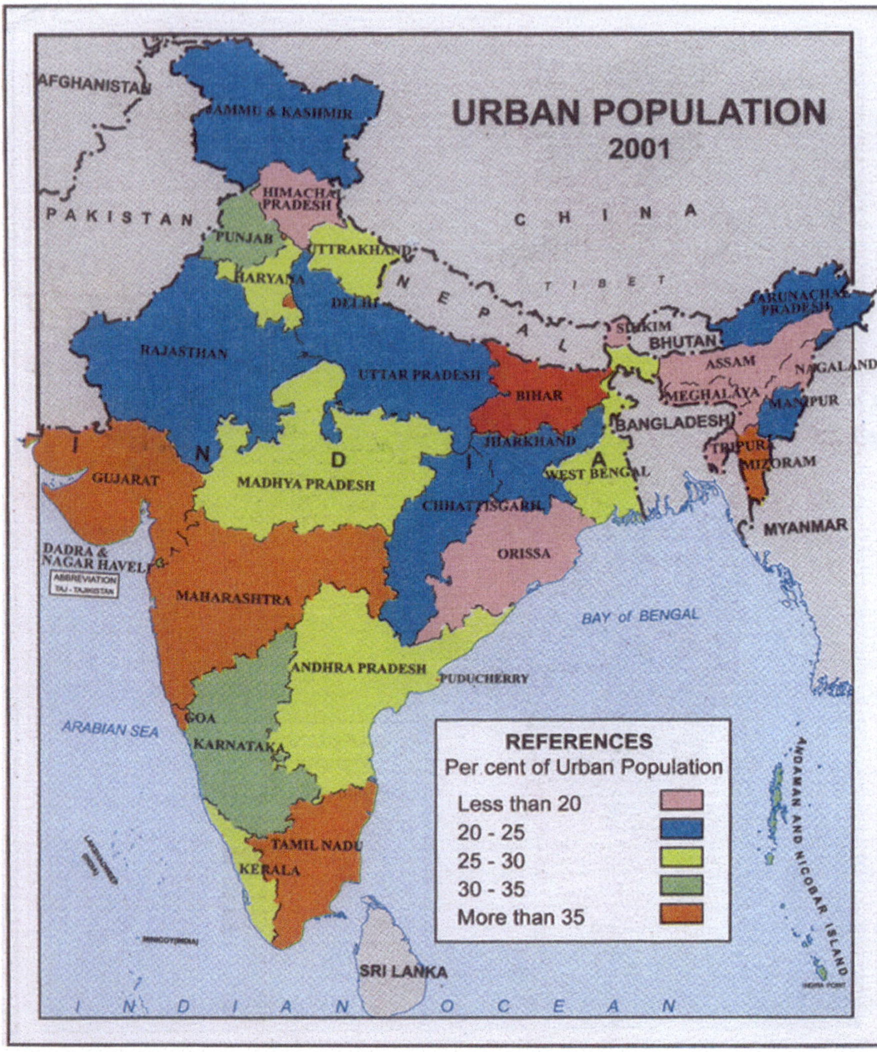

Fig. 12.3 Map of India displaying urban population on 2001, NATMO (Govt. of India under P. Nag)

development, it seeks to achieve uniformity in their well-being and enhance it by the allocation and dissemination of the range of benefits accruing from it (Tables 12.1, 12.2, 12.3, 12.4 and 12.5).

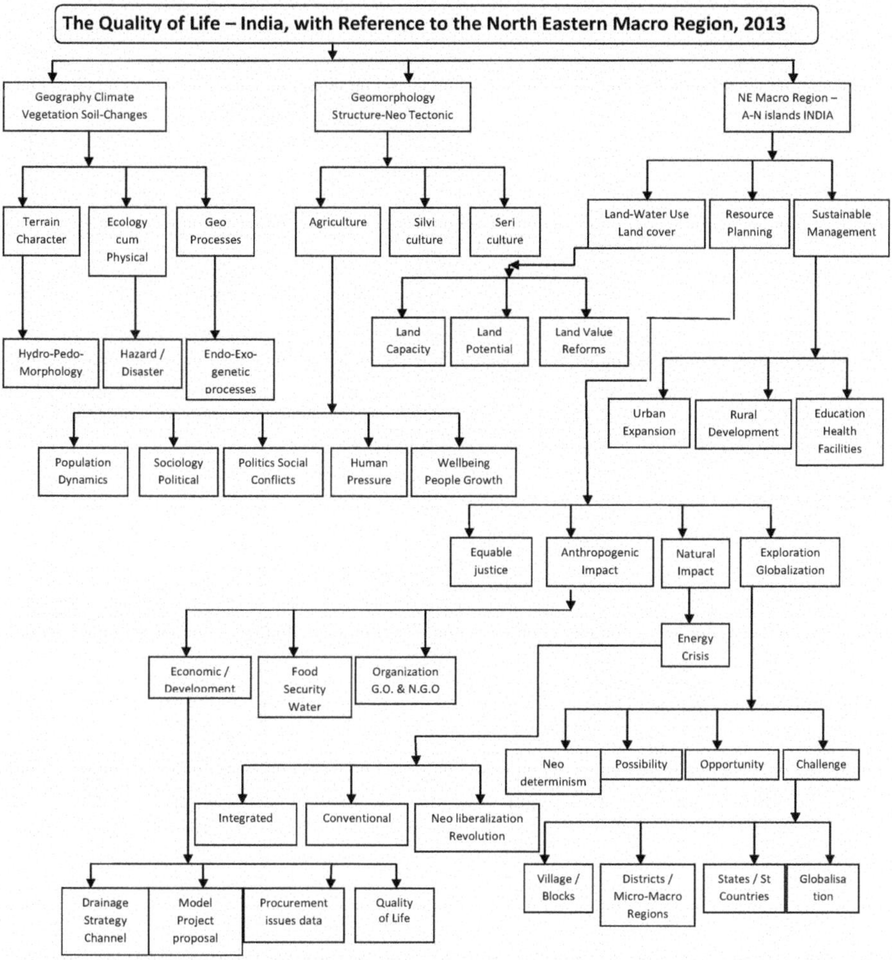

Fig. 12.4 Flow chart of the different aspects of quality of life in India, and Northeastern Macro Region including Andaman and Nicobar Islands

12.2 Status of Quality of Life, Especially in the Northeastern Macro Regions

Nowadays a large section of the population in the developing countries remained socially deprived, culturally marginalized and economically deprived in spite of the governmental efforts. In a pluralistic society like India, the problem of deprivation among minorities and backward communities such as scheduled castes and scheduled tribes posed a great threat to the social fabric of the nation-state. So far as the socio-politico-economic and related conflicts are concerned. The philosophical thrusts for the development studies in Geography as an academic discipline came from several

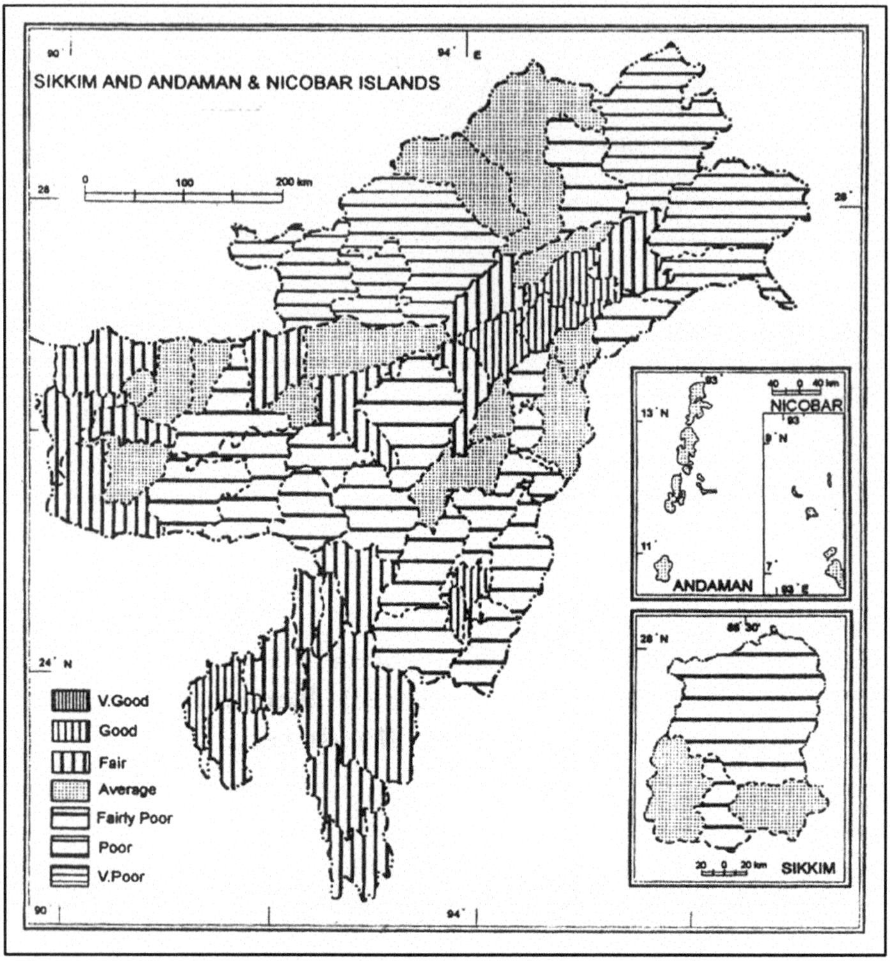

Fig. 12.5 The macro region of India and land use patterns with eight states and one union territory (UT), i.e. Andaman and Nicobar Islands in the eastern part exhibition land use patterns with the reflective status of very good, poor, very poor and the like

theoretical approaches among which, mention be made of Radical geography, Liberal views in geography, Humanistic geography and Geography of Welfare. These sub-disciplines individually and sometimes in accord with allied disciplines tried to focus on a theoretical basis of underdevelopment, for the country under consideration.

In a span of about sixty (60) years, the philosophy of development has undergone several paradigmatic shifts. It started with the need for development mainly in terms of economic growth. A quantitative approach was then replaced by qualitative transformation in terms of both time and space and still later a time–space compression, etc. The quality of life or geography of welfare is closely interrelated with devel-

Table 12.1 Present Borders along the Macro Region (State wise) including Andaman and Nicobar Islands (UT)

	International boundary percent to total state boundary (Approx)	State UT of area to total area (India)
Arunachal	70.12	2.55
Assam	18.58	2.38
Manipur	44.44	0.68
Meghalaya	33.89	0.68
Mizoram	71.66	0.64
Nagaland	22.64	0.50
Tripura	82.81	0.32
Sikkim	77.78	0.21
Andaman and Nicobar Island	100.00	0.003

Table 12.2 General status of qualify of life (2012) and sustainable as observed in the Northeastern States—a macro region including Andaman and Nicobar Islands up to Indira Point in the southeast of India

Country	Quality o life score	Sustainability
India	6.246	High
Mizoram	5.868	Mod. high
Meghalaya	5.068	Mod. high
Sikkim	5.093	Moderate
Tripura	5.007	Low
Assam	5.001	Low
Manipur	4.895	Low
Nagaland	4.877	Low
Arunachal Pradesh	4.826	Very low
Andaman and Nicobar Islands	3.327	Extremely low

opment economics although there are departures too in this respect. Several other themes such as geography of inequality, geography of hunger, and in later years gender-based issues in development geography, post-structural, post-colonial and post-modern views of the development of fragmented social groups in Third World metropolises have become very widespread in the literature of geography during the 1980s and 1990s. Uneven development which is a result of the capitalist system of production came to be regarded as the root cause of absolute poverty prevailing in the developing countries. All these focused on developmental issues particularly the differences between societies on the basis of caste, class, race, gender and ethnicity. During the post-1990s, again the focus shifted on human and social development as it was found that economic well-being alone could not bring equitable justice (Tuathail and Agnew 1992; Varshney 1991).

Table 12.3 Stages of development and quality of life by inputs, throughputs and outputs of India's societies

Inputs	Throughputs	Outputs
Environmental-Improvements	Biotic and Abiotic-Built-Environment	Environmentalism–Protection
Ecology–Feed Back	Nature-Concepts–Principles-Application	Ecosystems–Processes–Policy
Space ship Earth–Concepts-Planate	Time-Space-Energy, Agenda	Earth Environ–Geo-Sciences-Scarcity
Land-Ocean-Climate-Conference	Science-Technology-Productivity	Approaches-Methodology-Models
Landforms-Biogeo.-Chemical-Chronology	Cycles-Evolution-Basins-Spatial-Development	Slopes-Erosional-Depositional-Terraces
Resources-Land Bank-Values-Employment	Water-Soil-Vegetation-Fertility	Aesthetic-Conservation-Capability
Agri-Sylvi-Horti Culture, Hydrology	Industries-Chimney—Chimney less	Afforestation, Eco-Tourism-Dualism
Evolution–Thoughts–Equation	Population Dynamics-Tribal-Ethnic	Migration-National-International
Hazard-Disasters-Disciplines	Natural-Human-Impacts–Forests–Jt.-forest Man.	Mitigation-Challenges-Management
Plans-Index–Parity Progression-Equity	Interface-Sc-Eco.-Jet-streams-Behavioural	Basin strat.-Gen.-Biasness-Rad. Human Prob.
Civzn.–EAP–EIA–EFZ–Women-Emp.–Soc.	Socia-Politico-Conflict-Local-Global-Qualitative	Pollu.-Acid rain-Ecological Eco.. Colonization.
Env.-Move.-Irri.-Future-Possibilities	Industrialized–Eco.-Rural-Dev.-Scenario Modi.	Greenhouse Gases-man-Env. Relationship
Land Use–Actual–Potential-Initiatives	Society-Land Capability-Growth	Environ-Land Use, Conurbation Urbanization
Explosions. Inclusive-development	G.O.-N.G.O. (G.I.S.–R.S.) Sophisticate	Envr. Degradation Sustainable Develop
Revolutions-Welfare-Human Green	Rainbow Revolution–Wet-lands–Ramsar sites	Green-Blue-Red-White-Yellow, second Gr.-Brown
Global Warming, Socio-Spatial-Interaction	Sea level rises-Coastal Plains	Interdisciplinary knowledge, Geographers
Tools, Equipment Instrument-creation	Applied sense-Systems, Regions	Internets-Futuristic–Entrepreneurship

(continued)

Table 12.3 (continued)

Inputs	Throughputs	Outputs
Perspectives–Geographic-Quantitative	General-Physical-Cultural	Poverty–BPL-Crime
Examination–Stability-Security	Employment–Regional Imbalance	Techniques Diagrams-Maps
Liberal Views–Secretariat-expertise	Growth Development	Simulations Life–Neo-Determinism
Incomes–Gender equality	Education-Health-Multi-scalar-Institution	Fieldwork-RS-Softwares
Climate Landform–New Geographies	Intelligence Units–Mountain	Tropical–Monsoons–Drinking Water
Material Well-being,-Peace- & Happiness	Political Stability Freedom–Welfare	Political Freedom-Hills–Food Security
Family life-Human Resource Dev.	Community life Sanitation	Planners – Greening
Peri glacial-Glacial-Fluvial–Aeolian-Marine	Himala. Fore Deeps-Indo-Gangetic basin Plateau	Plains with facilities Coastal Plains.
Democracy–Municipal-Maya	Law-Order-Factors, Panchayats	Paradigm-Shifts-Aspirations-Neoliberalization
Global visualization–Time Space	Geopolitical Order–Discourse	Ideological–Enlargement-Geopolitical
Cybrogs–Dromological crisis situations	Spatial Representative-Modern Geopolitics	State Centred Terrestriality
Panchayat-Scales–Macro-Meso-Micro-Units	Quality of Life–Landscape Patterns	Global-Environmental-Governance

Table 12.4 Broad correlation matrix for land use variables of the macro region

Non-agricultural use	−0.8272	0.9385
	−0.7582	
Barren uncultivable	−0.6624	
Net sown area	−0.8674	

Correlation coefficients Significance level >0.714, 0.05 > 0.893, 0.01

Table 12.5 Aspects of qualify of life perspectives (physical and cultural) of India and eight states (2010–2011) including Andaman and Nicobar islands—a distinct macro region in India

Selected variables	Northern			Eastern			NE A & N Island		
	A	B	C	A	B	C	A	B	C
Land use (%)									
A: agriculture	30.2			41.5			5.24		
B: forest covers		45.0			49.3			38.2	
C: settlements			7.8			32.23			36.49
(i) Rural			98.6			79.56			82.36
(ii) Urban			29.3			38.42			34.87
Density of population (per sq. km)	980.00			913			503		
Average annual (%) growth	5.92			4.9			4.01		
GNI per capita (Dollars)	387.5			587.6			523.69		
Growth in per capita real wealth savings	1.7			0.87			1.82		
Population lying below the poverty line (BPL %)	Rural—31.25			Rural—29.47			Rural—22.34		
	Urban—6.34			Urban—36.23			Urban—12.58		
Genuine domestic saving (% of GDP)	4.92			8.27			3.82		
Adult literacy (%) of people 15 and above	79.31			79.49			40.23		
Agricultural productivity agri. value added per agri. worker (dollar)	313.4			397.24			302.4		
Per capita agri. land (ha)	0.91			0.42			1.08		
Per cent change in forest and woodlands	3.24			2.79			3.12		
Freshwater resources per capita (m^2)	1800			2000			1998		
Under 5, mortality rate per 1000	80			82			88		
Rank of socio-economic (comp Z score) quality of life (cultural)	5 (low moderate)			8.64			3 (moderate) 8.92		
Conservation index statistical method	0.93			0.86			0.43		

Source Based on Sample Survey, 2012: Primary source (fieldwork 2010–2012), Central Water Commission (CWC 2011). Population Census Report (2009), NIRD: Rural Development Statistics (2010–2011). Indian Economy, Sept. (2011). CMIE. Mumbai Ministry of Environment and Forest, G.O.I., Dehradun (2004–2010). Indian Agriculture in Brief (2009–2011). National Remote Sensing Agency (NRSA). Hyderabad (2008–2011). Profile District (2009–2012). Centre for Monitoring Indian Economy. Mumbai Food Security and Agricultural Dev. Dept. Sikkim 92008), Economic Review. Bureau of Applied Economics and Statistics. Govt. of W. Bengal (2009–2010). F.A.O. and World Development Reports (2009–2012). World Resource Institute (2011). UNDP (Human Development Report 2010–2012). Brahmaputra Board (2009–2010), Mukhopadhyay (2009, 2011, 2012, 2013) and Fieldworks 2012

12.3 The Importance of Income on Quality of Life

There is no denying fact that real GDP has an ever-reaching impact on quality of life. GDP and satisfaction from well-being are interrelated and depicts a linear relationship where the variation of GDP per capita contributes to variation in life contentment within the country by 50%. More the income more is the satisfaction achieved from life as is evident from surveys conducted on rich countries, where people earning more are noticed to be contented with their life than others with lower earning. Among 28 member states of EU, material well-being is recognized as the most significant indicator of life satisfaction on the basis of a survey conducted by Eurobarometer.

Though there has been a constant and notable increase in average income of developed nations, average life satisfaction growth trend is somewhat moderate and satisfactory. The existing contradiction between rising level of income and slow-moving level of life satisfaction cannot be explained due to lack of enough evidence that support the proposition of increasing income on one hand and diminishing state of community welfare on the other. On the basis of the present estimates, variation in levels of income poses least or no influence on the level of life satisfaction, where the latter is seen to be influenced more by absolute status than relative one associated with one's state of mind and level of aspiration. There is co-existence of factors of modernization that perfectly balance the positive impact emerging from it. The decline of traditional institutions is evident from the decline of religious faiths associated with the dwindling of trade unions that has given rise to social discrepancies in the form of crime, drug and alcohol addiction followed by the decline in public involvement that exists in form of politics thereby the reduction of trust and belief in public institutions and the continued waning of family and marriage institutions. This is also indirectly apparent from the increasing unreliability causing a great deal of personal risk associated with the gradual rise of income and associated higher choices. Stable family life and community are also on the verge of severe decline though being highly valued. Economists from all over the world have attached more importance on eight determinants and related factors of quality of life in terms of their coefficients provided in the equation in 2005.

12.4 The 2005 Quality-of-Life Index

For the computation of quality of life index for the year 2005, the following indicators have been taken into consideration: GDP, life expectancy, unemployment rate, and political stability. Changes in these factors are gradual are their estimation relies on the latest available data. The forecast index for 2005 and GDP per capita at PPP have been summed up in the table considering 111 countries (Bhattacharyya 1997).

An extensive and electronic survey was carried out on around 3000 respondents for the whole world in 2005, available from www.economist.com on people's perception and opinion on the factors contributing to the quality of life. The survey mostly covers the affluent, rich, English speaking and the globalized people that cannot be considered as true representative for the whole world. However, the immediate survey responses being compared with the approach undertaken by the Government of India in 2002 yield differences which are less striking as what has been expected supporting and properly justifying the undertaken approach (Govt. of India 2002).

12.5 Accounting for the Difference

The basis for estimation of quality-of-life indices compares and differentiates the variations in sources of quality of life between countries and regions wherein, the values are multiplied by equation coefficients. The position of Ireland at the top in the international quality-of-life league table is better explained by the combination of tradition and modernity including low unemployment rates, political liberties, stable family life and confronting joint family structures. The scores on these factors are well above the average of EU-15 countries that counterbalances its lower scores in attributes such as health, climate and gender equality. The United Kingdom, on the other hand, is at 29th position in the same list and is near the bottom as compared to the scores of the EU-15 countries. The United Kingdom is characterized by high rates of nuclear family structure and community breakdown coupled with low performance of health, liberty and freedom of people and social security that essentially balances the high per capita income and a higher percentage of employment opportunities. Italy holds a secured position among these countries, whereas Germany and France lag far behind contradicting the fact that these European nations repay for their productivity and fall behind the quality of life in a better way than America.

Economic growth model advocates that all countries pass through continuous and sequential stages of development. However, this theory was replaced on two basic grounds; *first*, by economic theories which employ statistical techniques to analyse the inherent processes of changes that a country passes through, and *second*, by theories that are more rational and political in nature. The modern theory proposes underdevelopment as an interlink and tussle between the continuously changing international and national connections, inelastic organizational economies leading to the expansion of intra-regional and inter-regional dual economies and dual societies. This theory essentially calls for the eradication of poverty and reduction in income inequality by bridging the gap between employment and unemployment scenario. All these factors provided the impetus for a neoclassical counter-revolution that emerged during the 1980s involving the economists who emphasized on the role and benefits of free markets and the huge costs underlining the interference of government in the achievement of development.

The unequal power relation between haves and have-nots is detrimental for the development of poor countries. The scholars such as Frank and others are of the opinion that underdevelopment is a consequence of capitalist development. They advocated that underdevelopment is associated with colonization and is an off-shoot of the capitalist system of production. The theory of dualism in economics that tends to separate two different economies on the basis of development, technology and related factors considers three indicators in terms of their concurrence for the analysis of levels of underdevelopment prevailing within a nation: conventional and contemporary methods of production in urban and rural economy; affluent-literate elite class and impoverished-illiterate section; powerful industrialized economies and weak agrarian economies. There has been growing emphasis on uneven development within metropolitan areas of the developing nations, accentuation of inequality among classes in urban areas, pauperization of already marginalized groups, and resulting poverty and deprivation at a large scale both at intra- and inter-regional level. This creates a disparity in the eco-cultural and socio-political condition of the mainstream population and a deteriorating quality of life. The initiation of neoclassical counter-revolution in the 1980s emphasized on the privatization and decentralization of the public sector in developed countries of the world that called for the deconstruction of public planning and management of economic activities. In this context, mention must be made of utilitarianism that provides the sound base for social justice in the achievement of overall welfare. The proponents of this approach are better known as 'maximisers' owing to their tendency to find out the means to the greatest overall well-being. The main focus is the distribution and allocation of goods, services, rights, freedom and political power in such a way so as to maximize the benefit accruing from them.

In this theory there are two advantages; one goods are produced efficiently and distributed equitably. This theory is criticized by on the ground that 'maximizing the sum of individual utilities is supremely unconcerned with the interpersonal distribution of that sum'. After this, the Theory of Justice as propounded by Rawls in 1971 can be taken as a point of illustration. For Rawls the natural right, and hence the primary aim of the institution, is social justice: thus each person possesses an inviolability founded by justice that even the welfare of society as a whole cannot override. Rawls advocates:

(a) Democratic Equality, (b) Equality of Opportunity, (c) Formal Equality of Opportunity, (d) Economic Equality and (e) Equality of Functioning Capabilities.

UNDP and World Bank while defining well-being have put emphasis on the removal of six important factors that retard development: malnutrition, disease, illiteracy, slums, unemployment and inequality. As measured on the basis of aggregate growth rates, development of a nation stands at a successful position but it is only a partial outcome or a complete failure when the indicators of employment, social justice and poverty eradication is considered separately as indicated by the World Development Institute. Development in the contemporary world is not only confined to economic means, moreover, it associates a multitude of factors in its determination thereby replacing the single focus. According to the former President of United Nations University Tokyo, the development effort of a nation is the strategic interplay and interconnection between the international and domestic indicators involving the potential of human beings.

In India the current thrust on development and welfare and well-being is on; our participatory approach in planning, on Micro level development through decentralized planning, Community development projects, Social welfare through "Basic Needs" approach and Universal education and justice (Govt. of India 2002; Varshney 1991). According to Prof. Amartya Sen, efficiency and competence of people with the utilization of resources, being possessed by them presume the most significance and care should be undertaken to their proper functioning, thereby highlighting capability over functions (Mukhopadhyay 1997, 1998).

12.6 Other Views of Quality of Life

In the later years, the welfare views in geography have become very popular. The important profounder of welfare approach in understanding development and underdevelopment has been initiated. Dworkin defines equality on two grounds; equality of welfare and equality of resources. The first notion describes equality in terms of resource distribution and resource allocation in such a way that brings equal welfare in every person's life. The second one focuses on the equal holding of resources by each people that determine their 'option luck', depending on the individual assessment and functioning of the market. The approach for 'equal opportunity for welfare' seems to fluctuate among people depending on how someone perceives the idea of welfare or well-being for his or her own sake.

In an effort to uplift the condition of the poor the state has adopted a decentralized planning so that the voices of the poorest of the poor and the marginalized section are heard. In order to look into the gender-based issues affecting the women belonging to the backward class and minority sections of the population, an emphasis is put on their political and economic empowerment. After the model of development suggested by Dreze and Sen in 1995, attention is given towards achieving social opportunity, i.e. school enrolment of female and male children, reproductive health care, provision for greater work participation of women, etc. In other words, more efforts are given toward attaining a better quality of life and capability building at the grass root level. In India, we face a problem of imbalance in sex ratio in the northern states, steps are taken in this direction so as to improve the sex ratio through social awareness campaign. It can be said that the recent trend in development studies focuses on the development of the Third World on the basis of Participatory Model of the Marxist mould. This model takes cognizance of environmental protection that is, ecological sustainability of the environment in relation to development. It also recognizes the division and diversity of the Third World countries and stresses on mass participatory politics. It further points out that the resolution of the environmental crisis this essentially a global political solution. The tremendous development thrust in the Third World countries due to their desperate need for survival is a major concern for environmentalists. The Participatory model seems to be more feasible as it takes into consideration the collective human good. At the same time, this model of development conceives of overcoming the environmental crisis by transforming the society politically, on a world scale.

Thus, the 1990s became the era of globalization when armed with the IMF and World Bank the expansion of global capital permeated the entire World economy. At present no country developed or developing more developed or less developed is entirely free from the impact of the market economy. Many countries have undertaken economic reforms so as to heighten the process of globalization. India has also undertaken economic reform during the 1980s. Since then has introduced a series of measures, i.e. privatization, liberalization and de-licensing in industrialization process. The country has experienced the multi-dimensional impact of globalization. How far this has minimized the extent of disparity among the rich and the poor and been able to reduce intra-regional and inter-regional disparities is a matter of debate.

1. Material well-being—GDP per person, at PPP is \$. Source: Economist Intelligence Unit.
2. Health—Life expectancy at birth, years, Source: US Census Bureau.

3. Political stability and security—Political stability and security ratings. Source: Economist Intelligence Unit.
4. Family life—Divorce rate (per 1,000 population), converted into an index of 1 (lowest divorce rates) to 5 (highest). Sources: UN Euro monitor.
5. Community life—Dummy variable taking value 1 if the country has either a high rate of church attendance or trade-union membership; zero otherwise. Sources: 110; World Values Survey.
6. Climate and geography—Latitude, to distinguish between warmer and colder climes. Source: CIA World Factbook.
7. Job security—Unemployment rate, %. Source: Economist Intelligence Unit; 110.
8. Political freedom—Average of indices of political and civil liberties. Scale of 1 (completely free) to 7 (unfree). Source: Freedom House.
9. Gender equality—Ratio of average male and female earnings, latest available data. Source: UNDP Human Development Report.

GDP measures have, however, failed to quantify the various non-marketed activities such as changes brought about by environmental pollution. However, these non-valuation techniques have faced great difficulties in imposing monetary values to the ecosystem services that provide benefits to human beings and bring welfare to the community. However, all these measures reflect selection bias in the factors selected for the thorough determination of quality of life and more precisely on the weightage to be imposed on them. Considering GDP as a measure, though is subject to various flaws in the estimation of purchasing power parity, pose a clear-cut framework in assigning values to different indicators for the goods and services. The survey outcomes are positive and grab attention in the recent years in spite of the criticisms faced during the early years due to the presence of cultural contrast and its resultant impact of differences of language across nations. However, attempt to summarize the problems arising out of these surveys include the inadequacy of the responses to reflect what people feel about their lives; instead, they claimed about their expectation from the range of satisfaction. Non-response rates are very low and the basic measure is seen to have been associated more with advanced tests and rating schedule by others aware of the individual and behavioural patterns. The survey results proved to be genuine and valid more than it was expected. The UN's Universal Declaration of Human Rights sounds appropriate in the determination of the indicators that require immediate inclusion in a quality-of-life measure as reported by some researchers. But that does not provide information on the weightage to be put on each of these indicators thus resorting to an 'Expert opinion'.

Here, an attempt has been made to analyse the important aspects of quality of the in India thus correlating mainly the development of landforms, and drainage—channel patterns along with the related hazards or disasters by adopting the modern methodology and fieldwork both qualitatively and quantitatively. These are well illustrated in terms of maps, diagrams, photographic evidence and for the advancement of the Hindukush–Himalayan environment. Some suggestion are made like the more measures in the conservation of the flora and fauna, area with specific land use, trauma centres, pollution-free water, etc. as a part of the organized resource utilizations, establishment of more trade centre, wide roads, introduction of modern/rapid transport and communications, afforestation, arrangements for education, health keep and secured accommodations, tourist centres arrangements for Environment Impact Assessments Emergency Action Plans (EAP), to boost up economic development and the like.

12.7 Features of Ethnic People

In a general way, the people of the Northeast Micro Region belong to diverse stock who migrated to this region during different periods of history. For example, the Ahoms from the Shan State of Myanmar crossed over the Patkai range in the thirteenth century and occupied and ruled Assam for over 600 years. There were hordes of migratory tribes such as the Khampis, whose script and languages is identical to the people of Thailand. The Khasis of Meghalaya have brought with them the tradition of Indo-Chinese races, who established themselves in the area from very early times. Their language has outlived among the Mon Khmer dialect, which has a well-defined and well-marked correspondence to that of Khasi dialect that is found to be existing in Myanmar and Thailand. With the exception of the autochthonous plains, tribals of the Brahmaputra valley, the Assamese today are not all indigenous people. Waves of migratory people from Uttar Pradesh and Bihar have settled in Assam from time to time mainly for carrying out trades and establishment for Business Centres.

The latest conquerors were the British, who invaded Assam from their base in Bengal and annexed Assam to their Indian realm, in around 1626. The British were interested in the timber, ivory and silks (eri, muga, etc.) of the North-East and the East India Company developed trade relations with the area. For governance, a new system known as the Non-Regulated System was evolved.

12.8 The Current Economic Scenario

Figures 12.1, 12.2, 12.3, 12.4, 12.5, 12.6 and 12.7, Tables 12.1, 12.2, 12.3, 12.4, 12.5) given in the text illustrate the current development of the Macro Region in India—The Brahmaputra basin and surrounding including Andaman and Nicobar Islands. It was felt in 1972 that the Northeast region presented a single geographical unit, where people had common interlinked developmental problems and shared the same destiny for security, in this strategic sub-continent border of India. The geographical conglomerate of seven states has the potential of becoming the richest segment of the country. Industries based on tea, paper, wood, oil, electricity, as well as agro-based and cottage industries have immense potentiality. To plan and implement projects for all round development the North-East Regional Council Act was promulgated in 1972 (Mukhopadhyay 2009, 2011, 2013).

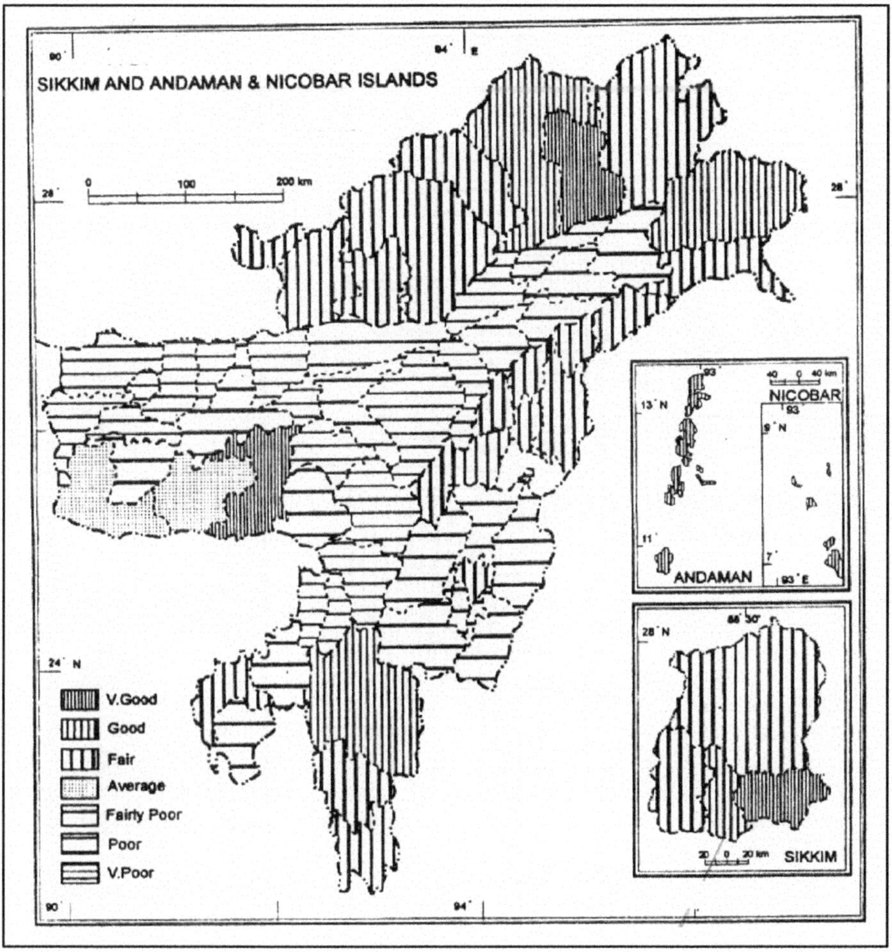

Fig. 12.6 Map of macro region displaying the degree of economic infrastructure in terms of good, poor, etc.

12.9 Locational Characteristics of the Northeast India

The states of Arunachal Pradesh, Assam, Manipur, Meghalaya, Mizoram, Nagaland and Tripura lie in the northeastern corner of India. The region is joined to the rest of the country by only a narrow neck of land hardly 80 km wide through the Terai region of West Bengal. The rest of its 3500 km boundary is shared with the neighbouring countries of Bhutan, China, Myanmar and Bangladesh. This gives the region its strategic significance.

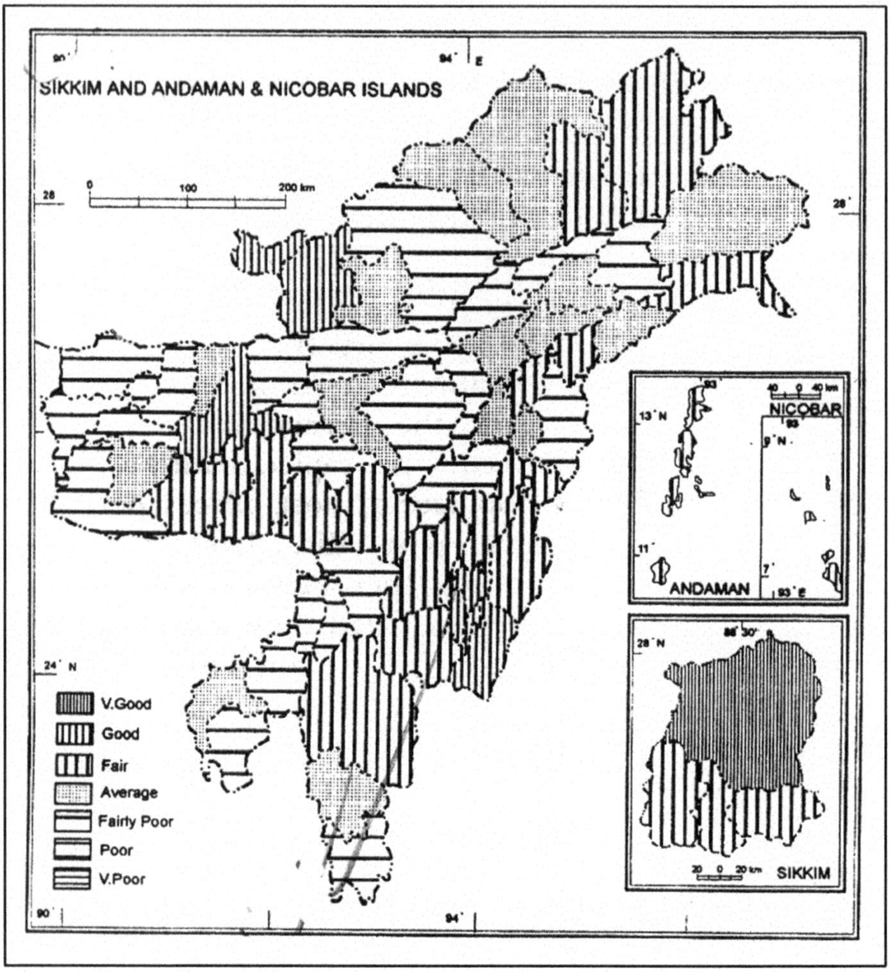

Fig. 12.7 Map of macro region showing the development of infrastructure

12.10 Physiographic Characteristics

Physiographically, the Northeast States can be divided into three units viz., the Assam valley—the continuation of the Indo-Gangetic trough; the Meghalaya Plateau—the eastern extension of the Chotonagpur Plateau; and the mountain ranges of Eastern Himalayas and its continuation southwards into the Patkai range, the Naga, Manipur and Mizo Hills (Figs. 12.1, 12.2 and 12.3).

Three main islands form the Great Andaman group. The Duncan passage separates the little Andaman from the Great Andaman. Off the main islands, lie numerous archipelagoes. Some of these like the Rutland and Cinque islands have been detached from the main islands by wave action, others like the Ritchie Archipelago are formed of newer rocks. The coasts of these islands are fringed with coral reefs (Fig. 12.2).

12.11 Important Demographic Characteristics

Since the quality of life is related to population and is expressed in terms of population, it is only imperative that the demographic component of the population is duly stressed. However, in the present study, it has not been possible to enumerate the levels of well-being of different cohorts of the population. Here the demographic component has been dealt with as an indicator of development or non-development. The purpose is to emphasize the actual situation, stressing on how the region differs from the rest of India. Generally, 14 parameters have been selected to study the demographic characteristics of these areas. These include population density, sex ratio, growth rate of population total, rural and urban, change in growth rate between 1971–81 and 1991–2001, percent of scheduled castes and tribes, population less than 5 and 14 years, main and marginal workers and the ratio between workers and non-workers (Figs. 12.2, 12.3, 12.4, 12.5 and 12.6).

India's population witnessed an overall increase of 17.7% equivalent to an increase of 181.96 million persons during 2001–11 as compared to 21.5% increase during 1991–2001 and rate of growth of female population (18.3%) surpassed that of the male whose percentage share stood at 17.1. However, rural areas accommodate more people (833.5 million) than the urban counterpart that houses 377.1 million people. As compared to 2011, the proportion of population residing in urban areas registered a growth of 1.8 times increasing from 17.3 to 31.2% in 2011. There has also been a positive change in literacy rate with respect to two census years of 2001 and 2011. Though male literacy rate (80.9%) is more than that of female (64.6%), the rate of growth in literacy stands more for females (10.9%) than males (5.6%).

12.12 The Ideas of the Macro Region and Related Socio-economic Features

The author has given some ideas on socio-economic features of the macro region. So far as the related socio-economic aspects are concerned, education is a basic human right and every individual must enjoy the privilege of being educated. Education determines the aspiration, technology, productivity and vertical and horizontal mobility of the people. It changes the perception of cost and values, which contribute to the economy of the household and the nation. But, in a developing country like India, the percentage of the literate population is often used as a measure of the level of education. As compared to the rest of India, the Northeast, Sikkim and Andaman and Nicobar Islands have a high literacy rate. Rural literacy is well above the all

India average of 30%, reaching as high as 72% in Mizoram, lowest being recorded in Arunachal Pradesh. The urban literacy rate is also much above the all India average of 57%. In no state is urban literacy less than 70% and reaches as high as 80–90% in some states. However, Arunachal Pradesh records the total literacy rate lower than the all India average of 52.21. This is true for both male and female literacy rates, as well. Meghalaya too has a literacy rate lower than the all India average. The present author has not discussed in details in the education of the area under study for obvious reasons (Luke 1996).

It seems reasonable to refer the 2011 Census of India in the context of Quality of Life which is found to develop mainly in the urban centres like Mumbai, Kolkata, Delhi, Bengaluru, Chennai, and Pune. According to the Census Report (2011) as referred elsewhere, India's total population as on 1 March 2011 stands at 1,210,726,932 or 1.21 billion which registered an increase of 181.96 million persons in total with an increase of 90.97 million males and an increase of 90.99 million females during 2001–11. Bihar (25.4%) experienced the highest decadal growth in population. India's population is noticed to be more concentrated in rural areas with 68.85% (i.e. more than two-thirds of the total population) and the remaining of 31.14% of the population residing in the urban area (Tables 12.3, 12.4 and 12.5).

12.13 Concluding Remarks

Different aspects of quality of life of India and its macro region, i.e. Northeastern states including one union territory—Andaman and Nicobar Islands have been elaborated with seven figures and six tables. These islands, Andaman and Nicobar islands, are indicative both of Physical especially climatological, i.e. southwest monsoon (burst of monsoon on may end every year). Its southern limit is called as Indira point (97° 35′ E, 6° 45′ N). This macro region consisting of eight states and one union territory—is known as Terra incognita. The physical and cultural features mainly are in support of the development of the quality of life in all the urban centres although some part, geographically and climatically, is not in favour for the growth equity and development of quality of life. The waves of urbanization are well observed in the capitals of eight states and one union territories as above. In general, in Asian countries (on the basis of the author's own fieldworks) the effects of urbanizations and in association with quality of life which are confined mainly in the urban can be found almost in all the nearby zones of the urban areas as above. The tables and the figures present also some aspects of the quality of life in India and also in the Northeastern Macro Regions along with Andaman and Nicobar islands. This author also likes to include environmental governance—which is (in the opinions of contemporary environmentalists) one of the most complex challenges in the context of the quality of life as discussed above (Figs. 12.1, 12.2, 12.3, 12.4, 12.5, 12.6 and 12.7, Tables 12.1, 12.2, 12.3, 12.4, 12.5).

Acknowledgements This author is grateful to Prof. S. C. Sarkar, of Geological Sciences (Retd.), Jadavpur University, Jadavpur and Dr. P. Nag (Retd.) Director, NATMO, Govt. of India, and Vice Chancellor of M. Gandhi Kashi Vidyapith University, Varanasi; who have extended their valuable advice and active co-operations in the preparation of this interdisciplinary paper on Quality of Life.

References

Bhattacharyya, B. (1997). *Sikkim: Land and people* (pp. 437, 102–142). New Delhi: Omson Publication.

Ghosh, A. (2009). *Environment and development* (pp. 32–248). New Delhi: A.P.H. Publishing Corporation.

Government of India. (2002). *NATMO national Atlas Thematic Mapping Organisation (NATMO)* (pp. 3–81). Kolkata: Department of Science and Technology, P. Nag. Atlas of India.

Luke, T. (1996). Identity, meaning and globalization: Dereaditionalization in post-modern time-space compression. In P. Heeles, S. Lash, & P. Morris (Eds.), *Dratraditionalization*. Oxford: Blackwell.

Mukhopadhyay, S. C. (1997). Hydro-resource of the North Eastern Indian Subcontinent and adjacent area, Kolkata. *Indian Journal of Landscape System and Ecological Studies, 20*(2), 166–189.

Mukhopadhyay, S. C. (1998). Geomorphology of the Sikkim Himalaya. In S. C. Rai, R. C. Sundriyal, & E. Sharma (Eds.), *Sikkim—Perspectives for planning and development* (pp. 1–15). Tadong, Sikkim: Sikkim Science Society.

Mukhopadhyay, S. C. (2009). People, environment and development of Upper Ganga Basin Area. In B Sinha (Ed.), *Environment and development, a global challenge for the 21st century* (pp. 305–318). New Delhi: New Century Publications.

Mukhopadhyay, S. C. (2011). Research methodology in geomorphological studies. In P. K. Sharma, R. S. Yadava, & V. N. Sharma (Eds.), *Research methodology: Concepts and studies* (pp. 345–363). New Delhi: R. K. Books.

Mukhopadhyay, S. C. (2013). Environment and development in the Brahmaputra Basin, India and China (Tibet) (pp. 1–13). In S. Chandra (Ed.). New Delhi: Mittal Publishers.

Tuathail, G., & Agnew, J. (1992). Geopolitics and discourse: Practical geopolitical reasoning in American foreign policy. *Political Geography, 11*, 190–204.

Varshney, C. K. (1991). *Population, environment and resources, population education* (pp. 1–37). New Delhi: NCERT.

Chapter 13
Quality of Life Among the Aged in India: Anthropological Insights

Reetinder Kaur and Rohit Kumar

Abstract The present study is an attempt to understand dimensions of life satisfaction and quality of life among the rural elderly. The data is collected from 160 elderly living in and around Naggar village situated in district Kullu of Himachal Pradesh. The results of the study reveal that elderly describe their life satisfaction in terms of financial self-sufficiency, social network and social support, religious disposition and satisfaction with their health conditions. It is suggested that a holistic all-inclusive policy must be drafted to address the life satisfaction and quality of life issues among the elderly in India especially the elderly women.

Keywords Elderly · Satisfaction · Integrated programme · Quantitative approach · Socio-demographic profile

13.1 Introduction

Ageing of the human population is one of the major demographic transitions of the twenty-first century. The proportion of elderly is increasing at an alarming rate and the aged constitute the fastest growing section of the population. According to Sample Registration System data, the population of aged in India has increased from 5.3% to 5.7% and from 6.0% to 8.0% from 1971 to 1981 and from 1991 to 2011, respectively. According to Census of India 2011, there are more elderly females in both rural (5.8%) and urban (5.5%) India as compared to males (5.1% in rural and 4.8% in the urban areas). The elderly population is expected to increase its share to more than 10% by the year 2021 (Central Statistics Office 2011). India is expected to become an ageing society by 2024, the focus would be on its preparedness towards meeting the ageing crisis from the present unstructured system (Lee et al. 2011). With the decline in fertility and mortality rates accompanied by the improvement in child

R. Kaur (✉)
Department of Anthropology, Panjab University, Chandigarh, India
e-mail: reetinder1986@gmail.com

R. Kumar
HelpAge India, New Delhi, India

B. R. K. Sinha (ed.), *Multidimensional Approach to Quality of Life Issues*,
https://doi.org/10.1007/978-981-13-6958-2_13

survival and increased life expectancy, a significant feature of demographic change is the progressive increase in the number of elderly persons. An important dimension of the ageing process in India is the rising share of females in the older age groups referred to as 'feminisation of older age' (Venkatesh and Vanishree 2014). Therefore, the government needs to initiate requisite programmes and policy interventions to ensure a life with dignity for the senior citizens of the country.

The Ministry of Social Justice and Empowerment, which is the nodal Ministry for this purpose focusses on policies and programmes for the Senior Citizens in India. Government of India adopted 'National Policy on Older Persons' (NPOP) in January 1999. The policy defines 'senior citizens' or 'elderly' as a person who is of age 60 years and above. In pursuance of the NPOP, a National Council for Older Persons (NCOP) was constituted in 1999 under the Chairpersonship of the Minister for Social Justice and Empowerment to oversee implementation of the Policy. The NCOP is the highest body to advise the Government in the formulation and implementation of policy and programmes for the aged. The Council was reconstituted in 2005 with members comprising of Central and State government representatives, representatives of NGOs, citizen's groups, retired person's associations, and experts in the field of law, social welfare, and medicine.

The Integrated Programme for older persons is a scheme that provides financial assistance up to 90% of the project cost to non-governmental organisations (NGOs). This money is used to establish and maintain old age homes, day-care centres, mobile and medicare units and to provide non-institutional services to older persons. The scheme also works towards other needs of older persons such as reinforcing and strengthening the family, generation of awareness on related issues and facilitating productive ageing. The Scheme for Assistance to Panchayati Raj Institutions, voluntary organisations and self-help groups for the construction of old age homes and multi-service centres for older persons has also been initiated. This scheme provides a one-time construction grant. The Central Government Health Scheme provides pensioners of central government offices the facility to obtain medicines for chronic ailments up to 3 months at a stretch. The National Mental Health Programme focusses on the needs of senior citizens who are affected with Alzheimer's and other dementias, Parkinson's disease, depression, and psychogeriatric disorders.

The Maintenance and Welfare of Parents and Senior Citizens Act, 2007 was enacted in December 2007 to ensure need-based maintenance for parents and senior citizens and their welfare. Indira Gandhi National old age pension scheme was launched by the Ministry of Rural Development. All persons of 60 years and above (revised downwards from 65 in 2011) and belonging to below the poverty line category according to the criteria prescribed by the Government of India time to time are eligible to be a beneficiary of the scheme. It is a part of National Social Assistance Programme (NSAP), which further includes Indira Gandhi National Widow Pension Scheme (IGNWPS), Indira Gandhi National Disability Pension Scheme (IGNDPS), National Family Benefit Scheme (NFBS) and Annapurna schemes other than Indira Gandhi National Old Age Pension Scheme (IGNOAPS). The pension amount, as of Union Budget 2012–13, is INR 200 per month per person from 60 to 79 years and

INR 500 per person for those above 80 years. The amount of Indira Gandhi National Pensions for widows is INR 300 per month.

13.2 Data and Methodology

Himachal Pradesh has the second highest percentage of elderly (10.3%) in India after Kerala (Census of India 2011). As ageing population in India is growing, there is a need to focus on issues that affect the elderly. In order to frame policies and to make the ongoing programmes and policies successful, data was required about various issues of the elderly. A combination of qualitative and quantitative approaches is required for a more comprehensive understanding of ageing issues. A number of disciplines such as anthropology, sociology, geography, psychology, social policy, law, economics and public administration can holistically deal with the issues related to ageing.

The present study is an attempt to holistically understand the life satisfaction among the rural elderly as it affects the quality of life. Quality of life is an individual's satisfaction with life, which he/she considers important. Historically known as 'life satisfaction' or 'subjective well-being', it is now sometimes referred to as 'overall quality of life' or 'global quality of life'. Moreover, the understanding of this quality of life or life satisfaction is essential to understand the gap between expectations of elderly and their fulfilment. The study was conducted with an aim to analyse the life satisfaction among the rural elderly in Himachal Pradesh. The data were collected from a rural sample of 160 elderly individuals (89 males and 71 females) living in and around Naggar village, district Kullu, Himachal Pradesh. To obtain data, a specifically designed schedule was used. The schedule contained the questions specifically on various aspects of life satisfaction and quality of life among the elderly. Life satisfaction among the elderly was measured using 'life satisfaction scale' given by Chadha and Willigen (1995). The scale has positively and negatively worded statements presented in 'likert-type' response categories with categories ranging from strongly agree to strongly disagree. Positively worded questions were scored from 7 to 1 for response categories of strongly agree to strongly disagree. Similarly, for the same response categories, negatively worded items were scored from 1 to 7. After scoring, the means and standard deviations for these categories were calculated. Sex differences in the scores were evaluated with the help of student's t-test. Apart from the quantification of data, the qualitative data are also presented to supplement the quantitative data.

13.3 Results

Table 13.1 clearly shows the socio-demographic profile (age, gender, educational and marital status) of respondents.

13.3.1 Life Satisfaction Among the Elderly

Life satisfaction is an important construct and one of the commonly accepted subjective conditions of quality of life and one of the important facets of ageing process. Both life satisfaction and quality of life are interrelated concepts and key elements in the understanding of ageing from a psychosocial perspective. Life satisfaction is a yardstick of 'psychosocial well-being' of the aged (Chadha and Willigen 1992). To determine whether the elderly have adapted to ageing, it is important to obtain their opinion about their condition. In this context, self-rating of life satisfaction is recognised as a principal measure of effective adaptation to ageing and well-being (Atchley 1998). Among the aged, it not only reflects their psychological adjustment but also their physical, social and financial adjustments (Chadha and Willigen 1992). The life satisfaction scores among the elderly are given in Table 13.2.

It is clear from Table 13.2 that at all ages the life satisfaction among males was higher as compared to females. There was a decrease in life satisfaction as the age progresses among both males and females.

Table 13.1 Socio-demographic profile of respondents

Socio-demographic indicators	Gender		Total
	Male	Female	
Age			
60–69	44.94	38.02	41.87
70–79	35.95	2.39	34.37
80–89	19.10	29.57	23.75
Educational status			
Illiterate	33.71	54.93	43.13
Able to read and write	4.49	2.82	3.75
Primary	15.73	12.68	14.37
Middle	25.84	16.9	21.87
Matric	13.48	8.45	11.25
Graduate	6.74	4.22	5.63
Marital status			
Living with spouse	79.77	66.2	73.75
Divorced	3.37	8.45	5.62
Separated	6.74	9.86	8.12
Widow/widower	10.11	15.49	12.5

Table 13.2 Life satisfaction scores among the elderly

Age group	Categories and number of respondents	Mean life satisfaction score	Standard deviation	t-values
60–69	Male = 40	125.80	15.94	1.876
	Female = 27	118.96	12.4	
70–79	Male = 32	110.21	16.84	2.103
	Female = 23	99.3	21.65	
80–89	Male = 17	85.05	24.42	0.195
	Female = 21	83.61	21.18	

Table 13.3 Sources of financial assistance among the elderly

Sources of financial assistance		Gender		Total
		Male	Female	
Dependent	Spouse	–	29.58	13.12
	Children	25.92	18.31	21.25
	Grandchildren	–	8.45	3.75
Self-sufficient	Pensions	40.74	12.68	26.25
	Business	11.11	5.63	8.12
	Agriculture	13.58	15.49	13.75
	Property rent	2.47	4.22	3.12
	Fixed deposits	2.46	–	1.25

13.3.2 Dimensions of Life Satisfaction Among Elderly

Knowledge of dimensions that are crucial to life satisfaction among the elderly is essential in order to improve the elderly care and address their issues (Borg et al. 2006). A number of attempts have been made by previous studies to understand these factors. The factors such as economic factors (Borg et al. 2006; Jung et al. 2010), health (Borg et al. 2006; Angelini et al. 2012), religiosity (Park et al. 2012), social support (Park et al. 2012), role in decision making (Onishi et al. 2010) and availability of health care facilities (Onishi et al. 2010) affect the life satisfaction among elderly. In the present study, the respondents described life satisfaction in terms of financial self-sufficiency, social network and social support, religious disposition and health status.

13.3.2.1 Financial Status of the Elderly

Economic conditions are the most important determinant of life satisfaction among the elderly (Jung et al. 2010). The sources of financial assistance among the elderly in the present study are presented in Table 13.3.

In the present study, the majority of elderly males were dependent upon their pensions followed by financial assistance from their children (25.92%). The percentage of males drawing pensions (40.74%) as compared to females (12.68%) was higher. The majority of female elderly were dependent upon their husbands (29.58%) or children (18.31%) for financial assistance. The dependency of females can be explained by the fact that the majority of female elderly were illiterate (54.93%) and around 43.8% were either widows or divorced or separated. Previous studies by Bloom et al. (2010) indicate that an overwhelming proportion of elderly live with their children in India (Bloom et al. 2010), and their economic security and well-being is largely contingent on the economic capacity of the family unit (Siva Raju 2011). In this scenario, females are more likely to depend on others, given economic dependency, lower literacy and higher incidence of widowhood among them (Gopal 2006). Moreover, in the present sample, elderly males were found to have a relatively higher life satisfaction score than the elderly females. The reason for lower life satisfaction score among elderly females can be attributed to their financial dependence on their husband and children.

13.3.2.2 Social Networks and Social Support Among Elderly

Social support is a concept that is generally understood in an intuitive sense, as the help from other people in a difficult life situation. One of the first definitions was put forward by Caplan (1974) who defined social support as an enduring pattern of continuous or intermittent ties that play a significant part in maintaining the psychological and physical integrity of the individual over time. Cobb (1976) defined social support as 'the individual belief that one is cared for and loved, esteemed and valued, and belongs to a network of communication and mutual obligations'. The definition of social support varies widely among those who have studied it. Lin et al. (1979) defined social support as 'support accessible to an individual through social ties to other individuals, groups, and the larger community'. Thoits (1986) defined social support as the form of coping assistance or as the active participation of the significant others in an individual's stress management efforts.

Social support is an important issue for elderly and research on social support has continued to be a dominant force in gerontological literature. It determines the subjective well-being in old age (Rathore 2009). In the present study, the data related to social networks and frequency of interaction with social network were obtained. The percentage distribution of the elderly feeling closer to their social network is given in Table 13.4.

The majority of the elderly in the present study felt closer to their spouses. Males felt closer to their spouses than females. Apart from their husbands, females felt closer to their children as well. These findings can be supported by the work of Antonucci and Akiyama (1987) who stated that females have a wider social network than males and males tend to heavily rely on their spouses for social support. Similar findings have been reported by other studies on sex differences in receiving social support among elderly (Antonucci and Akiyama 1987; Krause and Keith 1989). The

Table 13.4 Percentage distribution of elderly feeling closer to their social network

Person(s) the respondents felt closer	Male	Female	Total
Spouse	58.43	47.88	53.75
Children	14.61	29.57	21.25
Grandchildren	15.73	14.08	15.1
Other relatives	10.23	7.45	10.00

respondents were asked about the frequency of their interaction with a social network outside the family. Most of the male elderly visited their friends often followed by neighbours while the female elderly visited their neighbours more often than friends and relatives.

13.3.2.3 Religious Disposition

Religion is a powerful social institution, which plays an important role in shaping social behaviour. Religiosity involves organised worship and practice, as well as theology (Jenkins and Pargament 1995). Religiosity may be broadly defined as a search for the sacred that may include public as well as private and intrinsic dimensions (Miller and Thorsten 2003). Religiosity consists of two modes of religious involvement: the personal and the institutional mode. The personal mode is comprised of religious beliefs, feelings, and behaviour that find their source in personal and individualised religion. The institutional mode is comprised of the religious beliefs, feelings or behaviour related to formalised and institutionalised religion.

Numerous studies have suggested that religiosity is positively associated with life satisfaction among the elderly (Ardelt 2003; Koenig et al. 2001; Nelson-Becker 2005; Park et al. 2012). The gerontological studies reveal that elderly tend to get more religious as religion may provide them with social support (Dubey et al. 2011), means of interaction with social network (Dubey et al. 2011), companionship and counselling, coping mechanism and emotional support. The gender-wise distribution of places and frequency of prayer among the elderly in the present study are given in Table 13.5.

It is clear from Table 13.5 that the majority of elderly prayed twice at their home and visited the places of worship occasionally. The gender-wise distribution of changes in frequency of visits to places of worship in old age is given in Table 13.6.

Most of the elderly responded that their visits to places of worship increased with age and the decrease in frequency of visits to religious places was more among males than the females. These findings can be supported by the previous studies by Levin et al. (1994) and Dubey et al. (2011) which indicate that with increasing age, religiosity tends to increase.

Table 13.5 Places and frequency of prayer among Elderly

Places and frequency of prayer		Male	Female	Total
At home	Once a day	22.47	22.53	22.50
	Twice a day	57.3	64.79	60.62
	Occasionally	5.62	4.22	5.10
	Only on religious festivals	–	–	–
	No fixed schedule	14.61	8.45	11.87
At places of worship	Once a day	12.36	11.28	11.87
	Twice a day	22.47	8.45	16.25
	Occasionally	32.58	33.8	33.75
	Only on religious festivals	17.98	26.76	21.87
	No fixed schedule	14.61	19.72	16.87

Table 13.6 Changes in the frequency of visit to places of worship

Visit to places of worship	Male	Female	Total
Increased with age	64.04	74.65	68.75
Decreased with age	12.35	5.63	9.37
No change	23.59	19.72	21.87

13.3.2.4 Satisfaction with Health

Health is one of many dimensions contributing to the overall quality of life (Rathore 2009). It is a broad concept, which can embody a huge range of meanings, from the narrowly technical to the all-embracing or philosophical. To a layperson, health would mean a sound physical body. It is more so, a condition of a body that helps a person to perform his day-to-day activities to the expectation of others (Mehta 1992). To some people, health is a general sense of well-beingWell and feeling good. For others, health includes the expectations that they will not become ill or will be able to recover quickly. For most, health involves the ability to do what they want to do, with one's body not presenting difficulty in normal activities. For some, health has moral connotations, with the disease the consequence of immorality. People's prominent concerns with health generally encompass physical, psychological, emotional, and spiritual dimensions of well-being. The word health is derived from the old English word for heal which means 'whole', signalling that health concerns the whole person and his or her integrity, soundness or well-being. Only physical well-being no longer stands relevant in present context, a new conception of health has emerged within a broader state of complete physical, mental, social and spiritual well-being and not just the absence of disease and illness. Conceptions of what constitutes health vary widely. In the context of medical anthropology, Landy (1977) defined a state of health as 'the condition of an organism that permits it to adapt to its environment situation with relatively minimal pain and discomfort, achieve at least some physical and psychic gratification and possess a reasonable probability of survival'. While on the other hand, a state of disease, according to Landy 'is a condition of the organism that seriously obtrudes against these adaptive requirements and causes behavioural dysfunction'. Rao (1992) maintained that the aim and objective of health and medical science is to help achieve such a well-being that one can function at his choice not only as an individual, but also as a useful member of the family, social groups and community.

Health has two common meanings in everyday use, one negative and one positive. The negative definition of health is the absence of disease or illness. The positive definition of health is a state of well-being, interpreted by the World Health Organisation (WHO) in its Constitution as 'a state of complete physical, mental and social well-being, not merely the absence of disease or infirmity'. Assuring physical well-being by preventing disease, disability, dysfunction and premature death have been the primary focus of modern medical care. However, secondary social and psychological factors have also been recognised as having major influences on general health status (De La Carcela et al. 1998). Warren (1999) is of opinion that a more broadened description of the parameters of health may prove helpful and in that regard, health may be described as a relationship, a synergistic interplay between the physical, social, psychological and spiritual elements that create the well-being of individuals and/or groups in their physical and social environment.

In the present study, the data were collected regarding the occurrence of health problems among elderly, their satisfaction with their health and life, and desire for longevity. The most common health problem among the elderly in the present study was hypertension (13.12%). Its frequency was slightly higher in males (14.08%) compared to females (12.35%). The most prevalent problem among the females was arthritis (21.13%) which was less frequent among males (3.37%). Heart problems (11.87%), cataract (11.87%) and renal diseases (11.25%) were the other common problems among elderly in the study area. As a part of self-assessment of health conditions, majority of respondents (58.75%) were satisfied, 21.87% were less satisfied and 19.37% were not satisfied. 65.62% elderly were satisfied with their lives in general and 61.25% elderly desired for longevity. The desire for longevity was more among males (62.92%) than that of females (59.15%).

13.4 Conclusion and Suggestions

The present study attempted to analyse the life satisfaction and dimensions of life satisfaction among the rural elderly. The findings of the study suggest that the respondents described their life satisfaction in terms of financial self-sufficiency, social network and social support, religious disposition and satisfaction with their health conditions. The scores of life satisfaction suggest that males have more life satisfaction as compared to females and life satisfaction decreases with the progressing age. The study further suggests that females benefit less from the pension schemes as compared to males and are more financially dependent. While drafting policies, special attention needs to be paid towards the betterment of elderly females in India especially rural elderly females. Moreover, the amount of old age pensions and the proportions of elderly who benefit from them have to be improved significantly. Inspite of financial dependency among females, they had a wider social network than the males in the present sample. Religion, too, provided elderly with the social support and religiosity among elderly increased with progressing age. Majority of elderly were satisfied with their health and their lives in general. The desire for longevity was more among males than females.

Quality of life is an overall sense of well-being: physical, personal and societal well-being (Sharma 2009). Life satisfaction among the aged is an important concept, as it has far-reaching implications and it can give an overall view as to how much adjustment an individual is, or how the person is 'ageing successfully' (Chadha et al. 2009). Life satisfaction is an important area of research among the elderly. It reflects certain direct (economic conditions, social support, satisfaction with health, etc.) and indirect concerns (policies and programmes for the elderly, availability of health care services, etc.) of the elderly. Thus, the understanding of this multidimensional construct is crucial from various perspectives. From the healthcare perspective, understanding of the concept of life satisfaction helps in making the health care appropriate as per the needs and perspectives of the elderly. From the policy perspective, understanding of this construct helps in making the policies and programmes sensitive and beneficial for the elderly. With the emergence of old age homes and day care centres for the elderly, the understanding of the needs of the elderly becomes even more essential. Understanding of social factors that affect the life satisfaction such as social support and religiosity helps in making the social services provided to the elderly through NGOs more beneficial.

It is suggested that the disciplines such as anthropology, sociology, geography, psychology, social policy, law, economics, public administration need to work together to generate more and more data on the issues that affect elderly and their life satisfaction. More focus on elderly issues will bring significant changes in policy, their social environment and health care. These significant changes are essential to make elderly life more dignified in our country.

Ethical Statement For the present study, informed consent was obtained from all the participants and due care was observed in order to secure information of the participants. As the study was part of a Masters dissertation project, ethical clearance was not obtained and moreover, there was no provision of ethical clearance for such projects. The Panjab University Institutional Ethics Committee was formed much later than the project was actually conducted and submitted. However, ethical consideration such as obtaining informed consent using a consent form in the vernacular language (for instance, Hindi in our study) and use of participant numbers in order to secure identity of the participants was taken into consideration. Similarly, care was observed in writing and reporting of the research findings.

References

Angelini, V., Cavapozzi, D., Corazzini, L., & Paccagnella, O. (2012). Age, health and life satisfaction among older Europeans. *Social Indicators Research, 105,* 293–308.

Antonucci, T. C., & Akiyama, H. (1987). An examination of sex differences in social support among older men and women. *Sex Roles, 17*(11&12), 737–749.

Ardelt, M. (2003). Effects of religion and purpose in life on elders' subjective well-being and attitudes toward death. *Journal of Religious Gerontology, 14,* 55–77.

Atchley, R. (1998). Activity adaptations to the developments of functional limitations and results for subjective well-being in later adulthood: A qualitative analysis of longitudinal panel data over a 16-year period. *Journal of Aging Studies, 98*(1), 19–39.

Bloom, David E., Mahal, A., Rosenberg, L., & Sevilla, J. (2010). Economic security arrangements in the context of population ageing in India. *International Social Security Review, 63*(3–4), 59–89.

Borg, C., Hallberg, I. R., & Blomqvist, K. (2006). Life satisfaction among older people (65+) with reduced self-care capacity: the relationship to social, health and financial aspects. *Journal of Clinical Nursing, 15*(5), 607–618.

Caplan, G. (1974). *Support systems and community mental health: Lectures on concept development* (p. 4). New York: Behavioral Publications.

Central Statistics Office. (2011). *Situational analysis of the elderly in India* (p. 4). Central Statistics Office: Government of India.

Chadha, N. K., Aggarwal, V., & Mangla, A. P. (2009). Hopelessness, alienation and life satisfaction among aged. In K. L. Sharma (Ed.), *Dimensions of ageing: Indian studies* (pp. 48–61). Jaipur: Rawat Publications.

Chadha, N. K., & Willigen, J. V. (1995). The Life scale: The development of a measure of successful aging. *Indian Journal of Gerontology, 9*(3&4), 83–90.

Chadha, N. K., & Willigen, J. (1992). Hopelessness, alienation and life-satisfaction among aged. *Indian Journal of Gerontology, 6*(3&4), 82–92.

Cobb, S. (1976). Social support as moderator of life stress. *Psychosomatic Medicine, 38,* 300–314.

De La Carcela, V., Chin, J., & Jenkins, Y. (1998). *Community health psychology: Empowerment for diverse communities*. New York: Routledge.

Dubey, A., Bhasin, S., Gupta, N., & Sharma, N. (2011). A study of elderly living in old age home and within family set up in Jammu. *Studies on Home and Community Science, 5*(2), 93–98.

Gopal, M. (2006). Gender, Ageing and Social Security. *Economic and Political Weekly*, 21October, pp. 4477–86.

Jenkins, R. A., & Pargament, K. I. (1995). Religion and spirituality as sources for coping with cancer. *Journal of Psychosocial Oncology, 13*(1–2), 51–74.

Jung, M., Muntaner, C., & Choi, M. (2010). Factors related to perceived life satisfaction among the elderly in South Korea. *Journal of Preventive Medicine and Social Health, 43*(4), 292–300.

Koenig, H. G., McCullough, M., & Larson, D. B. (2001). *Handbook of religion and health: A century of research reviewed* (pp. 97–117). New York: Oxford University Press.

Krause, N., & Keith, V. (1989). Gender differences in social support among older adults. *Sex Roles, 21*(9–10), 609–628.

Landy, D. (1977). *Culture, disease, and healing*. London: Collier Macmillan Publishers.

Lee, S.-H., Manson, A., & Park, D. (2011). *Why does population aging matters so much for Asia? Population aging, economic security and economic growth in Asia* (ERIA Discussion Paper Series 2011). ERIA-DP-2011-14.

Levin, J. S., Taylor, R. J., & Chatters, L. M. (1994). Race and gender differences in religiosity among older adults: Findings from four National Surveys. *Journal of Gerontology, 49*(3), S137–S145.

Lin, N., Simeone, R. S., Ensel, W. M., & Kuo, W. (1979). Social support, stressful life events and illness: A model and an empirical test. *Indian Journal of Health and Social Behaviour, 20,* 108–119.

Mehta, S. R. (1992). *Communication and development: Issues and perspectives*. Jaipur: Rawat Publications.

Miller, W. R., & Thoresen, C. E. (2003). Spirituality, religion, and health: An emerging research field. *American Psychologist, 58*(1), 24–35.
Nelson-Becker, H. (2005). Religion and coping in older adults: A social work perspective. In H. R. Moody (Ed.), *Religion, spirituality, and aging* (pp. 51–67). New York: The Haworth Press.
Onishi, C., Yuasa, K., Sei, M., Ewis, A. A., Nakano, T., Munakata, H., et al. (2010). Determinants of life satisfaction among Japanese elderly women attending health care and welfare service facilities. *The Journal of Medical Investigation, 57,* 69–80.
Park, J., Roh, S., & Yeo, Y. (2012). Religiosity, social support, and life satisfaction among elderly Korean immigrants. *The Gerontologist, 52*(5), 641–649.
Rao, M. S. (1992). *Health and hospital administration in India*. New Delhi: Deep and Deep Publications.
Rathore, S. (2009). Subjective well-being in old age. In K. L. Sharma (Ed.), *Dimensions of Ageing: Indian studies* (pp. 16–24). Jaipur: Rawat Publications.
Sharma, K. L. (ed). (2009). *Dimensions of Ageing: Indian studies*. Jaipur: Rawat Publications.
Siva Raju, S. (2011). *Studies on ageing in India* (BKPAI Working Paper No. 2) (p. 2). New Delhi: UNFPA.
Thoits, P. A. (1986). Conceptual, methodological and theoretical problem in studying social support as a buffer against life stress. *Journal of Health and Social Behaviour, 23,* 145–159.
Venkatesh, S., & Vanishree, M. R. (2014). Feminization among elderly population in India: Role of micro financial institutions. *Global Journal of Finance and Management, 6*(9), 897–906.
Warren, R. (1999). *Oral health for all: Policy for available, accessible and acceptable care* (p. 1). Washington, DC: Centre for Policy Alternatives.

Part III
Socio-cultural and Economic Dimension

Chapter 14
Strategic Infrastructure Supporting the Quality of Life in Dhaka

Nurul Islam Nazem and Md. Anwar Hossain

Abstract This paper explores the role of strategic infrastructure, which includes key physical, environmental and socioeconomic setup of a region that facilitates a good living environment to live a quality life. A wide range of literature shows positive relationships between key infrastructure and quality of life in a region. It has been argued that the presence of adequate service infrastructure with good accessibility by the people provides with a better quality life. Taking Dhaka City Region as an example, the paper highlights that there is a severe infrastructure deficit in the region. Lack of serious initiatives to provide adequate infrastructure, especially in the sectors, such as transport and communication, housing, and utility services add considerably to the costs of development. Especially, due to poor planning and governance, the city fails to achieve the desired level of infrastructure provisions. The study also shows that adequate and quality infrastructure supports required impulses toward better living of the people where they have been planned and provided. Among various infrastructure, social and economic infrastructure are also important along with physical infrastructure. Health and education facilities and services, which are highly inadequate in the region make Dhaka one of the poorly living city regions in the world.

Keywords Strategic · Accessibility · Infrastructure · Governance · Health and education · City regions

14.1 Introduction

Rapid urbanization is a dominant factor in transforming the lifestyle in most of the Asian developing countries. In South Asian countries, especially in Bangladesh, rapid urbanization is manifested in the rapid growth of the urban population. Rapid urban-

---

N. I. Nazem (✉) · Md. A. Hossain
Department of Geography and Environment, University of Dhaka, Dhaka, Bangladesh
e-mail: nazem.info@yahoo.com; nazem.geography@du.ac.bd

Md. A. Hossain
e-mail: anwar.geography@du.ac.bd

B. R. K. Sinha (ed.), *Multidimensional Approach to Quality of Life Issues*,
https://doi.org/10.1007/978-981-13-6958-2_14

ization merely by the increase of urban population in Bangladesh creates tremendous pressure on the strategic infrastructure that determines the quality of life in urban areas. Dhaka being the largest urban agglomeration and being located centrally in the country attracts huge migrants from all over the country. Most of these migrants are economically poor and therefore cannot afford to get required amenities and utilities to live a quality life. This paper explores from secondary data the kind of strategic infrastructure provided mainly by the public sector available to support the quality of life of the people in the Greater Dhaka Region (GDR).

Quality of life in Dhaka City (like that of any other city) is one of the important factors in its sustainability. A better quality urban structure, such as high income, low unemployment, high investment, and for that matter, high living standards depends largely on the necessary infrastructure, which runs smooth functioning of the City. For citizens to be more dynamic and vibrant in an economic and social context, it is essential that an enabling environment exists in the City (ADB 2012). The World Bank's "Cost of Doing Business Report 2012" ranks Bangladesh well behind other South Asian countries on many of the indicators, including strategic infrastructure. Factors for which Bangladesh, and by implication, Dhaka, rank poorly include physical infrastructures, such as transport, provision of electricity, water supply, sanitation, waste management, health, and education services and recreation facilities.

There is a severe infrastructure deficit in Dhaka City Region. Lack of serious initiatives to provide adequate infrastructures, especially in the sectors such as transport and communication, housing and utility services add considerably to the cost of development. Moreover, due to poor planning and governance, the city also fails to secure its future infrastructure provisions. An ADB (2012) study shows that compensation for acquisition of land for road construction becomes very high, up to 40% to the total cost, even if the constructed buildings are illegal. This results in constraints in getting fund for the development of new infrastructure.

Apart from lacking in physical infrastructure, social, and economic infrastructure are also insufficient in the region. Health, education, and recreational facilities and services are highly inadequate, although these are the key components of human development. The paper highlights some of these key issues related to strategic infrastructure development in the Greater Dhaka Region that shapes quality of life.

14.2 Greater Dhaka Region

The Greater Dhaka Region (GDR) has been chosen as the study area. It consists of six administrative districts: Dhaka, Narayanganj, Gazipur, Narsingdi, Manikganj, and Munshiganj (Fig. 14.1). A substantial part of the area is fully urbanized, while some pocket areas are semi-urban and some are still rural.[1] As a geographical unit, the

[1]Dhaka, Gazipur, and Narayanganj are fully urbanized; the other three districts are partially urbanized but are important since these districts provide transport corridors between megacity Dhaka and other important areas of the country.

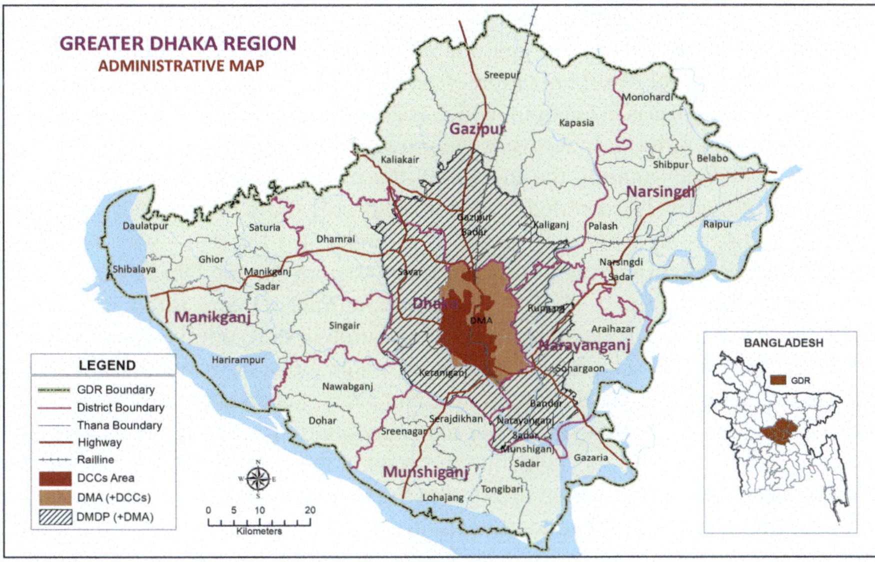

Fig. 14.1 The study area

area is difficult to define, as there is a number of entities that relate particularly to the region. At the core of the region is Dhaka Metropolitan area (DMA), which includes Dhaka city corporations (North and South) and some adjoining (nonmunicipal) areas, designated as Other Urban Areas, administered by Union Parishad.[2] The area of DMA is 306 km^2.[3] The second connotation is a planning area, called DMDP (Dhaka Metropolitan Development Plan) area. It covers an area of 1530 km^2, which is also known as the RAJUK area.[4] The third connotation is the present study area, known as the Greater Dhaka Region (GDR) or Dhaka Capital Region (DCR), which covers an area of 7,400 km^2 and can be considered to be Dhaka Metropolitan region in a wider sense (Fig. 14.1).[5]

The Greater Dhaka Region contains about 15.78 million urban populations, comprising over 35% of the national urban population. As a region, the level of urbanization in the GDR is the highest (67.28%) in the country. However, the level of

[2]Union Parishads are the lowest administrative units under the rural-local government structure. Like a municipality, the unions have an elected chairman and a certain number of ward councilors. This is rural-local government as opposed to urban-local government.

[3]Dhaka Metropolitan area is a jurisdiction of Dhaka Metropolitan Police. The area is truly urban, surrounded by four rivers, Buriganga on the south side, Turag on the north and west sides, and Balu-Sitalakhya on the east side.

[4]DMDP area includes DCC (north and south), DMA, other city corporations such as Narayanganj and Gazipur, Savar Municipality, and a large number of unions.

[5]GDR area was the study area for Dhaka Transport Plan (STP) and CCED study undertaken by ADB in 2009. The area also legally defined the jurisdiction of recently established Dhaka Transport Coordination Authority (DTCA).

urbanization varies substantially among the six districts of GDR. Dhaka District, which contains the largest urban agglomeration, has an urban population of over 10 million, with a level of urbanization of nearly 90%. The next largest concentration of urban population is in Gazipur, which is 2.2 million; followed by Narayanganj, which contains 1.9 million. In terms of the growth of the urban population, Gazipur accounted for 9% per annum, the highest in the region in 2011. Narayanganj and Munshiganj, respectively, recorded 4.8% and 4%—still above the national urban rate of growth. GDR, as an urbanized region, is growing at 4.1% rate—way above the national urban population growth. It is important to note that the Dhaka central area population is growing slowly (3.3%). The reason for this, perhaps, is that land prices and congestion discourage receiving more population in the central area of the City.

There are reasons for selecting GDR as a study area. First, the economic landscape of the area is undergoing rapid changes in recent years. Second, the concentration of industries is taking place along the major road network of the region, which gives the region the status of a very special economic zone in the country. Third, historically GDR was a capital region,[6] which means that the region was a seat of administration and various nonagricultural economic activities. Thus, the landscape of the whole area as a special economic zone is a justifiable concept.

14.3 Strategic Infrastructures in GDR

14.3.1 Transport Infrastructure

Dhaka is well connected by air, water, rail, and road networks to cities within the country and surrounding countries. However, the capacity of the modes of transport, particularly for passengers, is still low. The transport infrastructure of GDR is characterized generally by poor network planning, inadequate road capacity, poor road maintenance, and poor traffic management, undisciplined traffic management, overcrowding, slow movement, congestion, and frequent accidents (Islam 2005). Slow-moving cycle rickshaws, along with fast-moving motorized vehicles mix freely in the city streets, which are often chaotic and this creates congestion for unusually long periods (on average an hour for a short trip of about two kilometers). Apart from rickshaws, there are rickshaw vans and pushcarts and a few horse carts (in older Dhaka only), which ply regularly for business in the City. However, there are buses, CNG run three-wheeler "baby taxies", minibuses, and private cars to accommodate the limited road spaces in the City.

Road spaces within the Dhaka Metropolitan Area (DMA) will not be more than an estimated 15% of the city space.[7] Islam (2005) estimates that the total length of

[6]Dhaka was the capital of Bengal during the Mughal period since 1608. Besides Bikrampur (present Munshiganj), Sonargaon (present Narayanganj), and Savar (present Dhaka District) it had the status of capital at various point of time in history.

[7]Estimated by the study team, Detailed Area Plan reports of DMDP, Dhaka 2010.

the road network in DMA is approximately 3000 km, roughly one-quarter of these roads are of the primary type (main roads), with a width of more than 20 m. Although some of the new roads are wider, most of the roads in the City are narrow, ranging from 3 to 15 m.

The road transport system in Dhaka is operated by formal (public and private transport) and informal transportation systems. The most obvious negative conditions concerning the transport sector include poor transport management, using the same routes by both motorized and nonmotorized traffic and lack of provisions for parking facilities in the City. The problem further intensifies by the poor management and coordination among responsible organizations. This situation severely constraints smooth functioning of traffic and costs very high for sustainable economic development and the quality of life.

In Dhaka, transport development has been seriously neglected in the past and the budget has always been inadequate for development. On top of this, technical manpower was not adequately developed to face the challenges of growing demands created mainly by the City's increasing population. In the policy arena of city transport system, neither the participation of the private sector was encouraged, nor were the public agencies strengthened with trained and technical manpower.

Only recently, some initiatives have been taken to improve the transport systems of Dhaka. The most significant achievement to date is the preparation of a Strategic Transport Plan (STP) for the City Region (Louis Berger Group Inc. and Bangladesh Consultants Ltd. 2005). The STP has proposed a number of short, medium, and long-term measures to cope with the transport problem of Dhaka City. Some of the proposals have already been considered, such as the construction of new links between the existing networks, an elevated expressway, and a metro rail system. The ultimate target is to offer a multimodal, efficient, and integrated transport system in the city, which comprises a metro rail, an expressway, several circular roads, reducing traffic congestions and construction of a few dual carriageway roads to link important places in and around the City Region (Government of Bangladesh 2011).

14.3.2 Water Supply

The history of the water supply in Dhaka dates back more than 130 years. Modern pipe supply began in 1878, with the establishment of a treatment plant at Chandi Ghat on the bank of the River Buriganga in August 1874 (Akhtar 2009). It should be noted here that Dhaka was declared a municipality in 1864. The supply of pure water was the responsibility of Dhaka Municipality until Dhaka Water Supply and Sewerage Authority (DWASA, an autonomous body) was created in 1963, with responsibility for supplying water in Dhaka, Narayanganj, Demra, Tongi, Gazipur, and Savar. However, the authority could not manage all these areas and concentrated only on Dhaka City (360 km^2) (Sheesh 2010).

Dhaka WASA has a threshold population of 12.5 million to supply water. The water came from an underground aquifer (87%) and surface water (with treatment

13%) up to 2012. DWASA will be able to produce 2431 million liters every day, against a demand for 2560 million liters. However, a recently established treatment plant at Saidabad enhanced an additional production capacity of 220 million liters per day. This will reduce dependency on underground water from 87 to 78%. This thus reveals that only 22% of the demand for water can be met from treated surface water from DWASA's three water plants (DWASA 2012). However, demand is increasing due to population growth and the growth of industries and additional demands may be met by underground sources.

The present water supply infrastructure shows that the underground water is raised to the surface through deep tube wells. There are 490 such deep tube wells in operation. The overall length of water pipes in the City (DMA) is about 2600 km, providing water through more than 260,000 connections (Sheesh 2010). Of these, 92.7% of water goes for household use and the rest (6.54%) go to commercial and industrial uses. DWASA, however, supplies water to the low-income community almost free of charge, which is currently 0.68% of the total supply. It should be mentioned here that about one-third of the City population fall into the low-income category, receiving less than 1% of the water supply.

Average water consumption in the City is 130 L per person per day, of which 92% or 120 L is used such as for toilet flushing (22%), cleaning (7%), washing (2.2%), and bathing (41%). About 8% of water is used for cooking and drinking (DWASA 2013). The tariff for the domestic (household) water supply is heavily subsidized by the government and this encourages the misuse and overuse of precious water resources. On the other hand, the present tariff structure is flat for all categories of people. The authorities are thinking of introducing a progressive billing system to reduce the subsidy to those in the higher income bracket and heavy water users. Thus, increased revenue could be used for expanding the water supply service, improving quality, and making an investment in DWASA's other development plans. However, the main barrier in introducing such a progressive system of billing is that many user households are connected to one meter (account), especially in apartments, hostels, and communal worker accommodation, where segregation of consumption per household is difficult.

Access to drinking water coverage to GDR is shown in Table 14.1. It reveals that 98% of households had access to safe drinking water in the region. However, the proportion of households with access by various sources of water varies by district. It has already been indicated that the Dhaka district has provided 66.4% households with tap water. About 32% households who live in the slums use tube wells. The proportion of tube well users is high among other districts in the region. At least 5% of the households use water from sources other than taps and tube wells. Map A shows the spatial pattern of water supply in the region.

If compared with typical South Asian situation, Bangladesh's performance in providing safe drinking water and water for other uses for the country as a whole is little behind other South Asian countries. However, if considered water supply in GDR, its performance is better than South Asian countries. Water supply in Urban areas of Bangladesh shows 85% coverage, while GDR accounted for 97.8% coverage in the supply of water. India and Pakistan, respectively, covered 97% and 96% of

Table 14.1 Household sources of drinking water in greater Dhaka region

District	Proportion of households (%)		
	Tap	Tube well	Others
Dhaka	66.4	31.9	1.7
Gazipur	36.6	60.9	2.5
Manikganj	3.1	94.2	2.6
Munshiganj	2.9	93.8	3.4
Narayanganj	18.1	78.9	3.1
Narsingdi	3.2	94.4	2.5
GDR	42.2	55.6	2.2

Source BBS (2012)

their urban areas as a whole. Sri Lanka and Bhutan covers, respectively, 99% and 100%.

14.3.3 Sanitation

Bangladesh has made remarkable progress in providing better sanitary services. Access to sanitary toilets increased from 12.5% in 1991 to 63.5% in 2011 (BBS 2004, 2012). In urban areas, the situation coverage was found to be better. More than 80% of households in urban areas have access to improved sanitation, which is much higher than 58% in rural areas (BBS 2012). Dhaka megacity region (DMR) accounted for about 95% coverage. Sanitation conditions in GDR are better than the national urban scenario. About 86% of households in GDR have access to sanitary toilets. The sanitary conditions are worst in the slums and squatter areas of GDR. More than one-third of the population living in poor settlements and some poor households also enjoy sanitary toilets, meaning that conditions in Dhaka District are better than in the other districts of GDR. More than 93% of households have access to sanitary toilets in Dhaka, followed by 81.8% in Munshiganj, 81.5% in Gazipur districts (Table 14.2).

14.3.4 Access to Electricity

Electricity is possibly the most important factor contributing to a better living environment, quality of life and economic development. Among all the utility services, access to electricity is relatively good, but there is also an acute shortage of electricity supply and most areas experience frequent blackouts. The electricity coverage and supply for GDR is better than for the other areas in the country. In Bangladesh, little more than one-half of households (52.4%) have access to electricity, which is only

Table 14.2 Proportion of households having access to sanitation in GDR by districts in 2011

District	Proportion of households (%)			
	Sanitary (water-sealed)	Other sanitary	Non-sanitary	None
Dhaka	51.9	41.6	6.1	0.4
Gazipur	29.4	52.1	16.5	2.0
Manikganj	18.9	53.7	25.4	2.0
Munshiganj	23.7	58.1	16.6	1.7
Narayanganj	23.9	54.2	20.2	1.7
Narsingdi	20.2	40.9	30.4	8.5
GDR	**38.3**	**46.5**	**13.5**	**1.7**
Bangladesh	**24.8**	**38.7**	**28.7**	**7.7**

Source BBS (2012)

Table 14.3 Household electricity coverage in GDR by districts in 2011

Zila	Electricity coverage (% of households)
Dhaka	97.0
Gazipur	84.0
Manikganj	52.7
Munshiganj	90.1
Narayanganj	95.3
Narsingdi	72.8
GDR	**89.4**
Bangladesh	**52.4**

Source BBS (2012)

47% in rural areas and more than 85% in urban areas. In GDR about 90% of households have access to electricity (Table 14.3). In the central part of GDR, especially in Dhaka district, the proportion is about 97% (BBS 2012).

Due to rapid population and industrial growth, demands for electricity are increasing every year. At present, in the DESCO area, there are 0.59 million authorized consumers. In 2001, the number of consumers was only 0.11 million. However, the DESCO failed to supply the demanded quantity of electricity due to inadequate production. As a result, people face power shortages and power failures every day. People face load shading and frequent outages of electricity every day, but for longer in the summer, when the average power outages in Dhaka are four to five hours per day (BRAC 2012). On the other hand, the management of electricity supply is poor and as a result, government loses about 10% of revenue from this sector due to "system" losses, mainly through illegal connection (DESCO website 2013).

The poor and middle-income people face serious problems due to inadequate electricity supply. Most of the commercial, industrial consumers, and the upper-middle and upper-class residential consumers arrange backup sources of power in the form of acquisition and widespread use of IPS, generators, charger fans and lights. A study conducted by IGS (BRAC) shows that the use of backup facilities have become quite commonplace, though the extent of the use of backup options varies according to the abilities of households to pay (Choudhury 2012).

14.3.5 Telecommunication

Tele communication is an advanced way of enhancing the value of services. It increases the number of consumers by reducing physical mobility. It also plays a dominant role in economic growth and quality of life (Sridhar and Sridhar 2008). Recently, if compared with other traditional infrastructure, telecommunications is more pronounced due to its significant impact on generating economic growth. Information and Communications Technologies (ICT) infrastructure improves the efficiency of communication, marketing, reducing transaction costs, and times and thus increases the firms' output in various economic sectors (Roller and Waverman 2001). Increasing investment in ICT infrastructure and its derived services provide significant benefits to the economy. ICT is now considered as one of the key drivers of the economic competitiveness of cities.

Although the communication sector is relatively new in the country communication infrastructure is improving fast. At present, the total telecommunication transmission cable network is about 14800 km, connecting 59 districts out of 64 (BTRC 2013). There are more than 36 million internet users throughout the country (BTRC 2013) and a large proportion are from the GDR area. Urban areas, especially Dhaka, are enjoying this service the most. In Bangladesh, the number of mobile phone subscribers is about 110 million (BTRC 2013) and this number is increasing very rapidly. On the other hand, internet services are also expanding. In the ICT sector, Dhaka shows progressive growth. Within a decade, Dhaka has created its position globally as a productive and quality outsourcing city. According to some of the US-based leading companies and online agencies, Dhaka ranks third among the cities of the world where online jobs are outsourced from the West (BASIS website 2011). Dhaka wins in this competitive sector due primarily to its cheap labor and good communication command in English.

14.3.6 Health and Education

Healthcare facilities in Bangladesh are poor both in rural and urban areas. However, it is better in urban areas than its rural counterparts. Table 14.4 shows a variety of sources of treatment facilities available in the country. The use of the sources depends on the affordability of the patients.

It can be observed in the table that more than one-third of the patients receive treatment from medicine shops without prescriptions from qualified doctors, even in

Table 14.4 Sources of healthcare facilities in urban and rural areas, 2010

Facilities	Urban (%)	Rural (%)	National (%)
Government health worker	1.70	2.57	2.41
Government doctor (institution)	12.53	8.52	9.28
Government doctor (private)	19.57	13.11	14.34
Private doctor	22.0	25.04	24.46
NGO doctor	0.13	0.22	0.20
NGO health workers	0.64	0.31	0.37
Pharmacy/dispensary/shop	36.05	41.20	40.21
Homeopathic doctor	3.26	3.49	3.44
Traditional healers	0.97	1.44	1.36
Family and self-treatment	1.52	1.48	1.49
Others	1.63	2.62	2.43
Total	100.00	100.00	100.00

Source BBS (2010)

urban areas, where doctors and hospitals are available within very close proximity. It seems that going to a qualified doctor is beyond people's economic ability—a good number of patients even go to traditional healers. It can also be observed that there is a little variation between rural and urban areas. A larger proportion of urban patients (14.23%) avail themselves of government facilities than rural patients (11%).

Healthcare facilities have been increased under private sector development in Bangladesh. Most of these facilities are located in urban areas and Dhaka is the largest hub of such healthcare facilities under private sector. Patients from all over the country come to Dhaka for treatment and most of them go to private hospitals. Government facilities are limited and treatment is slow, thus the preference is for people to go to the private sector, though it is expensive. The poor cannot usually go to private sector hospitals and clinics. Their choices are reflected in the table above.

It is difficult to assess healthcare facilities in the GDR. LGED (2005) has found 114 hospitals and clinics in the Dhaka Metropolitan area. Most of these were developed under the private (formal) sector. All six district headquarters in GDR have at least one general public hospital, 250 beds each. Dhaka City has quite a good number of general and specialized hospitals in the public sector. However, the health infrastructure, whether in the public sector or private, has little accessibility for poor people.

14.4 Environmental Infrastructure and Threats of Climate Change

The physical infrastructure in GDR may face a serious challenge in the future due to the possible impact of climate change and natural disasters. The geological settings, geomorphological conditions, and easy river connectivity are some of the important controls for Dhaka and its growth. The older part of Dhaka is a wide natural levee and relatively at a higher elevation than the surrounding low lying areas in the east, west, and south. Over the past 40 years, the principles of geomorphological controls on urbanization of Dhaka have largely been undermined by the development process. Dhaka's fast-growing population and concentration of services and industries translate to higher consumption of natural resources such as wetlands, canals, and rivers. The City has already been facing pressures from natural disaster migrants in the city. About 20% of all migrants took shelter in the City due to natural disasters (Ishtiaque 2013). Most of these migrants were housed in informal settlements of the city and pressurizes on the available limited infrastructure.

14.5 Infrastructure and the Quality of Life

The paper looks at selected urban key infrastructure and services available in GDR (and in the country) to support the quality of life in Dhaka.[8] The urban population depends largely on the provision of some key infrastructure and basic services. It can be observed in the analysis above that strategic infrastructure, such as transport, water supply, sanitation, power, telecommunication, health, and education are not adequate for supporting the quality life and economy of GDR. Whatever infrastructure has been developed supports the rich in most cases (such as health, education, water, and sanitation). The poor have accessibility problems due to the cost of using facilities being much higher than their affordability.

Secondly, the most crucial condition can be observed in the cases of the transport and power sectors. Both of these sectors suffer from serious problems. The transport sector suffers from poor management and is in disarray as a result and the power sector suffers from supply shortages. It is necessary to develop the major strategic sectors for enhancing the quality of life in the City because:

- Better transport networks make accessibility easier, which reduces travel time and cost.
- Improved telecommunication services increase efficiency in communication, transaction, trade, and business.

[8]Infrastructure data were explored with a limited scope. This is a huge area of research to collate all the information. We have selected some important information to assess how it is related to the quality of life in GDR.

- Reduced utility costs and the availability of utility services increase the possibility of investments being made.
- Job satisfaction, quality of life, and social security increase efficiency as well as the productivity of workers.

References

ADB. (2012). *TA 7641-BAN: Strengthening regional planning and governance*, Unpublished project report. Asian Development Bank and Government of Bangladesh.

Akhtar, S. (2009). On the selection of Dhaka as the capital of Eastern Bengal and Assam 1905–1911. In S. U. Ahmed (Ed.), *Dhaka past, present and future*. Dhaka: Asiatic Society of Bangladesh.

BASIS website. (2011). Dhaka ranks third in global freelance outsourcing work. Dhaka: Bangladesh Association of Software & Information Services. Last browsed 26 March 2019. Available at https://basis.org.bd/media/whats_new_detail/10.

BBS (2004).*Population census-2001 national report (Provisional)*. Dhaka: Bangladesh Bureau of Statistics.

BBS (2010). *Report of the household income and expenditure survey 2010*. Dhaka: Bangladesh Bureau of Statistics.

BBS. (2012). *Population and housing census 2011*. Dhaka: Bangladesh Bureau of Statistics.

BRAC. (2012). *State of cities: Urban governance in Dhaka*. Dhaka: Institute of Governance Studies, BRAC University.

BTRC. (2013). *Mobile phone subscribers in Bangladesh*. Information collected from the official website of BTRC. Last browsed: 14 October 2013. Available at http://www.btrc.gov.bd.

Choudhury, L. A. (2012). Quality of urban life: Service realities. In Z. R. Hossain (ed.), *Bangladesh urban dynamics*. Dhaka: Power and Participation Research Centre (PPRC).

DESCO website. (2013). *Information collected from the official website of DESCO*. Last browsed: 14 October 2013. Available at http://www.desco.org.bd.

DWASA. (2012). *Dhaka WASA newsletter*. Issue no. 05 (July to December 2012). Dhaka: Public Information Department, DWASA.

DWASA. (2013). *Progressive water tariff potentials and challenges*. Unpublished office document presented in a workshop (March 30).

GOB. (2011). *The sixth five year plan 2011–2015*. Dhaka: Planning Commission, Ministry of Planning, Government of Bangladesh.

Ishtiaque, A. (2013). *Natural disasters and migration to Dhaka city*. Unpublished Masters Thesis, Submitted to the Department of Geography University of Dhaka.

Islam, N. (2005). *Dhaka now: Contemporary urban development*. Dhaka: Bangladesh Geographical Society.

LGED. (2005). *Paurashava statistics*. Dhaka: Local Government Engineering Department.

Louis Berger Group Inc. and Bangladesh Consultants Ltd. (2005). *Strategic transport plan for Dhaka*. Dhaka: Ministry of Communications, Government of the Peoples Republic of Bangladesh.

Roller, L. H., & Waverman, L. (2001). Telecommunications infrastructure and economic development: A simultaneous approach. *American Economic Review, 91*(4), 909–923.

Sheesh, K. M. (2010). Water supply in Dhaka in Bangladesh period. In M.A. Islam et al. (Eds.), *Environment of capital Dhaka*. Dhaka: Asiatic Society of Bangladesh.

Sridhar, K. S. & Sridhar, V. (2008). Telecommunications infrastructure and economic growth: Evidence from developing countries. *Applied Econometrics and International Development, 7*(2). Available at SSRN http://ssrn.com/abstract=1250082.

Chapter 15
Spatial Analysis of Educational Facilities and Quality of Life in Haveri District of Karnataka, India

H. Nagaraj, S. L. Karlawad and L. M. Pujar

Abstract Adequate and appropriate educational facilities are essential to the society. The society will no longer survive without education. The development of educational facilities in rural areas will help to improve the socio-economic life of the people as about 75% of the Indian population lives in rural areas. The quality of life has been measured in terms of a variety of suitable criteria; it includes health, education, social, economic and other aspects. These indicators among others reflect the quality of functioning of a social system and efficiency of its economic welfare. The existing educational facilities and socio-economic aspects of the region are necessary for the fulfilment of the aims of the quality of life. The purpose of this study is to examine taluk-wise distribution of such facilities, identify their different levels and suggest the priorities to reduce spatial disparities in the quality of life. The composite Z-score method is used to identify different levels of quality of life and summarizing the components of information. The spatial distribution of educational facilities is categorized into three levels.

Keywords Primary · Secondary · Educational facilities · Attainments · Socio-economic · Quality of life

H. Nagaraj (✉)
Mysore University, Mysore, Karnataka, India
e-mail: nagarajh66@yahoo.com

S. L. Karlawad
RR Women's College, Ranebennur, Karnataka, India
e-mail: slkarawad@gmail.com

L. M. Pujar
GFG College, Hirekerur, Karnataka, India
e-mail: laxmanpujarblr@gmail.com

B. R. K. Sinha (ed.), *Multidimensional Approach to Quality of Life Issues*,
https://doi.org/10.1007/978-981-13-6958-2_15

15.1 Introduction

Adequate and appropriate educational facilities are essential to the society. The society will no longer survive without education. The strong educational base of any society will have better prospect for its overall development. Today, the Science and Technology with Information Technology provides better avenues of employment to strengthen livelihood of the people. With this viewpoint everyone should avail the opportunity of achieving better quality education. The government or private sectors jointly make an attempt to provide education to the people; as a result, the educational institutions in India have emerged to gain much significance.

India being a developing country struggles to educate downtrodden and emerging as one of the most strong, stable and equalitarian societies of the world. The traditional order of social life in India till the beginning of the British rule was predominately rural or agrarian, based on caste and joint family systems, social structure. Vast majority of Indian population lived and made their livings in lakhs of tiny villages. The community of life was very rigidly organized on the basis of caste and sub-caste groups to provide with non-formal types of education. The children generation after generation continued to learn the traditional skills by pursuing from their respective family occupation.

Education is one of the important sectors of a region as it affects standard of living and employment and the sector is expanding rapidly due to the amazing growth of population. The real wealth of a country is its population (human resource) with good education which works as a base for development of the nation. People always think to satisfy their basic needs in the immediate vicinity. Wherever man lives, he has to adapt himself to his surrounding environment in order to meet the fundamental necessities. The first step for a 'regular development programme is to provide infrastructural facilities for rural development'. The development of educational facilities in rural area will help improve the quality of life of the people as about 75% of the Indian population lives in rural areas. In educational literature, 'educational development has been defined as the development of men in terms of knowledge and innovative skills'. In actual practice, the quality of life has been measured in terms of a variety of suitable criteria; it includes education, health, socio-economic aspects of people and infrastructural facilities, etc. These indicators among others reflect the quality of functioning of a socio-cultural system and efficiency of its economic welfare.

According to the World Bank 'Successful development entails more than investing in physical capital or closing the gap in capital. It also entails acquiring and using knowledge as well as closing the gaps in knowledge'[1]. India stands distinctly from the third world countries in implementing massive expansion of educational systems. The post-independent India has observed 'educational miracle' since the inception of economic plans, 1951.

[1]http://openknowledge.worldbank.org/handle/10986/5982.Lic.IGO.

The role of education in socio-economic development has been recognized ever since the days of Plato. Plato believed that education is indispensable for the 'economic health of a structured society'. Primary and secondary education is the major concern of all the nations. It is a base for a successful socio-economic transformation. Universalization of education is taken as a challenge by all the nations. School education is the base for the development of human resources.

Education is considered to be their most valuable socio-cultural asset and is an important indicator of lifestyle and socio-economic status. It focuses on the living standard of both the rural and urban people and access to the other amenities. Educational facilities reflect a human quality of life. It is an important goal of Indian development planning. Education is an important indicator of social welfare. Improvement in education is of pivotal significance to the development of traditional societies. Education helps an individual to improve his/her skill, to shed his/her ignorance and to understand the value of social justice. Education is more important in the case of socially deprived groups like the females and scheduled castes and tribes. Structural transformation of working force which manifests economic diversification of an economy may be taken as the barometer of economic well-being of the people of an area, and thus, form an important dimension of quality of life.

Among the various qualities of a population, educational attainment is essential to improve the quality of people. A low degree of literacy and lack of adequate facilities of education is serious obstacle to economic improvement in any region. Education is essential for eradicating poverty.

After independence, several plans and policies have been taken in India to drive out illiteracy completely but the disparity and discrepancy exist in many dimensions. 'India's progress in providing access to quality and relevant education to its children and youth is a story of mixed results, with some remarkable outcomes and some nonstarters. While India can contribute a large number of human resources to the pool of the world's most educated, scientifically and technically qualified people, it is equally appalling that the same country accounts for more than a third of the world's illiterates also (YOJANA January 2010, p. 35).[2]' This variation is mainly concerned with the inter-regional disparity in educational development.

Present study is an attempt to throw light on the disparity of education covering seven taluks of Haveri district. Educational attainments and facilities at primary and secondary levels and socio-economic factors reveal the quality of life.

[2]http://yojana.gov.in/cms/pdf/…/2010/January.p.35.

15.2 Objectives

i. Analyse the variations of primary and secondary education facilities and socio-economic status of Haveri district.
ii. Identify the spatial disparities in the quality of life of people in the study area.

15.3 Database

The primary and secondary data have been collected from district and taluka's head-quarters. In the present analysis, a set of 15 indicators from primary and 14 from secondary educational facilities have been taken into account to determine the levels of educational development at one hand and ten from socio-economic aspects on the other hand in the seven taluks of the district. In the first step, the raw data for each variable which determines the areal variations of educational facilities and socio-economic status have been computed into standard score (Table 15.1).

Table 15.1 Primary, secondary education and socio-economic indicators in Haveri district 2010–2011

Primary educational indicators	Secondary educational indicators	Socio-economic indicators
Enrolment ratio of students/1000 population (V1)	Enrolment ratio of students/1000 population (V16)	Literacy rate (V31)
No. of schools/1000 population (V2)	No. of schools/1000 population (V17)	No. of doctors/1000 pop (V32)
Students–teacher ratio (V3)	Students–teacher ratio (V18)	No. of beds/1000 pop (V33)
Students–school ratio (V4)	Students–school ratio (V19)	% of urban pop to total pop (V34)
Teacher–school ratio (V5)	Teacher–school ratio (V20)	% of SC/ST pop (V35)
% of dropout children (7–14 age group (V6))	% of dropout children (7–14 age group (V6))	No of post offices/lakh pop (V36)
% of SC/ST children in primary school (V7)	% of SC/ST children in primary school (V22)	No. of telephones/lakh pop (V37)
% of availability of toilet facilities (V8)	% of availability of toilet facilities (V23)	Road length/100sq.kms area (V38)
% of electricity supplies (V9)	% of electricity supplies (V24)	No of agri. Co-opp society/lakh pop (V39)
% of playground (V10)	% of playground (V25)	Average size of land holdings (V40)
% of ramp (V11)	% of compound wall (V27)	

(continued)

Table 15.1 (continued)

Primary educational indicators	Secondary educational indicators	Socio-economic indicators
% of compound wall (V12)	% of drinking water facilities (V28)	
% of drinking water facilities (V13)	% of library facilities (V29)	
% of library facilities (V14)	% of computer facilities (V30)	
% of computer facilities (V15)		

15.4 Methodology

The quantitative techniques as well as the statistical methods have been employed in the study. The distribution of primary and secondary school facilities has been studied by employing Z-score value method.

$$Z = \frac{Vi - Vm}{\delta}$$

where

Z Standard score of value.
Vi Actual value of ith unit.
Vm Average value of ith series of data.
δ Standard deviation of ith series.

To achieve objectives and spatial gaps have been discussed using tabular form. The reliable indicators are selected and grouped into three components, namely, primary education development, secondary education development and socio-economic development. These components aggregated to find the levels of quality of life.

15.5 Study Area

Haveri district has been named after the district headquarter "Haveri" city with creation of the new district in 1997[3] (GOK. RD, 42, LRD 87, 39) with Haveri as the headquarters. As per as the study area is concerned, it is situated in the cental part of Karnataka state and falls within the northern maidan. The district lies between 14° 19′ and 15° 9′ north latitudes and between 75°1′ and 75° 50′ east longitudes. The district is surrounded by Dharwad district in the northwest, Gadag in the north, Ballary in the east, Shivamogga in the south and North Canara district in the west. The

[3]Haveri was formed vide GOK Notification No. RD. 42. LRD. 87 (part-III) dated. 02.08.1997.

district is divided into seven taluks—Byadagi, Hangal, Haveri, Hirekerur, Ranebennur, Savanur and Shiggoun. It has a dimension of 111 km of length north to south and 87 km east to west. The district covers an area of 4848 square kilometres, Haveri district lies in the catchment area of the Varda, Kumadvati and the Dharma River. In the south-eastern and eastern sector, for a distance of about 130 km, the River Tungabhadra forms the natural boundary. As per as 2011 census is concerned, the population of Haveri district was 14.39 lakhs. It stands in twentieth ranks in terms of area and twenty-fifth in terms of population. The literacy rate of Haveri district is 77.6%. This is higher than the state average of 75.61%. The percentage of literates among male is 84.2% as against 70.7% of female literacy rate.

15.6 Development of Education in Haveri District

Haveri is an emerging district of Karnataka State. Progress in education and literacy rates are the most evolving factors for the overall development of the district. It is observed that socio-economic factors have a direct impact on the literacy level. Enrolments in schools have improved substantially because of the significant implementation of SSA and RMSA. It is also observed that the retention rate is very poor in rural areas. This is because many of the students are from agriculture families and the children inevitably have to associate their parents engaged in farm activities. There is a greater need to create literacy awareness among the parents.

15.7 Distribution of Different Levels of Educational Development

Among various qualities of a population, the education attainment and facilities are essential to improve the quality of life of people. Lack of adequate facilities of education is serious obstacles not only for the economic improvement but also for livelihood in any region. Therefore, primary and secondary school attainment and facilities are considered to identify the levels of educational development.

15.7.1 Levels of Primary Educational Development

Levels primary education development has been identified with the 15 indicators. Table 15.2 shown that there exist a spatial variation of primary education facilities among the taluks of Haveri district; based on the composite score value, taluks are categorized into three groups as high with more than 0.6091, medium with 0.1920–0.6091, and low with the less than 0.1920.

Table 15.2 Primary educational attainments (PEA) and facilities in Haveri district 2010–2011 (figures in the bracket are Z-score values)

Name of taluks	Primary educational attainments							Primary educational facilities								Composite value of Z-score
	X1	X2	X3	X4	X5	X6	X7	X8	X9	X10	X11	X12	X13	X14	X15	
Byadagi	99.77 (0.0153)	0.75 (0.0833)	22 (−0.8382)	133 (−0.1715)	6 (0.8690)	1.17 (0.5368)	32.86 (1.1856)	91.50 (−0.0924)	95.28 (−0.8783)	56.60 (−0.2137)	90.56 (0.0665)	86.79 (1.4378)	98.11 (0.7659)	87.73 (−2.0727)	15.09 (0.8631)	0.2224
Hanagal	109.33 (0.8310)	0.85 (0.8800)	25 (0.2641)	128 (−0.4573)	5 (−1.1519)	0.61 (−2.1961)	26.89 (−0.5663)	84.75 (−1.5440)	97.25 (0.4527)	65.91 (2.1552)	80.26 (−1.8916)	74.43 (−0.3482)	98.65 (1.1489)	96.41 (0.6740)	11.21 (−0.6121)	−0.1168
Haveri	89.74 (−0.8404)	0.57 (−1.3600)	25 (0.2641)	156 (1.1433)	6 (0.8690)	1.10 (0.1952)	29.74 (0.2699)	98.75 (1.4666)	99.37 (1.8851)	54.03 (−0.8676)	89.44 (−0.1463)	85.71 (1.2817)	98.13 (0.7801)	96.27 (0.6297)	16.14 (1.2623)	0.9761
Hirekerur	96.69 (−0.2474)	0.89 (1.2000)	20 (−1.5703)	108 (−1.6007)	5 (1.1519)	1.33 (1.3177)	30.44 (0.4754)	94.66 (0.5870)	95.63 (−0.6418)	58.78 (0.3409)	97.08 (1.3060)	75.24 (−0.2312)	96.11 (−0.6524)	94.17 (−0.0348)	10.19 (−1.0000)	0.0572
Ranebennur	78.31 (−1.8156)	0.57 (−1.3600)	23 (−0.4696)	137 (0.0571)	6 (0.8690)	1.11 (0.2440)	32.46 (1.0682)	94.27 (0.5032)	96.35 (0.1854)	54.68 (0.0610)	86.45 (−0.7148)	70.31 (−0.9436)	97.91 (0.6241)	98.43 (1.3132)	11.97 (0.0570)	−0.0459
Savanur	114.65 (1.2849)	0.69 (−0.0500)	29 (1.7317)	164 (1.6007)	6 (0.8690)	1.05 (−0.0488)	26.97 (−0.5429)	85.84 (−1.3096)	94.69 (−1.2770)	58.40 (0.2442)	92.03 (0.3460)	78.76 (0.2774)	94.69 (1.6595)	93.80 (−0.1518)	15.92 (1.1787)	0.8303
Shiggaon	108.65 (0.7730)	0.86 (0.9600)	26 (0.6310)	126 (−0.5716)	5 (−1.1519)	1.10 (0.1952)	22.41 (−1.8811)	93.78 (0.3978)	97.53 (0.6418)	53.70 (−0.9516)	95.67 (1.0380)	66.66 (−1.4710)	95.67 (−0.9645)	93.20 (−0.3417)	9.25 (−1.3574)	−0.5791
District	97.17	0.72	24	134	6	1.04	28.77	91.91	96.81	57.86	90.97	75.92	97.16	94.84	12.38	AM = 0.1319
Arithmetic Mean	99.59	0.74	24.28	136	5.57	1.06	28.82	91.93	96.58	57.44	90.21	76.84	97.03	94.28	12.82	
S.D	11.72	0.13	2.72	17.49	0.49	0.21	3.40	40.65	1.48	3.93	5.26	6.92	1.41	3.16	2.63	

Source Computed by author

Table 15.3 Levels of primary educational development—Haveri district

Category	Composite value	Taluks	Taluka name
High	>0.6091	02	Haveri, Savanur
Medium	0.1920–0.6091	01	Byadagi
Low	<0.1920	04	Hanagal, Hirekerur, Ranebennur, Shiggaon

Source Computed by author from DDPI annual report 2011–12. Haveri district

Areas of high level of primary education development are marked in two taluks, Haveri taluk which is situated in the central part and the Savanur taluk which is situated in the eastern edge of the district. Highest composite score value of primary educational status was observed in Haveri (0.9761) taluk followed by Savanur (0.8303) taluk (Table 15.3).

Only one taluk is identified in the medium category, namely, Byadagi which is situated in the central part of the district. The composite score of the taluk (0.2224) is recorded. The remaining four taluks found in low category, namely, Hirekerur (0.05720), Hangal (−0.1168), Shiggaon (−0.5791), and Ranebennur (−0.0459), which are formed low-level pattern due to lack of educational facilities (Fig. 15.1).

The high composite Z-score value in Haveri and Savanur taluks indicates good availability of primary educational facilities. This may be due to location of the headquarter of Haveri city itself in Haveri taluk where the urban influences and development of transportation network are better, whereas Savanur taluk has strong historical background, greater size of landholding, and low density of SC/ST population which leads to the development of primary education.

15.7.2 Secondary Education Development

Secondary educational facilities are playing an important role in improving the level of standard living and ability to face the social problems. The spatial distribution of secondary school facilities has been grouped into three levels. The level of development has been derived on the basis of 15 reliable indicators. Composite score is obtained by aggregating as indicated in Table 15.4. The taluks are categorized into three levels as high with value of more than 0.7113, and low level with less than 0.1539.

It has been observed that two taluks come under high-level category. The maximum educational facilities exist in Byadagi with 1.1623 followed by Ranebennur with 0.9170. It can, therefore, be concluded that the level of development is better in areas traversed by major transport arteries (Table 15.5).

Table 15.4 Secondary educational attainments (PEA) and facilities in Haveri district 2010–2011 (figures in the bracket are Z-score values)

Name of taluks	Secondary educational attainments							Secondary educational facilities							Composite value of Z-score
	X16	X17	X18	X19	X20	X21	X22	X23	X24	X25	X26	X27	X28	X29	
Byadagi	56.14 (2.0881)	0.26 (1.25)	27 (0.1164)	208 (0.7708)	8 (0.6735)	2.33 (0.9643)	48.20 (1.5899)	76.31 (−0.1879)	94.73 (0.4191)	89.47 (0.2810)	89.47 (0.4889)	92.10 (−0.6225)	89.47 (−0.6314)	92.10 (0.9363)	**1.1623**
Hanagal	41.14 (−0.7260)	0.21 (−0.3125)	26 (0.2850)	188 (−0.2569)	7 (−0.2619)	1.78 (−1.0756	45.94 (0.4809)	66.66 (−1.0814)	92.98 (0.1494)	87.71 (−0.1311)	84.21 (−0.5651)	92.98 (−0.2801)	92.98 (0.1573)	85.96 (−0.4590)	**−0.5824**
Haveri	39.69 (−0.9981)	0.21 (−0.3125)	22 (−1.8901)	185 (-0.4110	9 (1.6089)	2.22 (0.5563)	43.82 (−0.5594)	90.00 (1.0796)	100.00 (1.2311)	90.00 (0.4051)	86.66 (−0.0741)	96.66 (1.2996)	95.00 (0.6112)	90.00 (0.4590)	**0.4294**
Hirekerur	47.50 (0.4671)	0.29 (2.1875)	25 (−0.6865)	161 (−1.6443)	6 (−0.1973)	2.54 (1.7433	42.67 (−1.1237	75.00 (−0.3092)	92.64 (0.0970)	92.64 (1.0234)	89.70 (0.5350)	97.05 (1.3035)	92.64 (0.0808)	83.82 (−0.9454)	**0.2188**
Ranebennur	40.52 (−0.8424)	0.21 (−0.3125)	30 (1.3208)	189 (−0.2055)	6 (−1.1973)	1.97 (−0.3709)	42.51 (−1.2022)	95.83 (1.6194)	98.61 (1.0169)	91.66 (0.7939)	95.83 (1.7635)	95.83 (0.8287)	98.61 (1.4224)	95.83 (1.7840)	**0.9170**
Savanur	46.76 (0.3283)	0.20 (−0.6250)	29 (0.9193)	229 (1.8499)	8 (0.673.5)	1.81 (−0.9643)	44.44 (−0.2551)	63.63 (−1.3620)	81.81 (−1.5701)	87.87 (−0.0936)	84.84 (−0.4388)	90.90 (−1.0894)	93.93 (0.3707)	84.84 (−0.7136)	**−0.4243**
Shiggaon	43.36 (−0.3095)	0.22 (0.0001)	28 (0.5179)	194 (0.0513)	7 (−0.2619)	1.88 (−0.7047	47.15 (1.0746)	80.95 (0.2416)	83.33 (-1.3374)	78.57 (2.2716)	78.57 (−1.6953)	90.40 (−1.2840)	83.33 (−2.0112)	83.33 (−1.0568)	**−0.6434**
District	43.83	0.23	26	189	7	2.08	44.66	80.00	93.42	88.91	87.83	94.32	92.97	88.37	**0.0965**
Arithmetic Mean	**45.01**	**0.22**	**26.71**	**193.42**	**7.28**	**2.07**	**44.93**	**78.34**	**72.01**	**88.27**	**87.03**	**93.70**	**92.28**	**87.98**	
S.D	**5.33**	**0.03**	**2.49**	**19.46**	**1.06**	**0.26**	**2.03**	**10.80**	**6.49**	**4.27**	**4.99**	**2.57**	**4.45**	**4.40**	

Source Computed by author

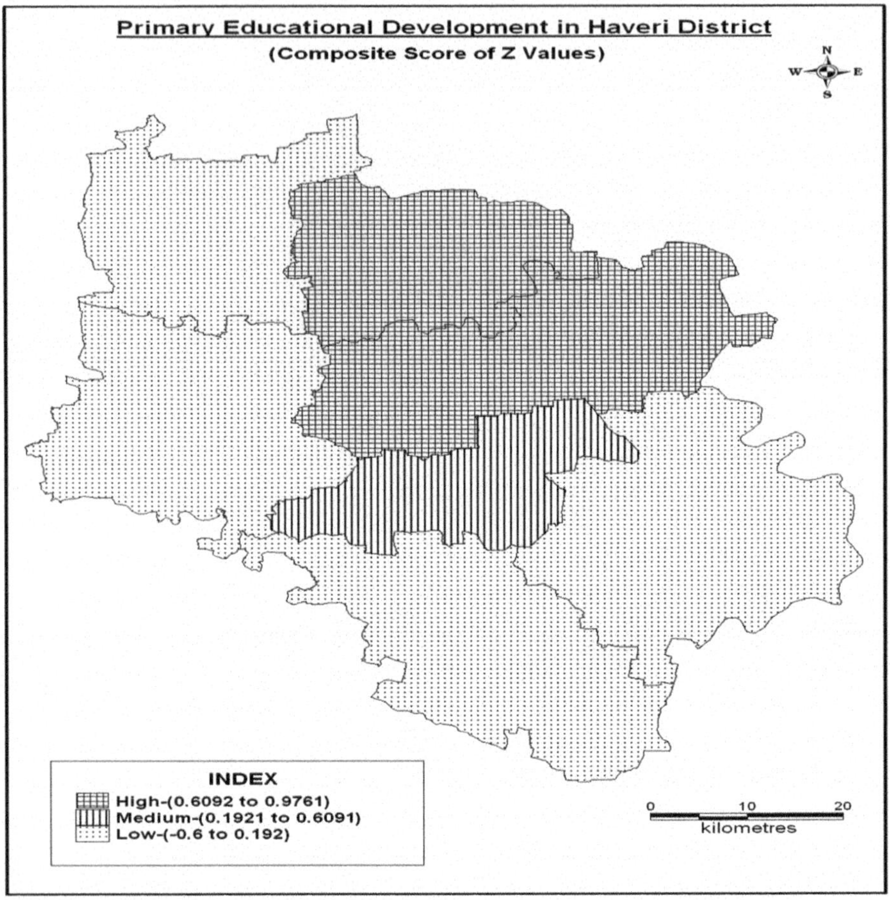

Fig. 15.1 Taluka-wise distribution of primary educational attainments and facilities. Taluks shown are based on composite Z-score value. *Source* Author. Data from DDPI Annual Report-2012, Haveri District

Table 15.5 Secondary educational development—Haveri district

Category	Composite value	Taluks	Taluka name
High	>0.7113	02	Byadagi, Ranebennur
Medium	0.1539–0.7113	02	Haveri, Hirekerur
Low	<0.1539	03	Shiggaon, Hanagal, Savanur

Source Computed by author from DDPI annual report 2011–2012 Haveri district

It has been observed that two taluks come under high-level category. The maximum educational facilities exist in Byadagi with 1.1623 followed by Ranebennur with 0.9170. It can, therefore, be concluded that the level of development is better in areas traversed by major transport arteries.

Figure 15.2 clearly shows that the medium category of educational development ranging between the composite Z-score value of 0.1539 and 0.7113 includes Haveri and Hirekerur taluks. The first one is located in the central part of the district and the second one lies at the eastern edge of the district. The low category (<0.1539) of secondary educational status was demarcated in three taluks, namely, Shiggaon (−0.6434), Hanagal (−0.5824) and Savanur (−0.4243) taluks formed pattern in northern part of the district, where there is dominance of agro-economic activities that lead to the lack of educational facilities and less number of secondary schools.

15.7.3 Socio-Economic Development

Socio-economic aspects are directed towards the improvement of standard of living of people. Socio-economic development is also multi-dimensional phenomena, which is governed by several factors of an area. It is important to assess the socio-economic development of Haveri district and to identify and classify taluks according to their aggregate level of development. For the socio-economic development, appropriate ten indicators were taken into consideration and combined into one component. The value of composite index of all the taluks has been given in Table 15.6, and on the basis of composite scores, taluks have grouped into three categories. It is pointing to high level (>0.4377), medium (0.0967–0.4377) and low (<0.0967) category. The higher socio-economic status was found in Ranebennur taluk (Fig. 15.3). This taluk is located in the south-eastern part of the district (Table 15.7).

Hirekerur (0.3022) and Haveri (0.2868) taluks are observed in the level of medium socio-economic development. These two taluks located in the central part of the district exist from west to east. There are four taluks in the low-level category. Out of theme Byadagi (0.0802) taluk was found at the lower portion of the development. This is followed by Shiggaon (−0.5236), Savanur (−0.1774) and Hangal (−0.1265) taluks in descending order. The taluks form its region in the north and western portion of the district.

15.8 Levels of Quality of Life in Haveri District

Quality of life is the result of interplay of economic, social, educational and institutional factors. So a comprehensive developmental plan incorporating the economic, social and educational components would be a visionary approach for the quality of life of people of this region.

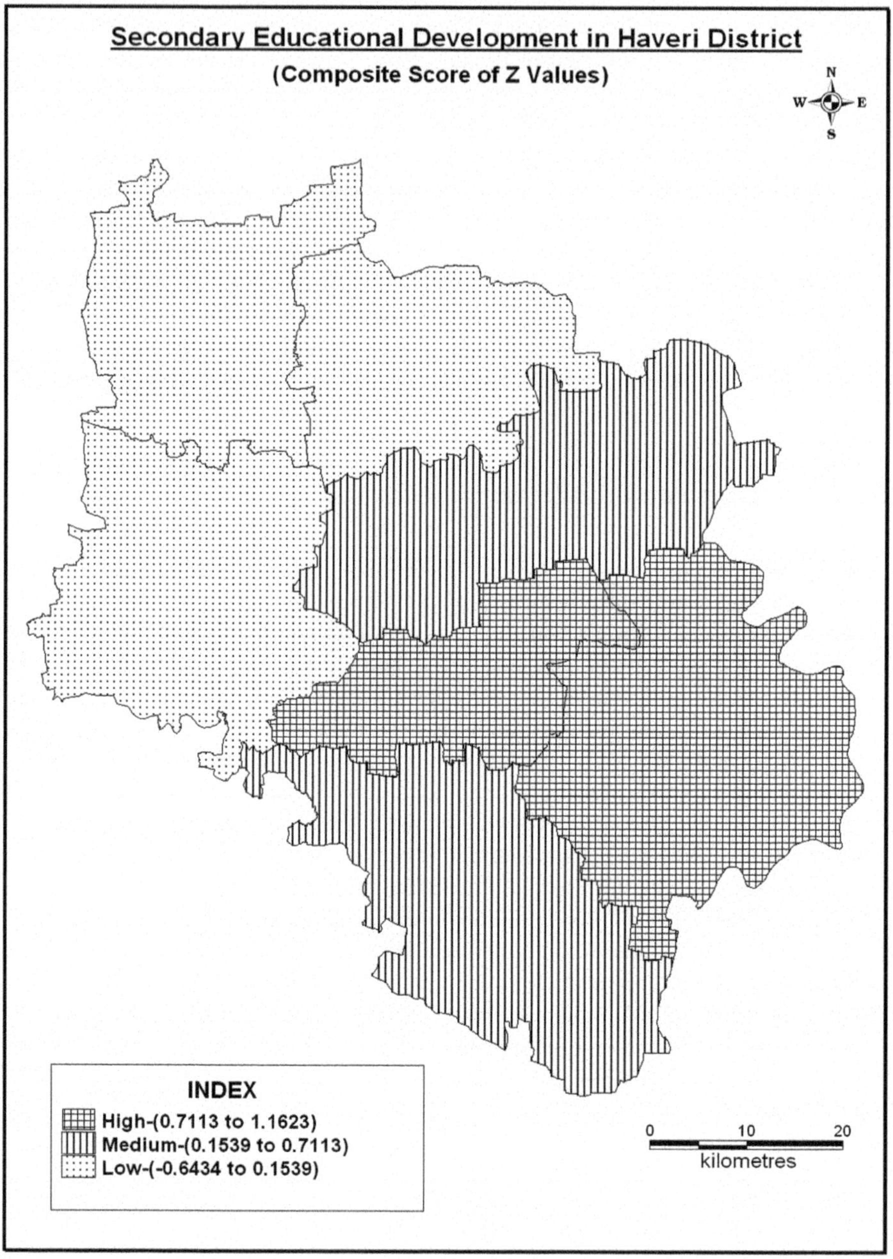

Fig. 15.2 Taluka-wise distribution of secondary educational attainments and facilities. Taluks shown are based on composite Z-score value. *Source* Author. Data from DDPI Annual Report-2012, Haveri District

Table 15.6 Socio-economic indicators of development in Haveri district 2010–2011

Taluks	X30	X31	X32	X33	X34	X35	X36	X37	X38	X39	Composite score of Z Value
Byadagi	77.5 (0.1830)	3 (−0.5590)	10 (−0.7601)	21 (−0.0800)	25.60 (1.6279)	16 (−0.2121)	893 (0.2476)	53.88 (0.7068)	19 (−0.0689)	4.76 (−0.5333)	0.0802
Hanagal	77.7 (0.2535)	3 (−0.5590)	11 (−0.4933)	11 (−1.2074)	22.90 (0.0581)	17 (0.2929)	770 (−0.0668)	56.24 (1.1975)	18 (−0.5615)	4.87 (0.2001)	−0.1265
Haveri	76.6 (−0.1338)	6 (1.8031)	15 (0.5733)	24 (0.2581)	22.01 (−0.4651)	14 (−1.2222)	1354 (1.4265)	49.25 (−0.2557)	20 (0.4236)	4.78 (−0.4001)	0.2868
Hirekerur	81.4 (1.5563)	3 (−0.5590)	12 (−0.2266)	08 (−1.5456)	24.01 (0.6976)	20 (1.8080)	436 (−0.9209)	54.99 (0.9376)	23 (1.9014)	4.61 (−1.5333)	0.3022
Ranebennur	78.4 (0.5001)	5 (1.0157)	21 (2.1733)	36 (1.6110)	21.90 (−0.5232)	14 (1.2222)	1335 (1.3779	41.10 (−1.9501)	20 (0.4236)	4.84 (4.84)	0.8357
Savanur	71.2 (−2.0352)	2 (−1.3464)	9 (1.0266)	25 (0.3709)	23.50 (0.4069)	18 (0.7979)	433 (−0.9286)	50.22 (−0.0540)	16 (−1.5467)	5.15 (2.0666)	−0.1774
Shiggaon	76.1 (−0.3098)	4 (0.2283)	12 (−0.2266)	27 (0.5963)	19.70 (−1.8022)	16 (−0.2121)	352 (−1.1357)	47.71 (−0.5758)	18 (−0.5615)	4.89 (0.3333)	−0.5236
District	77.4	4	14	22	22.60	16	878	50.14	20	4.83	0.0967
A.M	76.98	3.71	12.85	21.71	22.80	16.42	796.14	50.48	19.14	4.84	
S.D	2.84	1.27	3.75	8.87	1.72	1.98	391.05	4.81	2.03	0.15	

Source Computed by author

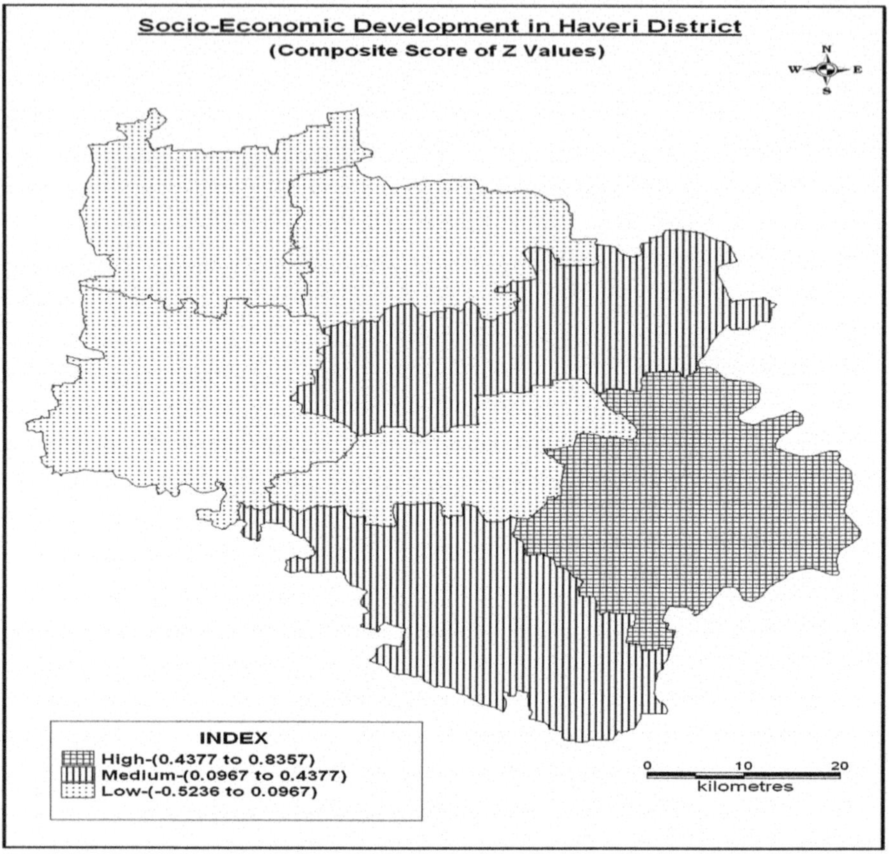

Fig. 15.3 Taluka-wise distribution of socio-economic factors. Taluks shown are based on composite value of Z-score. *Source* Author. Data from District Statistical and Economic Department- Report (District at a Glance)-2012. Haveri District

Tabel 15.7 Socio-economic development—Haveri district

Category	Composite value	Taluks	Taluka name
High	>0.4377	01	Ranebennur
Medium	0.0967–0.4377	02	Haveri, Hirekerur
Low	<0.0967	04	Byadagi, Hanagal, Savanur, Shiggaon

Source Computed by author from district at a glance 2011–2012 Haveri district

This unit of study deals with the measurement and analysis of the level of living at taluka level with a view to work out imbalance in the spatial distribution of educational amities regarding the quality of life in the district. For the purpose of micro-regional study, it would be desirable to combine various individual indices together to reflect the overall picture of the concepts of spatial distribution of amenities of quality life of population. The composite value of Z-scores was obtained by aggregating individual components of quality of life. For this purpose, primary educational attainment and facilities, secondary educational attainment and facilities and socio-economic aspects of population were taken into consideration to identify the quality of life of the people of the district.

15.9 Quality of Life Index Analysis

Here, the composite score of three components of quality of life was aggregated. Table 15.8 explains the positive value of the Z-scores which means high levels of living, while negative value means low level of living. The taluk-wise spatial distribution of educational facilities has been categorized at three levels, viz. high (>1.3772), medium (0.4427–1.3772) and low (<0.4427) level on the basis of availability of educational facilities in the concerned taluk. Table 15.9 clearly depicts the pattern of standard of living at taluka level and points the availability of educational facilities and progress of socio-economic development.

An examination of Fig. 15.4 reveals that there are three taluks that have very high composite score of quality of life. They are Ranebennur (1.7068), Haveri (1.6923) and Byadagi (1.4649) and have their position in the south and central part of the district. The taluks of high score value form a compact region, which is very well known as an urban and industrial centre. Developmental activities are agglomerated in and around the taluka's headquarters. The region has been benefited from the liberal private investment in educational, medical and other social sectors. The urban nodal activities located in the urban centres have influenced for high standard of living.

Areas of medium development have noted in Hirekerur (0.5782) taluk which is located in western part of the district and is benefited from expansion of industrial and tertiary activities centred in the taluk. Thus, the post-independence development in the socio-economic aspects has significantly been helpful to understand the micro-level development of quality of life.

There are three taluks in the low-level category of quality of life. They are Savanur (0.2286), Shiggon (−1.7461) and Hanagal (−0.8257) and are found located in the northern part of the district. This part is socio-economically backward dominated by primary nature of economic activities due to negligence of developmental activities.

Table 15.8 Indicators of educational facilities and regional development in Haveri district 2010–2011

Sl. No	Taluks	Composite scores of primary education			Composite scores of secondary education			Composite scores of socio-economic development	Composite scores of quality of life
		Attainment	Facilities	Total composite scores	Attainment	Facilities	Total composite scores		
1	Byadagi	0.2400	−0.0176	0.2224	1.0647	0.0976	1.1623	0.0802	1.4649
2	Hanagal	−0.3423	0.2255	−0.1168	−0.2667	−0.3157	−0.5824	−0.1265	−0.8257
3	Haveri	0.0773	0.8988	0.9761	−0.2865	0.7159	0.4294	0.2868	1.6923
4	Hirekerur	0.1038	−0.0466	0.0572	−0.0362	0.2550	0.2188	0.3022	0.5782
5	Ranebennur	−0.2009	0.1550	−0.0459	−0.4014	1.3184	0.9170	0.8357	1.7068
6	Savanur	0.6920	0.1382	0.8303	0.2752	−0.6995	−0.4243	−0.1774	0.2286
7	Shiggaon	−0.1493	−0.4298	−0.5791	0.0525	−0.6959	−0.6959	−0.5236	−1.7461
8	District mean	−0.0827	0.1319	0.1920	0.0573	0.0965	0.1539	0.0967	0.4427
	SD	–	–	0.41	–	–	0.55	0.34	0.93

Source Computed by author

Table 15.9 Levels of quality of life in Haveri district

Category	Composite value	Taluks	Taluka name
High	>1.3772	03	Ranebennur, Haveri, Byadagi
Medium	0.4427–1.3772	01	Hirekerur
Low	<0.4427	03	Savanur, Shiggaon, Hanagal

Source Based on author calculation

The drop-outs particularly of girls have been common phenomena in the district. This is noted as a result of poor socio-cultural development. The educational backwardness among weaker sections is more pronounced, and it is found that even when education is subsidized at all levels; the weaker sections are still away from education. Poverty is also one of the hindrances in the way of enhancement of quality of life.

15.10 Recommendations

Looking into the above picture, it can be said that there is need for formulation and implementation of the planning model; first preference should be given to investment in infrastructure and proper implementation of SSA and RMSA programmes. In order to develop the various components of quality of life, attention must be given to develop different taluks falling under low-level category. The 40 indicators of quality of life should be considered into care to less-developed taluks, so that the quality of life in such areas will also be of at most important with priorities.

15.11 Conclusions

Education facilities and socio-economic characteristics are needed for the betterment of any society or quality of life of people, and more so in case of the Haveri district. In most of taluks, where infrastructures have already in existence, display high level of quality of life. Included in such a category are Ranebennur, Byadagi and Haveri taluks influenced by urbanization and high concentration of educational facilities. Northern and south-western areas are acute distress in terms of quality of life. It indicates that the modern developmental programmes are ignored. From policy angle, such areas require the highest attention of the government to improve the level of quality of life.

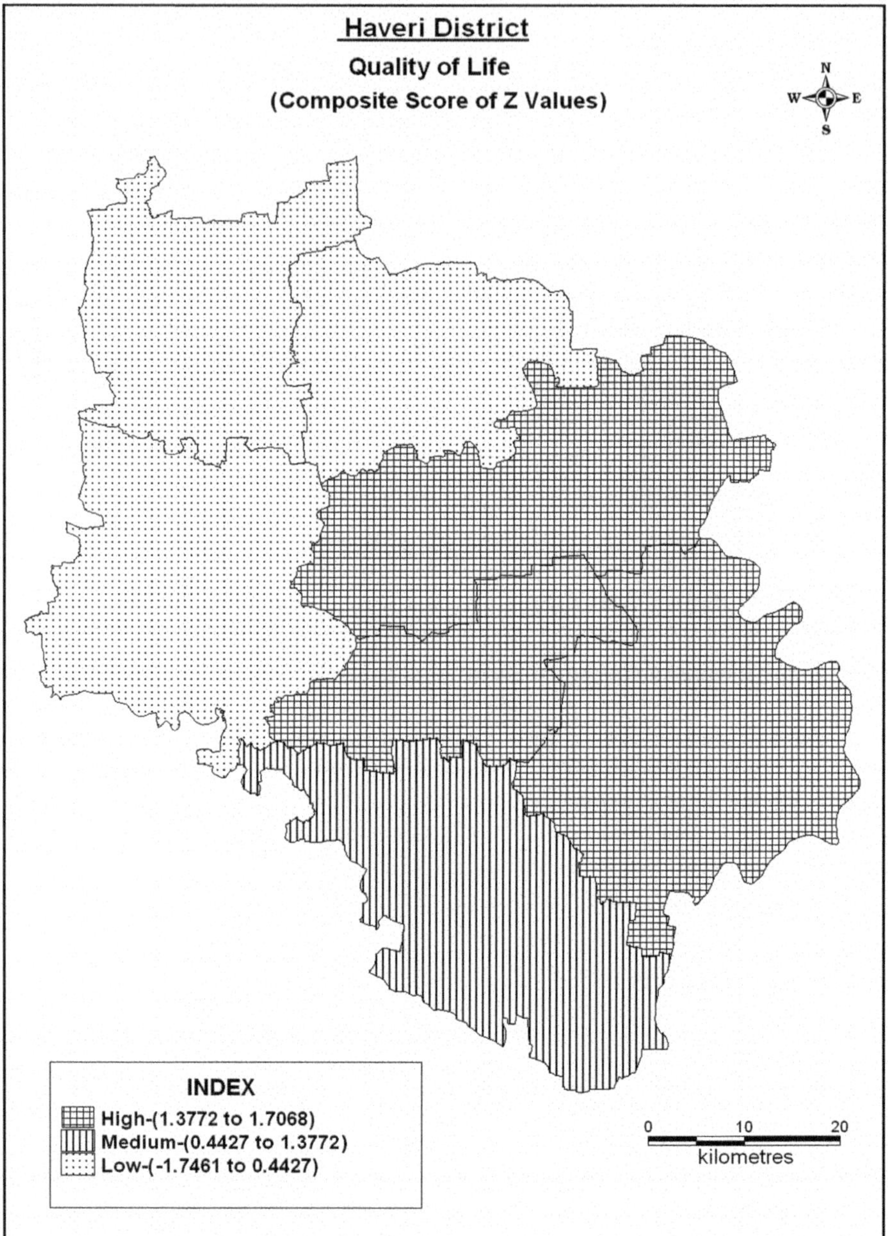

Fig. 15.4 Taluk-wise quality of life based on the composite Z-score value. *Source* Author. Data from DDPI Annual Report and District at a Glance-2011–12. Haveri District, Karnataka

References

Haveri was formed vide GOK Notification No.RD.42.LRD.87 (part-III) dated.02.08.1997.
http://openknowledge.worldbank.org/handle/10986/5982.Lic.IGO.
http://yojana.gov.in/cms/pdf/ 2010 January p.35.
www.censusindia.gov.in Primary Abstract 2011, p. 59.
www.censusindia.gov.in, DCHB 2.2011. p. 172.

Chapter 16
Vulnerability, Resilience and Quality of Life: A Micro Level Study of Ghoramara Island in the Sundarban Region of West Bengal, India

Angshumita Chakraborty and L. N. Satpati

Abstract Climate change has become a burning issue worldwide as the effects of it on the human beings are gradually increasing. The Millennium Development Goals (MDG) and Sustainable Livelihood (SL) are difficult to be achieved by the rural communities due to the climatic hazards in a socio-economically marginal area like the Sundarban. The study area is situated in a high-risk region of climatic accidents, which are occurring with increasing frequency and intensity day by day and generates fear, tension, stress, insecurity, social vulnerability as well as marginalization. As a result the quality of life, which can be viewed from the aspect of satisfaction regarding living conditions is deteriorating as some indicators of it are directly linked with vulnerability as well as resilience of people to the climatic uncertainties. The study area selected for the present problem is Ghoramara, an isolated island of the Sundarban which has already become popular as a vanishing island since parts of the island like Lohachara has been disappeared from the map. Frequent attack of different environmental hazards like cyclone, flood, tidal surge, periodic water logging arising out of extreme climatic events affects quality of life of the islanders. As a result, poor and marginalized people suffer the most resulting in poor living condition as well as outmigration of the inhabitants in a large number and emergence of environmental refugees. In this context, this paper throws light on different dimensions of resilience like human, financial, social, physical and natural capital of the people of the study area to deal with climatic shocks so that it helps to strengthen the adaptive capacity of the vulnerable community to sustain a decent quality of life of this fragile area.

Keywords Climatic hazards · Quality of life · Vulnerability · Resilience · The Sundarban

A. Chakraborty
Department of Geography, Mahishadal Girls' College, Medinipur, India

L. N. Satpati (✉)
Department of Geography, University of Calcutta, Kolkata, India
e-mail: satpati.ln@hotmail.com

B. R. K. Sinha (ed.), *Multidimensional Approach to Quality of Life Issues*,
https://doi.org/10.1007/978-981-13-6958-2_16

16.1 Introduction

Climate change has become a burning issue worldwide as the effects of it on the human beings are gradually increasing. The Millennium Development Goals (MDG) and Sustainable Livelihood (SL) are difficult to be achieved by the rural communities due to the climatic hazards in a socio-economically marginal area like the Sundarban. The study area is situated in a high-risk region of climatic accidents, which are occurring with increasing frequency and intensity day by day and generates fear, tension, stress, insecurity, social vulnerability as well as marginalization. As a result the quality of life, which can be viewed from the aspect of satisfaction regarding living conditions is deteriorating as some indicators of it are directly linked with vulnerability as well as resilience of people to the climatic uncertainties.

The issue of vulnerability can be viewed from different perspectives of the scholars of different knowledge domains, and even within the same domain (Fussel 2007: 155). Adger and Kelly (1999) outlined vulnerability as the state of individuals, groups or communities in terms of their ability to cope with and adapt to any external stress placed on their livelihoods and well-being. The concept of vulnerability has also been found in relation with social context 'to explore the key role played by socio-economic factors in creating a weakness in responding to, and recovering from, the effects of extreme natural events' (Armas et al. 2013: 1482). Sometimes vulnerability is being associated with 'resilience, marginality, susceptibility, adaptability, fragility and risk' (Fussel 2007: 155). Tesso et al. (2012: 871) mentioned that 'the resilience of households to climate change impact is another important issue in maintaining sustainable livelihood'. Resilient people can combat the climatic shock more successfully than non-resilient people. Adger and Kelly (1999) emphasized that a resilient community 'is able to maintain its core functions as a community despite those stresses'. Chambers and Conway (1992) included material as well as social resources as capabilities and assets within the livelihood concept and it has been accepted worldwide. Thus, livelihood becomes sustainable only 'when it can cope with and recover from stresses and shocks, maintain or enhance its capabilities and assets, while not undermining the natural resource base' (Chambers and Conway 1992: 6). On the other hand quality of life simply means the well-being of people which emphasizes on satisfaction level towards achieving happiness. Thus quality of life is a multidimensional concept which varies greatly according to space, time and human perception. Physical, cultural and social environment plays vital role in framing descent quality of life. Now, in a high-risk region of climatic accidents when vulnerability denotes the exposure of the community living there to different hazardous events, resilience refers to their capability to defend to those events or to cope with it. Therefore, quality of life of that community is deeply rooted within the interlinkages between vulnerability and resilience issues. Vulnerability is negatively linked with quality of life, whereas resilience is positively associated with it.

16.2 The Study Area

Ghoramara is an isolated island of West Bengal in the Sundarban region which has already become popular as a vanishing island since parts of the island like Lohachara has been disappeared from the map. Ghoramara village, a part of this island falls within Sagar C. D. block of South 24 Parganas district of West Bengal has been selected for this study. The village is located in an isolated island where tectonic, hydro-geomorphic, as well as climatic events play crucial roles in determining the fate of the islanders. Some portions of the island have already been disappeared. Climatic accidents, associated events and their effect aftermath like cyclone, flood, tidal surge, severe bank erosion, periodic water logging, increased salinity, economic instability create potential risk of social vulnerability of the inhabitants by affecting the indicators of quality of life like crisis of safe drinking water, sanitation, shelter, loss of farmland, dwelling.

16.3 Methodology

Household survey, field observation and interviewing of people are key sources of information for this study. Data has been collected through survey of 75 household through purposive sampling. Interview of selected informants from the village have also been taken into consideration. Data covered different aspects like educational level, population composition, age structure, economic condition, levels of poverty, income level, availability of drinking water as well as sanitation facility, house types, infrastructural facility, social support, buffer condition as all of these are well reflectors of the quality of life of the villagers. Simple cartographic representations have been used to display the findings.

16.4 Objectives

People of Sundarban are becoming more vulnerable and sensitive due to various events associated with climatic accidents which demands proper coping mechanism for sustainable living. Therefore, in this study attempts have been made to represent different dimensions of resilience like human, financial, social, physical and natural capital of the people of the study area to deal with climatic shocks so that it helps to strengthen the adaptive capacity of the vulnerable community to sustain a descent quality of life in this fragile area.

16.5 Findings and Discussion

Quality of life is not uniform everywhere. It varies spatially and depends on different aspects. There are many indicators of quality of life. But here, some indicators of quality of life have been highlighted, which are directly linked with vulnerability as well as resilience of people due to climatic events. Five important forms of livelihood assets have been mentioned by The International Institute for Sustainable Development in 2003 which forms the foundation of livelihood pattern like natural capital, social-political capital, human capital, physical capital and financial capital (Basar 2010: 13). All these have significant impact on people of the area of climatic accidents to respond, adapt and make proper recovery.

16.6 Human Capital

(A) ***Education***: This is one of the most effective human capitals as it is positively linked with higher level of resilience for long term. Illiteracy, low levels of education lead to ignorance, low level of perception as well as consciousness, prejudice which further obstruct them towards progressive thinking and adopt proper coping techniques. Level of education is low (Fig. 16.1). With the increase in educational level, the percentage of population is decreasing. 38% of the surveyed population had received primary education and 40% of them reached to upper primary level. On the other hand, 14% of them have completed secondary education, only 5% of them have reached to higher secondary level and 3% have reached to graduation level. In this study area, only 71% of the families were first learners and 24% of the surveyed population was illiterate; both of them unable to adapt the coping mechanism (Fig. 16.2).

(B) ***Gender***: Gender difference always creates a difference in quality of life between male and female, especially, after a climatic shock in rural areas of Sundarban. Women are mostly vulnerable due to 'their traditional roles as mothers and caregivers within the family; and when disaster is about to strike, they become

Fig. 16.1 Levels of education

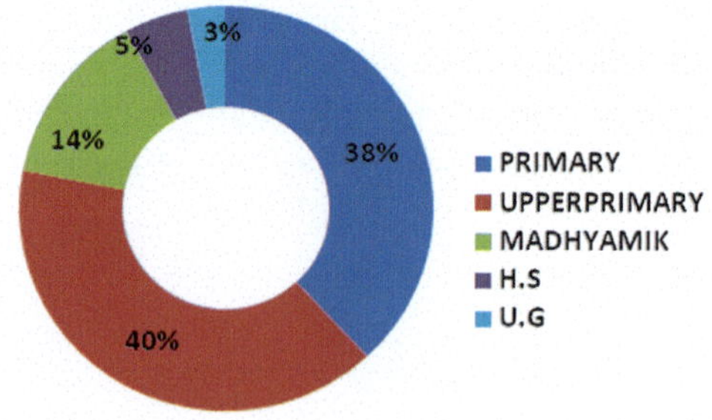

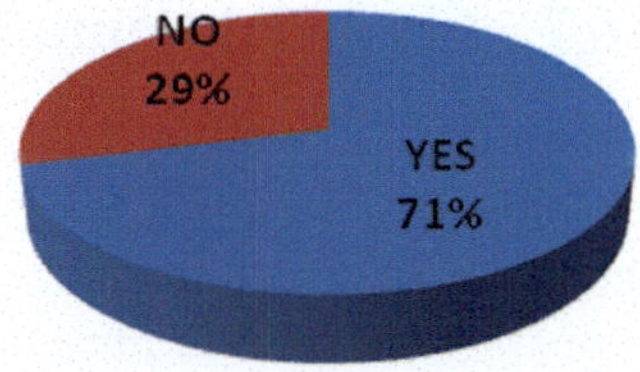

Fig. 16.2 First learner family. *Data Source Household Survey, 2013*

unable to seek safety as it restricted by their responsibilities to the young and the very old people' (Rygel et al. 2006: 748). Woman seldom possess equal position in the society as a result their right for basic needs is not being preserved. Their upbringing process lowers their confidence, consciousness and knowledge, power of expressing opinion and decision making power which creates crisis during disaster. Delaney et al. (2000: 14) also viewed that 'the usual role that women play as caregivers for the young, the elderly, and the disabled can also increase their vulnerability to disasters by limiting their mobility and doubling or trebling their workload'. Gender inequality has strong association with resilience. Mainly the gender division of work, social norms and traditional attire always create hurdles in building their resilience. As for example females are mainly engaged in cooking, collection of drinking water, cattle feeding, looking after the children and old aged family members. At the time of disaster as extra time and labour is needed to perform these activities, the females are being overburdened. Within the surveyed household, 49% population has been identified as vulnerable as they are females. The level of quality of life of women in such an area is always found to be lower than the men.

(C) ***Age***: The aged people as well as children are more susceptible to disasters and their quality of life. Vincent (2004: 13) opined that, 'populations with a low dependency ratio (high proportion of working age adults) and in good health are likely to have the widest coping ranges and thus be least vulnerable in the face of hazard exposure'. Their mobility is being restricted by their physical disability. Ngo (2001) mentioned that 'they are more likely to suffer health problems and experience a slower recovery'. They are the people who are financially dependent on others. Sometimes the older people deny shifting from their place of origin to another for making the evacuation process successful. Generally, lack of physical ability, financial support and will power stops the elderly people to respond quickly to evacuation process. The elderly people become anxious by the stress of leaving their own homes and living even on a temporary basis, in a group setting (Cutter et al. 2009: 21). The population that falls within the age group <5, 6–15 and >60 years are 10%, 21% and 8%, respectively, who have been marked as vulnerable. They have to depend on others for many reasons, especially, for economic help. Building resilience within the children, young adolescents and old-aged demands early warning and providing quick evacuation.

16.7 Financial Capital

People economically secure, stable and healthy are more likely to be resilient, and they have a capacity for anticipatory adaptation to reduce their vulnerability to (Vincent 2004: 14). Stable financial condition enables a family to withstand during climatic accidents. Financial capital is most critical dimension of resilience.

(A) ***Economy***: Most of the people of this area are engaged in work on a daily payment basis (Fig. 16.3). Apart from this, cultivation and fishing also occupy second and third position. Only 8% of them are engaged in different services. At the time of climatic accidents, agriculture and fishing become most affected due to salt water invasion, water logging and inundation of land. As a result, daily labourers also lose their work. Know-how strategy, introduction of salt-resistant species, alternative farming on the one hand and alternative income generation activities on the other can build resilience among them.

(B) ***Poverty***: People living below poverty line suffer badly during disaster. Fothergill and Peek (2004: 103) concluded that the poor are 'less likely to respond to warnings; more likely to die, suffer injuries, and have proportionately higher material losses; have more psychological trauma; and face more obstacles during the phases of response, recovery, and reconstruction'. Being poor is an obstacle for making better choices to recover from shocks of climatic events for existence. They are being unable to provide themselves the necessary equipment to combat or resist. In the view of Adger (2008: 9) 'poverty affects the coping and recovery from extreme events through directly constraining opportunities for coping and reducing the resilience to impacts'. 57% population is found to be within below poverty line who may act as weak in building resilience or adapting coping mechanism (Fig. 16.4). Leaving ancestral home and belongings along with asset like agricultural land, pond, betel garden in search of an alternative leaving is not at all easy for the poor.

(C) ***Income***: It acts as a strong indicator of resilience. People having a consistent and decent earning always hold a better position than the marginalized people (in terms of income) during climatic accidents. Low level of income (less than Rs. 3000) is found within 20% of the families. Another 25% of the families having monthly income within Rs. 6000 and they have been marked as vulnerable. As the levels of expenditure are nearer to the income levels, they cannot save much for the future.

Fig. 16.3 Occupational type

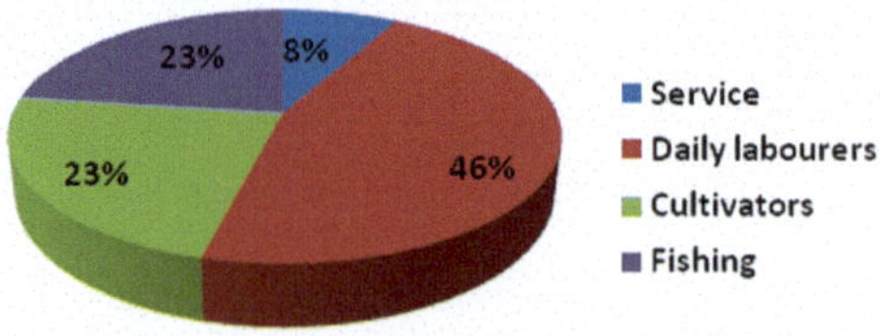

16.8 Physical Capital

(A) ***Drinking water***: This facility is also inadequate. Availability of safe drinking water depends mainly on deep tube well. Though they have tube wells, which are available within one kilometre (Figs. 16.5 and 16.6) but at the time of saltwater invasion and waterlogging, these tube wells are being submerged under the water and cannot meet the demand of drinking water. For making water usable again, people have responded in three manners, like some water cannot be purified, some portions can be through sweet water wash and through pumping out the saltwater.

(B) ***Sanitation***: Condition of sanitation is very poor. Most of the inhabitants (57%) still practice open defecation. Only 43% of the surveyed population avail sanitation facility (Fig. 16.7). Only 14% of them have a proper chamber within their house (Fig. 16.8). Rest of them have some semi-permanent structure like hole, pit. They do not pay any attention to the governments' initiatives like Nirmal Bharat Aviyan and Total Sanitation Campaign. Places of open defecation become limited after a cyclonic storm due to waterlogging. The basement of

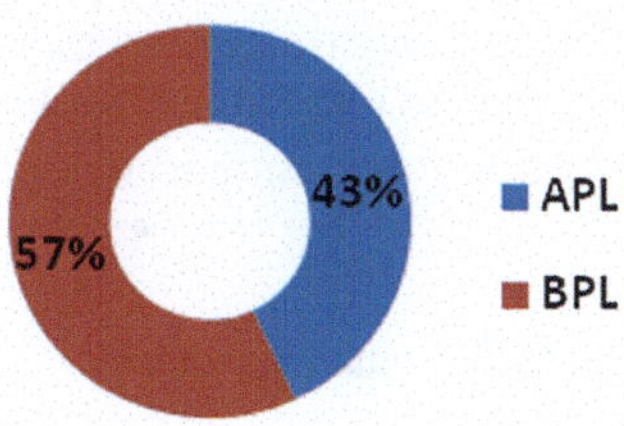

Fig. 16.4 Poverty level. *Data Source Household Survey, 2013*

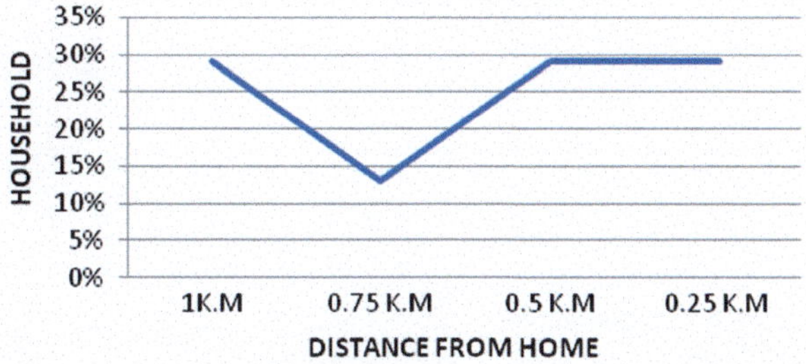

Fig. 16.5 Availability of drinking water

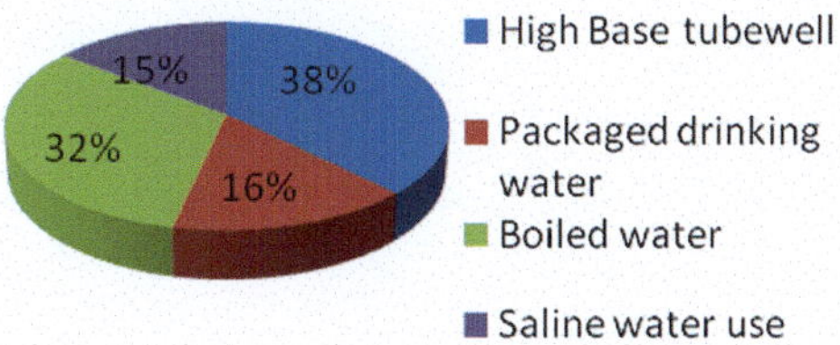

Fig. 16.6 Source of drinking water. *Data Source Household Survey, 2013*

latrines and tube wells should be raised above the embankment level to avoid the contamination. Both males and females use the river bank for defecation during disasters. In case of females, it leads to embarrassment, discomfort and lack of safety. Apart from that the waterlogged surroundings is also being further polluted and increases the scope of spreading water borne diseases. Thus, environmental hazard causes health hazards through unhygienic condition.

(C) **Housing profile**: Most (72%) of the houses are kachha in nature and another 28% are semi-pucca (Fig. 16.9). Only 14% of the roofs of the houses are pucca in nature. Most of the roofs (43%) are made of straws (Fig. 16.10). Lack of permanency, less durability, weak structure are the reasons behind the vulnerability of the population living in these houses. They are mostly exposed and marginalized. 25% huts are adapted to coping mechanism through raising the basement of huts. Kaccha houses should be converted in such a manner that it can resist disaster. As a result, they have to take shelter in a school building or any other high land during climatic hazard. Outmigration continues to happen in a huge volume and some people also get the rehabilitation facilities to the main Sagar land.

(D) ***Infrastructure***: This is an element that boosts up the resilience of the community. The condition of infrastructural facilities reflects quality of life. Infrastructure regarding health service and transport condition of the study area is very poor. During crisis period, people mainly get health services from local practitioners (quack doctor) and moving health team on vessels. Death also occurs due to unavailability of health service at proper time. On the other hand, it takes too much time to reach this island from the mainland and the boat journey is

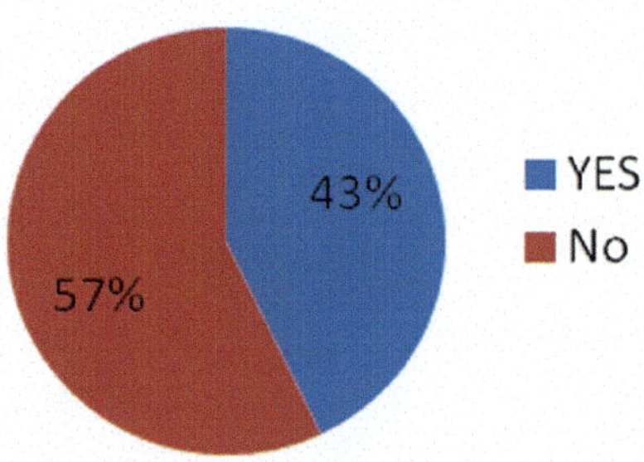

Fig. 16.7 Sanitation facility

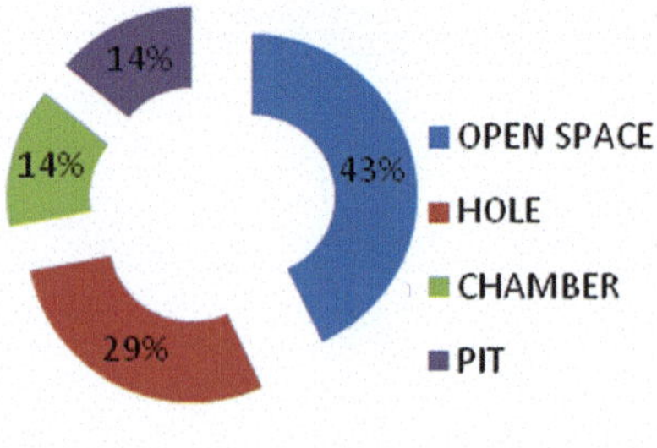

Fig. 16.8 Sanitation type. *Data Source Household Survey, 2013*

Fig. 16.9 House type

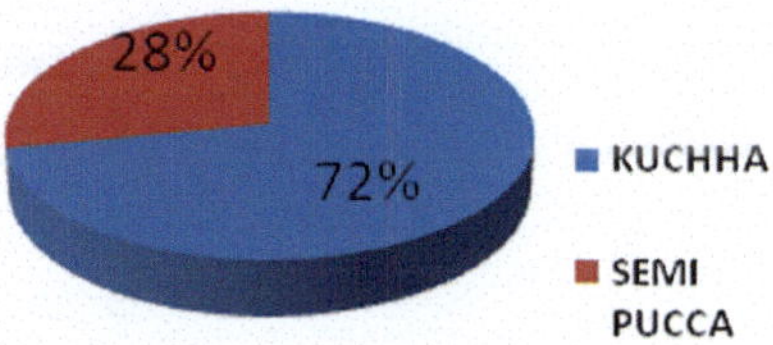

Fig. 16.10 Roof type. *Data Source Household Survey, 2013*

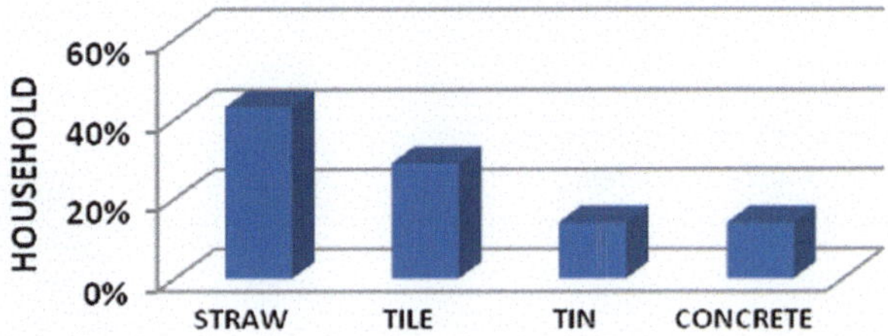

totally dependent on the time of tide. Some of the roads are muddy within the island.

16.9 Social Capital

(A) ***Social support***: Social network is associated with improved resilience as it acts as a buffer because it facilitates the way to easy recovery. Flood centre provides shelter to victimized people; emergency vessels rescue them to a safer place; radio broadcasting, and BDO/SDO send the alert immediately regarding the impending hazards. Television, newspaper, mobile message also provide information, but it takes time to reach (Figs. 16.11 and 16.12). Though it is a positive sign that most of them have mobile phone, but still there is a lack of provision of getting alert during calamities.

(B) ***Buffer scenario***: Buffering elements only includes assets and food stock. But when they have to migrate, leaving their home they cannot carry all food stocks or assets. So in true sense, the savings or insurance which can act as real buffer element is completely absent within the poor surveyed communities (Fig. 16.13).

Fig. 16.11 Social

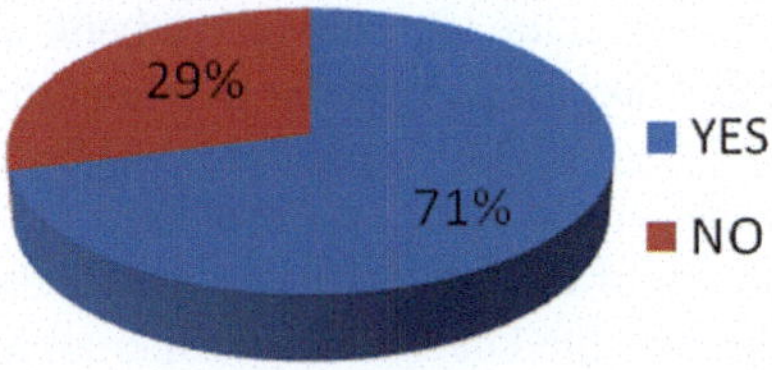

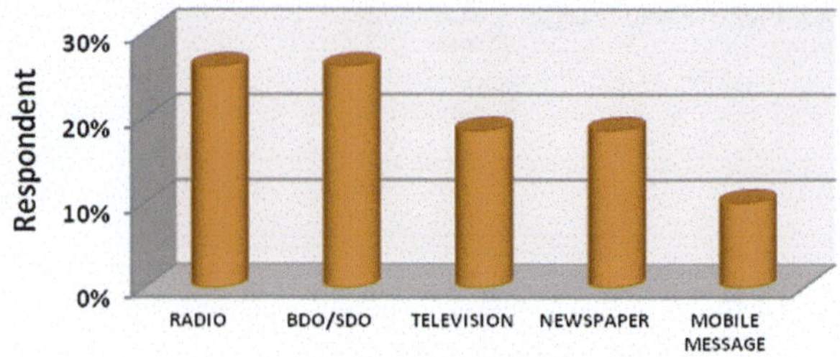

Fig. 16.12 Warning system. *Data Source Household Survey, 2013*

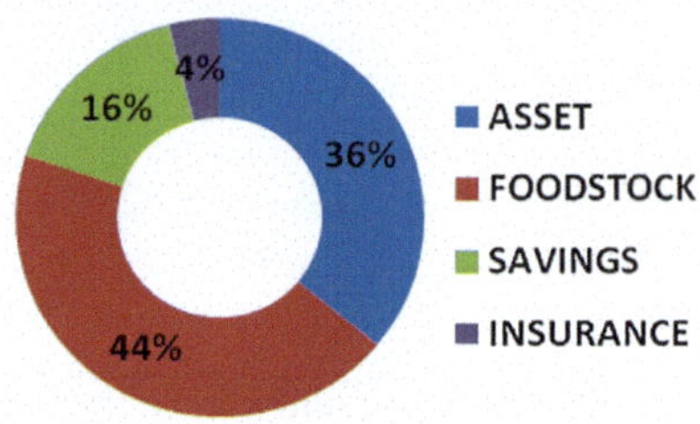

Fig. 16.13 Buffer elements. *Data Source Household Survey, 2013*

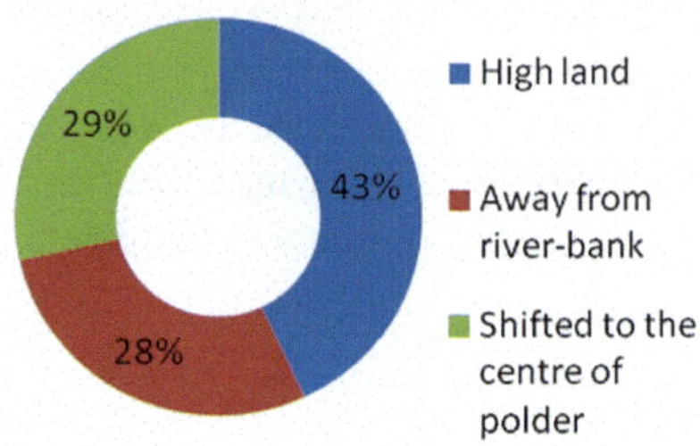

Fig. 16.14 Housing

16.10 Natural Capital

Agricultural field, water bodies, land of settlement, which seems to be the natural capital for the people of the study area get affected mostly by extreme climatic events. Maximum land loss is caused due to tidal surge and bank erosion. Proper maintenance of embankment and making them durable are needed. As it is going to be a vanishing island negligence of the government to invest here is a responsible factor. Most of the people are shifting towards the central land of the island as well as migrating to the main Sagar Island. Outmigration takes place in a huge volume and some people get the rehabilitation facilities to the main Sagar Island. People try to construct their houses on the high land, riverbank and shift to the centre of the polder (Fig. 16.14). They take shelter on the highland, flood centre, road and riverbank (Fig. 16.15).

Most of the respondents have idea on increasing temperature. They have also experienced late monsoon, irregular rainfall, water level rise, cyclone etc. Repeated attack of extreme climatic events damage crops, destroy their dwelling places and degrade the lands which further affects the food security of the local people. Malnutrition is also a very common phenomenon. As rice is their staple food and agriculture

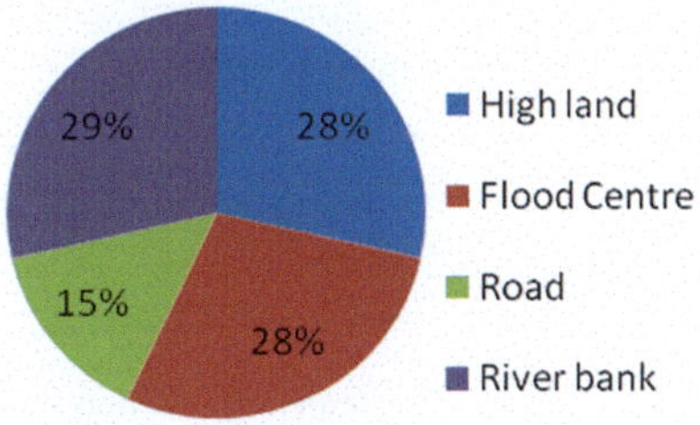

Fig. 16.15 Shelter. *Data Source Household Survey, 2013*

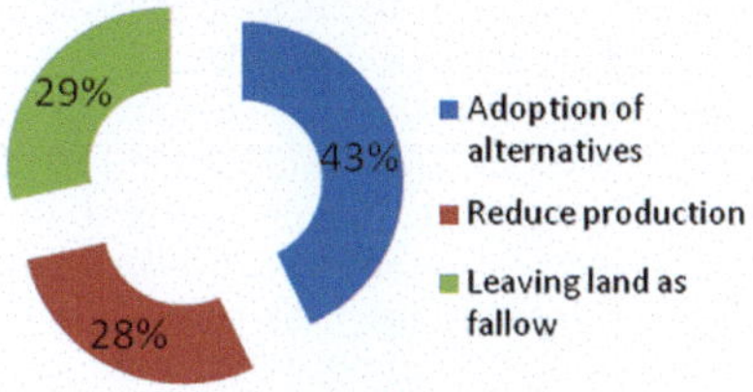

Fig. 16.16 Agriculture

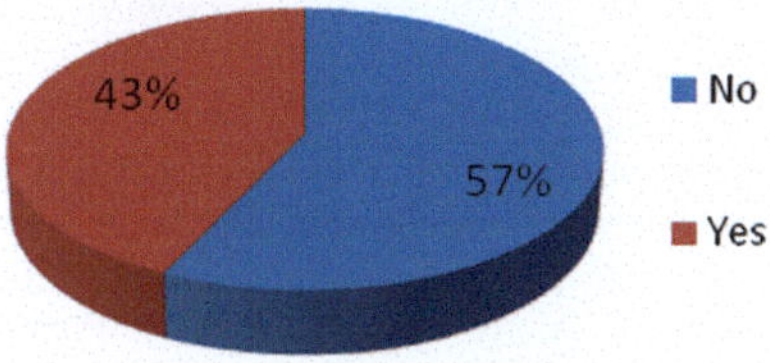

Fig. 16.17 Saline water fishing. *Data Source Household Survey, 2013*

is being disturbed, low production causes lower calorie intake. In case of agriculture, 29% of respondents reported that land remains as fallow, 28% of the respondents reported of reducing production and most of the respondents (43%) agreed that they adopt alternative methods to continue agricultural production (Fig. 16.16) after any hazard. In case of fishing due to the conversion of sweet water reservoirs into saline one, 43% of the respondents agreed (Fig. 16.17) to introduce saline water fishing.

16.11 Conclusion

It can be concluded that extreme climatic events have a definite impact on the quality of life of the inhabitants in this study area which further make them exposed, vulnerable, insecure and less resilient. In this part of Sundarban where people have to depend on nature's mercy for existence, mitigation through early warning, quick evacuation and suitable adaptive techniques are of utmost priority. Strengthening the community support system, empowering the womenfolk, betterment of social connectivity as well as communication is needed in building resilience. But topmost priority should be given in raising the level of consciousness of people through the provision of effective information and ideas about extreme climatic events, consequences, risks, coping strategies, etc. Initiatives in this regard should be taken at government, non-government, and community level in an integral manner for the benefit of the whole society.

References

Adger, N. W. (2008). *Indicators of Social and Economic Vulnerability to Climate Change in Vietnam*, CSERGE Working Paper GEC, pp. 1–16.

Adger, W. N., & Kelly, P. M. (1999). Social Vulnerability and the Architecture of Entitlements. *Mitigation and Adaptation Strategies for Global Change, 4,* 253–266.

Armas et al. (2013). *Social Vulnerability Assessment using Spatial Multi-Analysis (SEVI Model) and the Social Vulnerability Index (SOVI Model)- A Rumania*, pp. 1481–1493.

Basar, M. A. (2010). *Climate Change, Loss of Livelihood and the Absence of Sustainable Livelihood Approach: A Case Study of Shymnagar*, Bangladesh Centre for East and South-East Asian Studies, Lund University, pp. 1–68.

Chambers, R., & Conway, G. (1992). *Sustainable Rural Livelihoods: Practical Concepts for the 21st Century, IDS Discussion Paper 296* (pp. 1–33). Brighton: IDS.

Cutter et al. (2009). S*ocial Vulnerability to Climate Variability Hazards: A Review of the Literature*, Final Report to Oxfam America Hazards and Vulnerability Research Institute, Department of Geography, University of South Carolina Columbia, pp. 1–44.

Delaney et al. (2000). *Gender and Post-Disaster Reconstruction: The Case of Hurricane Mitch in Honduras and Nicaragua* (Decision Review Draft), pp. 1–60, Available at: http://www.anglia.ac.uk/geography/gdn/resources/reviewdraft.doc.

Fothergill, A., & Peek, L. (2004). Poverty and Disasters in the United States: A Review of Recent Sociological Findings. *Natural Hazards, Kluwer Academic Publishers, Netherlands, 32*(1), 89–110.

Fussel, H. (2007). Vulnerability: A Generally Applicable Conceptual Framework for Climate Change Research. *Global Environmental Change, 17,* 155–167.

Ngo, E. B. (2001). When Disasters and Age Collide: Reviewing Vulnerability of the Elderly. *Natural Hazards Review, 2*(2), 80–89.

Rygel, L., et al. (2006). A Method for Constructing a Social Vulnerability Index: An Application to Hurricane Storm Surges in a Developed Country. *Mitigation and Adaptation Strategies for Global Change, Springer, 11*(3), 741–764.

Tesso, et al. (2012). Analysis of Vulnerability and Resilience to Climate Change Induced Shocks in North Shewa. *Agricultural Sciences, Ethiopia, 3*(6), 871–888.

Vincent, K. (2004). Creating an Index of Social Vulnerability to Climate Change. *Paper, 56,* 1–50.

Chapter 17
Impact of Parks, Recreation, and Other Open Space Areas on Property Values and Quality of Life: A Case Study of South Middleton Township

Gary Greening and George M. Pomeroy

Abstract Parks, recreation, and open space activities generally provide numerous quality of life benefits and typically have positive impacts on property values. For a complete understanding of different dimensions of such benefits and impacts on quality of life, the South Middleton Township (a less studied suburban area) in South Central Pennsylvania was selected for a case study. To see the impact of adjacency and proximity of parks and open space on quality of life and on assessed property values regression analysis as a statistical technique was used. The results of the statistical analysis are not conclusive, suggesting a need for further consideration across a wider number of municipalities and open space types.

Keywords Recreation · Property value · Rural hinterland · Comprehensive plans

17.1 Introduction

Parks and open spaces are valued amenities in a community because they provide innumerable economic, environmental, social, psychological, and aesthetic benefits (Lindsey et al. 2004). All these aspects are closely related to quality of life. While many of these benefits are easy and obvious to describe qualitatively, the ability to describe the economic benefits of parks quantitatively is paramount in an age of fiscal responsibility and conservatism. One way of estimating the economic benefit of parks is through their impact on surrounding property values (Nicholls and Crompton 2005).

G. Greening
Transportation Planning Associate, Michael Baker International, Pittsburgh, USA

G. M. Pomeroy (✉)
Geography – Earth Science Department, Shippensburg University, Shippensburg, USA
e-mail: GMPome@ship.edu

B. R. K. Sinha (ed.), *Multidimensional Approach to Quality of Life Issues*,
https://doi.org/10.1007/978-981-13-6958-2_17

17.2 Discussion

Open spaces, particularly parks, bring a number of quality of life benefits. There are numerous studies that show how parks may help create social ties and develop a sense of community; bring health and fitness benefits to their users; and enhance property values (CMAP 2018). Using property values as the variable to determine economic impact assumes that the benefits of proximity to a park would be captured in the property value, which is called the proximate principle (Crompton 2005). Many factors influence the value of a property including structural, neighborhood, community, locational, environmental, and time-related characteristics (Table 17.1). Proximity to park or open spaces could be included in neighborhood, locational, or environmental attributes. In an empirical review of studies on the proximate principle, Crompton (2001) determined that 25 of the 30 studies found a positive correlation between distance or adjacency to a park and value of a property. However, most of these studies have taken place in urban settings and with community-level parks. Because state and national parks were not created to provide benefits to local residents, economic impact might better be measured through visitor expenditures rather than proximate property values. Nonetheless, the proximate principle should apply even though the impact may be perceived as "incidental" (Crompton 2001).

Nicholls and Crompton (2005) have summarized seven types of positive or negative impacts of rural regional parks on property values. These are clearly mentioned in Table 17.2. From this table, one can easily understand that parks in most cases had a positive impact except in case of public land in Michigan study area as explained by Nicholls and Crompton (2005).

At first, studies were focused on the impact of converting private property to parkland on the tax base. Barron and Jansma (1970) looked at a three-county region in rural northwestern Pennsylvania. They found that extensive public lands in this region did not decrease the tax base of local municipalities, and thus having public lands is "beneficial or at least not detrimental to the fiscal structure of local communities"

Table 17.1 Factors influencing property values

	Examples
Structural attributes	Number of bedrooms, bathrooms, fireplaces, garages; square footage of house, lot size; age of structure; the existence of pool
Neighborhood attributes	Socioeconomic characteristics of neighboring residents; quality of neighboring structures; ownership/rental; ethnic composition
Community attributes	School and tax districts
Locational attributes	Proximity and accessibility to various amenities including waste sites, power lines, highways, shopping centers, churches, schools, cultural opportunities, airport, public transportation
Environmental attributes	Views from property, noise levels, pollution levels, stormwater
Time-related attributes	Month and year of sale, number of days on market

Source Nicholls (2002)

Table 17.2 Impacts of regional parks on property values and property tax bases: a summary of previous studies

Authors	Year	Study area	Amenity(ies)	Impact on property values and/or tax base
David	1968	Wisconsin	Public land	Adjacency had a significant positive impact on land value
Barron and Jansma	1970	Pennsylvania	Public land	Increases in the amount of public land had no negative impact due to removal of property from the property tax base
Epp	1971	Pennsylvania	15 state parks and their and acquisitions	Location in a township containing a park was associated with an increase in value; the loss of taxable land caused by the establishment of these parks was more than offset by the increases in value on the remaining residential properties
Vrooman	1978	New York	One state park	Adjacency had a significant positive impact on land value
Gamble and Downing	1982	New England	State parks	Significant decline in value with distance
Brown and Connelly	1983	New York	Six state parks	Significant decline in value with distance in two cases, insignificant relationship for other four parks
Gartner et al.	1996	Michigan	Public land	Adjacency had a significant negative impact on property values

Source Nichols and Crompton (2005)

(Barron and Jansma 1970). They then began to look at the proximate impacts of state parks on property values. Such condition may have some kinds of effect on the life condition of the inhabitants of the area.

Vrooman (1978) looked at land prices of vacant land parcels proximate to Adirondack State Park in New York. The data used were concerning the sales of 284 vacant land parcels during 1971 through 1973. He found that a parcel of land that is adjacent to state land has a price that is about $20 per acre higher than a similar parcel that is not directly adjacent to state land. While Gamble and Downing (1982) were not specifically looking at the impacts of distance to state parks on property values while studying property values around nuclear power plants, they still included it as a variable. Their results showed a decline in price of $6.64 with each 100 feet, the property was located from a park. Though in some cases, there is also a positive impact and questions still remain. Nicholls and Crompton (2005) note the difficulty with rural parks:

Advantages such as country-like views and access to recreational opportunities appear to be counteracted in some instances by problems such as trespass, as well as residents' desire for relatively close human contact. In addition, lots of land in rural areas tend to be larger, thus offsetting to some extent the direct benefit of the large supply of open space nearby. Yet it is these larger parks, often located at the fringe of urban areas or in the rural hinterland, that are at the greatest risk from development pressure as suburban expansion continues.

17.3 Study Area

South Middleton Township is located west of Harrisburg, Pennsylvania, in central Cumberland County (Fig. 17.1) and was home of 14,663 people in 2010 (Census Bureau 2014). Harrisburg is the core for the census-designated Harrisburg–Lebanon–Carlisle Metropolitan Statistical Area. The township itself is among the fastest growing municipalities in one of the fastest growing counties within the state. The township owns 231.69 acres of parkland, broken into 9 units as shown in Table 17.3. Other parks and open spaces, not owned by the municipality, fall within the township boundaries include State Game Lands 305, Michaux State Forest, the Mount Holly Marsh Reserve, and the Appalachian Trail.

Article III Section 301, of the Municipalities Planning Code, states that Comprehensive Plans "shall provide a plan for land use to include park and recreation area," and that the plan "should include developing goals and objectives, establishing recreation needs, and identifying proposed location of future parks, trails, and recreation facilities" (Cumberland County Planning Department 2013). South Middleton Township's comprehensive plan does specify plans for the recreation area. However, their plans may be flawed. The comprehensive plan states that parks and recreation will be planned for in selected areas of need, not in small, fragmented areas (South Middleton Township Comprehensive Plan). However, more properties are affected

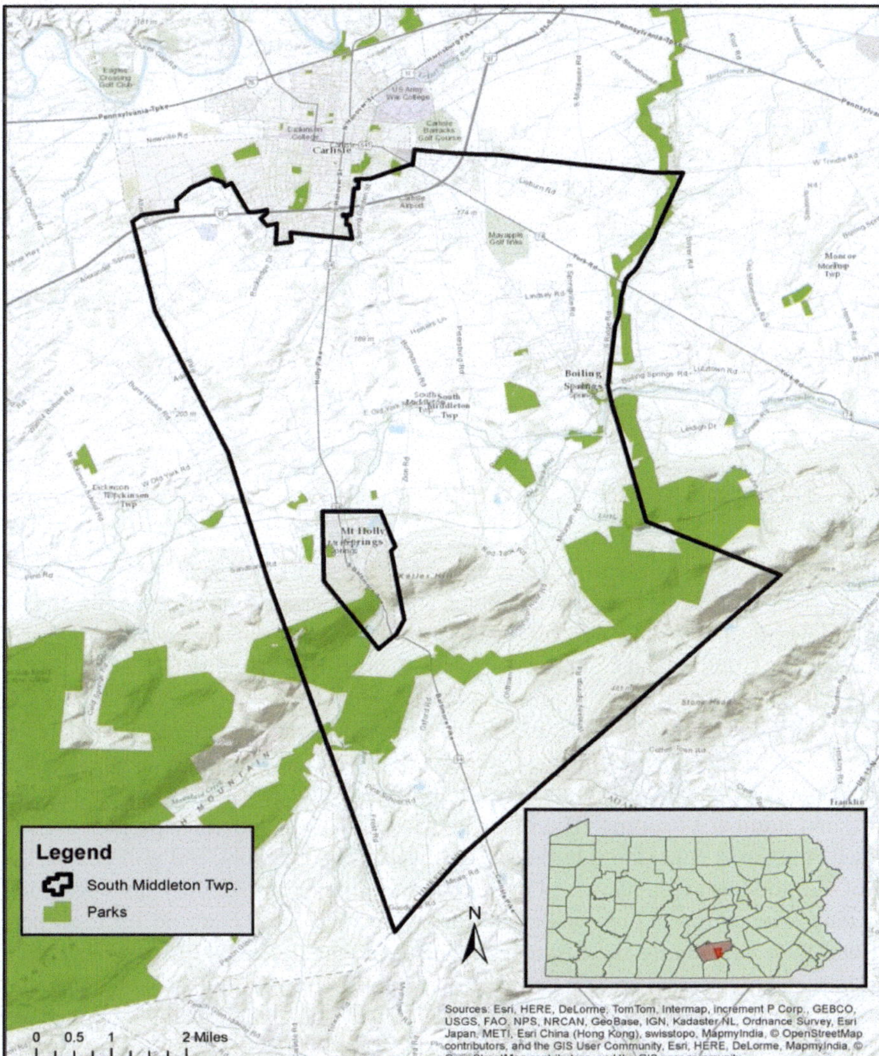

Fig. 17.1 South Middleton Township location and map (*Source* Authors)

when parkland is divided up into small, fragmented areas (Fig. 17.2). Furthermore, no recreational amenities are required when building single-family detached dwellings.

Table 17.3 Parks in South Middleton Township, Cumberland County

Park Name	Size (in acres)
Spring Meadows Park	90.00
Wittlinger Nature Reserve	50.00
South Middleton Park	40.00
South View Open Space	17.7
Seven Gables Park	9.66
Indian Hills Park	8.33
Bubble Park	7.00
Iron Works Park	5.00
Woodcrafters Park	4.00

Source South Middleton Township comprehensive plan (2007)

17.4 Data and Methodology

Data used in this research are related to ArcGIS formatted geospatial data pertaining to both parcel-level property attributes and to general community features. The parcel-level property data was obtained from the Cumberland County Assessor's office via the Cumberland County GIS Office (Cumberland County GIS). The parcel data set was for all properties within South Middleton Township. The statistical analysis was limited to using residential properties with detached single-family homes only. Variables contained within the parcel level data included acreage, square footage of residence, assessed land value, assessed building value, total assessed value, year built, and number of rooms. The other geospatial data included shape files for the parcels, the parks considered in the study, state forests, schools, and golf course for all of Cumberland County. The GIS Office of Cumberland County also provided this data. The data was then processed further by deriving a centroid for each parcel and then calculating the distances from each parcel centroid to the respective parks, recreation areas, and open space areas considered in the study. Descriptive cross-tabulations and regression analysis were employed to analyze the relationships between adjacency and proximity of properties with assessed values.

17.5 Analysis and Results

The first descriptive method used to analyze the parcel data for South Middleton Township was to find the mean of each variable that could possibly affect the property values of the parcels. In total, there are 4654 parcels. The data was categorized into "distance from park" subsets based on the literature cited earlier (Crompton 2005). Parcels that are adjacent to parks have the highest average acreage, the most square feet per building, the highest assessed land value, the highest assessed build-

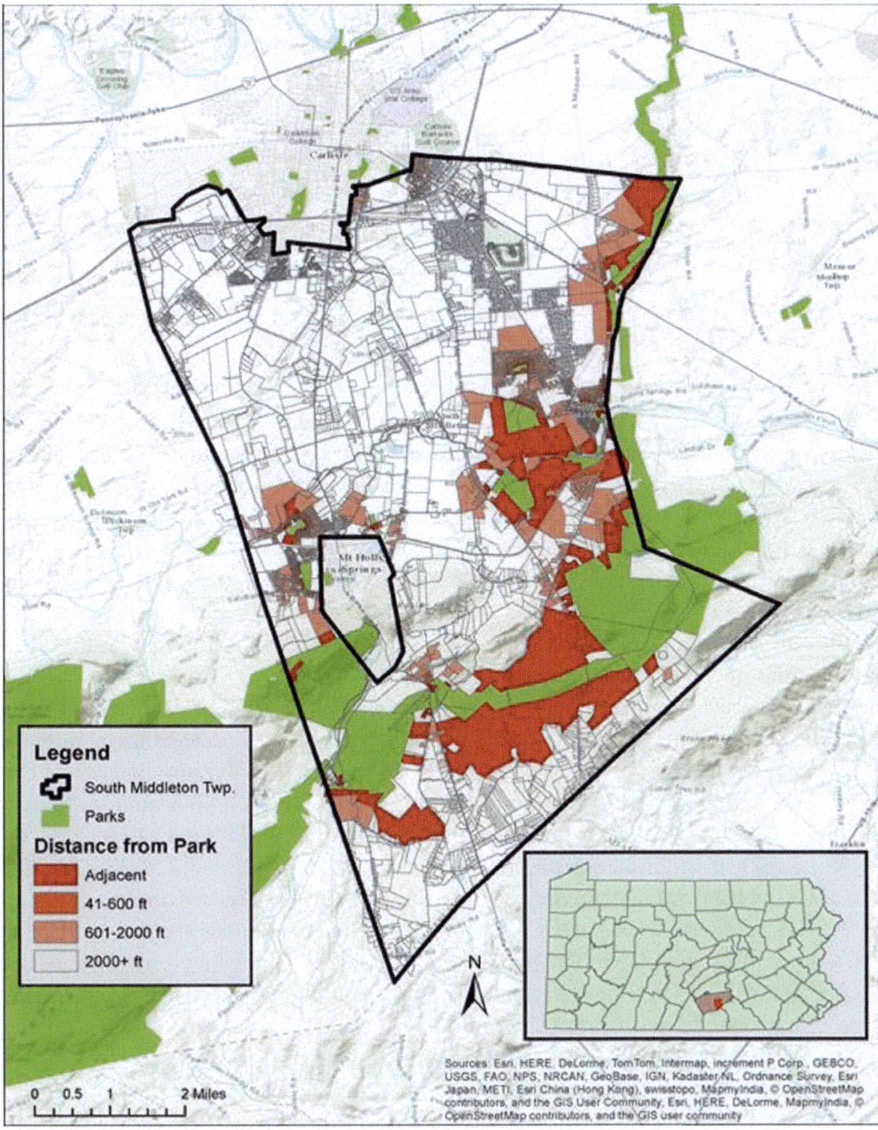

Fig. 17.2 South Middleton Township property parcels by distance from parks

ing value, highest total assessed values, and the oldest building completion date. While the acreage data is skewed by five properties that have over 1,500 acres, the other variables do not have such outliers. On the other hand, parcels with centroids 40–600 ft. away from parks have the lowest average acreage, lowest assessed land value, and the lowest assessed total value. The variables, including most notably total assessed value, as shown in Table 17.4, do not seem to have a linear relationship

Table 17.4 Mean values of variables for each parcel subset in South Middleton Township, Pennsylvania

Adjacency/distance	Acreage	Square feet	Assessed land value	Assessed building value	Assessed value	Year built	Number of rooms	Distance from park (ft.)
Adjacent to park	52.07	2061.75	$79,179.30	$186,429.11	$259,068.36	1952.13	6.82	0.95
41–600 ft. from park	0.76	1921.00	$56,047.93	$165,559.69	$201,680.00	1968.46	6.94	301.43
601–2000 ft. from park	2.78	1839.15	$60,635.33	$156,736.13	$217,371.46	1967.48	6.76	1084.83
2000+ ft. from park	6.41	1956.88	$68,211.69	$176,590.37	$244,802.06	1972.15	6.87	5480.98

Source Cumberland County GIS

when compared to the parcels' distance from a park. However, there does seem to be an impact on the assessed value due to adjacency based on this data.

Subsequently, mean assessed total value was compared to square footage of the house, acreage of the land, and total rooms within the house for each of the four "distance from park" categories. These categories help to make sure the comparisons are between parcels of similar properties.

The square footage categories used were (a) less than 1,500 sq. ft.; (b) between 1,501 and 2,500 sq. ft.; and (c) greater than 2,500 sq. ft. because that divided the data into an even number of parcels for each subset (see Table 17.5). While this was not done in the previous research, it seemed that this division is important to ensure the comparisons are of analogous properties. Within each of the distance from park categories, the mean assessed total value increases as the size of the residence increases, which is as expected, as larger houses should be worth more. In each of the three size categories, parcels that are adjacent to parks have a higher mean assessed total value than in any other distance category. Furthermore, for detached residences less than 1,500 sq. ft. and detached residences between 1,501 and 2,500 sq. ft., the mean assessed total value decreases as distance from park increases until the greater than 2000 ft. category, where value increases. Detached residences greater than 2,500 sq. ft. have a different pattern. The highest mean assessed total value is in the adjacent category but after 600 ft. the mean assessed total value increases. These data seem to agree that parcels, with houses of similar size, adjacent to parks have a higher property value than those parcels not adjacent.

Once again, even as none of the literature specifically divided the data based upon acreage of parcel, the data was divided into subsets based on the size of the property (Table 17.6). Again, this division is important to ensure the comparisons are of analogous properties. The four categories I used were (a) less than 0.5 acres; (b) between 0.5 and 1 acre; (c) between 1 and 5 acres; and (d) greater than 5 acres. These categories allow analogous comparisons between parcels. Each of the distance from park categories has a different pattern. For properties adjacent to parks and properties 2000+ ft. from parks, the mean assessed total value of residences with less than 0.5 acre is greater than the mean assessed total value of residences with between 0.5 and 1 acre. This statistic is surprising, as more acres should equate to higher property value. Besides those two statistics, the pattern is logical throughout the distance categories,

Table 17.5 Mean assessed property values, in US dollars, based on square footage of house and distance from park with number of properties in parentheses

Residences by sq. footage	Adjacent to park	41–600 ft. from park	601–2000 ft. from park	2000+ ft. from park
Detached residences less than 1,500 sq. ft. in area	164,015 (70)	155,035 (139)	152,087 (455)	170,038 (821)
Detached residences between 1,501 and 2500 sq. ft. in area	248,205 (127)	225,300 (271)	220,183 (591)	243,913 (1,318)
Detached residences greater than 2500 sq. ft. in area	397,760 (52)	320,483 (68)	354,821 (205)	366,130 (537)

Data source Cumberland County GIS Office (2013); compiled by authors

with more acres meaning higher total assessed mean value. In this Table (17.6), parcels that are adjacent to parks do not have the highest mean assessed total value throughout every acre category. In fact, those parcels that are 2000+ ft. away from a park have the highest mean assessed property value for residences with less than 0.5 acre, as well as between 0.5 and 1 acre. As a result, the adjacency does not seem to have an effect on mean property values with parcels of similar acreage.

As with the previous two comparisons, the next analysis also divided the parcels into categories based on the number of rooms within the single-family residential structures (Table 17.7). As before, this was done to ensure the comparisons are of analogous properties. The three categories used were 5 or fewer rooms, between 6 and 8 rooms, and 9 or more rooms. Within every distance category, the pattern is logical: more rooms correspond to higher mean assessed total property values. Except for residences with 5 or fewer rooms, parcels that are adjacent have a higher mean assessed property value. The pattern between distance categories is inconsistent until the 2000+ ft. from park category, where there is a spike in mean assessed total value. Adjacency seems to have an effect on mean values when comparing residences with similar numbers of rooms. Housing condition with number of rooms is also considered as one of the criteria for evaluating the quality of life. So, the analysis of adjacency and the number of rooms within the single-family residential structures is important.

When taking into consideration square footage of the house, acreage of the land, and total rooms within the house compared to mean assessed value of the parcel, adjacency, not linear distance from parks, seems to have the greatest impact on property value and quality of life. Almost every category in every comparison, the parcels that are adjacent have the highest mean assessed value. Meanwhile, there

Table 17.6 Mean assessed property values based on acreage of property and distance from park with number of properties in parentheses

Lot Size by acreage	Adjacent to park	41–600 ft. from park	601–2000 ft. from park	2000+ ft. from park
Detached residences with less than 0.5 acre	$222,481 (100)	$215,822 (349)	$199,589 (721)	$226,344 (1,286)
Detached residences with between 0.5 and 1 acre	$211,209 (52)	$215,479 (86)	$214,242 (247)	$221,897 (553)
Detached residences with between 1 and 5 acres	$256,441 (41)	$230,694 (37)	$250,187 (217)	$237,459 (500)
Detached residences with greater than 5 acres	$363,711 (56)	$335,033 (6)	$315,443 (66)	$361,877 (337)

Data source Cumberland County GIS office (2013); compiled by authors

Table 17.7 Mean assessed property values based on number of rooms and distance from park with number of properties in parentheses

No. of rooms per dwelling	Adjacent to park	41–600 ft. from park	601–2000 ft. from park	2000+ ft. from park
Detached residences with 5 or fewer rooms	$171,630 (53)	$146,507 (65)	$152,764 (309)	$178,525 (560)
Detached residences with between 6 and 8 rooms	$253,805 (167)	$237,979 (358)	$221,187 (771)	$247,969 (1,706)
Detached residences with more than 8 rooms	$381,822 (29)	$286,392 (55)	$316,913 (171)	$320,548 (410)

Source Cumberland County GIS

does seem to be a linear relationship between mean assessed value and distance from the park up to 600 ft. The mean values for parcels between 41 and 600 ft. were always less than those parcels adjacent to parks. However, the effect does not seem to be completely linear, as there are "spikes" in mean assessed values in 2000+ ft. away from parks category in nearly every comparison.

Considering more advanced statistics, the distance from park to assessed total value was compared using a scatter plot and found the R2 statistic as shown in Fig. 17.3, R2 = 0.0034. This statistic means that the distance from park variable accounts for 0.34% of the variation in the Assessed Total Value variable. This resultant R2 statistic is extremely low, as R2 can only range from 0 to 1, and thus the two variables have a weak relationship.

Finally, there is a preliminary regression using the Exploratory Regression tool in ArcGIS. While a few of the models had R2 values of 0.49, which means that 49% of variation in the dependent variable, Total Assessed Value, can be explained by the independent variable or variables, the models must have a R2 value of at least 0.5, and thus none of the models passed. As a result, the Exploratory Regression Global Summary is the first and most important to look at as shown in Table 17.8. As mentioned previously, this table shows those variables or combination of variables which are known and have a R2 over 0.50 and thus do not pass the test. 25 of the 31 models pass the max coefficient p-value test, with many having p-values of less than 0.001, and this shows that the variables are statistically significant. Every model

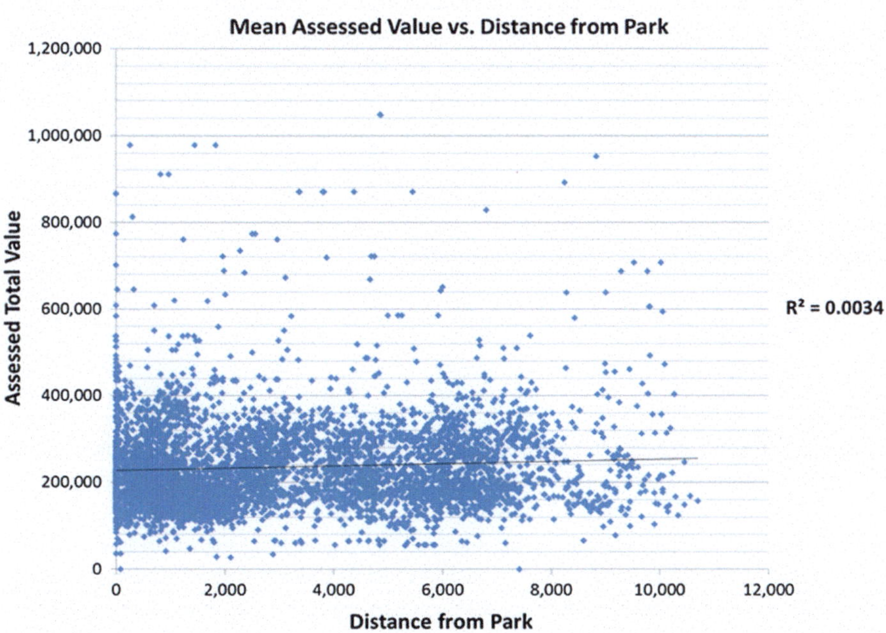

Fig. 17.3 Mean assessed values of parcels by distance from park (*Source* Calculated by authors)

Table 17.8 Exploratory regression summary

Search criterion	Cutoff	Trials	# Passed	% Passed
Min adjusted R_Squared	>0.50	31	0	0
Max coefficient p-value	<0.05	31	25	81
Max VIF value	<7.50	31	31	100
Min Jarque–Bera p-value	>0.10	31	0	0
Min spatial autocorrelation p-value	>0.010	14	0	0

Table 17.9 Exploratory regression results for optimal model

Model	+DEEDED_AC*** + SQFT*** + FULL_BATH_*** + NEAR_DIST***
AdjR2	0.49
AICc	118,709
JB	0
K(BP)	0.06
VIF	1.53
SA	0

passed the VIF value test which determines whether variables are redundant. None of the models passed the Minimum Jarque–Bera p-value test which could mean that the relationships are nonlinear or contain outliers. Likewise, all models failed the minimum spatial autocorrelation test because Number of rooms is not always statistically significant, and the model, in its current form, would be most useful for explaining the Assessed Total Value that would include acreage, square footage, number of bathrooms, and distance from park. The results of this model are shown below in Table 17.9. The model with these four variables has an R2 of 0.49. AICc is simply a comparison between models. It has a Jarque–Bera value of 0, which means that the relationships are nonlinear or contain outliers. Unfortunately, the Koenker value is 0.06, which is not statistically significant.

17.6 Conclusion

Several summary comments may be made concerning both the mechanics of the research and with respect to open space as it relates to quality of life. After looking into the mechanics of the research, it was found that no models passed the exploratory regression tests. So, changes must be made to the models. These results are a good first step in creating a functioning regression model. Potential fixes that could result in a successful model would add variables, getting rid of redundant variables, looking for outliers in the data, and determining the types of relationship between the dependent and independent variables. Furthermore, the inclusion of a dummy variable to represent adjacency would be essential to determining whether adjacency has an effect on property values and quality of life. Since there are no significant findings in this preliminary research, there are currently no implications for planning. Ultimately, while there are no advanced statistics indicating such a statistical significant conclusion, the authors do believe adjacency has an effect on property values. At first glance, Tables 17.5 and 17.7 show that the properties which are adjacent have a higher mean value than those up to 2000 ft. away. With further research, it is believed that the statistical significance can be obtained.

The first weakness in this research is using assessed value instead of sale price. The sale price would be the optimal dependent variable as it specifically shows the consumer's willingness to pay for a property. Assessed value is purely what the assessor believes a property is worth. The second weakness in this research is the limited number of explanatory variables. Solutions to these weaknesses are simple. Determine more independent variables and use sale price instead of assessed value. The second weakness is the arbitrary nature of placing each property into a specific category. As shown in Tables 17.5, 17.6, and 17.7 and explained previously, there is no literature to support those categories and the categories do not have an equal number of properties.

As to the question about the proximity of parks and the impacts they have on both property values and quality of life, there are methodological challenges in addressing these questions in low-density settings of small metropolitan areas. In the case of this research, the lower densities and the smaller number of residential properties make it difficult to isolate the variables being studied from other confounding variables.

Additionally, there is a clear need for further research that can examine connections between open space proximity and quality of life measures more broadly. Fortunately, greater attention is being paid to planning "healthy communities" by academicians and practitioners alike. The American Planning Association has begun an initiative related to healthy communities, which includes the development of a policy guide (American Planning Association 2018). Locally, in the area of South Middleton Township, there are active nonprofit groups, such as the Partnership for Better Health (2018). This speaks directly to these issues by funding trail projects as well as leveraging program that encourage the use of outdoors for purposes of physical and mental well-being and quality of life.

References

American Planning Association (2018). *Healthy communities policy guide*. https://www.planning.org/publications/document/9141726/. Accessed April 8.

Barron, J. C., & Jansma, J. D. (1970). Impact of public land programs on local government finances. *American Journal of Agricultural Economics, 52,* 365–371.

CMAP (Chicago Metropolitan Agency for Planning). (2018). *Quality of life benefits*. www.cmap.illinois.gov. Accessed April 7.

Crompton, J. L. (2001). The impact of parks on property values: A review of the empirical evidence. *Journal of Leisure Research, 33,* 1–31.

Crompton, J. L. (2005). The impact of parks on property values: Empirical evidence from the past two decades in the United States. *Managing Leisure, 10,* 203–218.
Cumberland County GIS Office. (2013). *GIS data.*
Cumberland County Planning Department. (2013). *Cumberland County land partnerships plan.* Obtained from http://www.ccpa.net/index.aspx?NID=942.
Gamble, H. B., & Downing, R. H. (1982). Effects of nuclear power plants on residential property values. *Journal of Regional Science, 22,* 457–478.
Lindsey, G., et al. (2004). Property values, recreation values, and urban greenways. *Journal of Park and Recreation Administration, 22*(3), 69–90.
Nicholls, S. (2002). *Does open space pay? Measuring the impacts of green spaces on property values and the property tax base.* Ph.D. dissertation, Texas A&M University.
Nicholls, S., & Crompton, J. L. (2005). Impacts of regional parks on property values in Texas. *Journal of Park and Recreation Administration, 23*(2), 87–108.
Partnership for Better Health. (2018). *Partnership for better health.* http://www.forbetterhealthpa.org/. Accessed April 8.
South Middleton Township. (2007). *South Middleton Township (Cumberland County) comprehensive plan.* Obtained from http://www.smiddleton.com/ordinances/comp_plan/compplan.pdf.
U.S. Census Bureau. (2014). *American factfinder, fact sheet.*
Vrooman, D. H. (1978). An empirical analysis of determinants of land values in the Adirondack park. *American Journal of Economics and Sociology, 37,* 165–177.

Chapter 18
Impact of the Restructuring of Romanian Automotive Industry on Demographic Change and Quality of Life: A Comparative Study Between S.C. Aro S.A. Câmpulung Muscel and S.C. Automobile Dacia S.A. Pitesti

Aurel Gheorghilaş

Abstract Industrial activities are known as an indicator of the urban environment and in many cases are identified as generators of urban phenomena. Undoubtedly, the two components, industrialisation and urbanisation are closely related, as they are in fact two different ways of achieving as well as expressing the level of social and economic development of a given society. In Romania especially, the industrialisation process has developed in close relationship with the urbanisation one, so that in many cases, the result was industrial urbanisation and the entire urban life revolved around the type of industry imposed by the communist regime. Industrialisation has had inevitable consequences on the features of the geographical space and the demographic structure: rural–urban migration, a concentration of population mainly in the urban areas, suburbanisation, expansion of the urban network, functional integration of rural settlements in metropolitan regions, etc. Based on all these facts, the present study aims to analyse the demographic changes and potential effects on quality of life components as a result of the industrial restructuring process once the market economy came into place, after 1990. Two representative cities for the production of automobiles during the communist period, Câmpulung Muscel (production of ARO-SUV) and Mioveni (production of the national car—Dacia) were chosen. After the 1989 revolution, the automotive industry proved to have overwhelming importance, with the decline or success of the social and economic life from these two urban centres depending on its capacity to adapt to the needs of the new market.

Keywords Industrialisation · Urbanisation · Economic restructuring · De-industrialisation · Demographic decline · Quality of life

---

A. Gheorghilaş (✉)
Department of Human and Economic Geography, University of Bucharest, Bucharest, Romania
e-mail: aghgeo@yahoo.com

B. R. K. Sinha (ed.), *Multidimensional Approach to Quality of Life Issues*,
https://doi.org/10.1007/978-981-13-6958-2_18

18.1 Introduction

The subject of urban restructuring caught the attention of researchers in social sciences, and geographers had their undisputed role (Stenning 2005; Turnock 2006; Popescu 2000; Ianoş et al. 2013). The urban restructuring was mostly linked, in a first stage, with economic changes and spatial transformation and, in a second stage, with the processes of regeneration and sustainability (Creţan et al. 2005). The urban and industrial restructuring process was correlated to the socio-spatial changes specific to former socialist states of Central and Eastern Europe (EEC). Significant industrial structural changes have characterised Romania as opposed to the other Eastern European countries (Jigoria-Oprea and Popa 2017). The economic and spatial transformations of urban centres in Romania can be linked to the urban shrinkage process, specific to the cities of the EEC; it can also be correlated with the downward economic processes, a phenomenon described by many researchers as a new pathway of urban development (Oswalt 2005, 2006; Großmann et al. 2008; Popescu 2014).

After the Second World War, the communist regime was introduced in Romania and it rapidly imposed a different social-economic development rhythm. Following the Soviet model, the subsequent communist leaders imposed a centralised system in all fields of activity. At the same time, the urbanisation process was multidimensional, complex, and contradictory. Between 1950 and 1989, the main element of the Romanian urban development was an accelerated, extensive, and socialist type of industrialisation, accompanied by explosive urbanisation and a systematisation of the rural and urban settlements. Thus, industrialisation has had a decisive role in the urban development of the country, and the industrial city constituted the symbol of an urban centre with an ascending evolution.

An important theme in building a socialist city was the nature of the relationship between cities and production processes. The industry presence in urban areas was considered a precondition for their future development. In this respect, Romania can be regarded as a particular case because it has faced a systemic crisis generated by an active disturbance of the inherited structures of the totalitarian period (Bănică et al. 2017). To attain the objective of an 'all-around developed' state, an ample process of industrialisation begun; that was followed by essential disturbances at the level of the socio-demographic structures of the country. Large enterprises from all industrial branches quickly developed in most urban centres, and in most of the smaller centres, industry becomes the dominant sector which led to the emergence of a new generation of urban centres—small cities having an economy based on one single type of industry—mono-industry based cities.

During the communist period, the automotive industry was seen as a 'key branch' of the Romanian industry and has been thus known as the largest amplitude in terms of territorial distribution and number of employees. Following a series of decisive factors among which we name: the presence of the raw materials and their valuing, centralised state policy, demographic potential, labour force and their specialisation, economic environment and marketplace, different sub-branches of the automotive industry developed such as: 1. Manufacture of machinery and machine tools—energy,

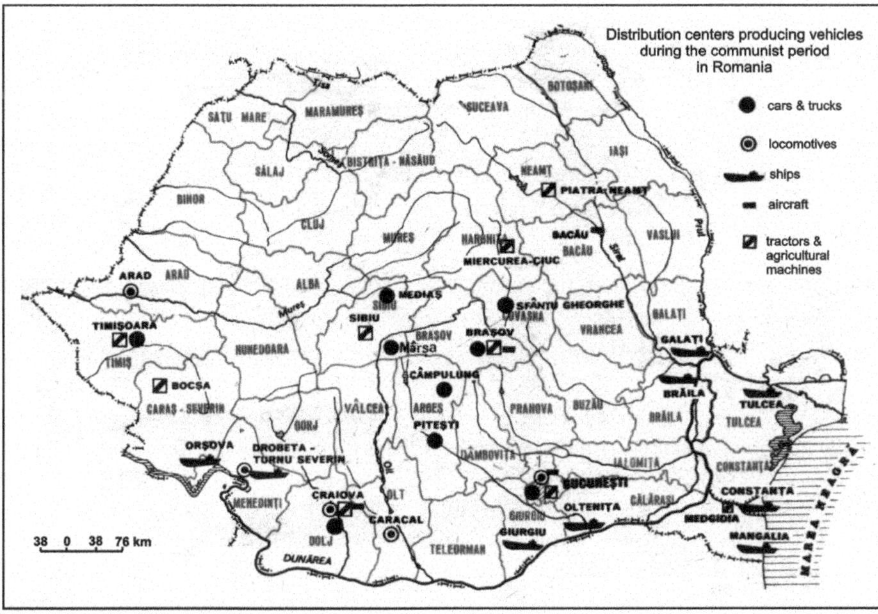

Fig. 18.1 Distribution centres producing vehicles during the communist period in Romania

oil, mining, technological, electronic and electro-technical equipment, tractors and agricultural machinery industry; 2. Transport industry that included locomotive and waggon enterprises, motor vehicles enterprises, shipyards and the aviation industry. Representative factories for the automotive production were established at Câmpulung Muscel—for the production of ARO-SUV and at Piteşti including the Colibaşi-Mioveni platform—for the DACIA model. These two entered into production in cooperation with the French group of Renault (Fig. 18.1).

The two urban centres Câmpulung and Mioveni are characterised mainly by an automotive, industrial profile, industry that developed after 1968. 'The great' industry attracted labour force from the surrounding rural areas, and the urban population continued to grow year by year which was also artificially fuelled by a positive migratory flow. After the fall of communism, the transition towards a market economy brought significant changes that enforced a complicated process of economic structuring. From this point onwards, the two urban centres experienced two different directions as far as social and economic development is concerned, which was required by the ability to adapt, or lack thereof, to the rigours of the local market industry. Thus, due to the collapse of the local automotive industry in Câmpulung, several new phenomena appeared such as demographic decline and an increase of unemployment. On the other hand, the fact that the Dacia enterprise in Mioveni managed to attract a strategic investor (the Renault Group) ensured the continuity of production and at the same time worked as a stabilising demographic factor. The presence of such phenomena brings with them visible changes in the labour force quality of life and implicitly the living standards of the inhabitants.

18.2 Romanian Automotive Industry: Production, Structures and Evolution

During the communist period, the automotive industry was one of the main pylons of Romania's economy; having employed large shares of population and contributing to increasing exports. Moreover, the development of this economic branch led to an increase in economic growth in the regions where they were located.

The success of the ARO and DACIA cars on the internal market and a relative increase in some external markets led to a growth in production, higher demand for workforce, development of auxiliary services which in turn helped sustain the local population and also attracted population flows from surrounding areas. The internal market success was explained by the fact that most of the population did not have access to other vehicles or to those produced abroad. The result was an increase in job supply and increased specialisation of the workforce in industrial activities while other economic branches were neglected. The development of this industrial sector contributed to the rise of quality of life of the local population through jobs supply, income increase, and access to improved facilities and goods which inhabitants of other regions lacked. The fall of the communist regime in December of 1989 and the transition from a centralised economy to a free market economy also influenced the economy of this region, as it had to go through economic restructuring, privatisation or even the complete disappearance of some industrial sectors or branches. This situation resulted in high unemployment, massive out-migration flows, and the overall economic decline of some towns or even the entire region. In the case of the automotive industry, there were different types of evolutions, from its revival in some cases to its disappearance in other, and as such, the population had to adapt, sometimes by leaving to other regions or even to other countries. In both cases, the population's quality of life was affected, reducing their access to certain goods and services, requiring them to change their work domains or move to other areas (large cities or the capital but even to rural areas). As a consequence, the number of total population decreased in the study area, and particularly the share of the young population also decreased. This led to demographic ageing, accelerated in turn by high out-migration and consequently low investments in infrastructure and services. Paradoxically, the process of deindustrialisation generated significant migration flows towards rural areas and increased the share of population employed to agriculture in the detriment of other sectors such as tertiary ones which saw only limited development.

Both the urban areas under study are the representatives for the Romanian automotive industry and faced the same situation, however, their evolution as well as the effects on them was different from economic as well as social standpoint point of view.

During the communist period, this sector of activity became the central pawn in the economic affirmation and development of the town of Câmpulung. Furthermore, Mioveni has developed once an automotive enterprise and it was established here in 1968. Nonetheless, a nucleus of the automotive industry was present long before this time. In 1935, at Câmpulung, there was a paper factory—I.A.R Braşov and it was fully equipped with aircrafts production with 400 employees. Between 1944 and 1948, several products such as locks, grape scissors, cookers, etc. were gradually manufactured here. In the same way, the foreshadowing of the Colibaşi factory started early in 1943 once the forests from the superior terrace of the village were cleared and the access roads were made. The first industrial halls were built and used for assembling the parts for the Romanian I.A.R 80 plains. After the war, the constructions began at Colibaşi and further attached with the administration of the Ministry of Transport which intended to establish here a depot for repairing locomotives.

From 1948, the enterprise in Câmpulung was renamed as 'The Câmpulung State Mechanical Enterprise' (C.S.M.E) and textile machinery like rings and flyers were produced here. In 1953, the plant was reconverted initially to provide motorcycles and then auto parts and in 1955 engines. In 1957, this was the location where the IMS-57 was assembled, and 2 years later, another model was launched—the M-59. Concurrent with the increase in production of the M-59 from 803 to 3222 pieces, in 1963, the design, trial, and preparation for the production of the M-461 model commenced, and it entered into the production line in 1964. 80,233 of the new and improved, both in design and in performance, M-641 SUVs were produced until the year 1975 out of which 46,549 were exported. After the year 1966, the design of the new SUV, the ARO-240 started and was the first in a series of 24. This model is the first, after the Range Rover, which used a curved chassis that allows for an increase of stability. An interesting fact is that in a test organised by Ford Europe in 1972 the ARO-240 came second after the Range Rover but ahead of established models such as Jeep—Willis, Ford, or Land Rover.

Following the 1973 oil crisis, the usage of Diesel engines on SUVs extended at a global level. In the beginning, at the Câmpulung plant, the engines on the ARO-240 were adapted for export and then in collaboration with the Braşov Tractor Enterprise the design for a Romanian Diesel (D.127) started. During next year, the ARO-240 was redesigned, and by the end of 1985, 125,000 more pieces were produced out of which 93,000 were exported in several countries. In 1980, after five years of designing, trial, and preparation, the ARO-10 model was launched. The export process started in 1980, and by 1985, 95% of production was being sent in countries such as Great Britain, Italy, France, Germany, Spain, Greece, and others. The engines used for these export models were the VW and Pegasso.

As per the Government Order No. 2004 dated September 16, 1966, the Colibaşi platform of an automotive plant for the placement was established in the vicinity of the 'VasileTudose' plant which was for a long time the leading supplier of parts and components for trucks and tractors. The investment for the new automotive plant was approved for a capacity of 55,000 pieces/year out of which 44,000 cars and 11,000 vans. On the 1st of July 1968, the first trials of the utilities and equipment started, and the first control car, after passing through all the 217 production posts, came out on August 3, 1968 with the inauguration of the plant and the series production of the Dacia 1100 taking place on August 20, 1968. In the year 1968, 2030 cars were produced with the estimations that the following year' production should be of 12,688 vehicles. The license contract for the Dacia 1100 meant at that point assembling the body (from pressed steel parts that came from France), painting, road testing, reception and delivery of the car. All the necessary parts and subassemblies necessary for these steps were imported.

In 1969, the production of the Dacia 1300 started, the car being simultaneously exposed at the EREN Bucharest in October 1969 and The French Automotive Salon under the brand Renault 12. Manufacturing began with parts made in France, but gradually it was entirely integrated into the Romanian industry. Thus between 1970 and 1973, many new plant sections were opened. Production evolved from 16,250 vehicles in 1970 to 55,511 cars in 1975 and 72,846 vehicles in 1978. In 1982, the Dacia 1310 model was launched and reached a production of 82,000 pieces/year in 1985. Between the years 1985 and 1989, new versions of the Dacia car entered the production line having a varied range of use: travelling, sports, racing, freight, ambulances, or vans. In the same time, the range of engines and gearboxes diversifies. The cars were mainly exported to China; countries from Latin America and Eastern Europe.

The automotive plant entered a new phase of existence with the December 1989 Revolution when the market economy was once introduced. The transition was a significant shock, and both enterprises registered drastic production decreases caused by faulty management that did not adapt to the market needs and requirements and the poor quality and lack of competitiveness of the cars on the leading external markets. The main Romanian automaker transformed after 1990 in S.C. AUTOMOBILE DACIA S.A. and registered a drastic decrease in production that reached its down-peak in 1992 followed by a production increase after 1993. The positive dynamic of the plant and market' absorption capacity enabled not only regular decent wages but also a sustained investment effort for the improvement and refurbishment of the production lines. New models like Dacia 1307, 1309, 1035 as well as the new Dacia Nova, which was entirely a Romanian design, were introduced.

Automobile Dacia S.A. merged in 1995 with others commercial firms from the industrial platform that will work as management and profit centres. The reunification of the platform was done based on the needs of the stage the automotive industry had to undergo and the positive results that it obtained proved that it was the viable solution that allowed for the survival of the company. The next stage confirmed the oscillating evolution of the newly formed company. Several problems like the lack of capital, narrowing up to annihilating of the external market, outdated technologies that in turn gave low production rates, and ever-decreasing demand for cars on the internal market due to the drastic reduction of the population purchasing power became acuter. At a later date, the enterprise passed through another restructuring phase in which the plant is divided into: one production and management company (S.C. Automobile

Dacia) and seven adjoining companies (S.C. Mecanica Dacia, S.C. Motoare Dacia, S.C. Utilaje Dacia, S.C. Transporturi Dacia, S.C. Maşini-Unelte Dacia, S.C. Matriţe Dacia, S.C. Servicii Comune Dacia). This phase was preceding the acquisition of the majority of the stock shares by the French group Renault, which was considered to be the most spectacular transaction that took place in Romania during the transition period. Later on, due to the reliability of the fusion of the Romanian company and French Group, the Romanian automotive industry registered substantial progress that ensured for more than a decade secure jobs and the development of related industrial branches. This, in turn, had a definite effect on improving the local population's quality of life.

The effects of the economic transition echoed into the opportunities of economic activities. The economically active participation rate of population at a national level suffered from essential oscillations. In 2015, the employment rate in Romania was 66% (the lowest one) compared to that of EU28 and other European countries passing through economic transition (Zamfir et al. 2017, p. 11). The example of the Renault group could be a positive one as it created economic development opportunities for the entire county.

The management of the Renault—Dacia group collaborated with different institutions and social actors (local councils, worker unions, and workforce occupation agencies) to create regional economic development strategies that would mitigate the impact of industrial restructuring and produce new jobs. Moreover, the plan in the short and long term was to transfer these strategies to other domains of social life (promoting the image of the local area, creating small and medium businesses, professional reinsertion of the unemployed population, etc.). This particular economic development strategy included a job quality dimension by considering employers opinions on employees job satisfaction and well-being.

As an important component of quality of life, the job quality dimension can only be analysed from a multidimensional perspective which needs to include several directions: skills and training opportunities, socio-economic security (decent wages and secure transitions), working conditions, work–life balance and family life (Schmid 2006; Eurofound 2008, 2017). Additionally, the economic growth, investments and profits of a multinational company such as the Renault—Dacia group contributed to the overall increase in quality of life and job opportunities. An improvement in economic prognosis and the county gross domestic product from 18,076 million lei in 2015 to 21,490 million lei in 2018 was also registered (Comisia Națională de Prognoză 2016).

A different situation characterised the ARO S.A. Company from Câmpulung. Production of SUVs has had a continuous downward trajectory during the transition towards a market economy period. The I.A ARO (transformed after the year 1989 in S.C. ARO S.A.) was affected by the low quality and lack of competitiveness on the external markets and Western Europe of the SUVs produced here like the ARO-35S, ARO-264 or ARO-80, which resulted in a yearly decrease of production. This was due to a faulty management policy that led to the loss of the Chinese, Vietnam or other Latin American markets. The management and production failure to adapt to the market' new standards entailed the loss of employees while production decreased.

Thus, if the 1978 production was of 13,104 units after the 90s, production dropped to 3.000 units in 1995 and 1.000 in 2002. The number of employees declined from 7.500 in 1978 and 8.300 in 1989 to 7.000 in 1990, to 4.580 in 1998 (when almost 3700 employees were let go) and in 2002 the company had 3480 employees. In 2003, a new privatisation programme stipulated further staff layoffs and the number of employees that remained at 1500 only.

After the restructuring programme, the ARO enterprise was divided into five companies: ARO S.A. (production and marketing), CESAR S.A. (Romanian Automobile Experimental and Study Centre), FPSA ARO S.A. (Parts and Auto Parts Factory), FSM ARO S.A. (Tools and Dies Factory) and CGC (The General Marketing ARO Centre). But neither the new organisational structure nor the sustained promotional efforts at the showrooms or specialised fairs produced significant changes, and the company has not been able to balance the production—sales ratio. With the lack of other privatisation offers and in the hope of a better future, the only survival method was the help provided by the state, which consisted of commissions by the National Ministry of Education (school buses) or the Ministry of National Defence.

The successful privatisation model of Dacia S.A. gave time for the hope to local authorities that privatising would mean the recovery of the enterprise and with this the industrial town where the ARO brand defined the life and prosperity of the inhabitants. Unfortunately, the decline became more evident, and the lack of a 'strategic investor' only worsened to an extreme of austerity conditions.

The majority of the stock shares were bought, in 2004, by an American company, Cross Lander, but they were more preoccupied with the production line opened in Brazil than the real recovery of the Câmpulung factory, so no dramatic changes took place. The 'death' of this industrial giant brought with it a dramatic situation and the town was more than once named in the local press as an 'industrial tomb' or 'dead town'. An economic recovery process was slow to emerge given the fact that inhabitants depended up to now on the SUVs manufacturer and the introduction of SMEs or small companies that would revitalise the economy of the town was insignificant.

18.3 Economic Restructuring, Geo-demographic Changes and Potential Effects on Quality of Life

Quality of life includes elements referring to physical conditions, social and economic environment, culture, politics, health, activities the population does, or goods and services population has access to (Marginean 2004), and their overall analysis is rather difficult. The economic restructuring also implies complex research and a multidimensional approach and their effects over the population's quality of life cannot be easily measured in the medium and long term (changing demographic patterns and behaviour, the emergence of a new migration pattern and residential mobility, deepening of social inequalities and poverty).

From an economic perspective, migration is evaluated through econometric models that consider income, advantages and attractiveness in the departure point and the destination point. In general, the migratory decisions depend on complex factors closely interdependent with the inequalities between the departure point and the destination point concerning the quality of life, standards of living, social costs, and costs of moving from location to another. More precisely it refers to net benefits of moving higher wages, lower housing costs and higher quality of life (Roback). Other factors that are usually closely related to societal opportunities or constraints are well-being, social inclusion or exclusion, which in turn are influenced by economic and political changes.

The technological, cultural and educational changes imposed by the communist regime were meant to change mentalities and the traditional demographic behaviour of a society that up to the beginning of the 60s was living mainly in rural areas (Ghinoiu 1978). This was the beginning of the period during which new urban civilisation values start surfacing and will eventually erase the existing traditional ones. In the same time, according to the urban society pattern, a new demographic reality is slowly but surely setting in (Florian and Sârbu 1997). Later on, with the strengthening of a different method of social, political and economic organisation, the excess of the labour force from rural areas is directed mainly towards those urban centres that were in the process of industrialisation—Câmpulung during the 70s and Colibaşi (nowadays Mioveni) during the 80s.

The location and development of the automotive industry in these towns have had similar demographic evolutions during the communist period with the population migrating from surrounding areas and increased their number of inhabitants. After 1990, the two municipalities evolved differently, the decline of the Câmpulung industry leading to the demographic decline of the city.

18.3.1 Economic Restructuring and Changes in the Demographic Size of Towns

After the Second World War, the number of inhabitants in Câmpulung increased spectacularly. In 1956, it reached to 18,880 persons; this was mostly correlated with the beginning of the industrialisation process and more precisely to the crystallisation of the automotive industry and the collectivisation. Events that accelerated the demography of Câmpulung were the birth rate as well a rural exodus to it. This town attracted the population from the surrounding rural areas. Continuous industrialisation of the town soon increased the inhabitants to 20,000. According to 1966 census, the population of Campulung reached to 24,877. In the next years, the town experienced a demographic boom. In 1966, abortions were banned as per the decree of 770/1966. In 1971, the population of the town reached to 26,828 and in 1977, this further reached to 31,533 inhabitants. The newly opened industrial units (factories for Synthetic Threads and Fibres as well as for Binders) and the diversification in

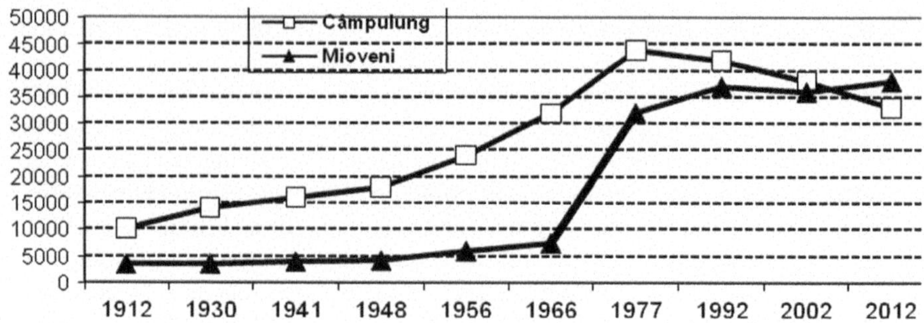

Fig. 18.2 Demographic evolution of Mioveni and Câmpulung

production at the ARO plant contributed to attracting more people living in the surrounding rural areas and implicitly to increasing the population number from 33,448 inhabitants in 1979 to 38,339 inhabitants in 1980 (Fig. 18.2).

During the last years of communism due to the gradual strengthening of the economic crisis, the town saw impacts on the evolution of its population, registering a slow increasing rate that led to some 42,678 inhabitants in 1989. The similar increase was also recorded and in 1992 census the number of inhabitants became 44,125 and this slowly reached to the maximum number of 44,560 inhabitants in 1995. The slight increase in population number during the first years of the transition period is justified on the one hand by the significant increase in home establishments and on the other by the relative diversification of the industrial branches which were at that moment in time productive.

The downward demographic curve is better defined especially after 1985 when Câmpulung's population was no longer capable of compensating for the decline of the surrounding rural areas, which were affected by an increase in the percentage of females, negative migratory balance and demographic ageing. On the other side, once the abortion law was abrogated at the beginning of the '90, the natural increase rate dropped significantly, becoming negative. The continuous industrial restructuration with the layoffs followed the downward spiral of the demographic evolution. At this point, a reverse migration phenomenon took place, a definitive return to the native rural localities, as the town was unable to provide wages or decent living standards to its inhabitants. The beginning of the 21st century did not bring with it a demographic revival of the town. The census from March 18–27 2002 showed a disastrous situation: Câmpulung had only 38,285 inhabitants, and its numbers continually decreased.

The economic decline that became ever acuter especially during the transition towards the market economy made for a long and slow.

Mioveni represents a particular case as it has had a continuous upward evolution with spectacular increase rates after the triggering of the industrialisation process. It was declared a town in 1989 under the Colibaşi name (called Mioveni in 1991), and the locality had for a long time fewer inhabitants than the neighbouring rural areas. In 1992, for example, together with its integrated villages it had only 3506 inhabitants which were even less than that of some other villages like Mihăieşti, Hârtieşti or Stâlpeni.

The demographic boom of the present day town of Mioveni happened by the end of 1960s, when the Dacia Automotive Factory, the leading car producer in the country, was opened. From some 9179 inhabitants in 1977, mainly due to a sustained migratory flow, the population reached to 33,897 between 1992 and 1997 and continued to rise to 36,193 inhabitants in 2002. Even though it was initially created as a satellite town for Piteşti, Mioveni soon became a demographically stable town compared to Câmpulung. A competition emerged between the two municipalities, and the population number, as well as other elements of economic and social infrastructure, had a crucial role in their future development.

The rise and fall of industrial influence mirrored the population's mobility both permanent and daily, respectively, in the increase and decrease of the daily flows of workers to these factories.

The daily migration flows or commuting was the dominant form of mobility during the communist period, with the consolidation of the urban centres based on productive industrial activities. The communist regime imposed commuting as the main migration method of the rural labour force based on the idea that sharing the working hours between urban and rural would maintain family balance, considerably increase the population's income and reduce the social distance between the two environments (Fig. 18.3).

The most important industrial centre that attracted labour force was Câmpulung. The rapid social-economic development of the town also determined the increase in number of employees from 1766 in 1950 to 23,500 in 1977.

The first of the geographic areas that provided labour force includes localities from the Câmpulung Depression followed by the villages that make out Schitu-Goleşti. These localities had, during the entire communist period, the same function, that of bedroom localities for the labour force employed in the industrial enterprises in Câmpulung, although they had assimilated or inherited several other economic functions (coal sorting and exploitation at SchituGoleşti, construction materials production at Valea Mare, limestone exploitation and processing at Albeşti, mineral springs exploitation at Bughea de Sus or tourism at Lereşti). The second area providing labour force to Câmpulung stretched between 15 and 32 km and included 11 villages (Berevoieşti, Aninoasa, Vlădeşti, Poienarii de Muscel, Boteni, Mihăieşti, Stoeneşti, Cetăţeni, Dragoslavele, Rucăr, Dâmbovicioara), that had either an agricultural profile (fruit-growing or livestock raising) or a manufacture one. The third supply area was situated at a distance of 50 km away and targeted the villages: Hârtieşti, Davideşti, Stâlpeni, Ţiţeşti, Bălileşti, Dârmăneşti and only remained at a project state as Piteşti, and later Mioveni exercised stronger attraction forces over this territory.

Villages from the northern part of the depression generated the maximum commuting flow with 1030 workers coming from Valea Mare Pavăţ, 1330 from Albeştii de Muscel and 1990 from Lereşti and the necessary staff was supplemented by workers from outside the Câmpulung depression from an area that overlaps with the former Muscel County. Daily movements of the population from inside the depression

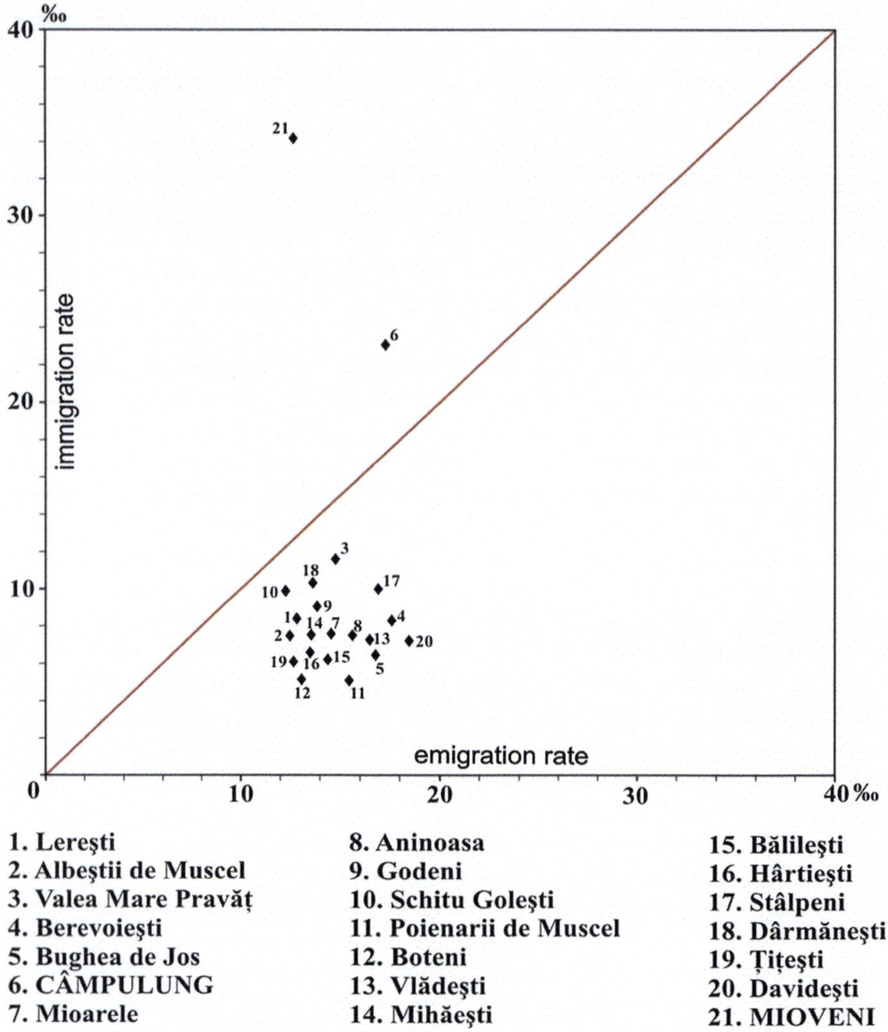

Fig. 18.3 Migration balance of urban centres in relation to neighbouring villages

towards other localities had a low intensity and were mainly represented by highly qualified workers travelling from Câmpulung to the Dacia enterprise of Mioveni (former Colibasi) or miners from the Mioarele village and the southern districts of Câmpulung going towards the lignite processing centres from Jugur, Poienari, Berevoieşti, Godeni, etc.

As far as definitive migration movements go, towards the 1980s, the increasing obstacles for rural exodus (governmental restrictions for real estate acquisition in the city as well as the dwindling job offer market) nullified any attraction that Câmpulung had for the surrounding rural area. In 1985, the villages from the close vicinity of

Câmpulung registered the lowest emigration rates (Mioarele 3.7‰, Poienarii de Muscel 3.9‰, Lereşti 5.5‰, Albeştii de Muscel 6.2‰, Godeni 7.7‰, Boteni 8.0‰, Berevoieşti 8.0‰, Bughea de Jos 8.2‰, SchituGoleşti 8.3‰). Mioveni was in a different situation; the town was reaching its peak development during this period, and the volume of home establishments was continually provided with inhabitants from the neighbouring rural areas. In 1985, the villages from around Mioveni registered the highest emigration rates (Davideşti 24.4‰, Ţiţeşti 14.7‰, Dârmăneşti 13.9‰, Stâlpeni 13.1‰, Bălileşti 13‰, Hârtieşti 12.6‰).

The analysis of the in-migration rate between 1970 and 2012 reveals large shares of new urban home establishments to the detriment of the nearby rural areas. The start of the industrialisation phase provided an increase to the urban in-migration rate so that in 1975, in Câmpulung, it had a value of 31.3‰ and of 32.3‰ in Mioveni. At that date, the rural areas registered much lower rates (less than 10‰), the exception being the localities with an agro-industrial profile (Stâlpeni 15.1‰, Aninoasa 13.5‰, SchituGoleşti 13.3‰, Valea Mare Pravăţ 11.2‰, Godeni 10.4‰). During the 1980s, the urban localities reached the first peak in in-migration rate (in 1980 Câmpulung registered 35.6‰ and Mioveni 58.7‰). During this period, the migration rate had different trends in the two towns. In Câmpulung, where industrialisation was triggered earlier, the in-migration started to decrease early on (15.1‰ in 1985), while in Mioveni, the volume of arrivals maintained at high values (the in-migration rate stabilised the same rates from the 1980s at 50‰). In the middle of the 8th decade, the rural areas registered the lowest in-migration rates values with almost 16 of them recording values of less than 5‰.

Up to the present day, the evolution of the migration rate kept the same trend it had at the beginning of the transition period. In the urban areas, it registered a significant decline which is understandable considering the economic decline of Câmpulung and the shrinking job offer in Mioveni, despite the revitalisation of the automotive industry (the immigration rate in 2012 was 10.9‰ in Câmpulung and 21.2‰ in Mioveni). The reverse migration phenomenon which was initiated by the massive layoffs and sustained by the clarification of a series of land ownership that lasted more than 10 years fuelled a high rural in-migration rate (Davideşti 23.9‰, Dârmăneşti 20.9‰, Berevoieşti 16.6‰, Ţiţeşti 16.5‰, Hârtieşti 13.8‰, Valea Mare Pravăţ 13.8‰, Stâlpeni 12.8‰, Mihăieşti 12.8‰, etc.).

The overall population balance between the natural increase rate and the migratory rates presents different dimensions and structures in the two analysed urban centres (Fig. 18.4). The comparative analysis and the interpretation of the graphic materials of the birth rates, death rates, immigration and emigration data between 1970 and 2012 gave two types of population dynamic specific to the two urban centres:

a. Mioveni recorded a highly accentuated dynamic, supported by increased birth rates and a large number of arrivals especially during the midsection of the analysed period. The town managed to achieve spectacular increase rates in a short time. During the first phase, increase was due to a favourable natural balance (in 1970 the birth rate was of 31.4‰), and during the second phase, the growth was explosive, its main motor being the volume of home establishments in the

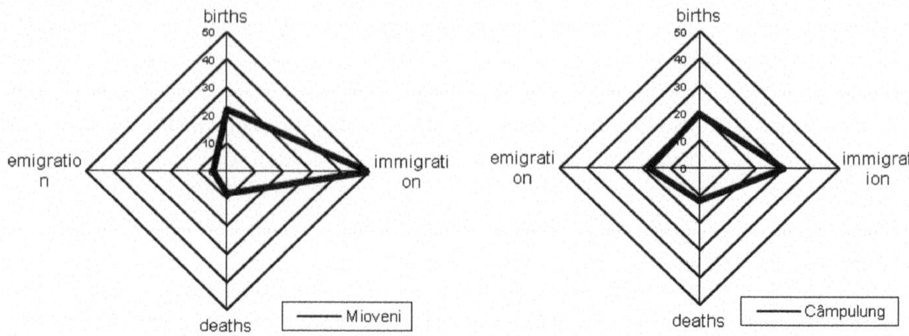

Fig. 18.4 Models of population dynamics

town (in 1980, the emigration rate was of 58.7‰). Presently, due to a decrease in immigration and during 2002 census, the first negative values of the migration rate were noted (−1.9‰), and there is a slight overall increase based on the natural balance (4.5‰);

b. Câmpulung registered an average dynamic, characterised by a relative equilibrium between the natural and migratory balance for the entire period analysed. Between 1970 and 2012, the town registered an overall balance of 12.6‰. The high values registered in 1980 (29.9‰) were compensated by the very low one from 1970 (6.1‰) to 2002 (−5.2‰).

18.3.2 Economic Restructuring and Changes in Demographic Structures of Towns

The decline in influence of industry for the Romanian urban development after 1991 is well portrayed by the evolution of the number of industry employees (Dumitrache et al. 2016). In the middle and medium-sized cities of Romania, urban restructuring and urban decline had negative effects generating spatial inequalities and lowering the living standard of the population (Jucu 2015). The lack of jobs and high unemployment are considered essential elements within the scope of life quality components. Several studies show that unemployment can have significant consequences for subjective well-being, with negative effects on the individual's personal life, by increasing anxiety, lowering confidence and generating the inability of solving everyday problems (Eurobarometer 2009, 2017; Theodossiou 1998).

The socio-economic phenomena that constitute the overall living conditions are numerous, complex and heterogeneous with specific manifestation and their quantitative and economic analysis and measurement must be differentiated for each case. The living standards can be correctly analysed only if an appropriate system of synthetic indicators that are meant to emphasise all essential aspects of the day to day life is used (Zamfir 1984). Thus, to statistically illustrate the socio-economic phenomena and processes that make out living standards, one has to study their essence and features and determine the suitable quantitative and qualitative methods. Encompassing research of all the phenomena vital for the living standards their trajectory can be adequately estimated, and their causes can be determined as well as all the factors that function during their progress.

18.3.3 Demographic Structure and Labour Force Renewal Rate

The economic changes that occurred had indirectly caused changes in the demographic structure of population, mostly resulting from the workforce migrating towards other cities or rural areas surrounding these towns. This process was mirrored implicitly in the increased weight of the elderly population. The demographic structure has significant implications demographically (birth rate, death rate and nuptiality) and economically, as the degree in which the population participates to the economic development is related to the physical and intellectual capacity of each age group (Erdeli and Braghină 1995). Large proportions of young population ensure demographic increase and the development of material and spiritual production while demographic ageing forecasts a demographic regression, decrease of the labour force and increase in the number of persons that will have to be economically supported by the society (Fig. 18.5).

The existences of large population segments that need to be supported economically determined a decrease in quality of life and affected standards of living due to a decrease in income, low access to goods and services, increased chances of social exclusions.

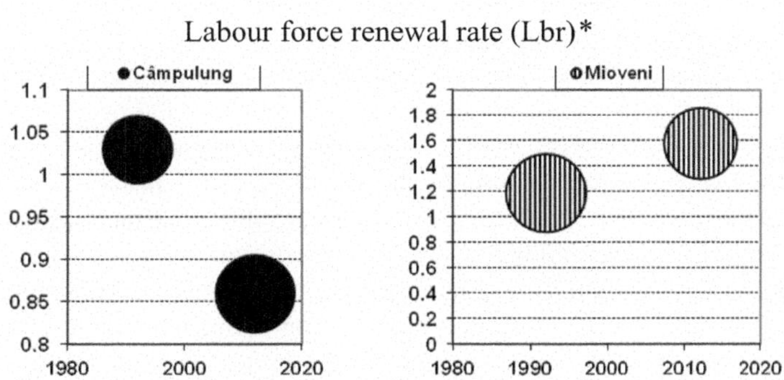

* **Lbr=Pop$_{15-29}$ / Pop$_{30-44}$** where: Lfr= labour force renewal rate;
Pop$_{15-29}$ = population aged between 15 and 29;
Pop$_{30-44}$ = population aged between 30 and 44.

Fig. 18.5 Labour force renewal rate

In order to determine the labour force potential as well as the active population but also to ensure the comparability of the data from different census years, the population was divided into five main age groups: 0–14 years, 15–24 years, 25–49 years, 50–59 years and over 60 years. The population was divided into two distinctive subgroups (0–14 years and 15–24 years) to better know the shape of the population segment that will ensure the change in the labour force but also the population segment that will give the future demographic evolution.

The adult population group was also divided into two subgroups (25–49 years and 50–59 years) to better quantify the group of adults that are close to retirement. The population segment over 60 years old (elderly population) offers interesting information regarding the demographic dependency rate. The discrepancies between the main age groups deepen the gap between the young, adult and elderly population groups and the central repercussions refer to the degree in which the active population is supporting the rest of the population.

The age and gender structural pyramids give specific quantitative and qualitative parameters that allow for the analysis of different age and gender groups, offering a relevant image of processes and phenomena like high or low birth rates, population flows, demographic ageing or existence of a young population (Erdeli and Dumitrache 2001). Analysing the age pyramids of the two urban centres, one can draw meaningful conclusions regarding the demographic ageing phenomenon and the labour force renewal rate for the next period (Fig. 18.6). Thus, the age pyramid for Câmpulung is stationary, having a narrow base due to a low birth rate and convex flanks because the adult population (that is no other than the 1955–1970 generations) is numerous and a flat top due to a numerous elderly population. An essential role in shaping this pyramid pertained to the 1970s migration wave when an important mass of people was attracted by the possibility of finding a better workplace in Câmpulung. This enforced the young and adult population segment and later contributed to the revitalisation of birth rates. Presently, due to the economic crisis and decline of the quality of life, the birth volume has decreased and there are no perspectives (at least not soon) of any changes to occur.

The town of Mioveni has a triangle shaped age pyramid with an excellent representation of the adult population (especially the one aged between 30 and 40) sustained by a large percentage of young age groups. This is because Mioveni is a young town supported mainly by the ample migratory flows that systematically supplied the town with 'fresh forces' during the 1980s. The narrowing shape showed on the graphic representation especially for the age groups 15–19 years and 20–24 years is due to the fact that these population groups are mostly still included in the educational system, are the most mobile and prefer to finish the high school and university studies in different centres because the town does not offer a diversified educational programme (both in terms of number of units as well as number of specialisations).

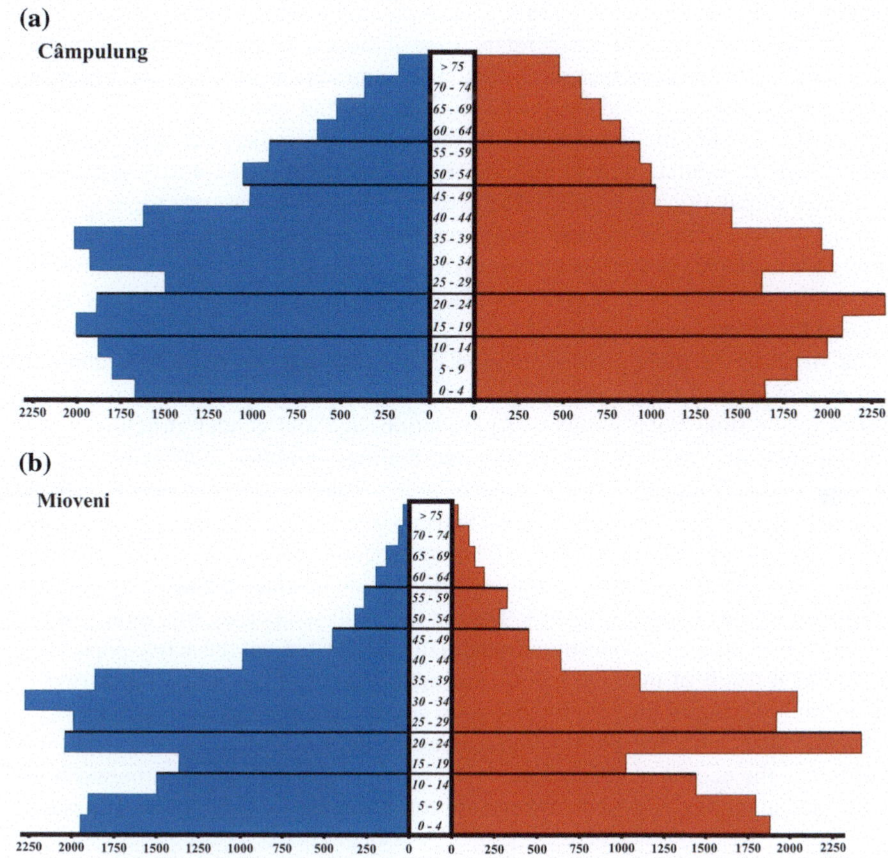

Fig. 18.6 Population age and sex structure (Types of age pyramids)

18.3.4 Active Population and Economic Dependency Rate

The changes that occurred in the demographic structure of the population as a result of the decline of the automotive industry incurred social changes and a deepening of the economic and social inequalities. The decrease of the active population as a result of industrial decline and respectively migration concluded in the increase of the economic dependency rate which had a negative impact on the population's quality of life.

The active population is estimated out of people who are performing an economically remunerated activity as well as those who are looking for a workplace, including employees, independent workers and also unemployed persons and young people looking for a job, because both of them are potentially active population segments (Erdeli and Dumitrache 2001).

At the level of the socio-economic structures, the active population has known fluctuant evolutions based on a general increase of those persons involved in an industrial activity up to 1989, and respectively their accentuated decrease in the following years as a consequence of the fall of the socialism and the subsequent economic restructuring. During the last decade, the difference in numbers between the active and the inactive population increased, among the causes of the explosive increase of the inactive population the author identified: the natural increase rate (demographic ageing), lowering of the retirement age in some activity fields (extractive industry and military for example) as well as early retirement of many people especially after the 1989 revolution. Also, in the past decade, the inconsistency between the demographic offer and the labour market demand increased, thus generating unemployment.

The structure of the active population could offer an image of the economic development level of the society as it is ultimately conditioned by the demographic realities of the time (total number of population, age and gender structure, living environments, etc.) as well as the economic realities (number of working places). The offer versus demand of working places makes balance which in turn is only the result of the economic development level that can be identified by analysing the active population structure. The occupation rate is an indicator calculated as a ratio between the active and total population and it shows the amount in which the active population participates in the economic activity. During the analysed period, this indicator has continuously decreased, proportionally with the diminishing of the active population segment as a result of massive layoffs and lengthening of the schooling period as well as the lowering of the retirement age in some socio-professional sectors.

Another indicator that shows imbalances in the population's socio-economic structures is the economic dependency rate which represents the ratio between the inactive and unemployed population and the active population (Fig. 18.7). The period

Economic dependency rate (Edr)*

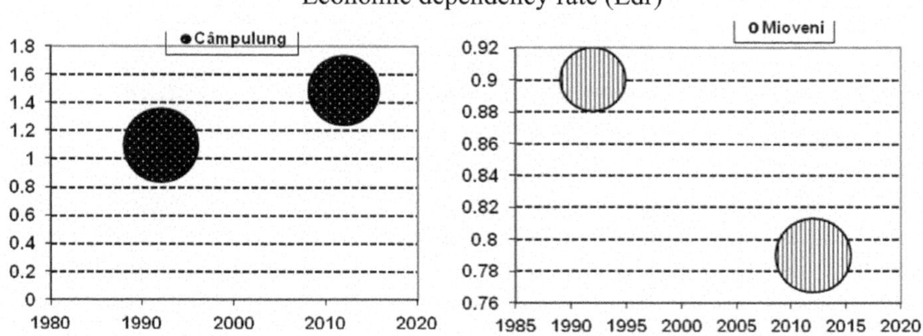

* **Edr = Ip + Up / Ep** where: Edr = economic dependency rate:
Ip = inactive population;
Up = unemployed population;
Ep = employed population.

Fig. 18.7 Economic dependency rate

of economic transition appears on the comparative graphs. Thus, in Câmpulung where the deindustrialisation process was more active, and it culminated with the ARO plant being shut down, the economic dependency rate increased, and the employed population had to sustain a substantial number of inactive and unemployed inhabitants. Mioveni, on another hand, went through successful privatisation of the Dacia car enterprise and had a significant share of the active population, so the economic dependency rate has significantly improved, with values of 0.90 at the start of the transition process decreasing to 0.79 in the present day.

To sustain an inclusive and intelligent development, the EU elaborated the 2020 Strategy in which employment played a crucial role in increasing quality of life, social inclusion and living standards (EC, 2010). Also, to sustain national economic growth and in the same time to improve quality of life, a 2020 objective of 70% employed workforce, aged 20–64 years old and an increase from the current level of 64% was set (Muncii 2015). The effects of rising old-age dependency ratio are numerous if adequate demographic policies do not support them. Workforce ageing has a direct impact on labour productivity and the abilities of an ageing workforce to adapt to the new demands of the global labour market.

18.3.5 Unemployment Rate

Employment represents an essential domain of the quality of life both nationally and a European level. In general, the deindustrialisation and economic restructuring phenomena are associated with high unemployment levels and a significant risk of poverty for the local households. These processes affected population's quality of life in the region, especially during the first years of the economic transition (1990–2004) when the active population was affected the most by the privatisation and restructuring of the automotive industry.

The inconsistency between demand and offer of labour force generates unemployment, a negative phenomenon that affects parts of the active population upon them losing their jobs (Erdeli and Dumitrache 2001). In Câmpulung, the unemployment rate at the beginning of the twenty-first century was 14.7%, a result of the layoffs generated by the 1997 and 1999 governmental orders. In Câmpulung, the labour force resources can include persons that receive unemployment payments during that period (4696 persons) and persons that stopped receiving social help but are still able to have a job (3786 persons). On October 31, 2001 in Câmpulung and in the surrounding areas, 1146 unemployed persons were receiving state help and 6000 unemployed persons were not, so a total of 7146 persons that did not have a job. On the other hand, the restructuring of Dacia company in 1999–2004 could have led to a significant decrease in job numbers (11,300 jobs), resulting in the onset of some socio-economic issues that could have affected the social balance of the area (Ciutacu and Chivu 2010, p. 61).

The fact that labour force offer does not coincide with demand which is emphasised by the age structure and professional categories of the unemployed segment of the population. Thus, the age structure shows that 415 persons have less than 25 years, 206 are aged between 26 and 30, 301 are between 31 and 40 years old, 144 are aged between 41 and 50 and 80 of them are older than 51. This situation determined a massive out-migration, people looking for a job, especially those aged up to 30 years old, with a higher degree of adaptability. The gender structure shows that unemployment among the male population in 2001 was 45.6% (523 persons) and 54.5% of the female population (623 persons).

The professional categories show that out of the total number of the unemployed population, 12.2% didn't have any qualifications, 78.5 had some qualification, 4.1% had a medium level of education, and 5% had a high level of education. Generally, the local labour force resources are qualified to work in the mining sector, in the manufacturing industry (welder, locksmiths, tool man—mould) and in other different jobs in constructions (building labourer, tile laying worker, plumber, mason, painter, decorator, civil engineer, etc.). A professional reconversion process was tried for all these unemployed categories (unfortunately without any success) for a new job like the autogenous welder, locksmith, carpenter, salesman, bartender, cook, and tailor.

Mioveni has registered a lower number (only 892) of unemployed people. The restructuration fever has also affected the leading employer of the town: S.C. Automobile Dacia S.A., and thus increased the number of unemployed population. At the beginning of 2002 after the layoffs from 1995 to 2001, there were some 655 unemployed (74.5%), and 227 persons were looking for a job (25.5%). The professional categories show that out of the total number of unemployed, 16.3% did not have any qualification, 39.1% of them did; 41.7% had a high school level of education and 2.9% of them finished university education. The age structure shows that the percentage of males is higher (53.7%) and most of them have a qualification (185) and 201 of them have a high school level of education. With the ending of the restructuring process in 2004, employment started to increase considering that the Renault Group determined a relaunching of production.

The 2008 economic crisis affected all types of qualifications required in the labour market, as the demand for low qualified jobs had decreased while other industrial branches including the automotive one required an ever-increasing level of qualification from its employees. Furthermore, one must also consider the issue of young workforce occupation as they are the most affected by economic crises and social exclusion. The EU specific strategy (Europe 202) is TineretulînMişcare (Youth on the Move) which includes new initiatives beneficial to the targeted social group: supporting entry to the labour market, promoting entrepreneurial spirit, consolidating a form of mobility that would help in acquiring the experience necessary for employment. The youth from the study area would benefit from programmes financed from priority axes such as '*Locuri de muncăpentrutineri*' initiative or the '*Inițiativa Educațieși competențe*' initiative (Ionescu 2017).

Overall at present times, the Sud-Muntenia (NUTS level II) Development Region includes the two towns in the study, registers medium level of economic development due to economic and service diversity as well as complex industrial activities, and the Renault Group had a significant role in increasing the living standard of the population and their quality of life. Projections regarding the evolution of employees between 2014 and 2020 demonstrate the interconnectivity between this indicator and phenomena associated with the economic crisis. Basing the analysis of data from the year 2014 as the year of rebound from the economic crisis the average number of employees has been rising (POR 2012). To diminish the adverse effects of unemployment, the authorities considered introducing policies for stimulating economic development and launching programmes focused on valuing the agricultural potential of the area, establishing SMAs and creating local commercial markets.

18.4 Impact of the Romanian Automotive Industry Restructuring on Quality of Life

Societal and economic evolutions can have a significant impact on the daily population life, with repercussions on their social, individual and collective well-being. As such, it is imperative to obtain a diagnosis of the economic situation as well as the evolution trends of the major economic indicators as they have a substantial social impact and affecting specific aspects or components of quality of life.

The economic restructuring phenomenon has substantial implications on the living standard and population's quality of life in the medium and long term. The most visible effects of this phenomenon are demographic and social, as the decrease in available workplaces and intensification of social processes such as unemployment and poverty caused demographic changes, urban decline and urban shrinkage. Other effects include physical degradation of industrial areas, increased derelict buildings, and the appearance of vacant brownfields due to lack of investments.

Measures that would diminish these social and spatial effects include urban regeneration strategies, physical renewal, and skills development. Socially, actions that would improve the situation should follow social development and urban poverty prevention programmes. Multinational companies are involved in activities that deal with the social reinsertion of their employees and unemployed population in general. A concept directly connected to the quality of life is that of corporate social responsibility (CSR). Based on competitiveness, performance and innovation, the automotive industry includes strategies for incorporating CSR components (Luo and Bhattacharya 2006; Butnariu and Filipeanu 2016; Madariaga-Garcia and Rivera-Rodriguez 2017).

According to the Renault Group director, Nicolas Maure, social responsibility is essential for an automotive company. The CSR policy respects international directives and is reflected by multiple actions and activities that deal with: environmental protection, natural resources conservation, human capital development, community development, investments in culture and education. An important objective of the CSR policy which also influences key domains of quality of life is increasing employability by offering professional development opportunities, through a programme called Drive for future. This program offers professional internships for college and master students thus giving them the opportunity to get a job inside a company. Another objective promoted is sustaining the community's social and economic development by offering access to education and mobility.

The 2020 European Strategy identifies multiple general objectives relevant to the social development and quality of life. These are relating to promoting workforce employability, supporting workforce mobility, fostering social inclusion and combating poverty and investing in education, competences and continuous learning.

In order to increase prosperity and population quality of life, certain consistent investments are aimed at the development of the human capital, cooperation between labour market actors, workforce and educational institutions by elaborating and coordinating policies that would mitigate the effects and provocations of demographic decline and migration.

18.5 Conclusions

Industrialisation remains the main sculptural factor of the geographic space that determined significant demographic mutations even though some blame this process for being the primary instability factor during the transition towards a market economy and at the same time, many people appreciate it as being the principal qualitative step in expressing human ingenuity. The analysed industrial centres are located relatively in close vicinity to one another in a geographic area polarised by the ancient town of Câmpulung. The town was founded and expanded as a great trading post and commercial centre thanks to the crafting traditions and long-standing business relationships with the surrounding regions, supported by ancient communication networks. Industrialisation as a process started at the beginning of the 20th century but experiences a peak during the communism period which amplified the role the town had, as a convergence centre for human and resource flows and information diffusion centre.

The development, increase and diversification of the industrial production, mainly of the ARO-SUV automotive industry led to changes in the demographic size of this town. Population number increased as a result of workforce in-migration flows while daily commuting flows from surrounding rural localities are also intensified.

Industrialisation was also responsible for modifying and overturning the urban hierarchy in the region.

The industrial enterprise Dacia is placed in a rural area (the villages Colibaşi—Mioveni) near the city of Piteşti, one of the principal urban centres in the region; during the 8th decade of the twentieth century, the former Colibasi village officially became a town and registered rather an impressive increase in population. During 2002 census year, the town had 35,849 inhabitants and it was almost equal to that of Câmpulung. A succinct overview of the statistics of population evolution number shows the role of the industrialisation process in the formation of a communist town compared to another one with 700 years of industrial tradition.

The most important changes in the active structure of population were due to the massive industrialisation during communism; the introduction of the automotive industry and the generated labour force deficit which was later supplemented by an accentuated commuting phenomenon. The polarising force of Câmpulung became more and more diffused over time as a result of the massive layoffs that took place at the ARO-SUV plant. On the other hand, the decrease in polarisation was accentuated by the effects of the Land Law, multiple waves of layoffs, a certain loosening of the pension's legislation which had the cumulative effect of an important number of persons stepping down from actively participating at the industrial process and redirecting towards agriculture and even moving in the rural areas.

At the first stage, the automotive industry had positive effects in the area, as increasing population numbers, through new job opportunities, expanding the labour force, growing the occupation rate, and of course rising incomes. The development of this industry generated a concentration of human capital and resources in these two urban areas; after 1990, the evolution of two towns diverged.

In Câmpulung, industrial restructuring led to unfavourable phenomena such as unemployment, a drop in workforce demand as the activities spectrum declined and automatisation increased, this increased social instability and decreased the population quality of life.

The industrial decline brought with it the decline of Câmpulung both demographically and socially while the revival of this industry after 1990 with the Dacia Mioveni enterprise resulted in the continuous development of that town.

Both evolutions affected directly and indirectly the local population and their living conditions. In case of Câmpulung, several negative effects can be noticed whereas, in case of Mioveni situation is entirely different.

An increase in unemployment and poverty as a result of massive layoffs and the reduced income led to increasing social inequalities and implicitly population vulnerability by limiting their access to specific services, including medical one, lack of investments in infrastructure, education and social amenities.

On the other hand, we concluded that a successful industrial restructuring has led to the revival of the automotive industry in the town of Mioveni which generated an increase in labour force occupation and income levels.

This different evolution of the two towns presented proves the necessity of development policies and investments correlated with adequate social strategies which can adjust certain social inequalities and generate economic growth having beneficial effects on the population quality of life.

References

Bănică, A., Istrate, M., & Muntele, I. (2017). Challenges for the resilience capacity of Romanian shrinking cities. *Sustainability, 9*(12), 2289.

Butnariu, A., & Filipeanu, D. (2016). Does CSR enhance market performance for automotive companies? *SEA-Practical Applications of Science, 4*(3), 431–441.

Ciutacu, C., & Chivu, L. (2010). Anticiparea şi managementul restructurării. Raport naţional, iunie 2010, ITC. Retrieved February 25, 2018, from http://ec.europa.eu/social/BlobServlet?docId=5748&langId=ro.

Comisia Națională de Prognoză (2016). Proiecția principalilor indicatori economico- sociali în profil territorial până în 2019. București. Retrieved March 5, 2018, from http://www.cnp.ro/user/repository/prognoze/prognoza_profil_teritorial_decembrie_2016.pdf.

Crețan, R., Nica-Guran, L., Platon, D., & Turnock, D. (2005). Foreign direct investment in Romania: progress in less—favoured areas. In D. Turnock (Ed.), *Foreign direct investment in Eastern Europe and the former Soviet Union*. Ashgate, Aldershot. Dumitrache L., Zamfir.

Dumitrache, L., Nae, M., Simion, G., & Stoica, I.-V. (2016). The urban nexus: Contradictions and dilemmas of (Post) communist (Sub)urbanization in Romania. *Human Geographies. Romanian Journal of Studies and Research in Human Geography, 10*(1), 39–58.

Erdeli G., & Braghină C. (1995). Efectele crizei economice în ţările aflate în tranziţie asupra forţei de muncă. Particularizarepentru România. *Terra*, nr. 1–4, Bucureşti.

Erdeli, G., & Dumitrache, L. (2001). *Geografia Populaţiei*. Bucureşti: Editura Corint.

Eurofound (2008). More and better jobs: Patterns of employment expansion in Europe. Retrieved March 5, 2018, from https://www.eurofound.europa.eu/publications/annual-report/2008/labour-market-business/erm-report-2008-more-and-better-jobs-patterns-of-employment-expansion-in-europe.

Eurofound (2017). European quality of life survey 2016: Quality of life, quality of public services, and quality of society. Publications Office of the European Union, Luxembourg. Retrieved March 5, 2018, from https://www.eurofound.europa.eu/sites/default/files/ef_publication/field_ef_document/ef1733en.pdf.

European Commission (2009). Perception survey on quality of life in European cities. Analytical report. Retrieved February 15, 2018, from http://ec.europa.eu/commfrontoffice/publicopinion/flash/fl_277_en.pdf.

European Commission (2017). Special Eurobrometer 467. Future of Europe. Social issues. Retrieved February 12, 2018, from http://ec.europa.eu/commfrontoffice/publicopinion/index…/80645.

Florian, V., & Sârbu, A. (1997). *Populaţie rurală în tranziţie – schimbare şi continuitate*. Economiirurale locale: Dimensiuni şi perspective, Editura Agris, Redacţia Revistelor Agricole S.A.

Ghinoiu I. (1978). *Populaţia şi aşezările depresiunii Câmpulung. Studiu de geografie şi etnografie*. teza de doctorat consultată în manuscris prin bunăvoinţa autorului.

Großmann, K., Haase, A., Rink, D., & Steinführer, A. (2008). Benefits and limits of a cross-national transfer of research approaches. In M. Novak & M. Nowosielski (Eds.), *Declining cities/developing cities: Polis hand German perspectives* (pp. 77–99). Poznań: Instytut Zachodni.

Ianoș, I., Petrișor, A.-I., Zamfir, D., Cercleux, A.-L., Stoica, I.-V., & Tălângă, C. (2013). In search of a relevant index measuring territorial disparities in a transition country. Romania as a case study. *Die Erde, 144*(1), 69–81.

Ionescu, I. (2017). Tinerii – grup exclus riscului de excluziun esocială: Analizarea factorilor care le îngreunează situația pe piața muncii și îneducație. *Calitatea Vieții XXVIII, 1*, 75–104.

Jigoria-Oprea, L., & Popa, N. (2017). Industrial brownfields: An unsolved problem in post-socialist cities. A comparison between two mono industrial cities: Reşiţa (Romania) and Pančevo (Serbia). *Urban Studies, 54*(12), 2719–2738.

Jucu, I. S. (2015). Romanian post-socialist industrial restructuring at the local scale: Evidence of simultaneous processes of De-/Reindustrialization in the Lugoj Municipality of Romania. *Journal of Balkan and Near Eastern Studies, 17*(4), 408–426.

Luo, X., & Bhattacharya, C. B. (2006). Corporate social responsibility, customer market satisfaction, and market value. *Journal of Marketing, 70*(4), 1–18.

Marginean, I. (2004). Modelul social românesc din perspectiva calității vieții populației. *Calitatea vietii XV, 3–4,* 203–218.

Madariaga-Garcia, J., & Rivera-Rodriguez, F. (2017). Corporate social responsibility, customer satisfaction, corporate reputation, and firms' market value: Evidence from the automobile industry. *Spanish Journal of Marketing -ESIC, 21*(1), 39–53.

Muncii, M. (2015). Strategia națională pentru promovarea îmbătrânirii active și protecția persoanelor vârstnice 2015–2020. Retrieved March 5, 2018, from http://www.mmuncii.ro/j33/images/Documente/Transparenta/Dezbateri_publice/2015-07-15_Anexa1_ProiectHG_SIA.pdf.

Oswalt, P. (Ed.). (2005). *Shrinking Cities 1: International research*. Ostfildern: Hatje Cantz.
Oswalt, P. (Ed.). (2006). *Shrinking Cities 2: Interventions*. Ostfildern: Hatje Cantz.
Popescu, C. R. (2000). *Industria României în secolul XX – analiză geografică*. București, România: Editura Oscar- Print.
Popescu, C.R., (2014). Dezindustrialization and urban Shrinkage in Romania What lessons for the spatial policy?. *Transylvanian Review of Administrative Sciences*, *42*, 181–202.
POR (2012). Studiu privind problemele sociale și calitatea vieții în RegiuneaSud-Muntenia. Regio. București. Retrieved March 5, 2018, from https://www.adrmuntenia.ro/download_file/…/studiu-social_adrsm_17122012_vfinala.
Schmid, G. (2006). Social risk management through transitional labour markets. *Socio-Economic Review*, (4), 1–33.
Stenning, A. (2005). Post-socialism and the changing geographies of the everyday in Poland. *Transactions of the Institute of British Geographers, 30*(1), 113–127.
Theodossiou, I. (1998). The effects of low-pay and unemployment on psychological well-being: A logistic regression approach. *Journal of Health Economics, 17*(1), 85–104.
Turnock, D. (2006). *The economy of East Central Europe, 1815–1989: Stages of transformation in a peripheral region*. London and New York: Routledge.
Zamfir, C. (1984). *Indicatori şi surse de variaţie a calităţii vieţii*. Bucureşti: Editura Academiei Române.
Zamfir, C., et.al. (2017). *Raport social al ICCV 2017. Starea socială a României Calitatea vieții: situația actuală și perspective pentru 2038*. Academia Română ICCV. București.

Chapter 19
Geographic Impact of Anthropogenic Activities on the Social Well-Being and Health Conditions of the Residents Living Around Wetlands/Lakes of Srinagar City, Kashmir (India)

Ishtiaq A. Mayer, Sheraz A. Lone and Manzoor A. Wani

Abstract Human well-being is generally considered as a unifying concept and varying characteristics of both objective and subjective factors which constitute health and quality of life. Stiglitz et al. (2010) in its report titled "Commissions of the measurement of economic performances and social wellbeing" identified eight key dimensions that need to be taken into account while defining human well-being. Some of the important key dimensions are income, health, education, economic activities, and environment. In this direction, human well-being indices like Happy Planned Index (HPI), Human Development Index (HDI), Gross National Happiness, Physical Quality of Life Index (PQLI), and Sustainable Society Index (SSI) are used by both the developed and developing societies to measure the level of human well-being. Statistical techniques are used in attaining desirable results. The present study on Kashmir has been carried out considering the above factors like geographic environment, income status, economic activities, housing pattern, and health profile (morbidity). The morbidity pattern has been calculated to project inequalities in the well-being of a particular section of people (boatmen) by calculating DALY to measure the level of well-being.

19.1 Introduction

The sustenance of all the living creatures on planet earth beyond any debate depends on the availability of water. Although more than 75% of earth's surface is covered

I. A. Mayer (✉) · S. A. Lone · M. A. Wani
Department of Geography and Regional Development, University of Kashmir, Srinagar 190006, India
e-mail: ishimayer@gmail.com

S. A. Lone
e-mail: sheraz.scholar@kashmiruniversity.net

M. A. Wani
e-mail: manzoorwani8559@gmail.com

B. R. K. Sinha (ed.), *Multidimensional Approach to Quality of Life Issues*,
https://doi.org/10.1007/978-981-13-6958-2_19

by water trapped in glaciers and accumulated in oceans, seas, lakes, rivers, and other wetlands/water bodies (Anil and Sreeja 2012). However, not more than 5% of it is suitable for human consumption because of varied and unstable water chemistry. After tropical evergreen forests, wetlands are one of the most productive ecosystems, in the biosphere to regulate ecological sustainability of a region (Carlos et al. 2005; Talukder et al. 2015). Archeological evidences reveal the establishment of earlier civilizations like Egyptian, Mohenjo Daro, Sind, and others on such wetlands/water bodies. They continue till date to meet the life-supporting system like drinking water, food production, water cycling and purification, terrestrial and extraterrestrial energy transfer, agroclimatic regionalization, and many more attributes. Across the globe, the aerial extension of wetlands are shrinking to near extinction due to manifold reasons, natural processes, and with strong anthropogenic interference like growing population, unplanned developmental policies, ambiguous management structure, and absence of national and international legislation and law to protect wetlands at regional and global levels (Julie et al. 2007). According to one estimate, about 50% of global wetlands have become extinct only in the last hundred years or so.

Srinagar city, the largest urbanized unit of Kashmir valley is famous throughout the world for its natural scenery as well as for its lakes, water bodies, meandering rivers, and wetlands such as Dal, Negin, Hokarsar, Jhelum, and others. Like other wetlands and water bodies, the degradation of wetlands of Srinagar city is not an exception. These wetlands and water bodies have suffered serious losses in terms of their aerial extent during the last few decades as a result of anthropogenic factors, urban sprawl, and the so-called agricultural technology and development. The urban population of Srinagar city has at present crossed one million persons (estimated on annual growth rate of 5.6% per annum, Census of India, 2001). These factors have put enough stress on wetlands/water bodies and lakes of Srinagar city. The waters of Dal, Hokarsar, Negin, and Jhelum have turned almost contaminated and polluted leaving a direct impact on disease causation and health conditions of the people residing on them. A high concentration of waterborne and other infectious diseases is prevalent in and around these wetlands. Therefore, in the backdrop of this, an attempt has been made to conduct a change detection analysis of wetlands and water bodies of Srinagar city and its environs taking the information of the last 35 years from 1971 to 2007 with a view to assess the quality of life and well-being of the people by studying the disease morbidity and mortality patterns using satellite images and geospatial tools.

The rapid growth in population, as well as consumerism, has speeded up waste generation thereby add up to waste loads vis-à-vis increase in pollutants and pollution level. Thus, in this way, quality of life imbalances, further man-made hazards are created causing harm to human well-being. Therefore, the environment is a matter of general concern. This is the basic attribute on which the human well-being and economy system are built up and hence is of vital importance. Similarly, the role of natural hazards cannot be underestimated in modifying the well-being aspects of the people in general (Burton et al. 1978; Summers et al. 2012). It is, therefore, interpreted into two complementary reactions; one is the influence of the environment upon man; the other is man's influence upon the environment. Hence, the environment contains man at its core or as an integral part of it. The distinction between physical and man-made environment is obvious. The physical world has been constantly modified at the advent of humankind as such the physio-economic geography at global level is undergoing a change with deteriorating ecological balance. Therefore, the man and environment are to be studied in an integrated manner (Dutta et al. 1986). The impact of anthropogenic agency is readily ascertained on the misuses of wetlands/water bodies at global level, although the sustenance of all the living creatures on the earth depends to a large extent on the availability of water that is preserved in various types of water bodies (Pierre et al. 2012).

The Himalayan region, spreading over a horizontal expansion of over more than 2500 mi known to have ample water resources, has shown declining trends in terms of its shrinking snow reservoirs due to natural climatic fluctuations and increased human intervention. One of its subregions of Jammu and Kashmir state has suffered more in its ecology and environment mainly due to socio-political, socio-cultural, and socio-economic attributes leaving adverse impacts on human habitation, human health, and health-related quality of life.

19.2 Study Area

Srinagar, the main city of the state of Jammu and Kashmir has its own image over time (Mayer 1992). The city extends from 33°53′ to 34° 17′ N latitude and from 74° 36′ to 75° 01′ E longitude (Fig. 19.1). It is situated at an altitude of 5200 ft above mean sea level and spreads over in the midst of an oval-shaped valley of Kashmir, tectonically in origin, and is prone to seismic activity.

The city as well as its hinterland is encircled by the natural wall of mountains with height ranging from 1800 to 4300 meters above mean sea level where human habitations with varying densities exist. These mountains are the sources of almost all water bodies including the artery river Jhelum which has unending importance in the drainage network as each and every fiber of the Kashmir Valley has been woven by its waters (Raza et al. 1978). Srinagar city has an area of 157 km^2, which includes the area under various wetlands/water bodies. Nature has gifted Srinagar city with the world famous Dal Lake which attracts both foreign and domestic tourists. River Jhelum divides Srinagar city into two parts and flows through the middle of it. Other important water bodies include the Anchar Lake, Hokarsar, Khushalsar, Brarinambal, and Negin Lake (Fig. 19.2). The total area under water bodies is 6,541 acres (16.84%). Dal Lake is situated in the north of the city extending from the Drugjan (Dal gate) area in the south to the Telbal in the north, this lake is very important from the tourist point of view. About 4% of the total population of Srinagar city resides on boats over the Dal and Negin Lakes and river Jhelum. However, there have been drastic changes in the areal extent of both the water bodies/wetlands of Srinagar City. A few small and medium-sized water bodies have disappeared entirely whereas many others are shrinking rapidly. Some of the major water bodies like Anchar Lake have reduced from 2.49 to 1.15 km^2, Hokarsar 1.63–0.92 km^2, and Negin lake 0.76–0.56

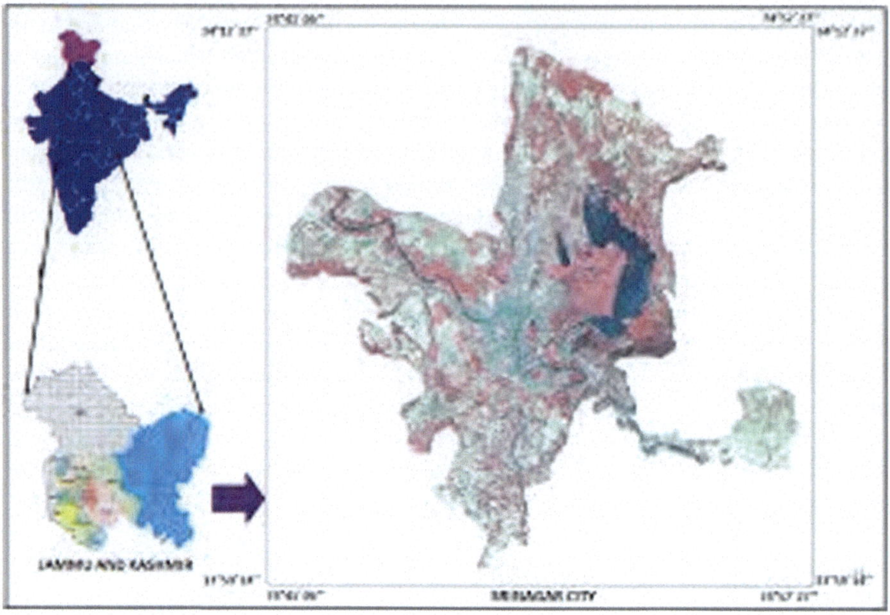

Fig. 19.1 Location map of the study area

km^2 from 1971 to 2004. Dal Lake too has witnessed aerial shrinkage and has lost much of its glory as well described by historians as "emerald in jewels". The total area of the wetland of Dal has reduced from 20.35 km^2 in1971–18.44 km^2 in 2004. This has mainly occurred due to encroachments by people for want of residential needs. Thus, illegal and unauthorized colonies have come up along shores of water bodies which by all means lack civil amenities. The residents of such areas dump wastes and flush sewerage into these water bodies causing ill health to them and at times epidemics of one or the other nature erupts from such sites as such the quality of life gets deteriorated.

19.3 Data and Methodology

The study is based on data collected from both the primary and secondary sources.

(I) Primary data has been collected through a range of methods which included:
(a) Household surveys.
(b) Personal narrations.
(c) Observations.

(II) Secondary data pertaining to population, number of households, disease reporting, and health facilities were collected from records of Sheri Kashmir Institute of

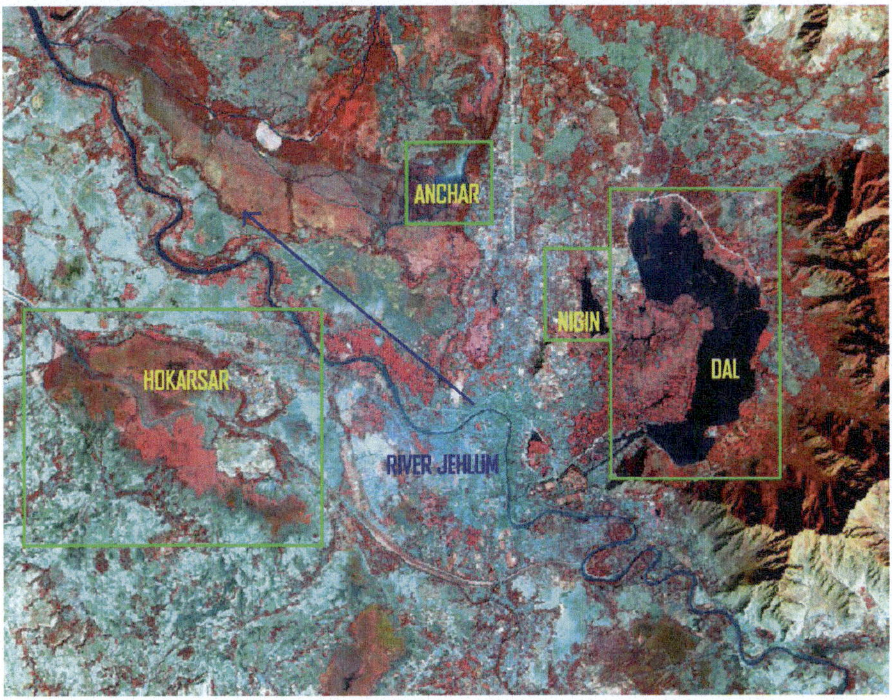

Fig. 19.2 Location map of water bodies/wetlands

Medical Sciences (SKIMS), S.M.H.S. Hospital, Srinagar, Statistics and Evaluation Department, Srinagar and census of India, series 8, J&K 2001. On the areal extension and location of Srinagar city, the Survey of India (S.O.I.) topographic map of 1:50,000 scale was used as a base map. The IRS-1D LISS-III images were used to generate multi-temporal land use/land cover maps of the wetland/water bodies. An area of 1.5 km buffer zone around wetland was taken into consideration, whereas a similar buffer zone of 1 km from territorial lake shores and 500 m from the banks of river channel of Jhelum was demarcated to assess the possible anthropogenic pressure on wetlands/water bodies; as a result, the water turns contaminated and its use injuries the human health and life condition. Statistical techniques (Z-Score, Composite index) were used to ascertain the level of human development for the selected section of population—the boatmen; living on water bodies of Srinagar City.

Table 19.1 Population growth in Srinagar city (1891–2011)

Census year	Total population	Density (persons/km^2)	Decadal growth rate
1891	1,18,960	–	–
1901	1,22,618	9579	+3.07
1911	126,344	9832	+3.04
1921	141,735	9788	+12.18
1931	173,573	9862	+22.46
1941	207,786	11,806	+19.71
1951	246,522	8351	+18.64
1961	285,257	6884	+15.71
1971	403,413	4867	+34.31
1981	606,002	2912	+40.13
1991[a]	788,680	3244	+30.14
2001	971,357	3492	+30.14
2011	1,147,617	3933	+18.14
2021(estimated)	22,78,000	–	–

Source District census Handbook, Srinagar district 1981
2. Census of India, J&K series (8) 2001–2011
3. Master Plan, Srinagar Metropolitan Area 2000–2021 (S.D.A)
[a]Population of 1991 was obtained through interpolation as census was not conducted in J&K

19.4 Discussion

The study reveals that population growth in Srinagar city is haphazardly expanding in linear and horizontal form. Population of Srinagar city shows a tremendous increase between 1891 and 2011 (Table 19.1).

The expansion of the city is more prominent in the western direction than in northern, northeastern, and southern directions. This is mainly due to the presence of geomorphologic barriers like hill-locks, reserved areas for sanctuaries, wetlands/water bodies, etc. The concentration of rural migrants is more in Srinagar city than in any other town of Kashmir Valley. These in-migrants have mostly occupied and encroached natural, agricultural, flood-prone area and water bodies as such they have constructed illegal and unauthorized dwellings. Therefore, these areas lack sewerage, sanitation, and other basic amenities and adversely affect the life support system and quality of life. Second, the preference of age-old tradition of joint family system in Kashmir is undergoing radical change into separate and divided family norms. Hence, the number of households has increased many folds during the last few decades. This has put an additional burden on land to offer the location for settlements or housing purpose.

Table 19.2 Generalized land use in Srinagar city

Generalized land use	Area in ha, 1971	Area in ha, 2001	Area in ha, 2006
Built up excluding 2 and 3	1925.20	2561.07	17,046.40
Residential area	1512.2	8772.93	9850
Commercial belts	38.4	193	729
Agriculture and forests, parks, and open fields	1538.1	22,940	14,549.76
Water bodies	6542.44	4855.00	2528.7
Total	17,542.60*	39,322*	38,868.2*

Source Srinagar Development Authority
* Includes the proposed area of Greater Srinagar city

19.5 Land Use Pattern

The land use patterns and their changes at times provide many social and economic benefits. However, these changes come at the cost of stability of natural environment. Land use depicts how different areas of land is being utilized under various activities which also help into overcome the problems of haphazard, uncontrolled development, deteriorating environmental quality, loss of prime agricultural lands, destruction of important wetlands (Anderson 1976). Urban land use pattern is one of the important attributes of urban planning which aims at orderly and balanced geographical distribution of all the uses of urban land. The land use pattern of a city or town is depicted its economic and social structure. Srinagar city can be broadly divided into five functional land use areas (Table 19.2).

19.5.1 Build up Area

The built-up areas covers 17,046.4 ha or 43.86% of the total land area of the city and includes government offices, educational institutions, industrial pockets, religious places, roads and streets, residential houses, and other buildings (Table 19.2). Being a capital city, Srinagar has always performed important administrative function. The administrative buildings perform district functional offices, such as the old secretariat complex, new secretariat complex, old high court complex, and new court complex. The main industrial pockets are found in Zadibal (Baghi Ali Mardan), Baghat-i-Barzulla, and Zanikot. The main educational institutions are located in the CBD although two of the main educational institutions, Kashmir University and the National Institute of Technology are located in the north of Hazratbal area, and the medical college is located in Karan Nagar (Kaksarai). There are several healthcare delivery institutions including some hospitals in the city. There are no appreciable industrial complexes in Srinagar. There are some stone crushers and brick kilns located on the periphery of Srinagar and are the main sources of pollution in the city.

19.5.2 Residential Areas

As far as the residential areas are concerned the central and south-central parts of the city have maximum concentration of residential houses. The eastern and the northern parts of the city have low density of residential houses due to the presence of the mountains and forests. This has given a high density of persons per room leaving direct impact on disease transmission process (Mayer 2006). There is a high dearth for residential areas compared to that of the growth rate of population. The need for residential land is projected at 63.35% of the total built area by 2021 AD as envisaged in Master Plan for Srinagar Metropolitan Area 2000–2021 (Srinagar Development Authority). Hence, wherever there is land availability, the human colonies come up. Most of these settlements do not fulfill the prescribed norms vis-à-vis health requirements. This is particularly observed in colonies which are situated along lake and river banks and around wetlands. As such, people suffer from various types of communicable and waterborne diseases and these diseases in turn adversely affect health and quality of life.

19.5.3 Commercial Belts

About 730 ha of Srinagar total area is under commercial use which comes to about 2% of the total area of the city. Almost all the important roads have commercial establishments on their flanks. The most important and the busiest retail shopping areas of the city are found in the hub of city—the residency road area, right from GPO in the east to Batamaloo in the west. All along the Maulana Azad road, measuring about 2 km has commercial units between Golf club in the east and Lal Chowk area. Another important commercial zone is located along either side of banks of river Jhelum popularly known as seven bridges from Amirakadal to Chhatabal (Veer). The important commercial centers established during residency era along this commercial belt are Fatehkadal (third bridge), Zainakadal, Aalikadal (fifth bridge) belt.

19.5.4 Land Under Agriculture, Forests, Parks, and Open Fields

Large chunks of the land within the municipal corporation boundary are under the use of agriculture, parks and playgrounds, forests, and hills. The total area under agriculture and forest comes to 14,549.76 ha which constitutes about 37% of the total area of the Srinagar municipal corporation (Table 19.2). This proportion is high due to the incorporation of new land by the corporation in 1981. The newly incorporated areas are agricultural farms, on account of which the proportion of land under this category has increased. The agricultural land is found on almost all sides of the city except the west, which is mostly forested and hilly. Besides, there are a number of public parks and open spaces; most important among them are the polo ground, Iqbal Park, Bakshi stadium, Sheri Kashmir stadium, golf clubs, and Mughal garden. These are located in different directions of the city.

19.5.5 Water Bodies

Srinagar city is gifted with the world famous Dal Lake which adjoins it. River Jhelum divides the city into two parts and flows through the middle of the town, other water bodies include the Khushalsar, Brarinambal, and Negin Lake. The total area under water bodies is 2528.7 ha. The Dal Lake, situated in the north of the city extends from the Dal gate area in the south to the Telbal in the north, this lake is very important from the tourist point of view. In the olden days, this lake and river Jhelum were the chief lines of transport and communication. About 3.93% of the total population of Srinagar city resides on houseboats over the Dal and Negin Lakes and river Jhelum. The Negin Lake is situated between Lalbazar and Saidakadal while the Khushalsar is located in the west of Hawal. In the light of above land use distribution, there is a high pressure of population on available land resources.

19.6 Results

It is now established fact that "Geogens" are responsible for "pathogeneses" of diseases. As diseases are the outcome of maladjustment of people to its environment and the etiology of the disease lies in the change of environmental parameters. Cultural, socioeconomic conditions and lifestyle changes are causative factors in various types of diseases. Population settled in and around the periphery of wetlands/water bodies of Srinagar city has been troubled severely by such environmental changes. To combat cold the house pattern and structure have developed here with least ventilation and with low ceilings. The city lacks well-developed drainage and sewerage disposal facilities. Most of it mingles with these water bodies thereby polluting and contaminating them. There is unchecked siltation from catchment areas of these water bodies resulting in their aerial shrinkage. Encroachment due to human habitation besides area distortion has adversely affected the ecology of these wetlands/water bodies. Boatmen population mostly use contaminated lake water for drinking and other domestic purposes thereby causing illness among them. The cumulative impact of such factors is seen on the health status of its people as reflected by disease com-

Table 19.3 Recommended drinking water standards (mg/l)

	World health organization (WHO)			
Characteristics	Highest desirable (mg/l)	Maximum permissible (mg/l)	Constituents	Recommended maximum limits of concentration (mg/l)
Turbidity	5.0	2.5	Antimony	0.005
Taste/odor	Nothing	Disagreeable	Arsenic	0.01
Color	5.0	50.0	Barium	0.7
PH	7–8.5	6.5–9.2	Boron	0.3
Total solids	50	150	Cadmium	0.003
Magnesium	30.0	150	Copper	2
Chloride	200	600	Cyanide	0.07
Sulfide	200	400	Fluoride	1.5
Nitrate	45	45	Lead	0.01
Fluoride	1.0	1.5	Manganese	0.5
Ammonia	0.2	1.0	Mercury	0.001
Cyanide	–	0.05	Molybdenum	0.07
Lead	–	0.1	Nickel	0.02
Cadmium	–	0.01	Selenium	0.01

Source Mishra and Mishra (2007), WHO

bination and morbidity pattern. All these deteriorate the overall health status and successively quality of life. Tables 19.3 and 19.4, reflect the deviation in admissible level of drinking water recommended by World Health Organization and the water available to these people living on such water bodies.

The changes in the physico-chemical characteristics of water of different water bodies and wetlands show greater variations depending upon the season, geological substratum, soil type, vegetation, water depth, and the anthropogenic effects (Pandit 1999). The cumulative impact of such factors on the health status of its people as reflected by disease combination and morbidity pattern becomes clear from Table 19.5.

Table 19.6, depicts the communicable nature of hepatitis disease among the people residing on and along different lake waters. The highest percentage is found in the age group of 20–35 years and the maximum concentration is in the Dal Lake. Hokarsar wetland shows the lowest percentage of this particular waterborne disease.

On the whole, about 60% of the Dal lake population suffers from waterborne disease. The corresponding percentages for Negin Lake and Anchar Lake are about 25–32%, respectively, and for Hokarsar wetland people suffering from such diseases is about 40%. The impact of morbidity pattern on the economic development of the abovementioned sites of Srinagar city is reflected in Table 19.7. Those, who reside on water bodies or on the periphery of wetlands lose more working days in a year

Table 19.4 Physicochemical analysis of water bodies of Srinagar city

Characteristics	Physicochemical characteristics of Srinagar water bodies			
	Dal lake average	Negin lake average	Anchar lake average	River Jhelum average
Alkalinity (mg/100 g)	105	110	125	95
PH	8.1	8	8.7	7.8
NO_3-N	675	500	305	–
Dissolved oxygen	6.9	7	6.1	6.6
Calcium (mg/100 g)	4	4	5.5	4.8
Magnesium (mg/100 g)	0.2	0.1	–	0.5
Chloride (mg/100 g)	11	13	17	12
Potassium (mg/100 g)	15	14	18	15
Nitrate (mg/100 g)	10	9.5	14	11
Phosphate (mg/100 g)	5	5	7.5	4
Fe (ug/l)	500	500	800	350

Source Lakes and waterways development authority, J&K Government, 2006
Urban environmental engineering department Srinagar, 2005–06

due to illness and other health-related problems. These are not a good sign from the point of view of health and health-related quality of life.

19.7 Conclusion

The study was undertaken to find out the geographic impact of anthropogenic activities on the social well-being and health conditions of people living on wetland/water bodies of Srinagar City, Kashmir, (India). The study was framed in such a way that it incorporates parameters like population expansion with time, land use dynamics in the past decades, basic amenities available (drinking water) and health-related problems associated with the people residing on the exhumed wetland and water bodies of Srinagar city, Kashmir. In Srinagar city huge population expansion has been witnessed during the past decades as shown in the above discussion which simultaneously affected the land use pattern, pattern of built up area, residential area, and commercial areas from 2001 to 2006 as shown in Table 19.2. The growth of population expansion extends to the inner skirts of the wetlands and along the banks of water bodies which do not affect the quality of water bodies only but also increased

Table 19.5 Pattern of waterborne diseases, 2006–07

Water body/wetland	No. surveyed localities	No. of household and boat population surveyed	No of persons surveyed			% age of persons suffering from waterborne diseases				% age of other diseases
			T	M	F	Typhoid	Diarrhea	Hepatitis	Gastroenteritis	
Dal Lake	15	45	267	135	132	19.5	9.6	14.6	12.8	40.5
Negin	8	30	151	80	71	3.5	4.2	8.4	9.2	74.7
Anchar	3	19	90	45	53	3.9	5.5	11.4	10.4	68.8
Hokarsar	10	50	205	101	104	4.5	5.4	20.1	10.9	59.1

Source Compiled from SKIMS, Srinagar; SMHS Hospital, Srinagar; Field survey

Table 19.6 Hepatitis disease in wetlands/water bodies by age and sex of Srinagar City 2006–07

Age group	Dal lake			Negin lake			Anchar lake			Hokarsar wetland			Total		
	T	M	F	T	M	F	T	M	F	T	M	F	T	M	F
<19 years	3		3	1	1	–	4	2	2	–	–	–	8	3	5
20–35 years	9	3	6	3	1	2	6	6	–	1	–	1	19	10	9
40–49 years	5	4	1	1	1	–	2	1	1	–	–	–	8	6	2
50–59 years	1	1	–	–	–	–	2	2	–	1	–	1	4	2	2
>60 years	–	–	–	1	–	1	–	–	–	–	–	–	1	–	1
All ages	18	8	10	6	3	3	14	11	3	2	–	2	40	21	19

Source SKIMS, Srinagar; SMHS Hospital, Srinagar

Table 19.7 Socio-economic impact of waterborne diseases in wetlands and water bodies of Srinagar City, 2006–07

Water bodies/wetlands	Average loss of working days of an individual worker per year	Crowding index no. of persons sharing one room
Dal lake	50 days	5.5–6.5
	70–95 among boat population	
Negin lake	20 days	5.5–5
Anchar lake	60 days	5.5–6
Hokarsar wetland	20 days	3–4

Source Field survey

the disaster vulnerability like devastated floods, and prolonged health problems in the presence of various water quality assessments revealing thereby suitable for drinking water as per WHO and BIS norms. The contaminated water adversely affects the health conditions of the residents of all age groups, and also have a direct impact on their socioeconomic life and social well-being. The study concludes that due to unplanned growth of urban centers and non-logistic intervention by the concerned administration the wetlands and water bodies continue to depleting constantly and it impacts the ecosystem of the area.

19.8 Suggestions

A large section of the rural population of Kashmir lives under the shadow of poverty, unemployment, ill health, unhygienic settings, socioeconomic disparities, spatial infrastructural imbalances, and extremes backwardness. The Srinagar district, one of the major administrative divisions, ranks highest in terms of total population and high proportion of urban population (>78%). Its rural population is largely engaged in horticulture using high dose of pesticides and fungicides which get mingled with underground water and surface water sources. Since the Srinagar district is nestled with some of the world famous lakes like Dal Lake, Negin, and Anchar and rivers like Jhelum and others, the water of these gets polluted and contaminated by pesticides and other chemicals. The water quality of these sources gets further polluted and damages at some locations of human refuse and domestic wastes are directly dumped into them. The leading health care institute of Jammu and Kashmir State, SKIMS also put hospital waste into Anchar lake untreated form. These all account for the percentage of waterborne diseases and consequently affect their quality of life. The crowding index of these sites can be ascertained by the fact that as many as 5.5–6.0 persons share one room/boat. As a result, numerous diseases are encountered in the densely populated areas compared to those with sparse populations in the city. The incidence of diseases is encountered in both high and low altitude areas. So, there is a need to ascertain geomedical causes that produce variations in the spatial pattern of diseases. Besides, the distribution pattern, health care needs to be analyzed in order to assess the levels of imbalances in their distributional pattern. Therefore, a holistic policy needs to be formulated for the future location/allocation of health care facilities taking into account the physical accessibility so that population of Srinagar city is duly served with these facilities and well-being or quality of life of the people can be promoted and maintained.

References

Anderson, J. R. (1976). *A land use and land cover classification system for use with remote sensor data* (Vol. 964). US Government Printing Office.

Anil, K., & Sreeja, S. (2012). *Ecosystem approach to disaster reduction*. New Delhi: National Institute of Disaster Management.

Burton, I., Kates, R. W., & White, G. (1978). *The environment as hazard*. New York: Oxford University Press.

Carlos, C., Simon, H., & Anthony, M. (2005). *Ecosystems and human well-being: Health synthesis: A report of the Millennium Ecosystem Assessment*. WHO Library Cataloguing-in-Publication Data. ISBN 92 4 156309 5.

Dutta, L., & Das, M. M. (1986). Regional variation in land use and agriculture in North East India. *North Eastern Geographer, 18*(1–2), 21–25.

Julie, L., Jason, D., & Linda, B. (2007). *Living downstream: Potable water and human health, my environment, my health, my choices*. University of Rochester.

Mayer, I. (1992). Creation of service centers in Jammu and Kashmir: An approach towards balanced and urban development. *The Geographic Review of India, 54*(3), September, 1992.

Mayer, I. (2006). Impact of physical environment on human health-An example from Kashmir Division. *Journal of Social Sciences, 1*(1), 78–90 2006.

Mishra, A., & Misra, A. K. (2007). Study of quaternary aquifers in Ganga Plain, India: Focus on groundwater salinity, fluoride and fluorosis. *Journal of Hazardous Materials, 144*(1–2), 438–448.

Pandit, A. K. (1999). *Fresh water ecosystems of Himalaya* (Vol. 13). New York: The Parthenon Publishing Group Inc.

Pierre, H., Finlayson., & Philip, W. (2012). Healthy wetlands, healthy people: A review of wetlands and human health interactions, Ramsar Technical Report No. 6, Ramsar Convention Secretariat 2012. ISBN 2-940073-32-5.
Raza, M., Ahmad, A., & Mohammad, A. (1978). *The Valley of Kashmir: A Geographical interpretation, Vo 1 The Land*. New Delhi: Vikas publishing Home Pvt. Ltd.
Stiglitz, J., Sen, A., & Fitoussi, J. (2010). *Report by the Commission on the measurement of economic performance and social progress*. Paris: Commission on the Measurement of Economic Performance and Social Progress
Summers, J., Smith., Case, J., & Linthurst, R. (2012). A review of the elements of human well-being with an emphasis on the contribution of ecosystem services. *Ambio, 41*(4), 327–340.
Talukder, B., Nobukazu, N., & Rashid, M. (2015). State and management of wetlands in Bangladesh. *Landscape and Ecological Engineering, 5*(1), 81–90.

Chapter 20
The Big Cat and Quality of Life: The Case of El Salvador

Michael O'Neal Campbell

Abstract Human quality of life (QOL), a vital aspect of human habitation of landscapes, is influenced not only by societal relations and the physical environment but also by human–animal relations. Large carnivores affect QOL negatively, through people's fear of threats and attacks, and actual observations of aggressive behavior. Such carnivores may also make contributions to QOL, though aesthetic viewing of biodiversity and conservation values. In Latin America, the largest carnivores are the jaguars and the cougars. In El Salvador, these species are nearly extinct or totally extinct. However, people are aware of the impacts of their presence, due to the media, generational communications and the nearby, reduced ranges of these species within the surrounding Mesoamerican Biodiversity Hotspot. This chapter examines the links between QOL and possibilities for big cat—human reintroductions in El Salvador. There is evidence of societal support for big cat reintroductions as supportive of QOL and conservation. However, there may be serious impacts on QOL from such reintroductions, as El Salvador is not a large country, and it has a large population. Also, favorable habitat has been reduced due to the historic civil war. The remaining habitat is close to farmland and urban centers, and the population of prey animals has declined. Isolated forests, excessive human hunting of prey animals and the devastating effects of the recent civil war also militate against a successful reintroduction. This study contributes to knowledge of QOL and conservation issues.

20.1 Introduction

Human quality of life (QOL) is affected by many factors, including people's perceptions of animals. Animals may evoke pleasure, a sense of conservation responsibility, repugnance or fear, based on real or imagined factors. The precise impact these relationships have on QOL depends on the definition of the parameters of QOL. These have been debated and are determined to be "multidimensional" (Felce and Perry 1995). Several parameters of QOL have been abstracted from numerous studies

M. O. Campbell (✉)
Michael Campbell, Simon Fraser University, Burnaby, Canada
e-mail: ecol55@hotmail.com

B. R. K. Sinha (ed.), *Multidimensional Approach to Quality of Life Issues*,
https://doi.org/10.1007/978-981-13-6958-2_20

(Felce and Perry 1996; Hughes and Hwang 1996; Cummins 1997a, b; Schalock 1997, 2000; Schalock et al. 2002). For example, Felce and Perry (1995) suggest five themes for QOL: these are physical, material, social and emotional well-being, as well as human life improvement or development and activities. Crucially, these dimensions are affected by regional and temporal factors such as gender, age, culture, and the socioeconomic situation of the people and social groups concerned (Elorriaga et al. 2000).

These points are crucial for the examination of any relation between people and other actors, especially large animals that interact strongly with people. Large carnivores have increased contacts with people, because more people live in proximity to their habitats, and the carnivores enter human life spaces for food, breeding sites and refuge, and to urban and agricultural land use expansion into carnivore habitats (Whittaker and Burns 2001; Treves and Karanth 2003; Gore et al. 2006). The key issues between people and large carnivores are competition for areas of high QOL, such as forests, watered, and/or high biodiversity landscapes. People use such areas for recreation, residence and economic activities, while animals forage, feed, and even breed in such areas. Relations between people and animals are changing, as human presence expands into wildlife habitats. Although large carnivore ecology is a critical area of research in the ecological sciences, their role in QOL requires more research (Herrero and Higgins 1999; Treves and Karanth 2003; Kleiven et al. 2004; Loe and Roskaft 2004).

QOL may be affected by the presence of large carnivores, especially physical (through physical attacks and predation), emotional (individual fear) and social (avoidance of areas due to carnivore presence) well-being. Perceived or real impacts on QOL may influence reduced public support for carnivore conservation, resulting in their decimation or even extinction. This is further complicated by the requirements of large carnivore conservation, which include acknowledgment of high carnivore mobility, complicated habitat requirements, large ranges and wide-ranging prey species (Grumbine 1990; Cardillo et al. 2004; Campbell and Torres Alvarado 2011). One solution concerns the development of conservation areas, but these may fail if the public is opposed. There may be conflicts over the use of land, as competing interests such as urbanization and agriculture may take precedence. Additionally, large carnivores may roam outside the conservation areas and contact with people (Grumbine 1990; Karanth and Stith 1999; Robinson and Bennett 2000; Balme et al. 2010). Public opinion on such matters may determine the success or otherwise of large carnivore conservation, alongside other ecological factors (Karanth and Stith 1999; Woodroffe 2000; Carbone and Gittleman 2002; Karanth et al. 2004; Karanth and Chellam 2009). This is a global issue, wherever there are large carnivores and human populations (Treves and Karanth 2003; Andersone and Ozolins 2004).

Lions, tigers, leopards, and jaguars (*Panthera* spp.) and other large cats are both rare and vulnerable to extinction and perceived as dangerous to people (Schipper et al. 2008; Karanth et al. 2010). Media information sources (some anecdotal others factual) document the dangers of human-large carnivore contacts. The “man-eaters” of the literature and news media have influenced the public mind and countered growing public sympathy with conservation (Campbell 2017). Despite this conflict, currently, dominant opinion states that adequate management with positive public support can preserve carnivore presence, in the face of human population increase, culturally variable tolerance levels and government intransigence (Woodroffe 2000; Linnell et al. 2001; Karanth and Chellam 2009). Therefore, the conservation of large carnivores is possible if there is comprehensive knowledge of relevant human behaviors, activities, and attitudes, and ecological information at species and population levels (Fonturbel and Simonetti 2011).

Currently, large carnivores locally extinct across the continents as pointed by (Weber and Rabinowitz 1996; Hayward and Somers 2009; Inskip and Zimmermann 2009). Several other large cat subspecies are already extinct. These include the Javan tiger *Panthera tigris spondaica* Temminck, 1844, which was extirpated during the 1970s. Java, the home of this species has an extremely high human population density, which may have played a role in its demise (Mazák and Groves 2006; Jackson and Nowell 2008). The Caspian tiger *Panthera tigris virgate* Illiger, 1815 is another extinct subspecies (Seidensticker et al. 1999; Jackson and Nowell 2008). The North African lion *Panthera leo leo* Linnaeus, 1758 is another well-known species that reached extinction, possibly after centuries of exploitation (Nowell and Jackson 1996). The Eastern Cougar *Puma concolor* Linnaeus 1771, previously common in the forests of eastern North America, was acknowledged to be extinct in 2011, this after several disputed sightings (U.S. Fish and Wildlife Service 2011). The jaguar *Panthera onca* Linnaeus, 1758 is considered rare or extinct n the United States, although some studies record some sightings in the southwestern United States, especially Arizona. Common reasons for the extinction of these subspecies are public opinion on their dangerousness, the spread of urban and agricultural land use, and the decline of habitats and prey species populations (Nowell and Jackson 1996; Jackson and Nowell 2008; Hayward and Somers 2009; Inskip and Zimmermann 2009; Campbell and Torres Alvarado 2011).

Considering the definitions of QOL and the status of variable human-large carnivore relations across regions, the relevant question is; *to what extent do large carnivores affect QOL, and what are the positive or negative impacts*? To answer this question, we must first acknowledge that we are concerned with both human attitudes to large carnivores (as beliefs, fears, and observations can impact on QOL) and actual attacks on people that may also affect QOL psychologically and physically. Because large carnivores can kill people, in addition to invading their life spaces, they potentially affect all the QOL dimensions listed. Carnivores that kill people obviously affect people's physical and social well-being. Knowledge of the close presence of dangerous animals also affects the emotional well-being of people. Where large carnivores affect human access to preferred areas, there are impacts on material well-being. These problems may also affect social developments and activities (Williamson 2002; Gore et al. 2006).

We are also concerned with an important, currently global conflict between: (1) the forces of conservation (which holds that large carnivores must be conserved for their own sake and for their ability to enhance QOL); and (2) those advocating safety, hunting or land use concerns, and the negative impacts of large carnivores on QOL (Schaltegger and Beständig 2012; Holthe and Baldus 2013). There are both positive and negative viewpoints on large carnivore presence, as the perception of the "problem" carnivore is counterbalanced with the view that such mammals must be tolerated, or even accepted, as part of a shared landscape and beneficial biodiversity, and may even contribute to increased QOL (Campbell and Lancaster 2010). Observation of large carnivores, either wild or in enclosures, may enhance the observer's emotional and social well-being, or therefore contribute to increase QOL.

We must also be aware that perceptions carnivores and QOL may vary according to the human observer, especially according to gender and age. Campbell's (2012) and Campbell and Lancaster's (2010) studies of large carnivores in North America hypothesized that: (1) women and older people fear large predators more than men and younger people; (2) women and younger people may support predator conservation more than men and older people, and may prefer that predators are tolerated, trapped or removed, rather than shot. These hypotheses were consistent with the relevant literature related to the study of (Hayward and Somers 2009). However, the findings of the first study were that more women than men thought cougar presence enhanced the quality of life, while majorities of men thought they decreased the quality of life, age being irrelevant. In the related study, people did not think that cougars reduced quality of life, regardless of gender or age (Campbell and Lancaster 2010).

20.2 The Situation in Central America

Central America is a zone where large predator conservation and human usage of land are in serious conflict. The Mesoamerican Biodiversity Hotspot dominates this region, because of the large expanse of dense forest, large volcanoes, and high human population density. The Central American region also serves as an ecological corridor between North and South America, and hence is home to species from both continents (Conservation International 2007). Local QOL and tourism are strongly based on this biodiversity, and volcanoes and beaches. QOL has also been damaged by marked environmental change, including: wars in El Salvador and other countries (Hecht et al. 2006), deforestation, partly associated with these upheavals (Weinberg 1991; Sloan 2007; Taylor 2007), agricultural intensification (Vandemeer 1990; Sanchez-Azofeifa 2000; Sloan 2007), land use conflicts (Schelhas 1996; Simmons 1997; Hoffman 1998; Southworth and Tucker 2001), and local mammal extinctions (Campbell and Torres Alvarado 2011). The impacts of these events on the populations of jaguars and cougars are uncertain (Silvius et al. 2004; Valenzuela-Galvan et al. 2008). However, there have been some serious consequences, as the jaguar is now extirpated El Salvador in Central America and is rare through the remainder of Central America (Caso et al. 2008). The cougar is commoner than the jaguar, but also extinct in El Salvador and quite rare in the rest of Central America (López-González and González-Romero 1998).

Both jaguars and cougars are considered dangerous to people, although they are usually recorded as killing and attacking fewer people than lions of tigers (Campbell and Torres Alvarado 2011). The jaguar is the largest cat in the world after the tiger and the lion, and in prehistory and recent history, it has been revered as a participant in indigenous religions in the Americas (Sanderson et al. 2002; Zeller 2007; McCain and Childs 2008). Although jaguars are feared as threats to people, there no evidence that they are as dangerous as tigers and leopards; therefore, their relations with people and their impact on QOL have been under-researched (McDougal 1987; Bailey 1993; Benson 1998; Saunders 1998; Santos et al. 2008). Jaguars are markedly less studied than other large cats (Brodie 2009), especially in Central America (Tôrres et al. 2008; Campbell and Torres Alvarado 2011).

The cougar is slightly smaller than the jaguar, generally a little larger than the old-world leopard (López-González and González-Romero 1998; Campbell and Torres Alvarado 2011). The cougar ranges over most of North and South America and usually shares its range with wolves brown and black bears, and jaguars (López-González and González-Romero 1998). The cougar, possibly because of its smaller size, is often assessed as less of a threat to people and livestock than the jaguar. This may be one reason that it is less hunted than the jaguar (Conforti and Azevedo 2003; Campbell and Torres Alvarado 2011). Cougars may sometimes kill livestock, but these killings may be blamed on jaguars, especially were jaguars have a worse reputation (Polisar et al. 2003; Scognamillo et al. 2003; Rosas-Rosas et al. 2008; Campbell and Torres Alvarado 2012; Rosas-Rosas and Bender 2012).

The habitat requirements of these cats may create conflicts with people, and affect QOL, even as their aggressive nature is exaggerated. They require large contiguous forest cover, forested corridors for movement, water and in some cases livestock which may substitute for natural prey. The range of both the jaguars and cougars widely varies, hence their habitats are very sparsely populated, especially near human habitation (Silver et al. 2004; Cullen 2006; Paviolo et al. 2008). Favorable habitats are usually dense forests or mixed vegetation, close to water sources but away from human presence (Núñez et al. 2002; Sunquist and Sunquist 2002; Navarro-Serment et al. 2005; Monroy-Vilchis et al. 2008, 2009a, b; Campbell and Torres Alvarado 2011). Perhaps, in addition to their avoidance of human presence, the two cats may avoid each other, with the smaller, more adaptive cougar varying its prey species and habitats to avoid the jaguar (Rabinowitz and Nottingham 1986; Emmons 1991). Both cats, especially the cougar may adapt to mixed environments, and human and livestock presence (Emmons 1987; Aranda and Sanchez-Cordero 1996; Taber et al. 1997; Scognamillo et al. 2003). Where the prey species are rare or extirpated, then both the jaguar and the cougar may prey on livestock (Schaller and Crawshaw 1980; Yáñez et al. 1986; Swank and Teer 1989; Emmons 1990; Farrell et al. 2000; Saenz and Carillo 2002).

20.3 The Unique Case of El Salvador

El Salvador (Fig. 20.1) has a population of just over six million people in an area of 21 041 square kilometers, and population density 288 per square kilometers (Campbell and Torres Alvarado 2011). This makes it the most densely populated country in Latin America. There are serious environmental problems in the country that may affect the quality of life of the people and affect their relations with wild animals. The most serious environmental issues concern deforestation and the contributory factors that also influenced other environmental and social change. The small size of the country and the large population increase the impacts of the environmental (Food and Agricultural Organization, Hecht et al. 2006). The complexity of the environmental issues is underscored by the fact that both deforestation and reforestation have occurred, creating more open yet patch dynamic landcover, with possible negative impacts on forest species (Hecht et al. 2006; Hecht and Saatchi 2007; Campbell and Torres Alvarado 2011). The long civil war affected the landcover, as fires and intense fighting contributed to deforestation, while land abandonment through farmer recruitment into the fighting forces, the movement of cultivators as refugees and the high death rate in rural areas precipitated reforestation of some cultivated land. Additionally, there are serious environmental episodes, including hurricanes from the Caribbean area, with consequent flooding and landslides, in a landscape heavily used for thousands of years (Pohl et al. 1996; Dull 2001; Sheets 2002; Rose et al. 2004).

In terms of QOL, the main issue concerns the extent to which environmental change, especiallydeforestation, population growth and hunting of prey species, has narrowed the opportunities for QOL, as preferred areas were reduced and competition with wildlife may have increased. Other countries record substantial conflicts and social concern in such situations. (Farrell et al. 2000; Polisar et al. 2003; Rosas-Rosas and Bender 2012). However, in El Salvador, there is some support for big cat reintroductions (Campbell and Torres Alvarado 2011). Campbell and Torres Alvarado (2011) found that most people believed that the big cats had a beneficial impact on QOL. Additionally, women more than men asserted that the big cats negatively affected QOL and men more than women believed that QOL improved with big cat presence, or there would be little effect. Young people were more likely than older people to think that big cat presence would have no effect on QOL but had similar opinions to older people on whether the big cats would either improve or degrade QOL. Women were more frightened of jaguars and cougars then men were, but younger and older people had similar opinions on this topic (Campbell and Torres-Alvarado 2011).

Men and women, and younger and older people, had similar opinions on the unrestrictcdreintroduction of the big cats, in that all the groups supported such reintroductions into the general forested areas or special areas. Most people (men, women, older and younger) also argued that big cats should be protected, as the absence of protection was one reason why the cats reached extinction (Campbell and Torres-Alvarado 2011). Other studies have found similar results, in that people expressed

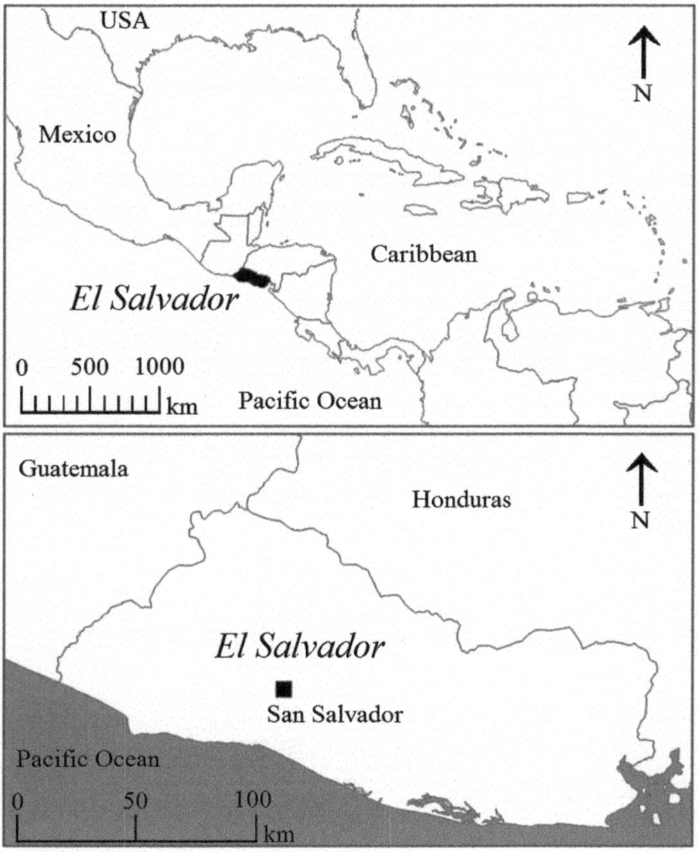

Fig. 20.1 Political map of El Salvador's location

widely differing opinions on the big cats on different topics (Conforti and Azevedo 2003). However, the sympathy for reintroductions does not negate some important issues important for human—cat relations in El Salvador. These are assessed in turn below.

20.4 The Small Size of El Salvador

Big cats require very large ranges for adequate food. These ranges must be composed of suitable habitat, and possibly similar landcover connect habitat patches. Serious problems emerge when human land use intrudes into such landscapes, as the big cats must traverse cultural landscapes such as cultivated or urban land to reach favorable hunting or breeding grounds. Where such conflicts emerge, there are impacts on human QOL (Campbell and Torres-Alvarado 2011). According to Sanderson et al. (2002) and Torres et al. (2008), one jaguar requires at least 40 km^2 of forest to survive, hence only about 500 could survive in El Salvador. This would be on the assumption that El Salvador was entirely forest, and it was well connected to the other forests of Central America. In reality, the forested area of El Salvador is very small, and it is also unconnected by corridors to any other forests in Central America. The forested landcover of El Salvador is generally distributed in patches, surrounded by intensely cultivated plots or urbanized areas. The border of El Salvador and the surrounding countries have not been studied in detail regarding their impact on wildlife, hence it is uncertain whether large cats can cross them in such of better habitat (Campbell and Torres-Alvarado 2011). Jaguars and cougars can cross many types of landcover (Rosas-Rosas and Bender 2012). However, there are few studies that review this ability in El Salvador (Campbell and Torres-Alvarado 2011). Based on the studies of jaguars and cougars in other countries, it may be concluded that the reintroduction of the big cats into the restricted environments of El Salvador will spark some conflicts, which may erode the support of the local people for the conservation of the big cats (Campbell and Torres-Alvarado 2011).

20.5 The Concentrated Human Population

El Salvador has a very high population density; in fact, it is more than double that of any of the other Central American countries (292 people per square kilometer, compared with Guatemala (129), Costa Rica (90), Honduras (67), Nicaragua (44), Panama (44) and lastly, Belize (13). Although it may be speculated that the high human population density was responsible for the decline of the big cats, there is no evidence presented in the literature to date (Campbell 2017). Hatten et al. (2003: 22) challenges such an hypothesis, arguing that human-dominated landcover can serve as a corridor for the passage of large wildlife, "provided that other habitat components (cover, water, prey) are available and the landscape has not been severely altered or degraded by human activities." Ibanez et al. (2002) found that densely inhabited cultural landscapes do not necessarily exclude big cats. For example, in the Panama Canal watershed, the human population increased by 500% from 1950 to 1990, but the big cats were not extirpated, perhaps due to the existence of corridor forest (Ibanez et al. 2002). Numerous studies have also recorded cougars, normally assessed as elusive, in Canadian urban areas (Campbell and Lancaster 2010). This evidence contrasts with documented avoidance tendencies (Monroy-Vilchis et al. 2008, 2009a, b).

20.6 Civil War

Another debated issue is the El Salvador civil war. The war reduced QOL in the rural areas and destroyed both potential carnivore habitats and human landscapes, through bombing and burning (Dudley et al. 2002). However, there are counter-arguments concerning the possible impact of this war on the ecology of the big cats (Campbell and Torres-Alvarado 2011). For example, the other Central American civil wars such as those in Guatemala and Nicaragua, which was a war with greater duration and more general damage, the big cats were still in existence after the wars but were rarer (Zeller et al. 2011). Of course, it must be noted that these countries are larger than El Salvador, with more forest and more connected forested corridors (Campbell and Torres-Alvarado 2011). Although war would not be the only factor for the populations of the big cats, the populations of jaguars and cougars are higher in those Central American countries with more stable, nonmilitary histories and less environmental degradation. These countries are Belize, Costa Rica, Honduras and Panama (Rabinowitz and Nottingham 1986; Ibanez et al. 2002; Foster et al. 2010). Other under-researched topics concern public attitudes towards the big cats in these countries and the possible differences in the occurrence of prey species (Campbell 2017). It is also uncertain if the link between the war and the occurrence of the big cat would be based on the damage inflicted on the environment, such as forest fragmentation, connectivity of forest stands and decline in forest stand quality, or it should be based on the actual shooting or disturbance of the big cats during the war (Campbell and Torres-Alvarado 2011). More research would be required to decide on a link between the war and big cat ecology and presence. Actual research on the other factors such prey species presence may be required, as currently the links are based on only theoretical inferences from studies elsewhere (Swank and Teer 1991; Sanderson et al. 2002).

20.7 Deforestation

Deforestation as an issue for big cat population change is linked to the issues above, as forest fragmentation and stand decline is one of the possible outcomes of the war. However, based on the evidence presented so far, it appears unlikely that the adaptable cougar could be extirpated from forest fragmentation alone (Rabinowitz and Nottingham 1986; Emmons 1991). The answer appears to be largely due to the extent to which the big cats compensate for forest habitat losses by occupying human-dominated landscapes and impacting upon QOL. The cougar is very versatile and inhabits areas of low QOL for people, where conflicts are unlikely. Therefore, other factors aside from war and forest fragmentation may influence its extirpation. In the United States and Canada, cougar presence in urban areas has been increasing markedly in recent time, and there are disputes as to the reasons for this occurrence. For example, some urban areas, such as San Diego, Los Angeles, Denver/Boulder and

Missoula, in the United States and some parts of Vancouver Island in Canada have recorded significantly more aggressive interactions between cougars and humans in the last 40 years than other areas with equivalent cougar populations (Spencer et al. 2001; Shuey 2008; Campbell 2014).

Jaguars appear to be more specialized in habitat preferences, mostly foraging in denser vegetation (Campbell 2017). As argued by Salom-Perez (2007) the deforestation in Central America is now of such magnitude that there may not be enough to support several hundred jaguars. Moist lowland forest is the preferred jaguar habitat, an example being the Guatemalan, Mexican and Belizean Selva Maya. There is also a forest corridor that extends from Honduras to the Choco-Darien of Panama and Colombia. There are areas outside the prime forest that can also harbor a jaguar population. These may be drier with lighter vegetation, but suitable prey species for a moderate jaguar or even cougar population. These may include parts of Costa Rica and Panama. There are also much drier or sparsely vegetated areas, or coastal areas with few prey species. For example, jaguars were formerly recorded in such drier areas in Arizona and other southwestern states (Campbell 2017). Other examples are some grassed areas coastal mangroves (Sanderson et al. 2002). Many drier, more open areas are also occupied with human activities, which may also reduce the available prey species and encouraging avoidance behavior in the big cats (Campbell and Torres Alvarado 2011).

There is some evidence of reforestation in El Salvador, but this is not a deliberate strategy to increase QOL. Generally, denser growths of trees emerged when land users moved, ceased cultivation or died during the long civil war. QOL was reduced in the rural areas, which in conflict zones were mainly occupied fighters, transients, and refugees. People in rural areas also moved to urban areas, largely per the industrialization in the country that resulted in increased global contacts and infused more technical, less labor-intensive systems into agriculture (Campbell and Torres-Alvarado 2011). Labor-intensive, traditionally organized cultivation patterns were steadily abandoned in favor of more capital-intensive models. Additionally, environmental policies gained traction, which fostered the development of some conservation areas (Perfecto et al. 1996; Deere and Leon 2000; Hecht et al. 2006; Hecht and Saatchi 2007). These in totality contributed to the regrowth of some forests, with some approaching former levels of density (Campbell 2016).

20.8 Excessive Human Hunting

Hunting in this sense refers to people killing of carnivores for their own or livestock protection, due to real or imagined reasons, or the killing of prey animals for food. Both types of hunting may affect carnivores, as the carnivores rely on the prey animals for their existence (Karanth and Stith 1999; Carbone and Gittleman 2002; Karanth et al. 2004; Karanth and Chellam 2009; Karanth et al. 2010). Both types of hunting may raise QOL, as prey animals are an important part of the human diet especially when livestock must be preserved for later consumption of sale and crop cultivation is strongly seasonal. Additionally, carnivores affect not only human security but also kill the livestock and prey animals that are part of the human diet and therefore reduce QOL (Campbell and Torres-Alvarado 2011). Jaguars and cougars may change their prey base and hence react to contextual changes, this behavior affecting human activities including livestock rearing and hunting (Karanth and Sunquist 1995; Hayward and Somers 2009). Prey selectivity is usually studied using indices that emphasize prey availability, and selective foraging (Griffith 1975; Chesson 1978; Stephens and Krebs 1986; Manly et al. 2002; Karanth and Chellam 2009). In El Salvador, herbivores that are prey species are popular for human consumption but are of low conservation or tourism concern. These include deer and peccaries, which are important for QOL through the food they provide as wild meat (Campbell and Torres Alvarado 2011).

20.9 Conclusions

This chapter has reviewed the importance of QOL for human–big cat relations, taking El Salvador as an example. The evidence shows that there are strong links between human perceptions of QOL, land use and conservation and reintroduction of big cats. QOL is a crucial issue because it influences or determines land use conflicts, especially when people and carnivores select similar landcover or food sources, and there is reduced support for conservation. It is imperative that conservation strategies assess the potential impact of species on QOL. For example, to what extent do the species preferences of the big cats' conflict with areas of high QOL? In this case study, it is apparent that areas of high QOL for farmers, tourists or hunters, such as watered forests of high biodiversity, would be considered prime jaguar habitat. There is evidence that cougars are more adaptive and cosmopolitan, but even they may intrude into areas of high QOL, such as grassland for cattle herders, or villages with small livestock. Detailed studies of the spatial configuration of areas of high and low QOL, the factors that may affect QOL and the adaptive abilities of big cats is necessary to support conservation strategies.

References

Andersone, Z., & Ozolins, J. (2004). Public perception of large carnivores in Latvia. *Ursus, 15,* 181–187.

Aranda, M., & Sanchez-Cordero, V. (1996). Prey spectra of jaguar Panthera onca and Puma Puma concolor in tropical forests of Mexico. *Studies of Neotropical Fauna and Environment, 3,* 65–67.

Bailey, T. N. (1993). *The African leopard: A study of the ecology and behavior of a solitary felid.* New York: Columbia University Press.

Balme, G. A., Slotow, R., & Hunter, L. T. B. (2010). Edge effects and the impact of non-protected areas in carnivore conservation: leopards in the Phinda-Mkhuze Complex, South Africa. *Animal Conservation, 13,* 315–323.

Benson, E. P. (1998). The lord, the ruler: Jaguar symbolism in the Americas. In N. J. Saunders (Ed.), *Icons of power: Feline symbolism in the Americas* (pp. 53–76). London: Routledge.
Brodie, J. F. (2009). Is research effort allocated efficiently for conservation? Felidae as a global case study. *Biodiversity Conservation, 18,* 2927–2939.
Campbell, M. (2014). Urban planning for cougar presence in North America: Practices, challenges and benefits. In M. P. Amado (Ed.), *Urban planning, practices challenges, benefits* (pp. 19–32). New York: Nova Science Publishers.
Campbell, M. (2016). The factors for the extinction of jaguars and cougars in El Salvador. *Journal of Biodiversity, Bioprospecting and Development, 1–7.* https://doi.org/10.4172/2376-0214.1000154.
Campbell, M. (2017). *Conservation biology in the 21st century: A conservation biology of large wildlife*. New York: Nova Science Publishers.
Campbell, M., & Lancaster, B. (2010). Public attitudes towards black bears Ursus americanus and cougars Puma concolor on Vancouver Island. *Journal of Society and Animals, 10*(1), 47–51.
Campbell, M., & Torres-Alvarado, M. (2011). Public perceptions of jaguars Panthera onca, pumas Puma concolor and coyotes Canis latrans in El Salvador. *Area, 43*(3), 250–256.
Carbone, C., & Gittleman, J. L. (2002). A common rule for the scaling of carnivore density. *Science, 295,* 2273–2276.
Cardillo, M., Purvis, A., Sechrest, W., Gittleman, J. L., Bielby, J. & Mace, G. M. (2004). Human population density and extinction risk in the world's carnivores. *PLoSBiology 2*(7), 0909–0914.
Caso, A., Lopez-Gonzalez, C., Payan, E., Eizirik, E., de Oliveira, T., Leite-Pitman, R., et al. (2008). "Panthera onca". In *IUCN red list of threatened species. version 201).1.* International Union for Conservation of Nature, Gland.
Chesson, P. L. (1978). Predator-prey theory and variability. *Annual Review of Ecological Systems, 9,* 323–347.
Conforti, V. L., & Azevedo, F. C. C. (2003). Local perceptions of jaguars Panthera onca and pumas Puma concolor in the Iguacu National Park area, south Brazil. *Biological Conservation, 111,* 215–221.
Conservation International. (2007). *Biodiversity hotspots: the most remarkable places on Earth are also the most threatened. CI, Arlington, Virginia.* Retrieved from http://www.biodiversityhotspots.org.
Cullen, L. Jr. (2006). *Jaguar as landscape detectives for the conservation in the atlantic forest of Brazil.* Ph.D. thesis, University of Kent, Canterbury.
Cummins, R. A. (1997a). Assessing quality of life. In R. J. Brown (Ed.), *Assessing quality of life for people with psychiatric disabilities (116–150).* Cheltenham, England: Stanley Thornes (Publishers).
Cummins, R. A. (1997b). *Comprehensive quality of life scale – Adult.* School of Psychology: Deakin University, Melbourne.
Deere, C., & Leon, M. (2000). *Genero, propiedad y empoderamiento: tierra, estado y mercado en America Latina.* Bogota: Tercer Mundo Editores.
Dudley, J., Ginsburg, J., Plumptre, A., Hart, J., & Campos, L. (2002). Effects of war on civil strife on wildlife and wildlife habitats. *Biological Conservation, 16*(2), 319–329.
Dull, R. (2001). *El bosque perdido: A cultural-ecological history of Holocene environmental change in El Salvador.* Ph.D. Thesis. University of California, Berkeley.
Elorriaga, J., Garcia, L., Martinez, J., & Unamunzaga, E. (2000). Quality of life of persons with mental retardation in Spain. In K. D. Keith & R. L. Schlock (Eds.), *Cross-cultural perspectives on quality of life.* Washington, DC: American Association on Mental Retardation.
Emmons, L. H. (1987). Comparative feeding ecology of felids in a neotropical rainforest. *Behavioral Ecology and Sociobiology, 20,* 271–283.
Emmons, L. H. (1990). *Neotropical rainforest mammals: A field guide.* Chicago: University of Chicago Press.
Emmons, L. H. (1991). Body size and feeding tactics. In Seidensticker J. & Lumpkin, S. (Eds.) *Great cats,* (p. 62). Emmaus: Rodale Press.

Farrell, L. E., Roman, J. & Sunquist, M.E. (2000). Dietary separation of sympatric carnivores identified by molecular analysis of scats. *Molecular Ecology*, *9*, 1583–1590.
Felce, D., & Perry, J. (1995). Quality of life: Its definition and measurement. *Research in Developmental Disabilities, 16*(1), 51–74.
Felce, D., & Perry, J. (1996). Assessment of quality of life. In Schalock, R. L. & Siperstein, G. N (Eds.), *Quality of life volume I: Conceptualization and measurement* (pp. 63–70). Washington DC: American Association on Mental Retardation.
Fonturbel, F. E., & Simonetti, J. A. (2011). Translocations and human-carnivore conflicts: Problem solving or problem creating. *Wildlife Biology, 17,* 217–224.
Foster, R., Harmsen, B. J., & Doncaster, C. P. (2010). Habitat use by sympatric jaguars and pumas across a gradient of human disturbance in Belize. *Biotropica, 42,* 724–731.
Gore, M. L., Knuth, B. A., Curtis, P. D., & Shanahan, J. E. (2006). Education programs for reducing black bear-human conflicts: Indicators of success? *Ursus, 17*(1), 75–80.
Griffiths, D. (1975). Prey availability and the food of predators. *Ecology, 56,* 1209–1214.
Grumbine, R. E. (1990). Viable populations, reserve size, and federal lands management: a critique. *Conservation Biology, 4,* 127–134.
Hayward, M. W., & Somers, M. J. (Eds.). (2009). *Reintroduction of top-order predators*. Oxford: Wiley-Blackwell Publishing.
Hecht, S. B., & Saatchi, S. S. (2007). Globalization and forest resurgence: changes in forest cover in El Salvador. *BioScience, 57,* 663–672.
Hecht, S. B., Kandel, S., Gomes, I., Cuellar, N., & Rosa, H. (2006). Globalization, forest resurgence and environmental politics in El Salvador. *World Development, 34*(2), 308–323.
Herrero, S., & Higgins, A. (1999). Human injuries inflicted by bears in British Columbia: 1960–1997. *Ursus, 11,* 209–218.
Hoffman, H. (1998). Land conflict and Mayangna territorial rights in Nicaragua's Bosawás reserve. *Bulletin of Latin American Research, 17*(1), 17–34.
Holthe, V., & Baldus, R. D. (2013). CIC position paper: Management of large carnivores in Europe. International Council for Game and Wildlife Conservation (CIC), Budakeszi.
Hughes, C., & Hwang, B. (1996). Attempts to conceptualize and measure quality of life. In Schalock, R. L. (Ed.), *Quality of life. Volume. I: Conceptualization and measurement* (pp. 51–61). Washington, DC: American Association on Mental Retardation.
Ibanez, R., Condit, R., Angehr, G., Aguilar, S., Garcia, T., Martinez, R., et al. (2002). An ecosystem report on the Panama Canal: Monitoring the status of the forest communities and the watershed. *Environmental Monitoring and Assessment, 80,* 65–95.
Inskip, C., & Zimmermann, A. (2009). Human-felid conflict: A review of patterns and priorities worldwide. *Oryx, 43,* 18–34.
Jackson, P., & Nowell, K. (2008). Panthera tigris. *IUCN red list of threatened species. Version 2011.1*. International Union for Conservation of Nature, Gland.
Karanth, K. U., & Chellam, R. (2009). Carnivore conservation at the crossroads. *Oryx, 43,* 1–2.
Karanth, K. U., & Stith, B. M. (1999). Prey depletion as a critical determinant of tiger population viability. In Seidensticker S. C. & Jackson P. (Eds.), *Riding the tiger: Tiger conservation in human-dominated landscapes* (pp. 100–113). Cambridge: Cambridge University Press.
Karanth, U. K., & Sunquist, M. E. (1995). Prey selection by tiger, leopard and dhole in tropical forests. *Journal of Animal Ecology, 64,* 439–450.
Karanth, K. U., Chundawat, R. S., Nichols, J. D., & Kumar, N. S. (2004). Estimation of tiger densities in the tropical dry forest of Panna, Central India using photographic capture-recapture sampling. *Animal Conservation, 7,* 285–290.
Karanth, K. U., Funston, P., & Sanderson, E. (2010). Many ways of skinning a cat: tools and techniques for studying wild felids. In W. Macdonald & A. J. Loveridge (Eds.), *The biology and conservation of wild felids* (pp. 197–216). Oxford: Oxford University Press.
Kleiven, J., Bjerke, T., & Kaltenborn, B. P. (2004). Factors influencing the social acceptability of large carnivore behaviors. *Biodiversity and Conservation, 13,* 1647–1658.

Linnell, J. D. C., Swenson, J. E., & Anderson, R. (2001). Predators and people: conservation of large carnivores is possible at high human densities if management policy is favorable. *Animal Conservation, 4,* 345–349.
Loe, J., & Roskaft, E. (2004). Large carnivores and human safety: A review. *Ambio, 33*(6), 283–287.
López-González, C. A., & González-Romero, A. (1998). A synthesis of current literature and knowledge about the ecology of the puma (Puma concolor). *Acta Zoologica Mexicana, 75,* 171–190.
Manly, B. F. J., McDonald, L. L., Thomas, D. L., McDonald, T. L., & Erickson, W. P. (2002). *Resource selection by animals: Statistical analysis and design for field studies*. Boston: Kluwer.
Mazák, J. H., & Groves, C. P. (2006). A taxonomic revision of the tigers (Panthera tigris). *Mammalian Biology, 71*(5), 268–287.
McCain, E. B., & Childs, J. L. (2008). Evidence of resident jaguars (Panthera onca) in the southwestern United States and the implications for conservation. *Journal of Mammalogy, 89,* 1–10.
McDougal, C. (1987). The man-eating tiger in geographical and historical perspective. In R. I. Tilson & U. S. Seal (Eds.), *Tigers of the world*. Park Ridge: Noyes Publications.
Monroy-Vilchis, O., Sanchez, O., Acuilera-Reyes, U., Suarez, P., & Urios, V. (2008). Jaguar (Panthera onca) in the State of Mexico. *Southwestern Naturalist, 53,* 533–537.
Monroy-Vilchis, O., Gómez, Y., Janczur, M., & Urios, V. (2009a). Food niche of Puma concolor in Central Mexico. *Wildlife Biology, 15*(1), 1–9.
Monroy-Vilchis, O., Rodríguez-Soto, C., Zarco-González, M., & Urios, V. (2009b). Cougar and jaguar habitat use and activity patterns in central Mexico. *Animal Biology, 59,* 145–157.
Navarro-Serment, C. J., Lopez-Gonzalez, C. A., & Gallo-Reynoso, J. P. (2005). Occurrence of Jaguar (Panthera onca) in Sinaloa, Mexico. *The Southwestern Naturalist, 50*(1), 102–106.
Nowell, K., & Jackson, P. (Eds.). (1996). *Wild cats: Status survey and conservation action plan.* Gland: IUCN/SSC Cat Specialist Group.
Núñez, R., Miller, B., & Lindzey, F. (2002). Ecología del jaguar en la reserva de la biosfera Chamela-Cuixmala, Jalisco, México. In R. Medellín, C. Equhua, C. Chetkiewics, P. Crawshaw, A. Rabinowitz, K. Redford, J. Robinson, E. Sanderson, & A. Taber (Eds.), *El Jaguar en el Nuevo Milenio* (pp. 107–126). México: Fondo de Cultura Económica-Wildlife Conservation Society-UNAM.
Paviolo, A., De Angelo, C. D., Di Blanco, Y. E., & Di Bitetti, M. S. (2008). Jaguar *Panthera onca* population decline in the Upper Paraná Atlantic Forest of Argentina and Brazil. *Oryx, 42,* 554–561.
Perfecto, I., Rice, R., Greenberg, R., & van der Voolt, M. (1996). Shade coffee is a refuge for biodiversity. *BioScience, 46,* 598–608.
Pohl, M., Pope, K., Jones, J., Jacob, S., Piperno, D., & de France, S. (1996). Early agriculture in the Maya lowlands. *Latin American Antiquity, 7,* 355–372.
Polisar, J., Maxit, I., Scognamillo, D., Farrell, L., Sunquist, M., & Eisenberg, J. F. (2003). Jaguars, pumas, their prey base, cattle ranching: Ecological interpretations of a management problem. *Biological Conservation, 109,* 297–310.
Rabinowitz, A., & Nottingham, B. (1986). Ecology and behavior of the jaguar in Belize, Central America. *Journal of Zoology, 210,* 149–159.
Robinson, J. G., & Bennett, E. L. (2000). *Hunting for sustainability in tropical forests*. Irvinton: Columbia University Press.
Rosas-Rosas, O. C., & Bender, L. C. (2012). Population status of jaguars (Panthera onca and pumas (Puma concolor) in northeastern Sonora, Mexico. *Acta Zoologica Mexicana, 28*(1), 86–101.
Rosas-Rosas, O. C., Bender, L. C., & Valdez, R. (2008). Jaguar and puma predation on cattle calves in northeastern Sonora, Mexico. *Rangeland Ecology and Management, 61,* 554–560.
Rose, W., Bonner, J., Lopez, D., Carr, M., & Major, J. (Eds.). (2004). *Natural Hazards in El Salvador*. Boulder: USGS.
Saenz, J. C., & Carrillo, E. (2002). Jaguares depredadores de ganado en Costa Rica: ¿un problema sin solucion? In R. Medellín, C. Equhua, C. Chetkiewics, P. Crawshaw, A. Rabinowitz, K. Redford, J. Robinson, E. Sanderson, & A. Taber (Eds.), *El Jaguar en el Nuevo Milenio* (pp. 127–138). Mexico: Universidad Nacional Autonoma de Mexico and Wildlife Conservation Society.

Salom-Pérez, R., Camillo, E., Sáenz, J. C., & Mora, J. M. (2007). Critical condition of the jaguar Panthera onca population in Corcovado National Park, Costa Rica. *Oryx, 41*(1), 51–56.

Sanchez-Azofeifa, G. A. (2000). Land use and cover change in Costa Rica. In C. Hall (Ed.), *Quantifying sustainable development* (pp. 477–505). New York: Academic Press.

Sanderson, E. W., Redford, R. H., Chetkiewicz, C. B., Medellin, R., Rabinowitz, A., Robinson, J., et al. (2002). Planning to save a species: The jaguar as a model. *Conservation Biology, 16,* 58–72.

Santos, F. R., Jácomo, A. T. A., & Silveira, L. (2008). Humans and jaguars in five Brazilian biomes: Same country, different perceptions. *Cat News, 4,* 21–25.

Saunders, N. J. (1998). *Icons of power: Feline symbolism in the Americas.* London: Routledge.

Schaller, G. B., & Crawshaw, P. G. (1980). Movement patterns of jaguar. *Biotropica, 12,* 161–168.

Schalock, R. L. (1997). Can the concept of quality of life make a difference? In R. L. Schalock (Ed.), *Quality of life volume II: Application to persons with disabilities* (pp. 245–267). Washington DC: American Association on Mental Retardation.

Schalock, R. L. (2000). Three decades of quality of life. *Focus on Autism and Other Developmental Disabilities, 15*(2), 116–128.

Schalock, R. L., Alonso, M. A. V., & Braddock, D. L. (2002). *Handbook on quality of life for human service practitioners.* Washington, DC: American Association on Mental Retardation.

Schaltegger, S., & Beständig, U. (2012). *Corporate biodiversity management handbook: A guide for practical implementation.* Berlin: Federal Ministry of the Environment.

Schelhas, J. (1996). Land use choice and change: intensification and diversification in the lowland tropics of Costa Rica. *Human Organization, 55,* 298–304.

Schipper, J., Hoffmann, M., Duckworth, J. W., & Conroy, J. (2008). The 2008 IUCN red listings of the world's small carnivores. *Small Carnivore Conservation, 39,* 29–34.

Scognamillo, D., Maxit, I. E., Sunquist, M., & Polisar, J. (2003). Coexistence of jaguar (Panthera onca) and puma (Puma concolor) in a mosaic landscape in the Venezuelan Ilanos. *Journal of Zoology (London), 259,* 269–279.

Seidensticker, J., Christie, S., & Jackson, P. (1999). Preface. Riding the tiger. In Seidensticker J., Christie S., & Jackson P. (Eds.) *Tiger conservation in human-dominated landscapes* (pp. X–XIX). Cambridge: Cambridge University Press.

Sheets, P. (2002). *Before the volcano erupted. The ancient cerén village in Central America.* Austin: University of Texas Press.

Shuey, M. L, (2008). The influence of landscape on cougar-human encounter hazard in Boulder and Colorado Springs, Colorado. ETD Collection for Texas State University. https://digital.library.txstate.edu/handle/10877/3004.

Silver, S. C., Ostro, L. E. T., Marsh, L. K., Maffei, L., Noss, A. J., Kelly, M. J., et al. (2004). The use of camera traps for estimating jaguar Panthera onca abundance and density using capture-recapture analysis. *Oryx, 38*(2), 148–154.

Silvius, K. M., Bodmer, R. E., & Fragoso, J. M. V. (2004). *People in nature: Wildlife conservation in South and Central America.* New York: Columbia University Press.

Simmons, C. S. (1997). Forest management practices in the Bayano region of Panama: Cultural variations. *World Development, 25,* 989–1000.

Sloan, S. (2007). Fewer people may not mean more forest for Latin American forest frontiers. *Biotropica, 39,* 443–446.

Southworth, J., & Tucker, C. (2001). The influence of accessibility, local institutions and socioeconomic factors on forest cover change in the mountains of Western Honduras. *Mountain Research and Development, 21,* 276–283.

Spencer, R. D., Pierce, D. J., Schirato, G. A., Dixon, K. R., & Richards, C. B. (2001). *Mountain lion home range, dispersal, mortality and survival in the Western Cascade Mountains of Washington.* Olympia: Washington Department of Fish and Wildlife.

Stephens, D. W., & Krebs, J. R. (1986). *Foraging theory.* Princeton: Princeton University Press.

Sunquist, M., & Sunquist, F. (2002). *Wild cats of the world.* Chicago: The University of Chicago Press.

Swank, W. G., & Teer, J. G. (1989). Status of the jaguar. *Oryx, 23,* 14–21.

Swank, W. G., & Teer, J. G. (1991). A proposed program for sustained jaguar populations. *Foundation for the study of physical, mathematical and natural sciences (FUDECI), Felinos de Venezuela: biologia, ecologia y conservacion* (pp. 95–106). FUDECI, Caracas.
Taber, A. B., Novaro, A. J., Neris, N., & Colman, F. H. (1997). The food habits of sympatric jaguar and puma in the Paraguayan Chaco. *Biotropica, 29,* 204–213.
Taylor, M. J. (2007). Militarism and the environment in Guatemala. *GeoJournal, 69*(3), 181–198.
Torres, N. M., De Marco Jr, P., Diniz Filho, J. A. F., & Silveira, L. (2008). Jaguar distribution in Brazil: Past, present and future. *Cat News, 4,* 4–8.
Treves, A., & Karanth, K. U. (2003). Human-carnivore conflict and perspectives on carnivore management worldwide. *Conservation Biology, 17,* 1491–1499.
United States Fish and Wildlife Service. (2011). *U.S. Fish and Wildlife Service concludes eastern cougar extinct.* Retrieved July 17, 2012, from http://www.fws.gov/northeast/ECougar/pdf/easterncougarnewsreleaseFINALR4.pdf.
Valenzuela-Galvan, D., Arita, H. T., & Macdonald, D. W. (2008). Conservation priorities for carnivores considering protected natural areas and human population density. *Biodiversity Conservation, 17,* 539–558.
Vandemeer, J. (1990). The political ecology of sustainable development: The Southern Atlantic Coast of Nicaragua. CICLAES, Michigan State University.
Weber, W., & Rabinowitz, A. (1996). A global perspective on large carnivore conservation. *Conservation Biology, 10*(4), 1046–1054.
Weinberg, B. (1991). *War on the land: Ecology and politics in Central America*. New Jersey: Zed Books.
Whittaker, D. G., & Burns, A. G. (2001). Black bear status in western North America: Summary of western state and province bear status report surveys. *Western Black Bear Workshop, 7,* 32–55.
Williamson, D. F. (2002). *Status, management, and trade of the American black bear (Ursus americanus) in North America*. Washington, DC: World Wildlife Fund.
Woodroffe, R. (2000). Predators and people: using human densities to interpret declines of large carnivores. *Animal Conservation, 3,* 165–173.
Yáñez, J. L., Cárdenas, J. C., Gezelle, P., & Jaksic, F. M. (1986). Food habits of the southernmost mountain lions (Felisconcolor) in South America: Natural versus livestocked ranges. *Journal of Mammalogy, 67,* 604–606.
Zeller, K. (2007). *Jaguars in the New Millennium data base update: The state of the jaguar in 2006*. New York: Wildlife Conservation Society-Jaguar Conservation Program.
Zeller, K. A., Nijhawan, S., Salom-Perez, R., Potosme, S. H., & Hinnes, J. E. (2011). Integrating occupancy modeling and interview data for corridor identification: A case study for jaguars in Nicaragua. *Biological Conservation, 144,* 892–901.

Part IV
Urban and Environment Related Dimension

Chapter 21
Effects of Rapid Urbanization on the Quality of Life

Keshav Bhattarai and Darlene Budd

Abstract This is a literature-based study on quality of life (QoL) that evaluates the environmental, physical, psychological, social, economic and political dimensions influencing the quality of life. QoL is also influenced by poverty, education, health, investment in various industries, social disruptions, psychology, urban greenery, and urban infrastructure. In the case of Nepal, rapidly growing municipalities are facing sustainability issues due to the lack of resources and essential infrastructure. Rural-to-urban migration and emigration to other countries have contributed to the separation of family members. Divided families have contributed to various serious social disruptions. Findings suggest that in order to improve the QoL, small and medium-sized cities need investment in infrastructure and basic services, while metropolitan cities require competitive development strategies, efficient policy-making, urban and regional planning, and environmental management. In rural areas, access to essential services can help improve the QoL.

Keywords Quality of life (QoL) · Urbanization · Migration · Environmental management · Essential services · Ruralopolis · Psychological dimension

21.1 Introduction

Today, over 50% of the global population lives in urban areas. Rapid urbanization continues in both developed and developing countries. According to the United Nations, the urban population of the world is projected to grow to 4.9 billion by

K. Bhattarai (✉)
School of Environmental, Physical and Applied Sciences, University of Central Missouri, Humphreys 223 C, Warrensburg, USA
e-mail: bhattarai@ucmo.edu

D. Budd
Department of Government International Studies and Languages, University of Central Missouri, Wood-204 C, Warrensburg, USA
e-mail: dbudd@ucmo.edu

B. R. K. Sinha (ed.), *Multidimensional Approach to Quality of Life Issues*,
https://doi.org/10.1007/978-981-13-6958-2_21

2030—an increase of 1.6 billion—while the rural population is likely to shrink by 28 million (UN-Habitat 2007).

Studies on the quality of life (QoL) in urban and rural areas are increasingly conducted in response to the many problems faced by urbanizing areas that aim to improve living conditions of communities or groups in a sustainable manner (Theofilou 2013; Lotfi and Solaimani 2009). Such studies often and to compare the QoL between urban and rural areas (Nzaku and Bukenya 2005). In many developing countries, urbanization has become synonymous with infrastructure improvements, increased life expectancy, a decrease in total fertility rates, more employment opportunities from various urban-based economic activities, and visible development in concentrated settlements. In rural areas, however, living conditions are mainly based on extractive or primary activities. To this end, cities can play a transformative role in a country's economic growth by capitalizing on opportunities created by the forces of globalization. Increased urbanization has shifted employment opportunities from primary to secondary and tertiary sectors, resulting in a reduction in urban poverty. For example, between 1990 and 2010, poverty rates in Nepal declined from 35 to 25% in large part due to increased urbanization (Khanal 2014).

Urban centers are commonly viewed as drivers of economic growth that will help reduce poverty at the local, regional and national levels. Such a notion continues to motivate many people to move to urban centers at an unprecedented rate causing excessive strain on urban services and resulting in acute housing shortages. As a result, many newcomers to urban areas live in unplanned settlements and suffer from poor accesses to basic services.

In the world today, over 750 million people live on $2 dollar per day and 290 million on $1 dollar a day presenting daunting challenges to sustaining and improving their QoL (World Bank 2013). In South Asia, one out of three urban dwellers lives in unplanned settlements on $1–2 a day, and Nepal's case is not much different (NLSS II 2011; World Bank 2013). Despite such poverty, outlying villages clamor to become part of new urban areas with the hope that their populations will live healthier lives, be better educated and become more prosperous than people living in the countryside. The reality is that urban poor are more likely to experience chronic and acute forms of hunger and disease, achieve less education, have access to fewer stable employment opportunities, and die younger than rural populations (UN-Habitat 2007).

Previous research evaluates QoL based on six dimensions: environmental, physical, psychological, social, economic, and political (Bhattarai and Conway 2010). Environmental QoL refers to the natural aspects of the neighborhood. Physical QoL assesses available facilities, urban land use, and infrastructure. Additionally, physical QoL considers accessibility to mass transportation as well as traffic issues. Social QoL addresses the social dimensions of the neighborhood including citizen interaction, involvement, and participation. Psychological QoL focuses on how citizens feel about their neighborhood. Economic QoL analyzes how individuals operate their businesses and manage their incomes. Finally, political QoL looks at ways in which urban development policies are implemented. These indicators suggest that improving the quality of life in urban areas is no longer a simple matter of bricks and mortar. Human satisfaction is influenced by a variety of urban attributes such as transportation, quality of public spaces, recreational opportunities, land use patterns, building densities, and ease of access to basic goods, services, and public amenities.

21.2 History of Urban Quality of Life (QoL)

Whether it is the Sanskrit word "*nagara*" for city or the Roman word "*civitas*" for citizens cities historically represent the highest form of socio-cultural achievement in human civilization (Dahiya 2014). Historical records reveal that quality of life in urban centers was discussed in ancient times. Aristotle (384–322 BC) spoke of the "good life", "living well", and the role of public policy. As early as 1889, the term "quality of life" was used in urban planning circles to improve the living conditions of urban communities (Marshall and Banister 2007). For over a century, "quality of life" has been the focus of many interdisciplinary studies (El Din et al. 2012). Such studies analyze and evaluate cultural traditions, political systems, human behaviors, neighborhoods, and the environment. Common to each study is a focus on how each of the topics affects the quality of life of individuals and communities and how people fulfill their aspirations and needs within a specific cultural context (Sun 2005).

Quality of Life (QoL) indicates the well-being of the people in the environment that they live and identifies the set of needs and wants that help people feel satisfied. There is no generally accepted social theory outlining the conditions of human wellbeing or the relative weights of each factor when defining urban Quality of Life (QoL).

Economic development is one of the most common factors associated with quality of life (Diener and Suh 1997) and is often measured by a country's gross national product (GNP) (Nzaku adn Bukenya 2005). However, some also consider such factors as social movements and "social belonging" the when measuringe of QoL (Sen 1981). Various types of indicators suggest that the concept of QoL revolves around the complex inter-relationships among economic, social, psychological, technological, and environmental factors. National and international relations matter, as do those of individuals and groups within a society. Housing quality, levels of urbanization, efficient governance, and social cohesion are non-material factors that are also quite significant (Costanza 2005; Eurostat Survey 2013; Nzaku and Bukenya 2005). A majority of citizens consider access to public facilities such as schools, hospitals, public transport, and state pension systems as good measures of quality of life (Nzaku and Bukenya 2005).

Studies also consider how individuals participate in society—physically, socially and psychologically—when measuring quality of life. The degree of participation in leisure activities compared to time spent engaged in obligatory occupational activities such as work, self-care and sleep all effect quality of life. Research reveals that leisure activities significantly predict the quality of life of the elderly in an urban environment (Lee et al. 2014).

Wirth (1938) studied QoL from a human ecology perspective while Milgram (1970) studied QoL from an environmental perspective. Barker (1968) studied it from various human behavior settings. Andrews and Withey (1974) argue that QoL may be measured by asking people how they view their own state of well-being. Koelle (1974) argued that the priorities of politicians and professionals are congruent with QoL. Campbell et al. (1976) discussed QoL in terms of health care provision, crime, education, leisure facilities, and housing. Lefcourt (1976) studied QoL as a function of human behavioral constraints. Fischer (1984) analyzed subcultures to evaluate QoL. Clark and Kahn (1988) estimated peoples' willingness to pay for urban cultural amenities such as museums, theater, dance, instrumental music and zoos to maintaining high QoL.

Pacione (1990) and Michelson (1997) argued that QoL could be evaluated based on urban-based spatial associations—specifically, how urban dwellers live in their surroundings. Pacione (2003) observed that QoL improves with technological progress that brings improvements in the social, political and environmental health of a nation through the increase in gross national product (GNP). Technology spurs innovation in the development of products, processes, and new ways of serving people though it also contributes to harmful impacts on society and the environment. Further, Pacione (2003) discussed QoL based on the environment (e.g., air and water pollution, poor housing) in which people live, along with individual attributes such as health and educational achievement. Song and Knaap (2004) studied urban QoL based on an analysis of single-family houses in neighborhoods with mixed land use. Chor, Chin and Foog (2006) explored the relationship between the accessibility to prestigious schools, residential property values and QoL. Richards et al. (2007) investigated various factors associated with informal housing while evaluating QoL. Adair et al. (2000) discussed the pricing structure and accessibility of residential property, while Lora et al. (2010) analyzed policy actions for improving QoL in rapidly growing cities. Throughout the history of urban development, urban planners have tried to create urban spaces that also incorporate elements from nature (Rodenburg et al. 2001). Some even include biophilic structure to mimic ecological environs that integrate economic (green gardening) and sociological (healing and recreational) structures.

The description of QoL is a complex and nonlinear. Studies on QoL suggest that a wide range of social, economic and environmental needs must be addressed on a spatial scale due to the fact that a city is linked to regional, national and international systems.

21.3 Case of Nepal

Nepal, one of South Asia's least urbanized countries until 1972 has been experiencing rapid urbanization. For example, in 1990 16% of the country was considered urbanized. This percentage rose to 38.6% in 2014 (GoN 2014). Since 1972, the percentage of urbanized terrority in Nepal has climbed to over 65%. Urbanization has contributed to a reduction in the poverty level from 33% in 2000 to 25% in 2010 (NLSSII 2004, 2011).

Due to the rapid increase in the urban population (acknowledged in the Constitution of Nepal 1972) urban planning has become a topic of national interest for Nepal as the country is transforming socio-economically as well as politically under the new federal structure and many elected representatives are aspiring to develop multiple megacities to improve the quality of life (QoL) for citizens. Urban areas are already playing a major role in the economic transformation of the country; however, the current situation is very chaotic. With the recent reorganization of Nepal's federal structure urban areas are increasing in number and creating a *ruralopolis*, while creating hopes for employment generation, market linkages, financial institutions, and basic services to improve the QoL. Complicating matters is the fact that the Nepali urban environment is characterized by increasing inequalities in accessing services such as financing, urban governance, and urban health services. Future development programs must consider accessibility of basic services and resources.

Urban development and planning at the federal level demands thorough research from socio-economic, political, infrastructural and environmental perspectives to improve QoL. There are suggestions to improve the QoL through proper urban planning using geospatial technology to lay the foundation for congestion-free, environmentally friendly, sustainable "Smart Citie". However, such planning requires an understanding of the historical processes of urban planning and development in the context of the recently restructured federal system in Nepal. A study that identifies the strength, weakness, opportunities and threats (SWOT) gaps and constraints for the sustainable economic and environmental development of urban areas through improved planning processes is needed.

Specifically, an analysis of the spatial distribution of urban centers in the recently federated Nepal (Fig. 21.1) and examining how smart cities will help public officials and businesses build smart cities and improve QoL.

Under the new federal structure, Nepal now ranks among the most urbanized South Asian countries n urbanization with over 65% of the population living in urban areas. Accordingly, there are over 250 municipalities, 9 sub-metropolitan and 6 metropolitan centers. Many rural areas are annexed to meet the population threshold to qualify as a municipality, sub-metropolitan, or metropolitan area. Such actions have increased the cost of land beyond affordable limits and the urban inequalities are widening unexpectedly. The majority of Nepal's municipalities are unplanned, exposed to possible seismic vulnerabilities and health hazards. Because of the annexation of many village *Palikas* (village administrative units) into *Nagarpalikas* (municipalities), Nepal's urban areas are characterized by "*ruralopolises*", where rural-based communities with high population densities compete for collective urban facilities. Increasing urban sprawl spatially through unsustainable rural–urban implosion has blended rural economic and social systems with metropolitan spatial organizations, where spatially well-organized infrastructures are missing and low-income people are living in various destitute conditions, yet, urbanization is increasing. The political leaders at all levels continue to expand urban areas and develop megalopolises by annexing many urban patches all over Nepal.

Though politicians are aspiring to create several megalopolises for quick social transformation through urbanization and improving the QoL, Nepal faces challenges

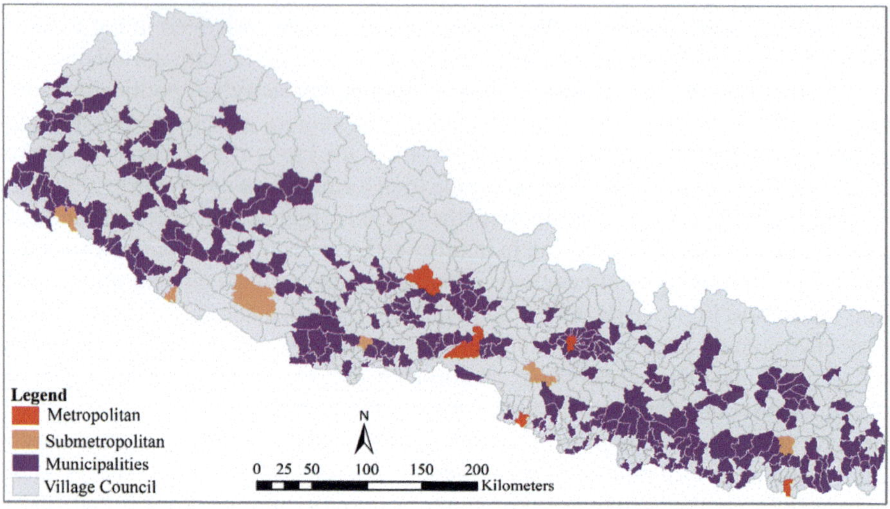

Fig. 21.1 Spatial distribution of municipality, sub-metropolitan, and metropolitan areas

of resource scarcity, severe poverty and socioeconomic inequality (World Bank 2017). Yet these newly defined cities exhibit significant opportunities in economic developments and in improving QoL. Urban planners, especially the newly elected representatives, are struggling to understand urban issues and opportunities while formulating appropriate programs and plans to achieve social justice and redistribution of development benefits. Detailed studies using geospatial technologies might be helpful to spatially relate different components that are related to the QoL.

21.4 Components Related to Quality of Life (QoL)

21.4.1 Environment and Quality of Life

Good QoL needs access to clean air, and water, while maintaining biodiversity, and maintaining lands free of toxins and wastes. Utilizing energy-saving technologies to create clean energy sources and efforts to reduce energy demands are necessary to maintain and improve QoL from an environmental perspective.

Urban populations and the physical area they occupy continue to grow. Unplanned urban growth triggers a number of environmental problems at multiple levels, including the loss of natural vegetation, open spaces, biodiversity and microclimate while exerting pressures on water, energy and infrastructure. As the population increases in urban areas, the needs for transportation also increases. The increasing number of vehicles pollutes urban air, contributes to different levels of noises, produces greenhouse gas emissions, and an ever-growing number of road accidents and deaths.

A growing population needs more water. With access to water supplies limited to a few days and hours per week, unregulated use of private pumps and the practice of leaving taps permanently open, exacerbates problems of low pressure, leakage, and infiltration in many systems. As a result, the use of shallow tube wells in residential areas has become common practice, in many parts of Nepal. Many water sources are contaminated with high levels of fecal matter from septic tanks and pit toilets, and organic and inorganic pollutants. Due to the poor quality of water supplies in many towns, low-income families are unable to boil water due in part to high fuel costs, and consequently, are at constant risk. As a result, the most prominent public health problems among the poor are largely preventable, gastrointestinal diseases caused by non-potable water.

The institutional framework for the disposal of solid and industrial (including hazardous) waste in many towns is ineffective. In most towns, solid waste collection is a local government responsibility and accounts for a significant proportion of the local budget. Insufficient financial resources prevent local governments from maintaining equipment and hiring trained technicians. Municipal garbage dumps are inadequately sealed from infiltration, and pose a potential environmental hazard throughout their lifespan. Most agencies responsible for waste disposal are unclear as to the nature and quantities of the waste they handle. In some areas, landfills contain unprocessed toxic waste and septic tank effluent. With an increasing population and changing consumption patterns, solid waste volumes—both biodegradable and nondegradable—will continue to increase in urban areas.

Waste volumes may be reduced through community awareness and education campaigns aimed at minimizing waste and increasing recycling programs. Though some municipalities have introduced innovative programs to involve unemployed youth in city clean-up programs, municipalities lack the financial and technical resources to maintain recycling vehicles, equipment, and facilities. One possible way to raise money for such programs is to impose a tax on all products that contain non-biodegradable packaging materials that have been categorized as dangerous by the Environmental Protection Agency (EPA).

21.4.2 Physical Aspect and Urban Quality of Life

Eco-friendly housing, safe neighborhoods, interconnected streets, and a transportation system that is accessible to all citizens are the factors considered when assessing the physical urban quality of life. Sidewalks and designated bike paths provide alternative modes of transportation for pedestrians that are safe and environmentally friendly. A well-planned infrastructure that incorporates built and non-built areas, creates fewer environmental hazards, and can be sustainably managed.

In the interconnected global economy, cities compete for business and investment. Such businesses influence the quality of urban life. Cities with efficient modes of transportation that function in an integrated system are more likely to evolve and prosper as centers for trade, commerce, and industry, than cities that cannot provide residents, workers, and business owners accessible and efficient mass transportation as well as safe roads.

As the number of private vehicles in many cities that do not have a well-managed road system, continues to grow, the number of fatalities also increases. At the global level, each year, road accidents result in 1.3 million deaths, and injuries to 20–50 million people. Forecasts estimate that by 2030, road traffic fatalities will be the fifth leading cause of death in the world (Bloomberg 2012). In Nepal, the number of private vehicles is increasing and lifestyles are changing in urban areas. More driving and less walking have contributed to air pollution, increased greenhouse-gas emissions and higher rates of obesity. Many "lifestyle diseases" such as stroke, hypertension and heart disease have increased in urban areas. For example, heart-related diseases killed 6,102 people in 1990 and more than 20,000 people in 2013 in Nepal (Neupane 2014). A sustainable transportation system in addition to maintaining green spaces, cultural centers and sports facilities could improve physical urban quality of life. Education campaigns to promote walking and cycling as elements of healthy living and to reduce vehicular emissions are essential. Many important quality-of-life benefits also arise when cities promote non-motorized transport.

21.4.3 Psychological Dimension and Urban Quality of Life

Historical evidence suggests that in order to maintain (or create) psychological urban quality of life, human beings must be close to nature. Ancient Egyptian towns, Persian settlements and medieval Chinese villages were all characterized by extensive and elaborate gardens based on the notion that quality of life was a function of a human being's proximity to nature (Kellert 1993). Japanese gardens of the ninth to twelfth centuries emphasized the orderly arrangement of trees and shrubs, streams and ponds, and open spaces (Wilson 1984). These artistic designs were considered symbols of a good quality of life. Today, the practice is termed *biophilia.*

The popularity of *biophilia* has increased recently due to the rapid disappearance of the green "living environment" in urban areas, and has generated a call for a better understanding of human nature and a more convincing environmental ethic (Kellert 1993). The present-day *biophilic* city incorporates innovative ways of maintaining nature and greenery—known as "green spaces"—to connect urban dwellers with nature (Wilson 1984).

Green spaces play an important role in sustaining the social, economic, cultural and environmental aspects of societies (Atiqul Haq 2011; Chiesura 2004). Green spaces are believed to help relieve stresses (Ulrich 1986) and improve children's cognitive functioning (Wells 2000). Parks not only offer venues for social interactions (Kazmierczak 2013; Peters et al. 2010), but also help in mitigating urban heat (Bowler et al. 2010; Quattrochi and Luvall 1999; Sailor 1995; Yu and Hien 2006) while enhancing biodiversity (Irvine et al. 2009).

In the case of Nepal, the historic town of Kathmandu had a rich cultural heritage amid unparalleled natural beauty. The intangible heritage that flourished in the cities—art, music, dance, and elaborate public celebrations and religious observances—used to add vitality and meaning to the buildings and urban fabric. However, this fabric has been damaged with the rapid expansion of urban areas. A rapidly increasing population and unmanaged urbanization have severely degraded the urban environment resulting in a dense urban area with few green spaces, narrow streets, and alleys. As a result, air, water, and land pollution have increased, severely affecting human health conditions. The lack of green spaces has increased the distance between human and nature.

Today, the Kathmandu Metropolitan Area has only 0.04% (2 sq. km) of public green space (DUDBC 2013). The city has only 15 parks, which are located on the outskirts of the city. The conservation of unique heritage sites and spaces, both tangible and intangible, can be a catalyst for urban revitalization, city livability, and creating a wide range of income-earning opportunities. Today, many residents of Kathmandu are making every effort to apply the *biophilic* concept with the hope that their efforts will inspire people to conserve and protect nature (Gurung 2014).

21.4.4 Social Aspects and Urban Quality of Life

The social aspects of urban QoL include equal access to affordable housing, employment and business opportunities, health services and education. Barriers that constrain the elderly, disabled, women, children and minority groups from participating in daily life activities must be overcome. Essential to social integration is the provision of a wide range of housing options to citizens across the socioeconomic spectrum. Public access to civic buildings and an adequate number of public gathering places will help to promote good relations and interactions between residents.

Prior to the incorporation of villages into urban areas, many villages served as the social unit that provided a forum for resolving family and kinship issues. Such local governance by village elders helped to sustain social cohesion. The social and economic bonds that were formed created an informal safety net for the community. However, demands for a higher standard of living believed to be found in urban areas have made it difficult for traditional leadership structures to respond adequately to the changing needs of families. An increasing percentage of urban youth have never visited their traditional village communities and have not developed strong bonds with the village and extended family members. Thus, the traditional safety net developed over hundreds of years is weakened. Many communities grapple with the transition from subsistence to cash-based livelihoods in growth-oriented economies. As a result, the gap between the rich and poor is increasing, as is the social distance between urban and rural family members.

As the number of citizens who live off the land has decreased, cash dependency has increased. The proliferation of overcrowded squatter and informal settlements, coupled with increasing unemployment rates have resulted in a number of social problems. The division of families and the consequent breakdown of the extended family, has led to an increase in crime and vandalism committed by unemployed, urban youth. Domestic violence has increased as have divorce rates, the number of single-parent households, and suicide rates. In Nepal, the number of suicides increased from 75 in 1990 to 6,512 in 2013 (Neupane 2014).

Private rental housing, where available, has been insufficient to meet rapidly increasing demand from lower income families. Overcrowding is common, with small rented rooms often accommodating families of 5–11 people. The rent for a single room shared by one or more families, accounts for 60–70% a family's annual income, leaving little money for food, clothing, education and health care. As a result, the number of illegal settlements without electricity, clean water, and proper sanitation is growing. These areas as well as the individuals and familes, are especially hard hit during extreme weather and natural disasters.

21.4.5 Economic Aspects and Urban Quality of Life

Historically, urbanization has been viewed as a growth mechanism to produce and increase the quality of life of urban residents for two reasons. First, urban growth and urbanization have been invariably associated with industrial growth—at least such was the case in Western Europe, North America, and Japan—where cities served as centers of employment for agricultural workers seeking manufacturing jobs and increased income. Second, urbanization led to reduced population growth rates, due to the fact that, unlike in rural-agricultural settings, children were no longer seen as an economic asset (Shrestha and Bhattarai 2003). In recent decades, many cities have followed similar patterns of growth. The urban quality of life has increased following a demographic transition producing a decrease in fertility rates.

Without a doubt, well-planned urban centers offer opportunities to manufacturing industries that contribute to improving QoL. In the case of Nepal, shortages of energy, agitating labor unions and high interest rates have been the major impediments to industry and growth. Excessive government interferences and centralization of power with the Prime Minister's Office have not helped in development. Despite Nepal's industrial sector contributing 62% of the GDP, Nepal's urban areas are characterized by unemployment and underemployment (Khanal 2014). Tax reform, better protection for workers' safety, low interest loans, and a less interfering government would undoubtedly attract local and foreign businesses.

A widening gap in the distribution of wealth, unequal access to services, and limited economic opportunities continue to inhibit economic growth. In the case of Nepal, international donors have helped to conduct policy studies and analyses, as well as provide financial services to implement employment generating programs. However, the lack of economic stimuli combined with the insecure political situation has resulted in a massive exodus of the Nepal's productive workforce seeking employment in other countries (World Bank 2000). Nepal's economy is increasingly reliant on highly volatile external remittance flows, rather than internal competitiveness (Khanal 2014). Remittances accounting for nearly 29% of the country's GDP have become instrumental in keeping the current account deficit under control in spite of a negative trade balance. However, remittances are only a temporary solution, and in the long run, lead to inflation and greater inequality among households.

In many urban areas, economic activities are stagnant and cottage industries are producing at low levels. Nepal needs to prioritize the "where, what, and how" of public investments and enhance the competitiveness of strategic clusters—such as cultural tourism, handicrafts, and agro-processing—to foster sustainable growth and create economic opportunities in urban areas. Cities are important centers for developing and promoting Nepal's handicrafts, because they are the places where many artisans create and produce, and wholesalers and retailers reside.

21.4.6 Political Aspect and Urban Quality of Life

Theoretically, urbanization enhances secondary and tertiary sector activities (including manufacturing, tourism, restaurants and hotels, and government services) and contributes substantially to foreign exchange earnings. However, government and politics greatly influence such activities. Nepal's political instability over the past two decades has affected its urban quality of life. First, the insurgency between 1996 and 2005 pushed many rural residents into urban areas. Second, newcomers were supported clandestinely by some political parties to occupy open spaces. Third, inadequate policing and security have led to an increase in criminal activities committed in large part by unemployed youths. Despite these problems, urbanization in Nepal has been an inevitable response to stagnating conditions in rural areas, few if any of which can offer the employment opportunities provided by the urban economy.

Nepal plans to advance to a "developing country" status by 2022 (Bhusal 2014). In order to advance, Nepal needs to meet at least two goals of three goals recommended by the United Nations during two triennial reviews of the Committee for Development Policy. First, per capita gross national income needs to reach US$1,190. Second, the Human Development Index (HDI) that includes an indicator for education and health must increase to 66. Third, the Economic Vulnerability Index (EVI) should be no more than 32. Records suggest that Nepal has made steady progress in Human Development Index (HAI); for example, in 1990 the HDI was 0.34, 0.424 in 2005, 0.455 in 2010, and 0.458 in 2011, but it is still low compared to the 0.548 average for the South Asian region for 2011 (UNDP 2011). Nepal achieved an HDI score of 59.83 and an EVI score of 27.80.

As Nepal slowly progresses toward a peaceful democracy, it is hoped that there will be some improvements in urban quality of life in two ways. First, the broadened sphere of urban governance will recognize the vital role of civil society. Second, local governments will focus on the principles of good governance such as democratic participation and representation, accountability and transparency, and the increasing use of new technologies and e-governance.

In 2015, Nepal hosted a South Asian Association for Regional Cooperation (SAARC) conference in Kathmandu. The event compelled Nepal to take steps to ameliorate urban blight and environmental degradation. Due to increased awareness and advocacy to clean up urban areas, some improvements were made in the Kathmandu Valley's environment and its infrastructure. In theory, the government is making continuous efforts to accelerate partnership with private, corporate, and non-governmental actors, but the current Communist government is without any clear vision whether to follow the neoclassical model or socialist model of economic policies. Though Nepal's new constitution includes a provision for investment by private entrepreneurs, investors are confused by the economic policy of the Communist led government. Though Communist leaders have committed to democracy and the involvement of the private sector in economic development, leaders do not appear certain about their exact economic policy plan or how it will contribute to the improvement of urban quality of life (QoL).

21.4.7 Conclusion

Based on the survey of the literature, this paper discussed the various aspects of urban quality of life (QoL). It discussed how various factors such as economic growth, employment opportunities, per capita income, remittances, industry and agriculture, water supply, the environment, and manufacturing services can influence the quality of life. It also provided an overiew of urban life quality in Nepal. A review of the literature suggests that there is no single factor that influences the quality of life significantly more than other factors. A country's urban infrastructure, access to technology, and level of education of its worker all influence quality of life.

Based on the review of the various dimensions of urban QoL, Nepal has the history and culture to improve the quality of life of residents living in urban areas throughout the country. The potential for improvements lies in a new constitution that will help guide federal and provincial governance. Strategic planning and infrastructure improvements in urban centers will attract domestic and foreign investments. A focus on Nepal's natural beauty, abundant resources, and vibrant culture will increase tourism. More investment and more tourists will create job opportunities that are essential to consistent economic growth.

Environmental protection regulations and associated taxes on products harmful to the environment will help to improve urban QoL. Planned development that prioritizes green spaces, public spaces, and safe neighborhoods are necessary to improve the quality of life. Access to clean water and proper sanitation is tantamount to keeping citizens healthy and productive. Trash collection, recycling programs, and the proper disposal of waste will decrease instances of gastrointestinal diseases through water-borne diseases. Efforts to improve roads and increase mass transportation options will help decrease the number of cars on the roads and subsequently the number of injuries and fatalities resulting from various vehicular accidents.

The *biophilia* movement taking hold in urban centers is a positive step toward bringing back all-important green spaces. Such efforts by residents and business owners contribute to the "intangible heritage" of Nepal's urban centers and rich culture. A stable government with firm urban industrial and environmental policies will create investment in environment and minimize pollution from new manufacturing facilities. Increased employment opportunities will reduce the number of Nepalese workers seeking employment overseas, this will also improve the quality of life through social cohesion.

References

Adair, A., Mcgreal, S., et al. (2000). House prices and accessibility: The testing of relationships within the Belfast urban area. *Housing Studies, 15*(5), 699–716.

Andrews, F. M., & Withey, S. B. (1974). Developing measures of perceived life quality: Results from several national surveys. *Social Indicator Research, 1,* 1–26.

Atiqul Haq, S. (2011). Urban green spaces and integrative approach to sustainable environment. *Journal of Environmental Protection, 2*(5), 601–608.

Barker, R. (1968). *Ecological psychoatelogy*. Stanford: Stanford University Press.

Bhattarai, K., & Conway, D. (2010). Urban vulnerabilities in the Kathmandu Valley, Nepal: Visualizations of human/hazard interactions. *Journal of Geographic Information System, 2*(2), 63–84. https://doi.org/10.4236/jgis.2010.22012.

Bhusal, Y. R. (2014). *Nepal's graduation strategy from LDC to DC: An appraisal*. 25 Years of Nepal German Association: Silver Jubilee Special Issue, Nepal German Academic Association (NEGAAS), pp. 42–46. http://www.negaas.org.np/portal/, December.

Bloomberg, M. R. (2012). *Leading the world wide movement to improve the road safety: Bloomberg global safety program*. Bloomberg Philanthropies. http://www.bloomberg.org/content/uploads/sites/2/2014/04/Bloomberg_Road_Safety_Midway_Report_Final.pdf. Accessed January 7, 2015.

Bowler, D. E., Buyung-Ali, L., Knight, T. M., & Pullin, A. S. (2010). Urban greening to cool towns and cities: A systematic review of the empirical evidence. *Landscape and Urban Planning, 97*(3), 147–155.

Campbell, A., Converse, P., & Rogers, W. (1976). *The quality of American life*. New York: Russell Sage Foundation.

Chiesura, A. (2004). The role of urban parks for the sustainable city. *Landscape and Urban Planning, 68*(1), 129–138.

Chor Chin, H., & Wai Foog, K. (2006). Influence of school accessibility on housing values. *Journal of Urban Planning and Development, 132*(3), 120–128.

Clark, D. E., & James Kahn, R. (1988). The social benefits of urban cultural amenities. *Journal of Regional Science, 28,* 363–377.

Costanza, R. (2005). Quality of life: An approach integrating opportunities, human needs, and subjective well-being. *Ecological Economics, 61,* 267–276.

Dahiya, B. (2014). Feature essay: Southeast Asia and sustainable urbanization. *Global Asia, 9*(3).

Diener, E., & Suh, E. M. (1997). Measuring quality of life: Economic, social, and subjective indicators. *Social Indicators Research, 40,* 189–216.

DUDBC. (2013). *Urban landscape guideline for Kathmandu Valley, final report*. Kathmandu: Department of Urban Development and Building Construction.

El Din, H. S., Ahmed, S., Farouh, H. E., & Elariane, S. A. (2012). Principles of urban quality of life for a neighborhood. *Housing and Building National Research Center (HRBC) Journal, 9,* 86–92.

Eurostat Survey. (2013). *European cities, quality of life in cities perception survey in 79*. European commission, Luxemburg publication office of the European Union.

Fischer, C. (1984). *The urban experience*. New York: Harcourt, Brace Janovich.

GoN. (2014). *Ministry of urban development*. Government of Nepal. http://www.moud.gov.np/. Accessed January 08, 2015.

Gurung, M. M. (2014). *Expanding Biophilic city design theory: A study of incorporating nature into the urban design elements of Kathmandu*. A Masters thesis in Architecture Engineering submitted to The Graduate School College of Arts and Architecture; The Pennsylvania State University.
Irvine, K. N., Devine-Wright, P., Payne, S. R., Fuller, R. A., Painter, B., & Gaston, K. J. (2009). Green space, soundscape and urban sustainability: An interdisciplinary, empirical study. *Local Environment, 14,* 155–172.
Kazmierczak. (2013). The contribution of local parks to neighborhood social ties. *Landscape and Urban Planning, 109*(1), 31–44.
Kellert, S. R. (1993). The Biophilia basis for human values of nature. In S. R. Kellert & E. O. Wilson (Eds.), *The Biophilia hypothesis* (pp. 42–69). Island Press/Shearwater Books.
Khanal, D. R. (2014). *Contemporary issues on global and Nepalese economy: Mainstreaming the real policy agenda*. New Delhi: Adroit Publishers.
Koelle, H. (1974). An experimental study on the determinants of a definition for the quality of life. *Regional Studies, 8,* 1–10.
Lee, J. H., Lee, J. H., & Park, S. H. (2014). Leisure activity participation as predictor of quality of life in Korean urban-dwelling elderly. *Occupational Therapy International, 21,* 124–132 (John Wiley & Sons, Ltd).
Lefcourt, H. (1976). *Locus of control*. New York: Halsted Press.
Lora, E., Powell, A., et al. (2010). *The quality of life in Latin American cities, markets and perception*. Washington, DC: The Inter-American Development Bank.
Lotfi, S., & Solaimani, K. (2009). An assessment of urban quality of life by using analytic hierarchy process approach. *Journal of Social Science, 5,* 123–133.
Marshall, S., & Banister, D. (2007). *Land use and transport*. Elsevier: Amsterdam.
Michelson, W. (1997). *Environmental Choice, Human Behaviour and Residential Satisfaction*. New York: Oxford University Press.
Milgram, S. (1970). The experience of living in cities. *Science, 167,* 1461–1468.
Neupane, S. P. (2014). Life expectancy and new challenges. *Setopati*. http://setopati.net/opinion/4680/Life-expectancy-and-new-challenges/. Accessed December 20, 2014.
NLSS II. (2004, 2011). *Nepal living standards survey 2003/04 and 2011: Statistical report* (Vol. II and I). Central Bureau of Statistics, National Planning Commission Secretariat.
Nzaku, K., & Bukenya, J. O. (2005). Examining the relationship between quality of life amenities and economic development in the Southeast USA. *Review of Urban & Regional Development Studies, 17*(2), July.
Pacione, M. (1990). Urban liveability. *Urban Geography, 11*(1), 1–30.
Pacione, M. (2003). Urban environmental quality and human wellbeing—A social geographical perspective. *Landscape and Urban Planning, 65,* 19–30. http://www1.geo.ntnu.edu.tw/~moise/Data/Books/Social/06%20social%20security/uban%20environmental%20quality%20and%20human%20wellbeing.pdf; https://doi.org/10.1016/s0169-2046(02)00234-7. Accessed January 8, 2015.
Peters, K., Elands, B., & Buijs, A. (2010). Social interaction in Urban parks: Stimulating social cohesion? *Urban Forestry and Urban Greening, 9*(2), 93–100.
Quattrochi, D. A., & Luvall, J. C. (1999). *High spatial resolution airborne multispectral thermal infrared data to support analysis and modeling tasks in the EOS IDS Project Atlanta*, NASA. (Online) http://wwwghcc.msfc.nasa.gov/atlanta/. Accessed January 8, 2015.
Richards, R., O'leary, B., & Mutsunziwa, K. (2007). Measuring quality of life in informal settlements in South Africa. *Social Indicators Research, 81,* 375–388.
Rodenburg, C., Baycan-Levent, T., van Leeuwen, E., & Nijkamp, P. (2001). Urban economic indicators for green development in cities. *Green Management International, 36*(Winter).
Sailor, D. J. (1995). Simulated urban climate response to modifications in surface albedo and vegetative cover. *Journal of Applied Meteorology, 34*(1694), 1704.
Sen, A. (1981). Public action and the quality of life in developing countries. *Oxford Bulletin of Economics and Statistics, 43,* 287–319. https://doi.org/10.1111/j.1468-0084.1981.mp43004001.x.

Shrestha, N. R., & Bhattarai, K. (2003). *Historical dictionary of Nepal*. Lanham, MD; Oxford: Scarecrow Press.
Song, Y., & Knaap, G. (2004). Measuring the effects of mixed land uses on housing values. *Regional Science and Urban Economics, 34*(2004), 663–680.
Sun, Y. (2005). *Development of neighborhood quality of life indicators*. Saskatchewan, Canada: University of Saskatchewan.
Theofilou, P. (2013).Theoretical contributions quality of life: Definition and measurement. *Europe's Journal of Psychology, 9*(1), 150–162. https://doi.org/10.5964/ejop.v9i1.337.
Ulrich, R. (1986). Human responses to vegetation and landscapes *13,* 29–44.
UNDP. (2009). *Nepal human development report 2009*. http://www.np.undp.org/content/nepal/en/home/library/human_development/nepal-human-development-report-2009/. Accessed January 8, 2015.
UNDP. (2011). *UNDP annual report 2011*. 28 June 2012. http://www.np.undp.org/content/nepal/en/home/library/annual_report/UNDP_annual_report_2011.html. Accessed January 8, 2015.
UN-Habitat. (2007). *Global report on human settlements 2007—Enhancing urban safety and security*. Nairobi: UN-HABITAT. http://www.unhabitat.org/pmss/listItemDetails.aspx?publicationID=2432. Accessed January 8, 2015.
Wells, N. (2000). At home with nature: Effects of "greenness" on children's cognitive functioning. *Environment and Behavior, 32*(6), 775–795.
Wilson, E. (1984). *Biophilia*. Cambridge, MA: Harvard University Press.
Wirth, L. (1938). Urbanism as a way of life. *American Journal of Sociology, 44*.
World Bank. (2000). *Cities in transition*. Washington, DC: World Bank.
World Bank. (2013). Managing Nepal's urban transition. http://www.worldbank.org/en/news/feature/2013/04/01/managing-nepals-urban-transition. Accessed December 29, 2014.
World Bank. (2017). *Nepal - urban governance and development program: Emerging towns project (English)*.http://documents.worldbank.org/curated/en/686631502720248497/Nepal-Urban-Governance-and-Development-Program-Emerging-Towns-Project. Accessed December 17, 2017.
Yu, C., & Hien, W. N. (2006). Thermal benefits of city parks. *Energy and Buildings, 38*(2), 105–102.

Chapter 22
Land Use Patterns: Key Element of Quality of Life in the Metropolitan Area of Bucharest

Gabriel Simion and Marioara Rusu

Abstract This paper aims to characterise different land use patterns and identify the goods and services related to quality of life (QoL) and to assess the influence of urban planning policies on land cover changes in the Bucharest metropolitan area (BMA). Topographical map of the year 1970 and CORINE Land Cover (CLC) maps of 1990 and 2012 are used to detect land cover changes. A survey in two selected settlements (one urban and one rural) provides primary data on socio-economic transformation and planning policies related to suburbanisation processes of the analysed area. The investigations were completed by field observations, questionnaires and interviews with local stakeholders. Secondary data on population were obtained from the National Institute of Statistics. The results suggest that land use pattern has undergone profound changes over the last 50 years, particularly regarding the conversion of agricultural lands and forests and into areas with residential, industrial and commercial uses. Local development policies combined with the positive effects of suburbanisation phenomena have improved the QoL of population living in the area. The urban expansion of Bucharest increased the pressure on farmers to sell the agricultural land, but at the same time contributed to the improvement of QoL for the landowners. The analysis of how land use in urban areas influences QoL can be a starting point in urban development policies. They can assist policymakers and practitioners in improving the balance between urbanisation and living environment.

Keywords Land use pattern · Bucharest metropolitan area · Ecosystem services · Quality of life · Suburbanisation

---

G. Simion (✉)
Faculty of Geography, University of Bucharest, Bucharest, Romania
e-mail: gabriel.simion@geo.unibuc.ro

M. Rusu
Institute of Agricultural Economics, Romanian Academy, Bucharest, Romania
e-mail: rusu.marioara@gmail.com

B. R. K. Sinha (ed.), *Multidimensional Approach to Quality of Life Issues*,
https://doi.org/10.1007/978-981-13-6958-2_22

22.1 Introduction

Quality of life (QoL) is a broad term to define, and experts have not agreed on a single and inclusive definition of this concept. It is considered as a multidisciplinary term found in the current use (Farquhar 1995a, b) and a vague term 'used by many, but with nobody clearly knowing how to use it' (Campbell et al. 1976). It is a measure of social well-being and life satisfaction of individuals in an area (Bhatti et al. 2017). QoL is relative, resulting from the assessment of the individual's living conditions and his or her needs and aspirations and require a complementarity between what the society offers and the demands of citizens (Veenhoven 2000). QoL also depends on the individual's ability to cope with daily problems and economic growth does not automatically determine wealth and happiness in society or at the individual level.

QoL in the urban environment is one of the top concerns of contemporary society in the context of an increasing number of population and cities (Pacione 2013; Muller and Zeller 2002). More than half of the world's population lives in urban areas, and it tends to increase. The issues of QoL are significant for a wide range of academics in the field such as human geography, urban planners, urban sociologists and economics. Understanding the relationship between population and environment (natural or social) is one of the focus of human geography studies related to the QoL amid the development of critical social sciences (Held 1980) or debates around radical geography (Peet 1977). In the context of urban studies, the congruence between population and the surrounding urban environment is analysed (Keys et al. 2007). A particular attention has been paid to the social problems of QoL in urban areas, such as the decline of city centres, deindustrialisation which led to specific issues related to unemployment, demographic ageing, housing quality and high-income population leaving central areas.

The concept of land use can be defined as the totality of arrangements, activities and inputs that people engage within a particular type of land cover (FAO & UNEP 1999). The cities have to respond functionally and operationally to the flows generated by the population and its needs. Contemporary cities are more dynamic than in the past due to their numerous functions and increasing agglomerations of population. These aspects make it increasingly challenging to create local urban development policies, as well as to identify methods and practices for their implementation in order to ensure a balance between development needs and the quality of urban life.

The analysis of how land use in urban areas influences QoL can be a starting point in urban development policies. They can assist policymakers and practitioners in improving the balance between urbanisation and living environment (Bhatti et al. 2017). Land use planning and regulation at a basic territorial level (neighbourhood) can create the premises for ways to improve QoL in a city (Serag El Din et al. 2013). Proper urban planning through land use regulation can positively influence QoL.

The development of built-up areas within the city and its densification may have adverse effects on the population's health, but also on its mental state and QoL in general (Chiessura 2004). The management policies of green areas within cities are increasing in the hands of authorities, who need to take into account of new concepts in urban planning and land use related to sustainable and smart cities (Yubing 2015).

During the socialist period (1947–1989), Romania went through an intense urbanisation process by increasing the number of cities and encouraging the rural–urban migration (Dumitrache et al. 2016a). The transition period from the centralist system to that of the market-oriented economy has led to the emergence of new concerns related to the urban environment, particularly the requirements of the population for economic competitivity, as well as the provision of public services to a level that will improve the QoL (Dumitrache et al. 2016b). The urbanisation rate in Romania is approximately 55%, but it can be a little higher if we consider the population of the rural–metropolitan area as urban, and in this condition, the urbanisation rate could be of about 65%. The cities and regional planning are regulated by Romanian Law 350/2001, with the aim to promote a balance social and economic development across the country. The law covers the managing of natural resources, protecting the environment, spatial planning of land use, and promoting the coherence of different administrative levels.

QoL is seen as an evaluative concept that can be defined as the reporting resultant of living conditions and activities that make up human life, needs, values and aspirations. It refers both to evaluate the overall life (how much it is satisfying different individuals, social groups or collective people) and to assess various conditions for living or life satisfaction: environment, work, interpersonal relationships and family life. According to the MEA (2005), there are four types of services, vital to human well-being, namely: (a) supply services—providing goods such as food, water, wood; (b) regulating services—such as controlling climate, rainfall, floods, waste and spread of diseases; (c) cultural services—relating to recreation and spiritual welfare; (d) support services—including soil formation, photosynthesis and nutrient cycles, etc.

This paper provides a short overview on QoL as a phenomenon dependent on and firmly connected with ecosystem services. Ecosystems are the basis of life and all human activities (de Groot 2006). They provide a variety of benefits to people, that are known as 'ecosystem goods and services' (Costantza et al. 1997). This paper mainly focuses on mapping different land use patterns in the BMA and identifying the goods and services produced by land use in relation to QoL.

22.2 Study Area

Bucharest City, the capital of Romania, is the leading industrial, cultural and academic city. Geographically, it is located in the south-eastern part of the country, approximately 100 km south of the Carpathian Mountains, 200 km to the west of the Black Sea and 60 km north of the Danube River (Fig. 22.1).

The BMA analysed here is comprised of Bucharest City (which subdivides into 6 administrative sectors) and Ilfov County (8 towns and 32 municipalities-communes) (Fig. 22.2). The BMA is situated in the Romanian plain region. Natural conditions

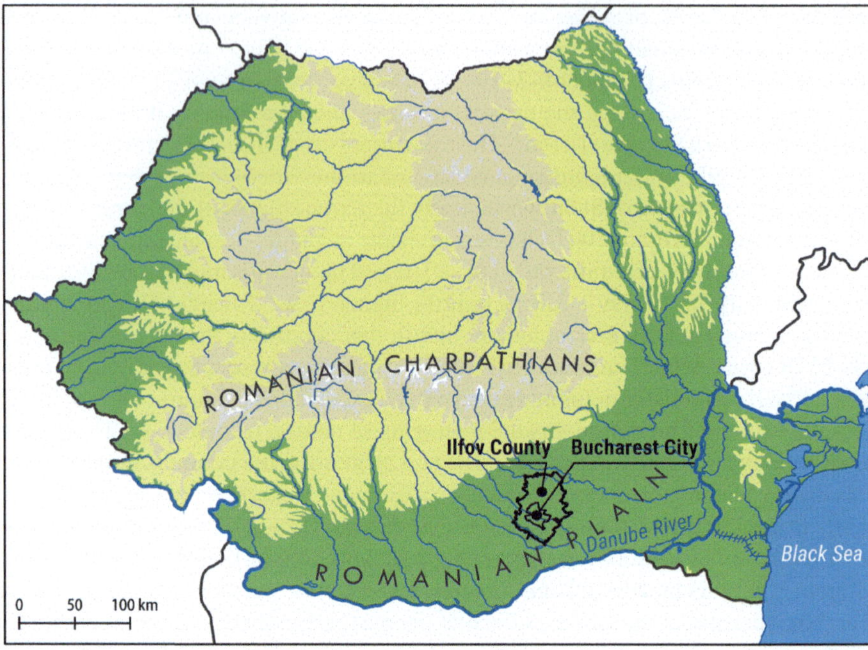

Fig. 22.1 Study area in Romania. *Source* authors

allow for the practice of agriculture due to soft slopes and do not require specialised equipment for crop management. Temperate climate features, with warm summers and cold winters, allow for the cultivation of cereals and vegetables, but lower rainfall makes irrigations a necessity/determined the use of irrigations. Soils have a high agricultural potential, most of them being very productive.

The total population of 2.3 million ranks the city 37th among all of the metropolitan regions in Europe. The population of Bucharest City declined from 2,067,545 to 1,883,425 during 1992–2011, but the population of Ilfov County increased to 35% between 1977 and 2011 pointing the absolute number from 287,738 to 388,738 (Table 22.1).

In the last decades, the population number evolved unevenly, both regarding time and space, according to the dynamics of the main demographic phenomena (Simion 2010). Evolution of population after 1990 shows a decrease in the number of the population due to the decline of birth rates and a high level of mortality rates. The demographic behaviour has changed by reducing the number of children per family. Also, a large number of Bucharest's population moved into new, single-family residences in the rural areas of Ilfov County.

The metropolitan spatial dynamic has been for a long-time spontaneous and uncontrolled: there has not been any indication of a broader development or changes of local master plans which would be correlated with a metropolitan strategy (Simion and Nistor 2012). Most investments in residential, commercial, industrial and service

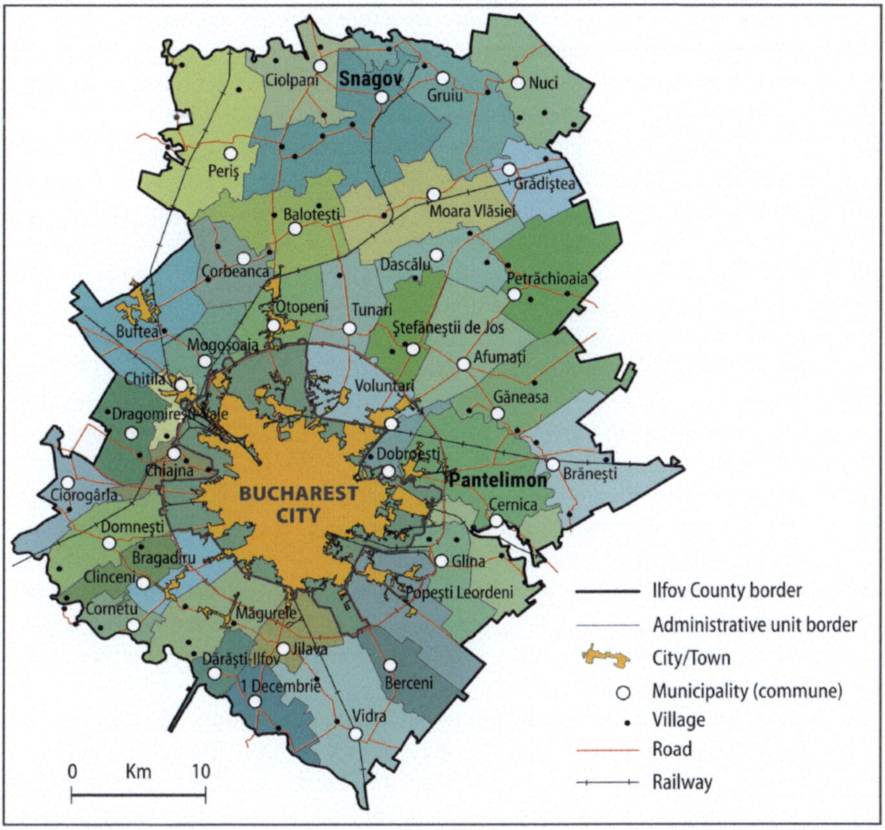

Fig. 22.2 Administrative map of the study area. *Source* authors

Table 22.1 Population evolution of the Bucharest metropolitan area

Areas	Year wise population			
	1977	1992	2002	2011
Romania	**21,559,910**	**22,810,035**	**21,680,974**	**20,121,641**
Ilfov county	287,738	286,965	300,123	388,738
Bucharest city	1,807,239	2,067,545	1,926,334	1,883,425
Bucharest metropolitan area	2,094,977	2,354,510	2,226,457	2,272,163
Bucharest metropolitan area national share (%)	9.7	10.3	10.3	11.3

Source Based on author's compilation from National Institute of Statistics, National Population and Housing Censuses (1977, 1992, 2002, 2011)

sectors were not connected with other infrastructure facilities such as transport and communication networks, water supply or sewerage. Currently, a new master plan for the City of Bucharest (*Planul Urbanistic General*—PUG) is undergoing, which will redefine and update the previous plan. According to Romania Planning Law 350/2001, PUG is a strategic and regulatory document, providing a legal framework for urban development and investments.

In the field of regional planning, three plans overlapping concerns the BMA: a. PUG managed by the Bucharest City Hall; b. a master plan for Ilfov County managed by Ilfov County Authority; c. Regional Development Plan for Bucharest-Ilfov led by Bucharest-Ilfov Regional Development Agency. The Regional Development Masterplan for Bucharest-Ilfov 2012–2020 aims to prioritised strategies on competitivity, social cohesion and sustainable development. Local strategies differ from city to city, reflecting exclusive local expectations. They have little clear focus on QoL, directing the investments in transport system or public infrastructures such as water and waste systems or disaster plans.

BMA has several significant competitive advantages that can contribute to improving QoL over the next decades. Its economic hinterland covers in a one-day drive by truck from the centre of Bucharest City a population of 11 million; within a two-day drive, it has access to a market of 83 million people. The region has the most educated labour force in Romania: 33% of the active population has vocational and tertiary education level compared to less than 15% in the rest of the country. Labour cost is the third lowest in Europe.

BMA dominates Romania regarding population and economy. It accounted for almost 25% of the national GDP in 2010, up from 11% in 2000. The region's share of the country population increased from 9.7% in 1977 to 11.3 in 2011 and is expected to continue over the next years. Raising income allows many people with Bucharest residence to move to the suburbs, despite poor public services like schools, mass transport system or retail facilities.

22.3 Methods and Data Sources

Several techniques have been used to obtain the datasets. Land use data are derived from the topographical map (1:50,000 scale) for the 1970s, and the CORINE Land Cover (CLC) maps for 1990 and 2012. The topographical maps were scanned and geo-referenced using GIS software, to allow overlapping with CLC maps for data comparison. To compare data from these different sources, a common classification system in eight classes was generated and counted the area and share for each category (Table 22.2). To calculate changes, the year 1970 was used as the base year for comparisons with the subsequent years. The methodology also involves empirical data gathered from two villages during field surveys and questionnaires applied in the metropolitan municipality halls. In addition, secondary data provided by Romania National Institute of Statistic were included.

Table 22.2 Land use classes share (%) in Bucharest metropolitan area

Land uses class	1970	1990	2012
Built-up areas	9.8	17.7	22.4
Urban green spaces and recreations sites	0.5	1.0	1.0
Arable lands	69.7	60.4	55.3
Vineyards	1.3	0.3	0.1
Orchards	1.9	1.2	1.0
Pastures	–	1.8	1.9
Forests	14.4	14.6	14.6
Water bodies	2.5	3.1	3.6

Source Based on author's compilation from Topographical map (1970) and CORINE Land Cover maps (1990, 2012)

22.4 Land Use Patterns

BMA has recently experienced a dynamic and complex reorganisation process, as a response to the political, institutional, economic and social changes. Land use patterns have undergone intense changes, particularly regarding the conversion of agricultural land and forests into residential, industrial and commercial uses (Figs. 22.3 and 22.4). The analysis of spatial dynamics of Bucharest shows that the area is currently going through the second phase of the urban lifecycle called suburbanisation, characterised by developing and enhancing the relationships between the metropolis and its metropolitan area (Plăcintescu et al. 2005: 9). Data derived from CLC2012 shows that 58.5% of the total BMA area is represented by agricultural land (arable, vineyards, orchards and pastures), 14.6% by forests and 22.4% by built-up lands (Table 22.2).

Over the last century, the landscape has transformed from mixed land use, characterised by houses with gardens, orchards and vineyards, to a socialist landscape, dominated by large residential areas with apartment blocks. The built-up landscape is marked by suburbanisation, with gated communities and transfer of several industrial activities in the metropolitan area (Mihai et al. 2015). In the area affected by urban growth, significant changes are the decrease of vineyards, orchards and arable land.

Agricultural land suffered intense pressure from urban growth and the primary income source for some of the landowners became the sale of their land properties. Arable lands shares in the total area slowly decreased from over 69.7% in the 1970s to around 55.3% in 2012. Once the land restitution process happened after the fall of the socialist regime, metropolitan farmers could sell their plots for different investments such as single-family homes or warehouses. The strategy on land use demonstrates the preference of landholders for arable land and led to the diminishing of vineyards and orchards.

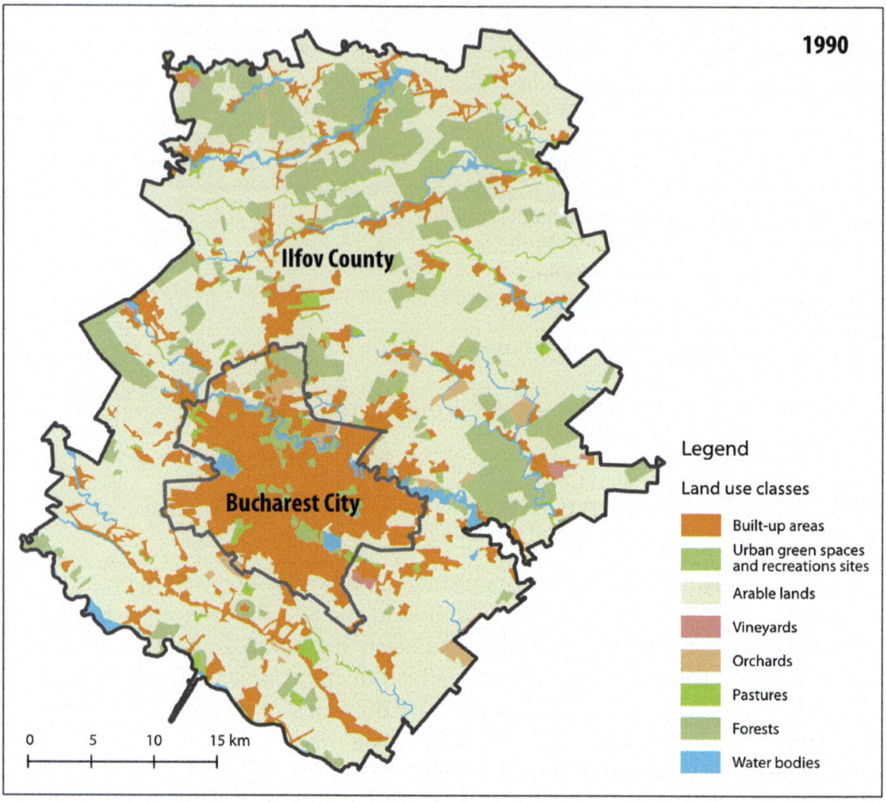

Fig. 22.3 Land use/land cover map (1990). *Source* Based on author's mapping from CORINE Land Cover maps (1990)

Vineyard cultivation has had a strong tradition in the past, but their spread decreased. Mainly, they are now cultivated in private gardens, in small plots near villages, alternating with other vegetables (onion, melon, cucumber and tomatoes). In 2012 on the CLC map, vineyards accounted for only 0.1% of the total area. The quality of vineyards is weak, as just hybrid grapes are predominantly cultivated. Orchards, based on CLC 2012, occupy an area which represents 1% of BMA. In the last 40 years, areas grown with fruit trees decreased at almost half. The existing data on pastures is not conclusive enough. Identifying their extension on topographical maps was not possible. The CLC showed a ratio of 1.8% pastures of the total metropolitan area in 1990 and 1.9% in 2012.

One example of reshaping geographical space as the effect of land use changes is Băneasa-Feeria commercial area, located in the suburban area, with a Carrefour hypermarket, Ikea, DIY stores (Dedeman, Brico Depot), cash and carry (Metro). The area's development is related to the several favourable elements such as the airports, residential buildings, forests and accessibility to the national road DN1.

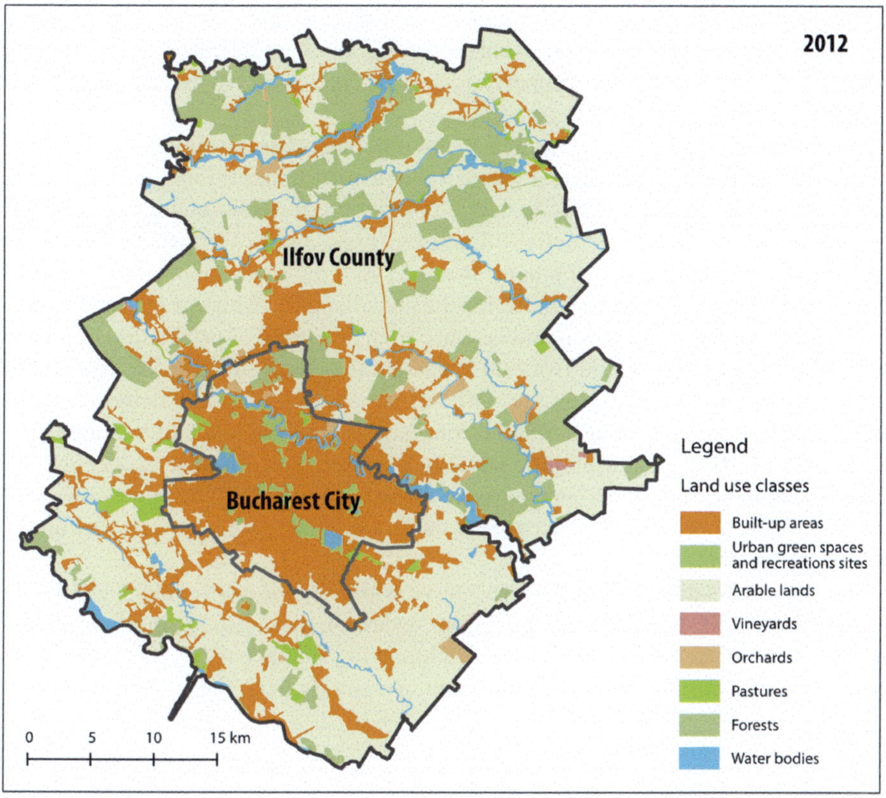

Fig. 22.4 Land use/land cover map (2012). *Source* Based on author's mapping from CORINE Land Cover maps (2012)

Pantelimon town is located near Bucharest City, being one of the largest settlements of BMA with 23,110 inhabitants in 2012. It has excellent natural resources—soils, land with development potential, water and forest landscapes and several cultural-historical sites—and human resources. During the socialist period, there were state farms and factories located here. The labour force was represented by local people but also people from the other areas of the country which transformed it into a bedroom town. After the fall of the socialist regime, the restructuring of the state industry resulted in the loss of jobs which has dramatically affected the local QoL.

Pantelimon Master Plan anticipates recent trends in rapid urbanisation and stipulates that almost all agricultural land would become buildable, only a small plot of forest remaining unaffected. Benefiting from low land prices and low taxes it attracted many new companies, some of them industrial. Services are also present, mainly commercial activities: wholesale warehouses, supermarkets and storage spaces. The development opportunities are given by the residential attraction, represented by two new residential areas located north and west of the city core. Agriculture is not a typical activity for the households, only a few farmers are certified as agricultural producers. The average land property is 1–2 ha, and some of the families grow vegetables mainly for domestic consume.

Snagov municipality went through a dynamic suburbanisation after 1989. It is located 30 km north of Bucharest City, in the area of Snagov Lake, and is one of the largest municipalities of BMA, with a population of 6,748 inhabitants in 2012, and a tremendous natural potential offered by forest and beautiful lake landscape attractive for residential development. Before 1990, the investments were oriented through recreation and leisure centre for the socialist elite. Most of the landowners are interested in the sale of farmland because of the increase of production costs and the diminishing profits, while from the land sale they earn much more than would gain from agriculture. The pressure on land market increased and determined the municipality to transfer the use of land from farming to available building area. The Masterplan of 2005 established the strategy for local development as a centre for services and leisure activities and approved the extension of building area with about 1,000 ha. Such development strategy was expected to have a positive impact on the QoL of inhabitants.

The suburbanisation process had a negative impact on the environment, especially during early 1990, when few people were aware of the need for minimal public infrastructure for extensive residential development. The lake water was polluted by spilling directly into the lake the wastewater and sludge from the house's toilets.

22.5 Services of Land Use Patterns

22.5.1 Subsistence and Commercial Agriculture

Land reform laws were passed after the fall of the socialist regime in 1989 and determined a return to the property structures existing before the socialist period, but the situation in agriculture and in the countryside had changed in the last seventy years. The single symbol of land restitution for farmers was regaining their sense of ownership and had little to do with their ability to cultivate the land. In fact, the land owners only recuperated their property, while the other components of the production chain remained the same or went through an extreme decline.

The landholders took back their lands from the socialist associative farms but they were missing the machinery needed for practising modern agriculture. The first crops affected by this situation were vineyards and orchards, which from an economic point of view are high maintenance crops.

Rusu (2005: 79) claims that most of the agricultural labour is operated inside self-contained households: self-employed (farm leader) and unpaid family members. Self-employed workers are predominantly seniors, 2/3 from among them are over 50 years old and 1/3 have exceeded the age of 65. Only very few farms are

Table 22.3 Income sources and migration rates of the BMA population

Indicator	Total
Which is the main income source for the household in this municipality?	1. Wages 2. Sell off the own land 3. Agriculture 4. Pensions
Estimative number of persons living abroad	52
What percentage of households receives money from relatives working abroad (%)?	11.2
Average number of families which get social aids from the state	127

Source Based on author's calculation from questionnaires sent to BMA municipality halls

controlled by young farmers (less than 34 years). The primary income sources of households are in order of prevalence: wages, sell off the own land, agriculture and pensions (Table 22.3). The spatial differentiation is related to the remote rural areas where the primary household incomes are wages, pensions and agriculture. The situation is profoundly different in the municipalities surrounding Bucharest City, where suburbanisation is the most intense; here the prevalence of income is represented by salaries and land transactions. The current situation of household income is determined partially by their dependence on financial aid from the government, dependence on family members who work abroad and from alternative income sources. There is a correlation between the degree of population ageing and reliance on government aids.

Changes in land ownership give new characteristics to crop cultivations. Natural features have determined differences regarding the importance placed on certain crops (regarded as a percentage) as opposed to others. For instance, the increasing shares of cereals (wheat and corn) compared to other crops, especially the industrial plants, are best illustrated by the percentage of areas cultivated for sugar beet, but due to some economic problems the sugar factories has significantly decreased resulting in situations where cultivation is completely stopped.

A significant impact on the type of farming is given by the role of neighbouring, meaning the cultivation together of the same crops to promote a lower cost of planting and harvesting. Both crops and livestock are also influenced by national and international market and the financial capacities of farmers or government agricultural policies.

Geographical distribution of the settlements in the proximity of Bucharest City defines two contradictory attitudes of the landowners. On the one hand, in some settlements agriculture has lost its importance, farmland being sold and occupied by built-up areas (residential, offices, warehouses logistics). On the other hand, further away from Bucharest City, subsistence agricultural practice is the main feature, determined by the high share of population ageing, and higher transport cost to markets.

Farmers cultivate mainly cereals with the opportunity to sell the product in one trail, often to traders who buy directly from the farm.

One aspect that questionnaire sent to BMA municipalities was focused on the percentage of household which cultivated wheat, corn, sunflower, potatoes and vegetables. The responses showed that in most of the metropolitan municipalities, households are characterised by multi-cropping, meaning a mechanism of subsistence based on sequentially cultivating different crops, to both trade out and consumption within the family. Moreover, this system covers risk management, i.e. if a particular yield will be affected by natural events or low prices, investments can be recovered partially from another plant/crop, which will prevent bankrupting the farm and ensure farming in the next year.

Farming is a source and a resource for local development in the BMA. Bucharest as the main city in Romania has been for a long time a massive market for agricultural products. This was enhanced by its increasing number of inhabitants who consume and demand a more complex variety of food. The importance of the settlements from suburban areas as vegetable suppliers for the city is emphasised by the number of people with farmer certificates. Farmer certificates are issued by local municipalities for those who want to sell their farm production in urban markets (Table 22.4).

The indicator regarding farmer certificates might very well be mirrored by the percentage of farms which consume more than 50% of the production within the household. The questionnaires revealed that on average more than half of families' household absorbs most of the products. In close relation to the above question is the one concerning the percentage of farmers who sell over 50% of total products directly to consumers. The result revealed that there are less spatial differences within the metropolitan area. An additional question included in the questionnaire has shown as a predominant response to the fact that trading would take place directly in markets between producers and consumers. Fieldwork has also revealed enough evidence that there are plenty of cases where intermediaries are involved.

Table 22.4 Indicators of agricultural products commercialisation

Indicator	Total
People with farmer certificate	96.7
Estimative percentage of agricultural operations which consume more than 50% of production inside the households	55
Estimative percentage of households which sell more than 50% of farm products directly to consumers	33.6
Where do the municipality' farmers sell their products?	In the city, directly in the market

Source Authors' compilation based on questionnaires sent to BMA municipality halls

22.5.2 Housing, Real Estate and Land Market

So far, land acquisition for agricultural use purposes has been limited. This is because agriculture has limited importance in the metropolitan economy and land is subject to accelerated urban growth and landowners prefer to wait for their property to be marked by municipalities' master plans as a built-up land, meaning an increase of land prices.

Agricultural land transactions are regulated with the pre-emption right established by the law, which can be carried out by the co-owners, landlords and tenants in the immediate neighbourhood. Implementation of pre-emption right is made in all cases by the local council in the jurisdiction in which the land is situated. Most of the agricultural lands included in the built-up areas are used for residential or commercial sites, industrial spaces or warehouses. The agricultural to built-up land conversion takes place mostly in the surrounding area of Bucharest, predominantly in the northern and north-eastern parts due to their proximity to the city as well as due to the presence of the transport infrastructure and lower land prices. For such kind of development project (residential, industrial, commercial) at least 10–25 ha of agricultural land is required.

Suburbanisation specific to the early 1990s was characterised by promising to the new suburban residents something that we might call the illusion of rural life but with city convenience. The houses previously built have all the internal standards, in opposition to the exterior shared public spaces such as streets, which can hardly accommodate two cars/lanes, resulting in street congestion. The lack of sewerage networks led to water and air pollution as well as contamination of the surrounding lakes. Later, some of the mentioned problems have begun to be corrected by building residential gated communities that have own adequate infrastructure for housing.

Bucharest reached a new phase of its urban evolution that can be named as 'development of new urban economies and gated communities'. This phase makes the transition from a centrally planned economy of the socialist period to a market-oriented economy of the present or the development from a communist industrial city to a service-based city. It concentrates the permanent headquarters of multinational companies both in the city centre and at the peripheries in the shape of business parks.

The agricultural activities producing fresh food supply for the city has decreased and still activate a lower scale away from the city. Residential projects were developed both in the city, mainly replacing the industrial platforms, and in the suburban area, predominately in the north. Land prices, in general, reached the highest values during the period 2005–2008 and this particularly in the northern region reached to about 2,000–2,500 €/m^2. For parcels smaller than 1,000 m^2. This is considered as a giant leap compared to the prices in 2003 when investors had to pay 200–400 €/m^2. (Colliers International 2006: 72). The context of economic crisis started in 2008 that determined a collapse of the real estate market and consequently, land prices dropped considerably (Grigorescu et al. 2012).

The suburban area continues to attract investments in the real estate market, mainly in the northern region, facilitated by its proximity to one of the main roads of the country. Investments localisation in BMA, mostly close to Bucharest, was facilitated by the lower price of the land, affordable labour market and some tax facilities from local municipalities. There was a wave of urban decongestion of industry and services activities that have been relocated in the suburban area, and these activities transformed and diversified the economy and increased household income and local budgets.

The agricultural land, due to its availability close to the city, became after the 1990s the most attractive area for houses and as a result, many persons even living in the city centre like to have a second home. A representative case in this sense is Pipera, located in the north-eastern part of Bucharest where an entire quarter has been developed and the former agricultural land and pastoral activities were replaced or abandoned. Another example of suburbanisation is Snagov, an exclusivist area, attractive for rich people. This area was developed mainly after the 1950s when it saw investments in tourism and sports facilities. The newcomers preferred private houses, built-up in the region bordering Lake Snagov or isolated dwellings located further in the agricultural fields.

Most of the industrial areas located in the city were abandoned or converted to other uses because of the pressure of land prices, which made the land more profitable for sale than for industrial purposes, due to the environmental regulation that forced the factories' management to close some of the more polluting activities. Retail centres represent the first major foreign investments in Bucharest's local economy. These centres contributed to the reconfiguration and reorganisation of urban spaces, large areas of agricultural land being converted for retail, alongside with amusement parks or/and residential.

22.5.3 Semi-natural Habitats

Forests and surface water were considered as part of semi-natural habitats. Table 22.2 shows that lowland forests cover 14.6% of the BMA, consisting mostly of different species of quercinee and elm, linden, ash, etc. in smaller shares. Lakes and rivers are adding up 3.6% of the total BMA and have specific features: lakes are mostly anthropogenic, and are, for the most part, ponds arranged along the river paths.

In the past, due to reduced population, the forestry operations were done traditionally within a system of sustainable land management. Since the mid-eighteenth century, population growth was followed by intensified forestry operation which reduced the area occupied by forests at the expanse of areas intended for agriculture, construction and infrastructure. Logging various timber species is occasional. Operations regarding other forest products—fuelwood, medicinal plants, berries, mushrooms, materials for crafts, are sporadic. Thus, the data available to measure income generated by the goods and services produced by semi-natural ecosystems or the number of goods produced are limited or non-existent. Their most important role is leisure services. From an economic and social point of view, these services, if well managed, can be an indispensable source of income, mainly, for rural households.

22.6 Conclusions

Land use plays a key role in the development of rural areas of BMA and in achieving an increased QoL. The economic growth together with diversity and complexity of the social dimension were deciding for the land use patterns. Thus, the primary land use patterns identified were: commercial and subsistence agriculture, infrastructure, housing, industries and services, natural and semi-natural habitats. The paper identifies critical relationships between the land use patterns and QoL. Land use patterns deliver a set of goods and services that are essential for the population's survival and welfare. The land plays a central role in the QoL of families and communities. Services provided by different types of land use are essential resources for many people. In addition to the economic value associated with these services, there are also historical and cultural values, which should not be ignored because, in time, they have shaped the communities' social organisation. Therefore, land, as the most important natural resource, should be considered and analysed in a natural, social, economic, and cultural context. QoL's implications show the need for public actions, residential mobility, economic growth and the sustainable use of natural resources.

References

Bhatti, S., Tripathi, K., Nagai, M., & Nitivattananon, V. (2017). Spatial interrelationships of quality of life with land use/land cover, demography and urbanization. *Social Indicators Research, 132*(3), 1193–1216.

Campbell, A., Converse, P. E., & Rodgers, W. L. (1976). *The quality of American life. Perceptions, evaluations, and satisfactions*. New York: Russel Sage Foundation.

Chiessura, A. (2004). The role of urban parks for the sustainable city. *Landscape and Urban Planning, 68*(1), 129–138.

Colliers International. (2006). *Analiza pieţei imobiliare*. Bucureşti.

Costantza, R., d'Arge, R., de Groot, R., Farber, S., Grasso, M., Hannon, B., et al. (1997). The value of the world's ecosystem services and natural capital. *Nature, 387*, 379–395.

de Groot, R. (2006). Function-analysis and valuation as a tool to assess land use conflicts in planning for sustainable, multi-functional landscapes. *Landscape and Urban Planning, 75*(3–4), 175–186.

Dumitrache, L., Zamfir, D., Nae, M., Simion, G., & Stoica, I. V. (2016a). The urban nexus: Contradictions and dilemmas of (post)communist (sub)urbanization in Romania. *Human Geographies, 10*(1), 39–58.

Dumitrache, L., Nae, M., Dumbrăveanu, D., Simion, G., & Suditu, B. (2016b). Contrasting clustering in health care provision in Romania: Spatial and aspatial limitations. *Procedia Environmental Sciences, 32*, 290–299.

FAO & UNEP. (1999). *The future of our land: Facing the challenge*, Rome.

Farquhar, M. (1995a). Elderly people's definitions of quality of life. *Social Science and Medicine, 41*, 1439–1446.

Farquhar, M. (1995b). Definitions of quality of life: A taxonomy. *Journal of Advanced Nursing, 22*(3), 502–508.

Grigorescu, I., Mitrică, B., Kucsicsa, G., Popovici, E. A., Dumitraşcu, M., & Cuculici, R. (2012). Post-communist land use changes related to urban sprawl in the Romanian metropolitan areas. *Human Geographies, 6*(1), 35–46.

Held, D. (1980). *Introduction to critical theory: Horkheimer to habermas*. London: Hutchinson.

Keys, E., Wentz, E. A., & Redman, C. L. (2007). The spatial structure of land use from 1970–2000 in the Phoenix, Arizona, metropolitan area. *The Professional Geographer, 5*(1), 131–147.

MEA–Millennium Ecosystem Assessment. (2005). *Ecosystems and human well-being. Current state and trends*. Washington: Island Press.

Mihai, B., Nistor, C., & Simion, G. (2015). Post-socialist urban growth of Bucharest, Romania—A change detection analysis on Landsat imagery (1984–2010). *Acta Geographica Slovenica, 55*(2), 223–234.

Muller, D., & Zeller, M. (2002). Land use dynamics in the central highlands of Vietnam: A spatial model combining village survey data with satellite imagery interpretation. *Agricultural Economics, 27*, 333–354.

Pacione, M. (2013). Quality-of-life research in urban geography. *Urban Geography, 24*(4), 314–339.

Peet, R. (1977). *Radical geography: Alternative viewpoints on contemporary social issues*. London: Methuen.

Plăcintescu, D., Nădejde, Ş., & Bădilă, A. (2005). *Zona metropolitan Bucureşti. Ghid de informare pentru autorităţile publice locale*. Bucharest: Proiect finanţat de Institutul pentru o SocietateDeschisă.

Rusu, M. (2005). *Dezvoltare arurală. Politici şi structurie conomice*. Bucureşti: Editura Expert.

Serag El Din, H., Shalaby, A., Farouh, H. E., & Elarian, A. (2013). Principles of urban quality of life for a neighbourhood. *HBRC Journal, 9*(1), 86–92.

Simion, G. (2010). The spatial changes of land use in the Bucharest metropolitan area 1970s–2000s. *Human Geographies, 4*(2), 115–123.

Simion, G., & Nistor, C. (2012). Spatial structure changes inside post-communist capital city of Bucharest. *Human Geographies, 6*(1), 79–89.

Veenhoven, R. (2000). The four qualities of life. Ordering concepts and measures of the good life. *Journal of Happiness Studies, 1*, 1–39.

Yubing, X. (2015). *Effects of land use and transport on quality of life: A life-oriented behavioral analysis*, Hiroshima University: Graduate School for International Development and Cooperation, (Doctoral Dissertation).

Chapter 23
Links Between Human Quality of Life and Gulls in Urban Areas

Michael O'Neal Campbell

Abstract Human–avian interactions in urban areas are an important aspect of human quality of life (QOL). Positive impacts on QOL include the aesthetic value of wildlife observation and nature bonding. Negative impacts on QOL include noise, waste material deposition, disease and attacks on domestic animals and people. In the QOL-conscious cities of North America and Europe, large gulls of the Genus *Larus*, the dominant urban foraging birds, have been extensively studied for their social and ecological impacts. This chapter examines the positive and negative roles of urban gulls in urban QOL. Gulls tend to select areas of high QOL. People and gulls select similar urban contexts (vegetated areas, car parks, roads, waterfronts, riverbanks, beaches, eating places, transport spaces). People use such areas for the enhancement of QOL; recreation, feeding, transport and social interaction. Birds use such areas for foraging, feeding, roosting and sometimes nesting, and actively adapted to human behaviour. The positive impacts of this close association include wildlife observation and conservation values. The negative impacts include predation of valuable animals, noise, building and vehicle damage, food theft, intrusive scavenging of human residences and even attacks on people and companion animals. In terms of QOL, the negative impacts outweighed the positive impacts. The positive impacts were nevertheless important enough for more effective management and further study. This analysis is useful for both QOL and conservation studies.

Keywords Gulls · Urban · Quality of life · Conservation · Conflict

23.1 Introduction

The relation between human quality of life (QOL) and wildlife is an intriguing and currently important topic of investigation for many scientists. Urban settings are particularly important in this regard, due to the large, condensed human populations and the presence of adaptive wildlife and vegetated areas (Campbell 2013a, b, 2017;

M. O. Campbell (✉)
Simon Fraser University, Burnaby, Canada
e-mail: ecol55@hotmail.com

B. R. K. Sinha (ed.), *Multidimensional Approach to Quality of Life Issues*,
https://doi.org/10.1007/978-981-13-6958-2_23

Konijnendijk 2017). Urban areas have been criticized for neglecting QOL issues, allowing the vices of social degradation such as overcrowding and psychological depression to proliferate (Campbell 2013a). Additionally, theoretical issues such as the definitions of QOL, animal ecology, conservation and wildlife conflict must be examined and related to urban case studies. Human quality of life is difficult to define, as it attempts relevance to many attributes of the human existence, sometimes through the lenses of multiculturalism, historical changes and environmental dynamics (Bradburn 1969; Schalock et al. 2002; Konijnendijk et al. 2006; Campbell 2017; Ludwig et al. 2017).

Many authors have studied definitions of quality of life, and attempted lists of QOL indicators sufficiently robust to withstand socio-environmental variation (Felce and Perry 1996; Hughes and Hwang 1996; Cummins 1997a b; Schalock 1997, 2000; Ludwig et al. 2017). Emerging from such studies are eight core QOL domains: (a) emotional well-being, (b) interpersonal relationships, (c) material well-being, (d) personal development, (e) physical well-being, (f) self-determination, (g) social inclusion, and (h) rights (Glatzer et al. 2015). Felce and Perry (1995) argue that QOL is "multidimensional" and offer five dimensions: physical well-being, material well-being, social well-being, emotional well-being, and development and activity. These domains or dimensions vary according to social variables such as age, culture and social outlook (Elorriaga et al. 2000; Ludwig et al. 2017). QOL is usually held to be a universal concept and hence to be relevant in any context, Hence, in a study of QOL concerning human–animal relations people may have some values regardless of the land cover or animal species involved. The animals' appearance and behaviour may still be relevant, important parameters being perceived attractiveness, adaptability, aggression and compatibility.

In this chapter, it is not intended to address the full range of QOL domains, or to challenge existing definitions, which are sufficient for our purpose. The objective is to examine the relationship between two important QOL domains (emotional and physical well-being) and urban environmental variables, based on the hypotheses that human emotional and physical well-being is enhanced by a quality environment, and that animals and nature contact may both enhance and degrade QOL (Campbell 2007; 2008a, b; Schaltegger and Beständig 2012). The relevant environmental variables, in this case, are the physical spaces in urban areas (vegetated areas, car parks, river banks, beaches, airports, recreational facilities) and the biological actors (in this case urban *Larus* gulls, the commonest and dominant animals in urban settings) (Campbell 2010, 2017).

Urban gulls are seen as both positive and negative indicators of QOL, due to their high populations, dominant, invasive and aggressive behaviour and aesthetic appearance in highly populated urban areas (Campbell 2007, 2008a, b, 2010; Ma et al. 2010). The intense engagement between gulls and people is based on the truism that gulls and people select the same areas (vegetated areas, car parks, roads, waterfronts, riverbanks, beaches, eating places, transport spaces). These areas are used by people for recreation, feeding, transport and social interaction, and by birds for feeding and sometimes nesting. This intensity of human and gull numbers in urban spaces creates conflicts, with both positive and negative consequences for human health, comfort and quality of life. Positive avian roles for human QOL include scavenging, aesthetics, feelings of closeness to nature, human recreational bird watching and feeding, and biodiversity values (Jones and Kress 2012). Negative effects concern invasive behaviour, including nuisance scavenging, roof colonisation and obstruction of human communications and transport (Campbell 2007; Camphuysen et al. 2011).

Considering these arguments, from the perspective of QOL there are arguments for both increased bird presence (bird conservation and even more extreme preservation) and bird eradication. Waterbird conservation is currently important, as visual biodiversity, bird presence and wetland and coastal conservation are seen as beneficial for ecosystem health and human emotional, physical and material well-being (Deluca et al. 2008; Esteve et al. 2008; Jones and Kress 2012). Simultaneously, there is increasing recognition of the pest status of some waterbirds, especially gulls, which have serious impacts on human safety and well-being (Cooper 2002; Rock 2002; DeLuca et al. 2008; Douglas et al. 2010; Camphuysen et al. 2011).

A key question is, *in terms of human quality of life, what are the conflicts between gull conservation and pest status?* The answer to this question lies in two main strands of literature: (1) those, which focus on the beneficial aspects of gull presence and conservation, especially in relation to ecosystems and people; and (2) those with a more negative stance. The literature is divided between these two research strands and few studies have attempted a balance between the opposed viewpoints. Here, some of the recent literature on both topics is reviewed and some insights for future research are offered.

23.2 Gulls May Enhance QOL

Gulls must be conserved for the benefit of ecosystems and people (Campbell 2013a). They provide a link between watered and non-watered ecosystems and may kill animals regarded as pests, including worms, insects, lizards and small rodents. They also perform scavenging roles for human refuse, provide people with opportunities for recreational feeding, are aesthetically pleasing to many people and contribute to the biodiversity of human recreational areas (Campbell 2010; Jones and Kress 2012). As already noted, biodiversity may contribute to QOL (Schaltegger and Beständig 2012). In coastal and wetland areas, gulls and other waterbirds may be considered indicators of ecosystem health (Boyd et al. 2006; Brinker et al. 2007; Heslenfeld and Enserink 2008; Parsons et al. 2008; Gremillet and Boulinier 2009; Oro et al. 2009; Wolf et al. 2010).

Some studies provide evidence for increased gull numbers in urban settings and document some of their positive, foraging activities (Harris 1970; Spaans 1971; Drury and Kadlec 1974; Vermeer 1992; Conover 1983; Belant and Dolbeer 1993; Belant 1997; Campbell 2013a). Other, generally more recent literature documents gull extinction, due to pollution, fish extinction, habitat destruction and hunting (International Union for Conservation of Nature (Boere et al. 2006; Stroud 2006; IUCN 2009). There has been a neglect of multi-species, comparative and seasonal studies of waterbird guilds such as gulls, ducks and marsh birds, and their responses to urban riverine dynamics, non-riverine environments and the human presence in such contexts (Marzluff et al. 2001; Rock 2005; Clark et al. 2007; Coulson and Coulson 2008). In such studies, coastal urbanized areas are often neglected in favour of riverine environments, but both contexts are important for QOL and represent important spaces for bird–human engagement (Traut and Hostetler 2004; Boyd et al. 2006; Parsons et al. 2008; Gremillet and Boulinier 2009; Campbell 2010; Wolf et al. 2010; Schippers et al. 2011). Important topics for avian research would include water proximity, littoral and riverbank vegetation and the relation of these to seasonal and human-induced disturbances and presence (Campbell 2008b; Hostetler et al. 2011).

Urban areas are important for waterbird habitation and hence for studies of waterbird conservation (Traut and Hostetler 2004; DeLuca et al. 2008; Thrush et al. 2008; Bulleri and Chapman 2010; Campbell 2010). Colonization may occur in areas of high social amenity and QOL, such as buildings, treed avenues, gardens, vegetated and concrete parks, sports fields, tree plantations riverbanks, beaches and cemeteries; and in areas with lower value, such as rubbish dumps, transport networks, bridges, rooftops, road potholes and gutters. In such areas, gull presence may also attract bird watchers and nature observers (Campbell 2008a, b). For the conservation objective, urban features that repel gulls may be factors for reduced QOL (Campbell 2010). These include visual, acoustic, chemical and physical disturbances, from building and mechanical construction, vehicular, aerial and water traffic, and noisy human presence and movements (Rock 2005; Lotze et al. 2006; Studds et al. 2012). Urbanization also contributes to habitat fragmentation and a loss of habitat connectivity, changes in the nutrient and contaminant levels, and reductions in invertebrate and fish populations (Baird et al. 2004; Shriver et al. 2004; Bilkovic et al. 2006; Scavia and Bricker 2006; DeLuca et al. 2008; Scheffer et al. 2009; Erwin et al. 2011). The negative environmental variables may drive both people and birds to areas of higher value, contributing to the shared engagement that enables both higher QOL through recreational feeding and aesthetics.

An important aspect of QOL in areas of avian colonization is the feeding of birds. In some cases, as noted below, gulls may intrude into feeding relationships between people and other smaller birds, such as doves and crows. However, in some cases people deliberately feed gulls. In such cases, gulls may contribute to QOL. Gull feeding can be an important part of QOL in urban parks, beaches and even parking lots, roads and sidewalks. People respond positively to gull proximity and may be interested in observing the distinct species of gulls, their physical beauty and their intra- and inter-species interactions and competition. Examples include the feeding of competing herring, lesser black-backed and black-headed gulls in southern England, Scotland and Canada (Campbell 2007, 2010). In some cases, feeding of gulls is so popular that warning signs are erected to warn people against the practice, as per the health impacts on the birds and their increased presence in urban areas (Campbell 2010).

To support the positive variables, there may be urban vegetated area development, with additional positive implications for QOL (Campbell 2008a, b). There may also be increased sanitation, which may reduce disease and increase QOL, and encourage some avian scavengers attracted to human feeders (Campbell 2010). Restoration sites may also be developed, to which birds may be attracted using decoys, chick translocation, playbacks of acoustic vocalizations, scent attractive agents and research on the extinction factors of the locality. Necessary supports are the relocation of birds to more tolerable locations, the creation of multiple breeding sites for insurance, predator and competitor control and financial support (Kress et al. 2008; Jones 2010; Weiser and Powell 2010; Jones et al. 2011; Jones and Kress 2012). In the planning of conservation efforts, there are inter-species differences in adaptation. Gulls are among the most adaptable waterbirds, as may be seen by their local numbers and alert and flight distances (Fernández-Juricic et al. 2001; Traut and Hostetler 2004; Campbell 2008a; Evans et al. 2009). Most gulls are strongly attracted to people and may emerge from conservation projects dominant and relevant to QOL (Fuller et al. 2009; Campbell 2010; Stagoll et al. 2010; Fontana et al. 2011).

23.3 Gulls May Degrade QOL

Studies focussed on gulls as pests offer contrasted findings and opinions. Increased numbers of gulls, due to conservation or natural factors, may result in the excessive predation of valuable animals, noise, building and vehicle damage, food theft, intrusive scavenging of human residences and even attacks on people and companion animals (Ruiz-Olmo et al. 2003; Oro and Martinez-Abrain 2007; Campbell 2008a, b, 2010). Several studies document strong increases in gull numbers and invasive aggression in urban areas, even those far from water (Marzluff et al. 2001; Cooper 2002; Francois 2002; DeLuca et al. 2008; Douglas et al. 2010). Although few studies compare urban features that attract gulls with those that may repel them, it has been argued that the urban features that repel some avian scavengers may not be sufficient to repel more adaptive gulls (Cooper 2002; Francois 2002; Kushlan et al. 2002; Traut and Hostetler 2004; Campbell 2008a, b, 2010).

One of the main impacts of gulls on QOL is roof-nesting, which harasses maintenance personnel and results in defecation on nearby vehicles, offensive smells, the attraction of rodents and insects, obstruction of roof drain systems and even chemical and structural damage to buildings (Belant 1997). Other impacts are human disease transmission though gull faeces (e.g. *Bacillus, Clostridium, Campylobacter, Escherichia coli, Listeria* and *Salmonella* bacteria) and general nuisance through noise, defecation and harassment of people, with examples being food theft from patrons of outdoor restaurants, fouling of tables and park benches and even frightening of tourists and residents (Belant 1997; Campbell 2010). Preventive measures include the redesign of roofing, where needle-like structures are placed on the perching sites of the gulls. These, however, may not drive the birds away, as they may resort to overhead hovering or soaring, or simply perching on the ground.

Campbell (2007, 2010) describes recreational feeding of urban birds as an important aspect of QOL, that is jeopardized by gulls that attack the preferentially fed birds (mallard ducks and rock doves) and human feeders. Such attacks resulted in leaving behaviour from the other birds, and in some cases human protection of vulnerable birds and people retreating from parks under gull attacks (wing flapping, pecking and defecation). People were also attacked when eating in parks, hampering their patronage of such areas. Studies have shown that repeated feeding of gulls encourages the more aggressive individuals and species to attack people, through close perching, diving, aerial defecation, p-pecking and loud calling. Such behaviour also affects companion animals such as dogs and cats and can even disturb children. People complained that aggressive gull presence disturbed their recreational experiences in parks and in some cases reduced the quality perception of recreational spaces. Some respondents compared aggressive gull behaviour with human antisocial behaviour and even crime (Campbell 2007, 2010).

Gulls are frequently documented as colliding with airplanes near airports, especially as many airports are located near large riverine or coastal cities with large waterbird populations (Mackinnon 1999; Campbell 2008a, b, 2010; Camphuysen et al. 2011). This may reduce QOL and even create fear among airline passengers, who may be worried about the safety of airplanes on take-off and landing. These fears may be based on the considerable media attention to airplane crashes brought about by collisions with birds. Consequently, research on bird–airplane conflicts, often termed Bird–Aircraft Strike Hazard (BASH), is an extremely important aspect of avian and applied social studies (Gard et al. 2007; Camphuysen et al. 2011). Mackinnon's (1999) study in Canada, recorded the following collisions involving airplanes: take-off (25%), landing (19%), approach (17%), and climb (10%), en route (4%), taxi (<1%) and others (2%) with 22% unreported). The U.S. Federal Aviation Administration recorded 57,702 bird–aircraft collision reports within the United States between 1990 and 2004, with over $600 million damage (Gard et al. 2007). "Large flocking birds and birds of large body size" are described as particularly susceptible to such collisions (United States Department of Agriculture 2003). Factors include bird migration patterns and bird attraction to the prey sources in the grassed areas near the airports (Gard et al. 2007). For example, New York's John F. Kennedy International Airport is described as a "model airport in managing its bird population", it recorded more bird strikes than any other major US airport (over 300 annually) before 1988 (Camphuysen et al. 2011).

Attempts to ameliorate these problems may either kill birds, or modify the environment. Killing birds may encounter public opposition, as gulls remain for some people at least, an important aspect of QOL. Environmental modification involves runway patrols discharging fire shotguns, loud shell crackers, propane cannons and recordings of bird distress calls, falconers using raptors to kill or chase gulls, spraying insecticides to kill gull food sources, shooting gulls (with permits from the U.S. Fish and Wildlife Service, cleaning refuse sites and closing landfills (Camphuysen et al. 2011). The referred study concludes that further research is required on slope soaring behaviour of gulls (which, occurring over some objects such as hills, may enable decisions about the location of such features near airways). The soaring height of gulls near airports, feeding ecology of gulls, the introduction of predatory mammals and birds, constant disturbances, runway patrols, and restriction of prey availability and human discards must also be studied (Camphuysen et al. 2011).

Attempts to control such events may conflict with conservation efforts for gulls, as repopulation efforts might create these very problems (Heslenfeld and Enserink 2008; Parsons et al. 2008). From this perspective, features that repel gulls may be positive, while negative for conservation (Campbell 2010; Studds et al. 2012). Therefore, it is important that the conflicting issues be evaluated, to encourage waterbird colonisation in less problematic areas, while preventing their colonization in other areas, e.g. near airports. The high mobility of gulls complicates these efforts (Campbell 2008a, b). Problems would include individual bird, flock or even colony dispersal, species and population recovery and adaptation (Francois 2002; DeLuca et al. 2008; Douglas et al. 2010). Other problems involve the impact of relocated gulls on QOL in less critical areas, such as urban vegetated areas and concrete parks (Campbell 2008a, b). Easier solutions include the control of the human discards which serve as food sources for gulls (Mitchell et al. 2004; Cadiou and Yesou 2006).

Another important problem of increased waterbird populations concerns the impacts of certain *Larus* gulls on other animals, which may be of social importance and affect QOL (Campbell 2010). In many cases, there is over-predation by gulls on other species (Blokpoel et al. 1997; Kress 1997; Anderson and Devlin 1999; Ruiz-Olmo et al. 2003; Igual et al. 2007; Schippers et al. 2011). For example, the yellow-legged gull *Larus michahellis,* which preys upon the young of other birds; e.g. greater flamingo, Balearic Shearwater, lesser black-backed gull and parasitic skua (Oro and Martinez-Abrain 2007). These predatory behaviours have important social relevance, as in many cases the prey species are popular with human observers and feeders and therefore a play a role in human emotional well-being and recreational spaces (Campbell 2010). Examples are cited of ducks and doves in the vegetated areas of Glasgow, which are important for park visitation, but are heavily exploited and in some cases locally depopulated by gulls (Campbell 2008a, b).

The incidence of predation on such species provides the rationale for the culling of gulls (Vidal et al. 2000; Ferns and Mudge 2000; Oro and Martinez-Abrain 2007). There are problems, however, including rapid gull population recovery, gull dispersal, and non-recovery of prey species (Guillemette and Brousseau 2001; Oro 2003; Martinez-Abrain et al. 2004; Somers et al. 2011). Oro and Martinez-Abrain (2007: 122) note “there has recently been increasing concern about the suitability of controlling predators to enhance the survival of threatened species.” In some cases, this may also not be politically acceptable, given the concerns of environmentalists and the public (Campbell 2007). An alternative suggestion is the control of refuse that attracts gulls (Mitchell et al. 2004; Cadiou and Yesou 2006; Oro and Martinez-Abrain 2007). However, such refuse may also threaten more socially preferred species (Arcos and Oro 2002; Campbell 2010). Also possible is large-scale habitat restoration for both predator and prey species, especially if linked to human recreation that attracts birds, provides aesthetic value and increases QOL (Oro and Martinez-Abrain 2007; Campbell 2008b).

23.4 Bird Adaptation and QOL

The enhancement of the positive human–gull relations, while reducing the negative relations is difficult because gulls may adapt to human behaviour. This may be termed co-dependent behaviour or even actancy on the part of the birds (Murdoch 1998; Campbell 2010). Here, actancy refers to individualist avian reactions to options, risking accusations of anthropomorphization of birds (Johnston et al. 2000). This makes inter-species assessments difficult, as both people and birds may exhibit strong individualism in location selection for optimal QOL, with innumerable opportunities and results for cohabitation and conflict. Campbell's (2010) study found that in areas of human feeding or presence, there were generalizable behaviours (gulls were more aggressive towards people than other species such as doves and mallard ducks), but gulls also exhibited variable behaviour, between violent diving and wing flapping, and passive calling or observational perching.

In that the individual variations in gull behaviour appeared linked to human behaviour, it could be defined as actancy. The gulls used such techniques to bully people to favour them in feeding, to the detriment of less aggressive species such as ducks. Such actions even included anticipatory attacks on people who had not even opened feeding bags or started eating their food. Further, co-dependence was evident in the observational perching, repetitive flyovers and low hovering in areas of known feeding, such as green and concrete parks, lawns on riverbanks and beach sidewalks, in some cases before people appeared. Bird numbers increased with human presence, even when there was no food (people eating with discards, or actual feeding of birds). Hence, as people sought places of QOL, birds fashioned their presence according to these human choices, regardless of their previous habitats. These reactions may be manifestations of the individual birds' memories of human actions. From the human perspective, the adaptation of the birds might ingrain bird presence into perceptions of QOL in different areas, which previously did not attract birds. Both positive and negative perceptions may result from this, attracting or repelling people from places previously identified as enhancing QOL.

23.5 Conclusions

The posed question was *in terms of human quality of life, what are the conflicts between gull conservation and pest status*? The answer appears to indicate that gulls both enhance and reduce QOL, through multiple behaviours, and the conflicts are principally concerned with aesthetics versus obstruction, contributions to both sanitary and insanitary conditions, and to both increased and decreased biodiversity (through attacks on other species) with QOL impacts. Aggressive, invasive behaviour, and gentler flyovers and soaring behaviour may occur wherever there are gulls. Although the conservation of gulls, like that of other species is an admirable goal, the evidence points to a need to discourage the dense presence of gulls in areas of high value for QOL. Therefore, where there is over colonization, these efforts must be geographically spread across areas of QOL. Simultaneously, attractants such as rubbish dumps may be placed in remote areas with lower QOL. It is apparent that areas of high QOL must be clearly mapped while areas of low QOL must have a minimum physical distance from such locations. Although this will not entirely eradicate the problem, due to high gull mobility and adaptability, more research appears to be the way forward. More comparison is required between regions, contexts and species, both for QOL research and planning evaluation. Evaluation of urban areas, airports, forests, grasslands and wetlands, and more attention to migration and dispersal possibilities is necessary. Inter-species comparisons between gull species may also be required.

References

Anderson, J. G. T., & Devlin, C. M. (1999). Restoration of a multi-species seabird colony. *Biological Conservation, 90*, 175–181.

Arcos, J. M., & Oro, D. (2002). Significance of fisheries discards for a threatened mediterranean seabird, the balearic shearwater puffinus mauretanicus. *Marine Ecology Progress Series, 239,* 209–220.

Baird, D., Christian, R. R., Peterson, C. H., & Johnson, G. A. (2004). Consequences of hypoxia on estuarine ecosystem function: energy diversion from consumers to microbes. *Ecological Applications, 14,* 805–822.

Belant, J. L. (1997). Gulls in urban environments: landscape-level management to reduce conflict. *Landscape and Urban Planning, 38,* 245–258.

Belant, J. L., & Dolbeer, J. L. (1993). Population status of nesting Laughing Gulls in the United States: 1977–1991. *American Birds, 47*, 220–224.

Bilkovic, D. M., Roggero, M., Hershner, C. H., & Havens, K. H. (2006). Influence of land use on macrobenthic communities in nearshore estuarine habitats. *Estuaries and Coasts, 29,* 1185–1195.

Blokpoel, H., Tessier, G. D., & Andress, R. A. (1997). Successful restoration of the island common tern colony requires on-going control of ring-billed gulls. *Colonial Waterbirds, 20,* 98–101.

Boere, G. C., Galbraith, C. A., & Stroud, D. A. (Eds.). (2006). *Waterbirds around the world.* Edinburgh: The Stationary Office.

Boyd, I. L., Wanless, S., & Camphuysen, C. J. (2006). *Top predators in marine ecosystems: Their role in monitoring and management*. Cambridge: Cambridge Universal Press.

Bradburn, N. M. (1969). *The structure of psychological well-being*. Chicago: Aldine.

Brinker, D. F., McCann, J. M., Williams, B., & Watts, B. D. (2007). Colonial-nesting seabirds in the chesapeake bay region: where have we been and where are we going? *Waterbirds, 30,* 93–104.

Bulleri, F., & Chapman, M. G. (2010). The introduction of coastal infrastructure as a driver of change in marine environments. *Journal of Applied Ecology, 47,* 26–35.

Cadiou, B., & Yesou, P. (2006). Evolution des populations de goelands bruns, argentes et marins Larus fuscus, L. Argentatus, L. Marinus dans l'archipel de Molene (Bretagne, France): Bilan de 50 ans de suivi des colonies. *Review of Ecology (Terre Vie), 61,* 159–173.

Campbell, M. (2007). An animal geography of avian ecology in Glasgow. *Applied Geography, 27,* 78–88.

Campbell, M. (2008a). An animal geography of avian feeding habits in Peterborough. *Area, 40*(4), 472–480.

Campbell, M. (2008b). The impact of vegetation, river, and urban features on waterbird ecology in Glasgow Scotland. *Journal of Coastal Research, 24*(4), 239–245.

Campbell, M. (2010). An animal geography of avian foraging competition on the Sussex coast of England. *Journal of Coastal Research, 26*(1), 44–52.
Campbell, M. (2013a). Issues of importance in waterbird ecology, conservation and environmental policy. In E. Creighton & P. Danovich (Eds.), *Environmental policy: Management, legal issues and health aspects* (pp. 129–146). New York: Nova Science Publishers.
Campbell, M. (2013b). Biographical change and environmental policy in the western greenbelt. In E. Creighton & P. Danovich (Eds.), *Environmental policy: Management, legal issues and health aspects* (pp. 147–164). New York: Nova Science Publishers.
Campbell, M. (2017). *Biological conservation for the 21st century: A conservation biology of large wildlife*. New York: Nova Science Publishers.
Camphuysen, K., Verheij, J., & Cremer, J. (2011). *Risk assessment of bird strike hazards: gulls laridae*. Oosterend: CSR Consultancy.
Clark, H., Maughan, E. W. E., & Sellers, R. M. (2007). Survey of roof-nesting gulls in caithness. *Scottish Birds, 27,* 74–76.
Conover, M. R. (1983). Female–female pairings in Caspian Terns. *Condor, 85*, 346–349.
Cooper, D. S. (2002). Geographic associations of breeding bird distribution in an urban open space. *Biological Conservation, 104,* 205–210.
Coulson, J. C., & Coulson, B. A. (2008). Lesser black-backed gulls *Larus fuscus* nesting in an inland urban colony: The importance of earthworms (Lumbricidae) in their diet. *Bird Study, 55,* 297–303.
Cummins, R.A., (1997a). Assessing quality of life. In R. J. Brown (Ed.), *Assessing quality of life for people with psychiatric disabilities* (pp. 116–150). Cheltenham: Stanley Thornes (Publishers).
Cummins, R. A. (1997b). *Comprehensive Quality of Life Scale—Adult.* School of Psychology: Deakin University, Melbourne.
DeLuca, W. V., Studds, C. E., King, R. S., & Marra, P. P. (2008). Coastal urbanization and the integrity of estuarine waterbird communities: Threshold responses and the importance of scale. *Biological Conservation, 141,* 2669–2678.
Drury, W. H., & Kadlec, J. A. (1974). The current status of the Herring Gull population in the United States. *Bird-Banding, 45*, 297–306.
Douglas, I., Goode, D., Houck, M., & Wang, R. (2010). *The Routledge handbook of urban ecology*. Oxford: Taylor and Francis.
Elorriaga, J., Garcia, L., Martinez, J., & Unamunzaga, E. (2000). Quality of life of persons with mental retardation in Spain. In K. D. Keith & R. L. Schlock (Eds.), *Cross-cultural perspectives on quality of life*. Washington, DC: American Association on Mental Retardation.
Erwin, R. M., Brinker, D. F., Watts, B. D., Costanzo, G. R., & Morton, D. D. (2011). Islands at bay: rising seas, eroding islands, and waterbird habitat loss in Chesapeake Bay (USA). *Journal of Coastal Conservation, 15*(1), 51–60.
Esteve, M. A., Carreno, M. F., Robledano, F., Martınez-Fernandez, J., & Minano, J. (2008). Dynamics of coastal wetlands and landuse changes in the watershed: Implications for the biodiversity. In: R. E. Russo (Ed.), *Wetlands: Ecology, conservation and restoration*. New York: Nova Science Publishers.
Evans, K. L., Newson, S. E., & Gaston, K. J. (2009). Habitat influences on urban avian assemblages. *Ibis, 151,* 19–39.
Felce, D., & Perry, J. (1995). Quality of life: Its definition and measurement. *Research in Developmental Disabilities, 16*(1), 51–74.
Felce, D., & Perry, J. (1996). Assessment of quality of life. In R. L. Schalock & G. N. Siperstein, (Eds.), *Quality of Life Volume I: Conceptualization and Measurement* (pp. 63–70). Washington DC: American Association on Mental Retardation.
Fernández-Juricic, E., Dolores, M., & Lucas, E. (2001). Alert distance as an alternative measure of bird tolerance to human disturbance implications for park design. *Environmental Conservation, 28*, 263–269.
Ferns, P. N., & Mudge, G. P. (2000). Abundance, diet and salmonella contamination of gulls feeding at sewage outfalls. *Water Resources, 34,* 2653–2660.

Fontana, S., Sattler, T., Bontadina, F., & Moretti, M. (2011). How to manage the urban green to improve bird diversity and community structure. *Landscape and Urban Planning, 101,* 278–285.
Francois, R. (2002). Numbers and behaviour of roof—nesting herring gulls *Larus argentatus* and lesser black backed gulls *Larus fuscus* in Belgium. *Natuur. Oriolus, 68*(3), 123–126.
Fuller, R. A., Tratalos, J., & Gaston, K. J. (2009). How many birds are there in a city of half a million people? *Diversity and Distributions, 15,* 328–337.
Gard, K., Groszos, M. S., Brevik, E. C., & Lee, G. W. (2007). Spatial analysis of bird-aircraft strike hazard for moody air force base aircraft in the state of georgia. *Georgia Journal of Science, 65*(4), 160–169.
Glatzer, W., Camfield, L., Møller, V., & Rojas, M. (Eds.). (2015). *Global handbook of quality of life*. Dordrecht, Netherlands: Springer.
Gremillet, D., & Boulinier, T. (2009). Spatial ecology and conservation of seabirds facing global climate change: A review. *Marine Ecology Progress Series, 391,* 121–137.
Guillemette, M., & Brousseau, P. (2001). Does culling predatory gulls enhance the productivity of breeding common terns. *Journal of Applied Ecology, 38,* 1–8.
Harris, M. P. (1970). Breeding ecology of the Swallow-tailed Gull, Creagrus furcatus. *The Auk, 87,* 215–243.
Heslenfeld, P., & Enserink, E. L. (2008). OSPAR Ecological quality objectives: The utility of health indicators for the north sea. *ICES Journal of Marine Science, 65,* 1392–1397.
Hostetler, M., Allen, W., & Meurk, C. (2011). Conserving urban biodiversity? Creating green infrastructure is only the first step. *Landscape and Urban Planning, 100*(4), 369–371.
Hughes, C., & Hwang, B. (1996). Attempts to conceptualize and measure quality of life. In Schalock, R. L. (Ed.), *Quality of Life. Vol. I: Conceptualization and Measurement* (pp. 51–61). Washington, DC: American Association on Mental Retardation.
Igual, J. M., Forero, M. G., Gomez, T., & Oro, D. (2007). Can an introduced predator trigger an evolutionary trap in a colonial seabird? *Biological Conservation, 137,* 189–196.
International Union for Conservation of Nature [IUCN]. (2009). *2009 IUCN Red List of threatened species*. Gland: IUCN.
Jones, H. P. (2010). Prognosis for ecosystem recovery following rodent eradication and seabird restoration in an island archipelago. *Ecological Applications, 20,* 1204–1216.
Jones, H. P., Towns, D. R., Bodey, T., Miskelly, C. M., Ellis, J., Rauzon, M. J., et al. (2011). Chapter 11: recovery and restoration on seabird islands. In C. P. H. Mulder, W. B. Anderson, D. R. Towns & P. J. Bellingham, (Eds.), *Seabird Islands: Ecology, Invasion, and Restoration* (pp. 460–531). Oxford: Oxford University Press.
Jones, H. P., & Kress, S. W. (2012). A review of the world's active seabird restoration projects. *The Journal of Wildlife Management, 76*(1), 2–9.
Johnston, R. J., Gregory, D., Pratt, G., & Watts, M. (2000). *Human Geography*. Oxford: Blackwell Publishing.
Konijnendijk, C.C. (2017). Cities and nature: Urban forestry for greater biocultural diversity. In Biological Conservation. In M. Campbell (Ed.), *Biological Conservation in the 21st Century: A Conservation Biology of Large Wildlife* (pp. 15–30). Nova Science Publishers, New York.
Konijnendijk, C. C., Ricard, R. M., Kenney, A., & Randrup, T. B. (2006). Defining urban forestry—A comparative perspective of north america and europe. *Urban Forestry & Urban Greening, 4*(3–4), 93–103.
Kress, S. W. (1997). Using animal behavior for conservation, case studies in seabird restoration from the Maine Coast, USA. *Journal of the Yamashina Institute for Ornithology, 29,* 1–26.
Kress, S. W., Borzik, R. V., & Hall, C. S. (2008). *Egg rock update 2008*. Ithaca: National Audubon Society.
Kushlan, J., Steinkamp, M. J., Parsons, K., Capp, J., Cruz, M. A., Coulter, M., et al. (2002). *Waterbirds for the Americas. The North American Waterbird Conservation Plan, Version 1*. Washington DC: Waterbirds for the Americas Initiative.
Lotze, H. K., Lenihan, H. S., Bourque, B. J., Bradbury, R. H., & Cooke, R. G. (2006). Depletion, degradation, and recovery potential of estuaries and coastal seas. *Science, 312,* 1806–1809.

Ludwigs, K., Lucas, R., Burger, M., Veenhoven, R., & Arends, L. (2017). How does more attention to subjective well-being affect subjective well-being? *Applied Research in Quality of Life* (pp. 1–26). Retrieved from https://doi.org/10.1007/s11482-017-9575-y.
Ma, Z., Cai, Y., Li, B., & Chen, J. (2010). Managing wetland habitats for waterbirds: An international perspective. *Wetlands, 30,* 15–27.
MacKinnon, B. (1999). *Database for bird and wildlife collisions with Aircraft in Canada.* Internet Report. Aerodrome Safety Branch, Ottawa. Retrieved from http://www.tc.gc.ca/aviation/aerodrme/birdstke/info/about.htm.
Martinez-Abrain, A., Sarzo, B., Villuendas, E., Bartolome, M. A., Minguez, E., & Oro, D. (2004). Unforeseen effects of ecosystem restoration on yellow-legged gulls in a small western Mediterranean island. *Environmental Conservation, 31,* 219–224.
Marzluff, J. M., Bowman, R., & Donnelly, R. (2001). *Avian ecology and conservation in an urbanising world.* Boston: Kluwer Academic Publishers.
Mitchell, P. I., Newton, S. F., Ratcliffe, N., & Dunn, T. E. (2004). *Seabird populations of Britain and Ireland.* London: T. & A. D. Poyser.
Murdoch, J. (1998). The spaces of actor network theory. *Geoforum, 29*(4), 357–374.
Oro, D. (2003). Managing seabird metapopulations in the mediterranean, constraints and challenges. *Scientia Marina, 67,* 13–22.
Oro, D., & Martinez-Abrain, A. (2007). Deconstructing myths on large gulls and their impact on threatened sympatric waterbirds. *Animal Conservation, 10,* 117–126.
Oro, D., Perez-Rodriguez, A., Martinez-Vilalta, A., Bertolero, A., Vidal, F., & Genovart, M. (2009). Interference competition in a threatened seabird community: A paradox for a successful conservation. *Biological Conservation, 142,* 1830–1835.
Parsons, M., Mitchell, I., Butler, A., Ratcliffe, N., Frederiksen, M., Foster, S., et al. (2008). Seabirds as indicators of the marine environment. *ICES Journal of Marine Science, 65,* 1520–1526.
Rock, P. (2002). Roof Nesting Gulls in bath. Follow up survey conducted in April 2002 and summarising surveys from 1995. *Bath: Report to the department of environmental services.* Northeast Somerset Council, Somerset.
Rock, P. (2005). Urban gulls: Problems and solutions. *British Birds, 98,* 338–355.
Ruiz-Olmo, J., Blanch, F., & Vidal, F. (2003). Relationships between the red fox and waterbirds in the Ebro Delta Natural Park, N.E. Spain. *Waterbirds, 26,* 217–225.
Scavia, D., & Bricker, S. B. (2006). Coastal eutrophication assessment in the United States. *Biogeochemistry, 79,* 1878–2208.
Schalock, R. L. (1997). Can the concept of quality of life make a difference? In R. L. Schalock (Ed.), *Quality of life volume II: Application to persons with disabilities* (pp. 245–267). Washington DC: American Association On Mental Retardation.
Schalock, R. L. (2000). Three decades of quality of life. *Focus on autism and other developmental disabilities, 15*(2), 116–128.
Schalock, R. L., Alonso, M. A. V., & Braddock, D. L. (2002). *Handbook on quality of life for human service practitioners.* Washington, DC: American Association on Mental Retardation.
Schaltegger, S., & Beständig, U. (2012). *Corporate biodiversity management handbook: a guide for practical implementation.* Berlin: Federal Ministry of the Environnment.
Scheffer, M., Bascompte, J., Brock, W. A., Brovkin, V., Carpenter, S. R., Dakos, V., et al. (2009). Early-warning signals for critical transitions. *Nature, 461,* 53–59.
Schippers, P., Stienen, E. W. M., Schotman, A. G. M., Snep, R. P. H., & Slim, P. A. (2011). The consequences of being colonial: Allee effects in metapopulations of seabirds. *Ecological Modelling, 222,* 3061–3070.
Shriver, W. G., Hodgman, T. P., Gibbs, J. P., & Vickery, P. D. (2004). Landscape context influences salt marsh bird diversity and area requirements in New England. *Biological Conservation, 119,* 545–553.
Somers, C. M., Doucette, J., Chip Weseloh, D. V., Kjoss, V. A., & Mark Brigham, R. (2011). Interactions between double-crested cormorants and other ground—nesting species. *Waterbirds, 34*(2), 168–176.

Spaans, A. L. (1971). On the feeding ecology of the Herring Gull Larus argentatus Pont. in the northern part of The Netherlands. *Ardea, 55*, 73–188.

Stagoll, K., Manning, A. D., Knight, E., Fischer, J., & Lindenmayer, D. B. (2010). Using bird–habitat relationships to inform urban planning. *Landscape and Urban Planning, 98,* 13–25.

Stroud, D. A. (2006). Declining waterbirds: problems, processes and sites. Workshop Introduction. In G. C. Boere, C. A. Galbraith & D. A. Stroud, (Eds.), *Waterbirds around the world* (pp. 641–642). Edinburgh: The Stationery Office.

Studds, C. E., DeLuca, W. V., Baker, M. E., King, R. S., & Marra, P. P. (2012). Land cover and rainfall interact to shape waterbird community composition. *PLoS One, 7*(4), e35969.

Thrush, S. F., Halliday, J., Hewitt, J. E., & Lohrer, A. M. (2008). The effects of habitat loss, fragmentation, and community homogenization on resilience in estuaries. *Ecological Applications, 18,* 12–21.

Traut, A. H., & Hostetler, M. E. (2004). Urban lakes and waterbirds: effects of shoreline development on avian distribution. *Landscape and Urban Planning, 69,* 69–85.

United States Department of Agriculture. (2003). *Wildlife hazard assessment for Moody Air Force Base, Georgia.* Washington DC: US Government Print Shop.

Vermeer, K. (1992). Population growth of the Glaucous-winged Gull Larus glaucescens in the Strait of Georgia, British Columbia, Canada. *Ardea, 80,* 181–185.

Vidal, E., Medail, F., Tatoni, T., & Bonnet, V. (2000). Seabirds drive plant species turnover on small mediterranean islands at the expense of native taxa. *Oecologia, 122,* 427–434.

Weiser, E. L., & Powell, A. N. (2010). Does garbage in the diet improve reproductive output of Glaucous Gulls? *Condor, 112,* 530–538.

Wolf, S. G., Snyder, M. A., Sydeman, W. J., Doak, D. F., & Croll, D. A. (2010). Predicting population consequences of ocean climate change for an ecosystem sentinel, the seabird cassin's auklet. *Global Change Biology, 16,* 1923–1935.

Chapter 24
Post-socialist Urban Changes and Role Strain in Assessing the Quality of Life: The Case of Bucharest, Romania

Mariana Nae and Liliana Dumitrache

Abstract The changes through which the former socialist cities passed were depended on multiple driving factors and the expertise of many actors. Post-socialist cities have experienced significant transformations in the past three decades in terms of urban fragmentation, land use and economic restructuring. This article aims to extend its contribution to the quality of life literature, underpinning the post-transition urban changes that occurred in Bucharest, the capital city of Romania. The study focuses on the potential role strain in assessing the quality of life in this city after 28 years of post-socialist transformations. The research is based on a survey conducted by the authors: a number of 985 questionnaires have been administered in 26 census tracts in order to identify the potential role strain in assessing the quality of life. The authors applied binary logistic regression and found that the factors encompassing the role strain relate to personal health status and access to health care, unemployment and low wages, housing conditions and housing affordability as well as environmental risks. Overall, the post-socialist changes can be seen as a spatial–temporal container (Tuvikene, Int J Urban Reg Res 40: 132–146, 2016), but the alterations of hybrid mix physical spatial features still remain and are connected with the divergent tendencies of socio-spatial polarisation. Communities and decision makers must develop the quality-of-life strategies with reliable guidelines.

Keywords Quality of life · Post-socialist urban changes · Role strain · Multiple criteria · Bucharest · Romania

24.1 Introduction

The expression of 'quality of life' is a multidimensional, complex and elusive one. Quality of life is difficult to assess and does not have an agreed definition (Rosenberg 1995). Notions like 'quality of life', 'standard of living' 'welfare' or well-being

M. Nae · L. Dumitrache (✉)
Department of Human and Economic Geography, University of Bucharest, Bucharest, Romania
e-mail: dosaredumitrache@yahoo.com

M. Nae
e-mail: mirellanae@gmail.com

B. R. K. Sinha (ed.), *Multidimensional Approach to Quality of Life Issues*,
https://doi.org/10.1007/978-981-13-6958-2_24

appear easy to understand at first sight, and they are even used as synonyms, but they differ considerably. Specialised studies have substantially clarified that the analysis of the notion of quality of life changes with respect to different perspectives such as economic, social, psychological or geographical. *Grosso modo*, it would mean various aspects of living conditions for different people. Therefore, quality of life is a relative term and varies from individual to individual. This can explicitly be seen under the following heads.

First, apparently, it is being used in a comprehensive manner in all environments of social life, heavily promoted and debated in the media, becoming an 'increasingly slippery or complex construct over the course of its use' (Rapley 2003: 10).

Second, it represented the subject of much theoretical and empirical research in social science disciplines and 'the literature is now too vast for any individual researcher to fully assimilate' (Cummins 1997: 118).

Thirdly, urban design is linked to the quality of life (Myers 1988; Rowley 1998; Brown et al. 2004; Romice et al. 2017).

Myers (1988: 350) underlined the five stages in the recommended planner's method of measuring quality of life, so-called 'community trend or internal monitoring'. These are the literature review on quality of life, interviews with leaders of major interests groups, collection of data related to objective indicators of various dimensions of the community's quality of life; surveys that evaluate citizens perceptions on their quality of life; and outlining reports for public debates.

According to Rowley (1998: 154), 'the urban designers have difficulty defining urban design and agreeing what constitutes good urban design amongst themselves'. Rowley made a list which was not exhaustive, underpinning a range of competing views about what constitutes quality of urban design grouped into four categories: 'functional and social use considerations; natural environment and sustainability considerations; visual considerations; and the urban experience.'

Many of these studies emphasised the importance of quality of life and focused mainly on urban areas both for urban competitive issues and spatial inequalities determined by the segregation and gentrification processes (Hamnett 1994, 1996; Marcuse and van Kempen 2000, 2002) as well as on (quality) urban design *problématique*.

The diversity of definitions depends on the scientific criteria; there is a consensus among specialists on two approaches: an external one (objective approach), that concerns the physical environment and an internal one (subjective approach), related to persons or individuals.

Objective quality of life is linked to living conditions, in relation to financial standing/constraints and living safety environment (Pacione 1982). Subjective quality of life is defined in terms of effective and cognitive reactions regarding an individual's private life (Diener et al. 1999; Myers and Diener 1995; Das 2007).

There is no consensus regarding the core QOL dimensions; many scholars suggest several possible domains covering all aspects of life (Haggerty et al. 2001; Massam 2002; Pacione 2003; Philips 2006; Nae 2009).

These components (constituents) are determined by the relationships between spatial environment and territorial factors, which in turn interrelate at different scales: global (global economy), regional and local factors (persons/individuals). Many of these components could be purely descriptive and placed into a frame to design a feature (overlapping or interfering with the notions of 'standard of living' or 'lifestyle').

Depending on the criteria used for defining quality of life, the studies elaborated by researchers or international organisations (WHO, UN, OECD) base themselves on different domains of living: the material well-being (ownership, employment); well-being and human capital (economy, labour, health care); physical well-being (health, mobility, wellness); living environment and urban services (public spaces, transport, dwellings); legislation and prerogatives (regulations, norms and civic responsibilities). At European level, the Eurostat national-scale feasibility studies cover multiple domains: physical livings standards, health, education, jobs, political voice, governance, freedom, physical environment, economic security, social connections (individual level) and subjective well-being. Following the same line of research, OECD launched in 2011 (OECD 2011) an interactive model of quality of life, '*Your Better Life Index*' that analysed 11 dimensions of well-being: housing, jobs, income, community, education, governance, safety, health, life satisfaction, environment and work–life balance.

The Romanian studies on quality of life have had a multidisciplinary perspective and covered a variety of domains (living standard, diagnosing poverty, living costs or social policies, and others). Significant studies on quality of life were performed (starting from 1990) mostly by sociologists under the aegis of the Romanian Academy, Institute for the Quality of Life Research. Rapid social changes, such as transitions, for example, are triggering favourable circumstances for social sciences; they can be used to emphasise the experimental side of such events or to verify new theories and hypothesis.

In Romania, these studies have mainly focused on the 'subjective' dimensions of quality of life, stressing on perceptions and evaluations. The essential themes addressed three issues: subjective well-being, economic resources, and social policies (Mărginean 2004; Mărginean and Bălașa 2004; Mărginean and Precupețu 2010; Codreanu 2012; Zamfir 2014). Considerable researches were conducted on the quality of life diagnosis (1990–2000; 2003, 2010, 2015) dealing with: dwellings and living conditions, health, living standards, public services, social services, family life, etc. These diagnoses were based particularly on socio-economic indicators and statistics on living conditions. Some research focused on specific population groups, according to age (young or elderly) or to their ethnic or social background (disadvantaged groups).

Romanian Geographer's interest on quality-of-life issues increased, although initially, they focused only on some aspects of the complex domains that QOL entails. These were transposed in the context of the existing relationships between components of the geographical environment and the quality of life components being presented at a national, regional, or local level.

For Bucharest, based on the premise that the geographical space plays a significant role in organising/planning the city, Nae (2009) analysed in an integrated manner quality-of-life domains such as housing, living standards, health, urban services, leisure and urban security. Besides, although a clear distinction between the two approaches of quality of life (objective vs subjective) is useful, this first geographical study aimed to combine both of them to achieve a more conclusive image of the phenomenon in the capital city.

24.2 Relativity Criteria in Assessing the Quality of Life: Research Programmes and Rankings

Due to multidimensional construct, the assessment of the quality of life requires the elaboration of sophisticated methods and tools that would encompass the integrated value of its specific domains, with the goal of making cities more sustainable. Several indicators centre on evaluating the sustainability of cities, but they also need to be able to ensure an integrated monitoring method to assess objectives and goals, and to incorporate recommendations that cities should follow.

In a broader sense, some studies and European programmes as Urban I (1994–1999) or Urban II (2000–2006) are linked to the quality of life's implications on economic policies that focused on sustainable development and urban social cohesion. Also, the Urban Audit Programme aims to collect comparable data, using 300 indicators.

Conversely, other researches were conducted on city ranking issues based on weighted QOL indicators. This typology of ranking cities has its roots in the work of Liu (1976); he used a simple statistical method, in order to compare the performance (so that cities could be ranked as substandard, adequate, good, excellent, or outstanding) of 240 metropolitan areas in the U.S.A. (Lambiri et al. 2007: 9).

Since 1990, Cushman and Wakefield (2010) published *European Cities Monitor Report* providing an overview of relative attractiveness for the business of cities across Europe. It analysed comparatively the evolutionary critical factors considered by organisations when assessing new locations; while also indicating how each European city is perceived to perform according to different criteria, including quality of life of employees.

Another example is *The Cultural and Creative Cities Monitor*, which was designed to help national, regional and municipal policymakers to identify local strengths and opportunities and comparing similar urban centres. Using both, quantitative and qualitative data as well as composite indicators, it shows the role of culture and creativity for the cities' social and economic well-being in the case of 168 selected cities in 30 European countries (EC 2017).

Several indicators and frameworks are applied to assess the sustainability of cities: Quality of Life Index (QLI), European Green City Index, Blue City Index (BCI), etc. The indicators for sustainability are different according to goals and objectives with specific methodologies (collecting data, data normalisation and construction of composite index). For example, European Green City Index (Siemens 2012) is framed on 30 individual indicators aiming to assess water consumption, greenhouse gas emissions. The EIUs Global Liveability Ranking (Conger 2015) is based on 30 indicators touching on different components (domains) of quality of life: health care, education, infrastructure, stability, culture and environment.

Establishing the criteria necessary for defining and evaluating the quality of life implies a system of objective and subjective indicators. They are determined by using methods acknowledged by specialised literature: Analytic Hierarchy Process (AHP), Aggregated Indices Randomization Method (AIRM), COPRAS, Analytic Network Process (ANP), Disaggregation–Aggregation Approaches, ELECTRE (Outranking), Goal Programming (GP), Grey Relational Analysis (GRA) (Kaklauskas et al. 2018).

An integrated database is NUMBEO, which developed the Quality of Life Index (Numbeo 2012). Out of 66 European cities considered, Bucharest was ranked by NUMBEO (2012, 2013, 2014) on the 53rd place and was overtaken by other Romanian cities like Cluj-Napoca and Braşov. Nonetheless, a comparative analysis of the methods mentioned above shows that there are differences when calculating these indicators; also, these frameworks do not provide automated guidelines for creating indexes and, therefore, are unable to provide reliable values that would permit a city to be ranked the best of the other ones analysed (Kaklauskas et al. 2018).

24.3 Post-socialist Changes in Bucharest: The Urban Design and the Quality of Life *Problématique*

After the fall of communism, the city of Bucharest, as well as other cities in Central and Eastern Europe were dramatically transformed. These cities have been continuously changing from a post-socialist city to a composite and eclectic one, as all the various meanings of urban functions (Castells 1983).

The relationship between post-socialist transformations and quality of life should be analysed in-depth and precisely because of the changes in the meaning of urban functions; however, not many Romanian researchers focussed on this type of approach.

With its population of 2,102,912 inhabitants in 2017 (NIS 2018), Bucharest is an important and dynamic South-Eastern European regional centre, with great business and investment potential. The city is part of the Bucharest-Ilfov NUTS 3 administrative region (with a total population of 2,510,417 inhabitants), and from its position of capital city, it represents an economic competitiveness pole.

The Bucharest-Ilfov Region registered a 4.3% economic growth in 2017, with a 39,400 € GDP per capita PPS in 2015, slightly surpassing the Berlin Region in Germany (34,400 €) or Attica in Greece (GDP 26,800 per inhabitant PPS) (Eurostat 2017). Unfortunately, merely highlighting statistics has no relevance, as the process of transition to the market economy deepened the gaps between regions and cities, without real outcomes in improving quality of life, well-being, or prosperity of the population, and does not guarantee a higher standard of living than other European capitals and regions. These differences could be explained by the lower prices specific to Romania (the level of prices is half the EU average in terms of purchasing power), and by the economic attractiveness of the Bucharest-Ilfov region, due to direct investments and high concentration of multinational companies, the existing institutional infrastructure and the highly qualified workforce. It is a well-known fact that there are national level differences in living standards and quality of life; these disparities often translated into significant gaps between regions, which led the experts to talk about Romania's multi-tiers economic development.

Bucharest's spatial development was distinctive; it was slower in the first years of the transition process, and more rapid after the year 2000, according to a pattern that followed divergent spatial trajectories (Ianoș et al. 2016) between the central, semi-central areas, and outskirts of the city, with a tentative un-cluttering of the centre and an increase in built-up area at the periphery.

The periphery has expanded mostly towards north and north-west due to urban transport corridors—the A1 and new projected A3 highways—as well as to the location in this area of retail spaces and logistic parks, growing less eastward and even less towards the south.

For the city of Bucharest, in its new socio-spatial frame of development, the challenges were mainly related to spatial planning which mostly followed the typology of the post-socialist transformations. Specific processes relating to the emergence of new spaces of production/consumption after the decline of industrial production, reconversion of former industrial zones, investments in office and retail spaces, brownfield and greenfield investments and investment in commercial areas and shopping malls have distinctly transformed the city's configuration. In addition, socio-residential differentiation in extensive development of new housing, rapidly rising property prices, the emergence of suburban enclaves and gated communities contributed to increasing polarisation of areas.

Other spaces changed their functions significantly by converting the obsolete industrial area to residential function and business centre or to mixed spaces forming landscapes of 'curios hybrid' like the Civic Centre area (Light and Young 2010). Despite the conversion and regeneration of former industrial sites and their transformation into commercial or residential spaces, the issues are linked to urban sustainability that needs to address: air pollution, road traffic congestion, loss of public green spaces.

Green areas is one of the important dimensions of quality of life. It works positively in the life condition of the population. From this standpoint, a synoptic view of green areas in Bucharest becomes important. The green areas in Bucharest have been found decreasing particularly after the year 1989 and this decline has been worsening the air quality by generating an increase in dust particles pointing to three times higher than European norms. Between 1990 and 2006 alone, green areas decreased from 3,471.2 to 2,274.4 ha (Iojă et al. 2008). The Green Areas Register (*Cadastrul Verde*) managed by the municipality contains contradictory data and showed that the proportion of green area per inhabitant in 2012 was 23.12 m^2 (this included private terrains too) compared to the European average of 26 m^2 per inhabitant. The distribution of green areas in Bucharest is uneven; however, the central and north-western parts of the city are the most advantaged.

Bucharest is a space of continuities and discontinuities in terms of housing as well. Its historical and urban evolution fell under two utopias which marked the construction and development of this European city intermingling its monarchy heritage with its socialist heritage. Dwelling construction was inextricably linked to the state property policy. After the Second World War, living in urban areas changed profoundly. In the political and ideological context, the rapid industrialisation and increasing urban population determined the construction of dwellings that did not respect any building or living norms as the socialist authorities focused on *quantity* rather than *quality*.

The period between 1950 and 1958 was marked by the major systematisation plans and sociopolitical changes, which translated into the mutilation of the urban landscape through massive reconstruction and reconfiguration campaigns. Since 1948, the socialist state has paid little attention to financing housing construction and focused primarily on investments in heavy industry (Nae and Erdeli 2008).

The periods between 1925 and 1955 was called as the époque of the high tower blocks of flats or blockhouses that had 6–10 floors. The most common type of apartments had two rooms and dependencies and the average of living space was 50–52 m^2. The present housing stock consists mainly of old collective flats located in blocks (built between 1970 and 1990 and considered inferior).

These dwellings offer a clear image of the current living conditions, as they require restoration, maintenance of common areas, seismic consolidation works and have low energy efficiency.

Over 80% of the dwellings were built before 1970 half of which dates from before 1944. The newer apartments, built after 1990, make out 7% of the total number (Suditu 2011). More than 60% of old buildings in Bucharest have a high seismic risk (approximately 370 buildings containing 6.480 flats) where most of these apartments are presently inhabited (Romania Regional Development Programme and World Bank 2015: 155).

The old dwelling stock, with low insulation levels, has started to be rehabilitated (by retrofitting buildings envelopes) through national and European programmes and investments, as all dwellings and residential buildings must now conform to the European directives on energy efficiency. All new buildings must be 'nearly zero energy standards', a requirement from 2020 onwards. The energy performance of buildings also has a significant impact on the affordability of housing (EC 2016a, b). Nationally, the living area is still below the European average (46.9 m^2 compared to 102.3 m^2).

After the year 1990, the population's residential preferences are changed as per the defined property rights. People started to opt for newer and larger dwellings or pavilion houses. The offer of new dwellings is rather homogenous but limited in terms of building standards and location (Suditu et al. 2014a). The newer and larger residential complexes do not capitalise on the semi-central dense areas, because of the lack of space and local urban regulations, however, instead of this the spread at the periphery of the city create suburban developments. The standards of living space should follow the Housing Law defining 58 m^2 for one-person apartments, 81 m^2 for two-person apartments with one bedroom and 102 m^2 for three-person apartments with two bedrooms. Due to high construction costs in new dwelling the private investors focused on building 1 or 2 rooms apartments or small-scale blocks of flats that can capitalise on the areas located inside the city with better accessibility to urban amenities.

The new societal context and economic restructuring led to urban challenges, including urban sprawl, failing infrastructure and social polarisation. During the second stage of transition (2000–2007), the big private companies invested in the inner city. More and more residential parks and shopping centres emerged, which were clustered especially in semi-central and peripheral areas. 'The office developments moved northwards to Dorobanţi and then expanded into the lake land zone particularly in Pipera along with Băneasa, Floreasca and Tei, with a complementary growth around Piaţa Unirii and other inner city areas' (Nae and Turnock 2011: 218). New office buildings with a total of 265,000 m^2. GLA (gross leasable area, i.e. floor space to be rented for commercial use) were completed in 2016. The existing housing stock is concentrated in the northern area (56%), centrally (27%) and west (13%), while the eastern (2%) and southern (2%) areas have a very low distribution of office functions (Active Property Services 2017) (Fig. 24.1).

Infrastructure and essential amenities such as water supply, sewerage, transport, waste collection and processing, energy, gas, public lighting, street network condition the functioning of a city. These are generically called *public services*; the notion itself is quite ambiguous and differs depending on the country, which is why they are particularly difficult to compare. The characteristics and especially the disparities concerning accessibility are interesting and revealing when studying quality of life as it is a well-known fact that in qualitative terms service proximity is of utmost importance (Nae 2006). In order to improve quality of life, Bucharest municipality has launched the 2016–2030 transport strategy (*Planul de Mobilitate Urbană Durabilă*) which aims to develop public transport by extending the metro and tram networks, building 250 km of bike tracks, reorganising pedestrian spaces, creating park-and-ride-type areas located at the most important public transport stations.

Regarding healthcare infrastructure and medical services, Romania experienced necessary changes, which are mainly associated with the reform process, which gradually took place in all the CEECs countries, by replacing the centralised Semasko system with other organisational and financing models. In Romania, health reform started in 1990 and determined significant changes at the level of HCS financing—by introducing the social health insurance system (Bismarckian model) along with other sources of financing (Health Insurance Law—1998), at the level of HCS organising—by restructuring medical infrastructure and gradual directing health activities towards primary care—as well as the emergence of private health sector—mostly specialised medical offices, stomatology offices, pharmacies and after the year 2000—hospitals.

A lack of planning and long-term health strategies, HCS under financing and unequal health workforce distribution has led to limiting population' access to quality health care (Zamfir et al. 2015).

Despite a political commitment to invest for the improvement of Primary Health Care, Romania has not given priority and failed in strengthening PHC. There are

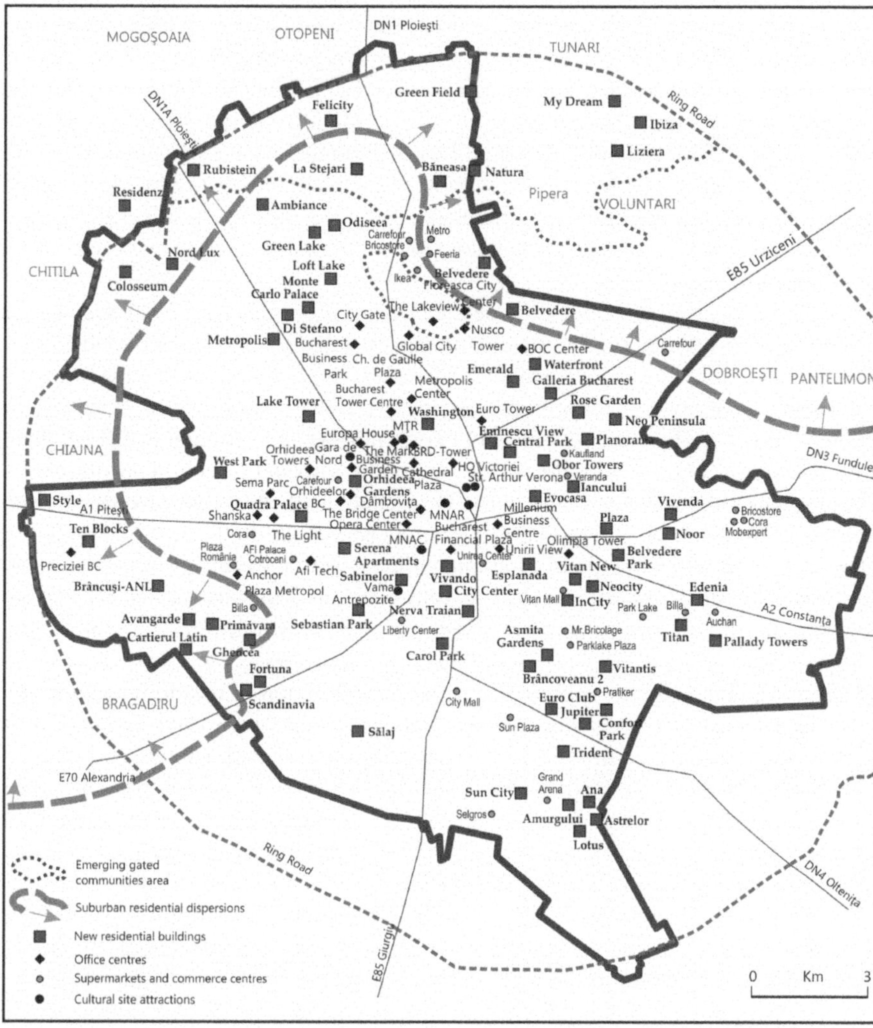

Fig. 24.1 Distribution of new residential parks and office centres

organisational malfunctions, lack of GPs in rural areas and weak delivery of primary healthcare services. All these have increased the rate of hospital use, population accessing hospitals for simple diagnosis or routine investigations raised the hospitals expenditure to 50% of total health expenditure. The *National Strategy for Hospital Rationalization* (2011) was supposed to transfer more diagnostic responsibilities to family doctors and to introduce copayment but this plan was criticised by both the hospital and family doctors. Many GP offices do not have the necessary equipment and similarly the population accessibility to primary care services is limited especially in rural areas. Thereby, in spite of sustained efforts on the part of authorities, hospitals remain *the polarising centre* of healthcare activities in Romania (Dumitrache 2014).

According to 2011 legislation, the total number of hospitals (467) has been classified into five categories based on the level of availability of necessary equipments and the number of specialists and specialities. Although, hospitals are numerous and relatively evenly distributed territorially most of them are unable to provide complex care due to lack of equipments or medical personnel and as a result, patients are generally transferred to a few regional hospitals or to major emergency or university hospitals in Bucharest.

The private sector has had a slow development before the year 2000 even being the stomatology offices, radiological centres, test labs, gynaecological and family planning offices the most predominant. Only after 2000, the private sector recorded a significant development through privatising sections of some public hospitals or building new private hospitals (76 in 2011). Even despite a continuous development in the private healthcare services, the private sector does not yet represent an alternative to the public healthcare sector, only in Bucharest and in other few largest cities private operators compete: Medlife, Medicover, Regina Maria and Polisano.

Private health insurances, which should support private health services, are modestly developed in Romania. These are optional and additional services. Recent attempts at introducing compulsory private insurances proved to be unpopular and have generated waves of protests including riots in January 2012.

Therefore, healthcare activity in Romania is mostly based on public sector and public funds, as 90% of hospitals and GP offices as well as the largest number of doctors remain mainly within this sector. The shortage of medical personnel due to emigration and its uneven distribution at national level increase the difficulties that Romanian healthcare system is facing. Providing medical care, given the acute lack of medical personnel (doctors and nurses as well) and limited financial resources is a continuous challenge for medical authorities.

The post-socialist changes have a specific background having taken place in a spatial and temporal container, but their long and short-term consequences on the population are difficult to pinpoint and have opposing tendencies and significances.

These changes have undoubtedly had positive effects on the development and spatial extension of the city. They contributed to the city's better organisation by redistributing state and private influence (the decentralisation of power), increasing the competitive advantages due to the market economy, consolidating private property, structuring social classes by slightly highlighting the middle class, and overall improving the population's quality of life.

The transfer of development resources and opportunities from the public sector to the private sector facilitated the individual options that the population gained in terms of living standards; it increased residential mobility and extended suburban developments although some of them lacked basic amenities and other were in fact structured as gated communities (Dumitrache et al. 2016a). At the same time, the social costs of the transition process from centralised to market planning led to sharpening the multiple social layers and gave rise to segregation processes.

The socialist state had diminished segregation by building large residential areas that were socially homogeneous (blocks of flats where the working class was living together with the highly educated population). The increasing costs of living corroborated with the social transformations occurring after the year 1989 resulted in increased income inequalities, as well as generating poverty, unemployment and social vulnerability (Suditu et al. 2014b). These social inequalities are avoidable or can at least be mitigated through targeted public policies. Increased costs of living affect all quality-of-life dimensions negatively, either objectively or subjectively. The way in which the population relates to these changes is relative and sensitive and constitutes the object of the next section.

24.4 Beyond the Objective Indicators for Quality of Life: The Role Strain in Assessing Quality of Life

Since the economic transition and the post-socialist transformations, the general elements of quality of life and well-being are not perceived from an immutable perspective. These changes in quality of life might occur in all the domains of social life in a city. While summarising the main post-socialist transformations during 28 years of post-economic transition, with numerous positive and negative effects on the quality of life of Bucharest's inhabitants, the authors have developed this section in terms of potential strains affecting the quality of life of residents, so it requires a subjective perspective. With this view point one theoretical perspective, i.e. the 'role strain' hypothesis, which proposes a negative association between multiple role obligations and well-being (Goode 1960) is required. The concept of quality of life is based on social and cultural factors and postulates that people could possibly receive and understand information about different living standards through the lens of their cultural and social background.

In general, in social sciences, role refers to a set of behaviours that are associated with a particular status or social position occupied by an actor. The role strain is assigned as difficulty experienced by an individual with incompatible behaviour, expectations or obligations.

The first level of analysis is based on identifying the 'role strain' when assessing the quality of life. The second level of analysis aims to identify the importance that residents give to city amenities and how they relate to the quality of life' dimensions. The responses related to different meanings for the quality of life could be affected by the order in which the questions appear due to specific general representations of the topic. To minimise the potential errors that appear in understanding the meanings for the quality of life from general to specific, we followed Sudman and Bradburn's (1982) advice and employed the technique of sorting the questions according to their level of generality and specificity. In doing so, we asked the general questions first and the specific ones last.

'What people see as the meanings of their lives and the living they consider desirable or undesirable are matters of personal choice' (Hofstede 1984: 389; Kahneman et al. 1999). At the same time, individual choices could be influenced by the cultural environment. The components of quality of life relating to their personal lives are very complex and usually correlated with several variables (education, age, socio-professional structure and sociocultural environment). Data collection consisted of the standardised survey (n = 985) in 26 census tracts within the city and secondary sources. The sample frame followed the 2011 census data. The sampling design complies with the methodological requirements for a general population representative survey. The survey captured the perspective of respondents with questions about their community, amenities and neighbourhood attachment. This sample has a confidence interval of ±3, with a confidence level of CI 95%. The average mean of the sample was 40.99 years old (lower bound was 39.05 years old and upper bound was 42.04 years). The statistical analyses were performed using SPSS Statistics 20 (IBM Corp 2011).

Quality of life is complex and multidimensional; its perception depends on many factors. Therefore, the assessment is difficult, and the measures are relative. In order to reveal the significance of quality-of-life criteria, starting with the cognitive experience of people, 14 criteria of the survey were analysed. The criteria cover the main domains or constituents of quality of life such as health, housing, employment, infrastructure, civic participation, environmental sustainability. In order to explore the significance of life domains and see the way in which the residents understand, feel, and live their everyday life, respondents were asked to mention from a list of 14 life condition-related items, which have an important value to their quality of life. The importance of these criteria was measured on a four-point Likert scale (0—low importance, 4—high importance). Is there an association between quality of life and access to good sanitation? Is there an association between the relationships with neighbours and the community and the city's infrastructure?

In order to understand which factors could influence the inhabitants' quality of life and play a potential role strain on their everyday life, we used binary logistic regression (Hosmer et al. 2013). The dependent variable is the satisfaction/dissatisfaction over their own quality of life while the explicative variables are the potential strain variable evaluated as being of high or low importance. The authors considered the following factors in their analysis: better access to healthcare services, job-related stress, work relations and social cohesion, attachment to their neighbourhoods, safety in their neighbourhoods, level of wages, pollution and air quality, decent living conditions, affordability of new housing, unemployment, capacity to find a new job, access to leisure amenities, noise level and noise pollution, water quality, connectivity to the transport network.

Forward stepwise method has been performed, and eight models have resulted, with the eighth one meeting the conditions and improving predictions (82.8%). The fitness of the model and the manner in which it predicted the outcomes by considering the Nagelkerke's R^2 coefficient was checked (Nagelkerke 1991; Hosmer et al. 2013). The results were interpreted using the odds ratio measure (about the change in the odds with a unit change in predictor) (Spicer 2005; Field 2009) (Table 24.1).

Table 24.1 Model parameters results

Model/summary	1	2	3	4	5	6	7	8	9
−2LL	1236.5	1203.2	1174.5	1162.9	1150.8	1145.3	1139.1	1140.7	1133.5
Cox & Snell R^2	0.072	0.103	0.128	0.139	0.149	0.154	0.159	0.158	0.164
Nagelkerke R^2	0.098	0.139	0.175	0.188	0.203	0.209	0.216	0.215	0.223

Cox & Snell R^2: has a theoretical maximum value of less than 1
Nagelkerke R^2: an adjusted version of Cox & Snell R square to assess the fit of the model (full range from 0 to 1; a value closer to 1 implies a better predictive power)
Source Based on authors' calculation

The resulting binary logistic regression model produced an 82.8% overall success rate of correctly predicted values for the factors that determine the dissatisfaction of personal life. Nagelkerke R^2 coefficient indicates that the model explained 21.5% of the variation in outcome. Adequacy of fit for a logistic regression model is assessed by the significance of the omnibus chi-square test of the model coefficients and the Hosmer–Lemeshow goodness-of-fit test (Hosmer et al. 2013), which groups cases into deciles based upon the predicted probability of each one; a non-significant chi-square goodness-of-fit test suggests a well-fitting model (Smith and McKenna 2013). A chi-square statistic is computed comparing the observed frequencies with those expected under the linear model. The model which is fit and acceptable χ^2 (8) = $6.037, p = 0.535$, indicates that our model predicts values not significantly different from what was observed in the field (Table 24.2).

Issues relating to pollution and other associated phenomena can represent potential strains when measuring the satisfaction level regarding personal life and quality of life in general. The odds ratios of environmental issues increased by a factor value of 2.141, the result of those people who considered this constituent of high importance

Table 24.2 Main factors associated with dissatisfaction about their personal life and quality of life

Variables	B	S.E	Wald	p-value	Odds ratios	95% C.I. for odds ratio	
						Lower	Upper
Environmental issues	0.761	0.190	16.027	0.000	2.141	1.475	3.107
Health status and access to healthcare services	1.115	0.185	36.155	0.000	3.051	2.121	4.388
Housing conditions and economic affordability of a new housing	1.786	0.204	76.301	0.000	5.966	3.996	8.907
Unemployment/potential strain in search of a new job	0.644	0.184	12.270	0.000	1.904	1.328	2.729
Low wages	1.446	0.167	74.635	0.000	4.247	3.059	5.896

(continued)

Table 24.2 (continued)

Variables	B	S.E	Wald	p-value	Odds ratios	95% C.I. for odds ratio	
						Lower	Upper
Stress and conflict at work	1.018	0.261	15.228	0.000	2.768	1.660	4.617
Constant	−4.420	0.527	70.252	0.000	0.012		

Wald Chi-Square statistic is used to test the significance of the variable in the model
B = regression coefficient is associated with the intercept as it is included in the model
SE = standard error of regression coefficient
Source Based on authors' calculation

in comparison with those who did not. The odds ratio of the respondents who were not satisfied with their life increased by a factor value of 3.051 when personal health and access to better health care were considered to be of high importance compared to those finding these as being of low importance.

The odds ratio of the respondents who were not satisfied with their personal life increased in case of those who considered their living conditions and economic affordability for new housing as being of high importance (OR = 5.966, $p = 0.000$). Also, the odds ratio of dissatisfaction with the personal life of those who perceived unemployment and potential strain in searching of a new job as a factor of high importance (OR = 1.904, $p = 0.000$) increased in comparison to those who considered this factor as a low importance. Finally, the odds ratio of dissatisfaction with personal life increased in case of those who perceived low wages as a factor of high importance (OR = 4.247, $p = 0.000$) in comparison to those who considered this factor as a low importance.

The odds ratio of dissatisfaction with personal life increased in case of those who perceived stress and conflict at work regarded this as a factor of high importance (OR = 2.768, $p = 0.000$) in comparison to those who considered this factor as low importance.

These results confirm that many potential strain factors that can affect, the quality of life of city residents are related to domains considered essential. The major factors having role strain in affecting quality of life are linked to dwellings and housing conditions, personal health and access to better health care, living standards and wages at a level considered sufficient.

Housing conditions are very complex and usually influence the quality of life. Unfortunately, social segregation and spatial inequalities are thriving; higher income differentiation contributed to a social polarisation among households. In the largest cities, even if the offer for old and new apartments is more varied, the issue of real estate is delicate. Romania occupies a medium-superior position on a hierarchy of European countries that measures the burden that households bear in the mortgages and other real estate-related type of credits (50% out of their total income compared to the EU average of 28–32%) (Eurostat 2016).

Accessibility to new dwellings in terms of prices can be a potential economic strain and could substantially contribute to a negative perception of the quality of life. The data and information provided by a series of studies seem to confirm multiple aspects regarding acquiring new dwellings (old or new) (Romania Regional Development Programme and World Bank 2015). Usually, the gaps in income by households are statistically expressed in deciles showing the average earnings for different social groups.

According to the latest results of the family budget survey (NIS 2014), the gap between average incomes per person of the ninth decile (1,520.3 RON, approximately 330 €) and the first decile (318.3 RON, approximately 69 €) have significantly increased. Moreover, new potential homeowners belonging to the third decile income/household (1,741.3 RON, 379 € equivalent) would be eligible for a bank loan, valued at 30,000 € (the equivalent of low-cost housing).

Housing affordability in Romania's larger cities is centred on accessibility in terms of pricing when buying a new home as a result of an extending credit programme, called *Prima Casă* (First Home Loan). The *Prima Casă* Programme was launched in 2009; it was a governmental programme that offered real estate loans to first-time home buyers at a price ceiling of 60,000 €. This price ceiling meant that middle-sized and large cities buyers had to turn in most cases to the old housing stock, built during the socialist era, as they could not afford the newer built apartments. As such, the public sector programmes did not encourage the building of a new stock of housing that could be available to lower income families. Studies, which combined bank statistics, real estate data and population income data from the NIS, have confirmed that most houses traded through this programme would be affordable for the population of the third decile average income/household.

In the case of Bucharest, based on family income and an advance payment of more than 5% (of the house value), all types of houses can be purchased under this government programme. Most of the dwellings bought through the Prima Casă Programme were affordable up to the third income decile; these are dwellings with a reduced living area (less than 40 m^2). More spacious, two-bedroom dwellings priced at 38,000 € could be affordable only for middle and upper middle-income deciles (MDRAP 2017: 51).

Personal health status is often related to the quality of life dimension. Specific to health-related studies, the term 'strain' is defined in many ways, always in relation with the caregivers as 'the caregiver's perception of enduring problems or an altered state of well-being' (Kane 2001; Thorton and Travis 2003; Dahlrup et al. 2015). In this study, we referred to a more general dimension of this indicator and not a very specific one.

According to a European survey (2016), the level of satisfaction with healthcare services shows large variations between cities. Nevertheless, at least half of the respondents are dissatisfied with this dimension in 16 cities, including 7 EU capitals (Athens, Warszawa, Budapest, Bucharest, Riga, Bratislava and Rome).

Studies have shown that people are accessing private/public healthcare sector according to their general assumptions about their health and not according to a real conceptual framework of clinical medicine. Although reforms and restructuring policies of the Romanian health system continued to improve access to better quality health care (Nae 2014; Dumitrache et al. 2016b), inequalities in healthcare access persist.

There are more than 70 hospital units in Bucharest. According to the Ministry of Health classification (2011), only 19 were included in the highest category of performance (Fig. 24.2).

Many public hospitals operate in ancient, non-functional buildings, classified in different seismic risk classes and would require renovation or consolidation works. (e.g. Colțea Hospital dating from 1887, Panduri Hospital dating from 1948).

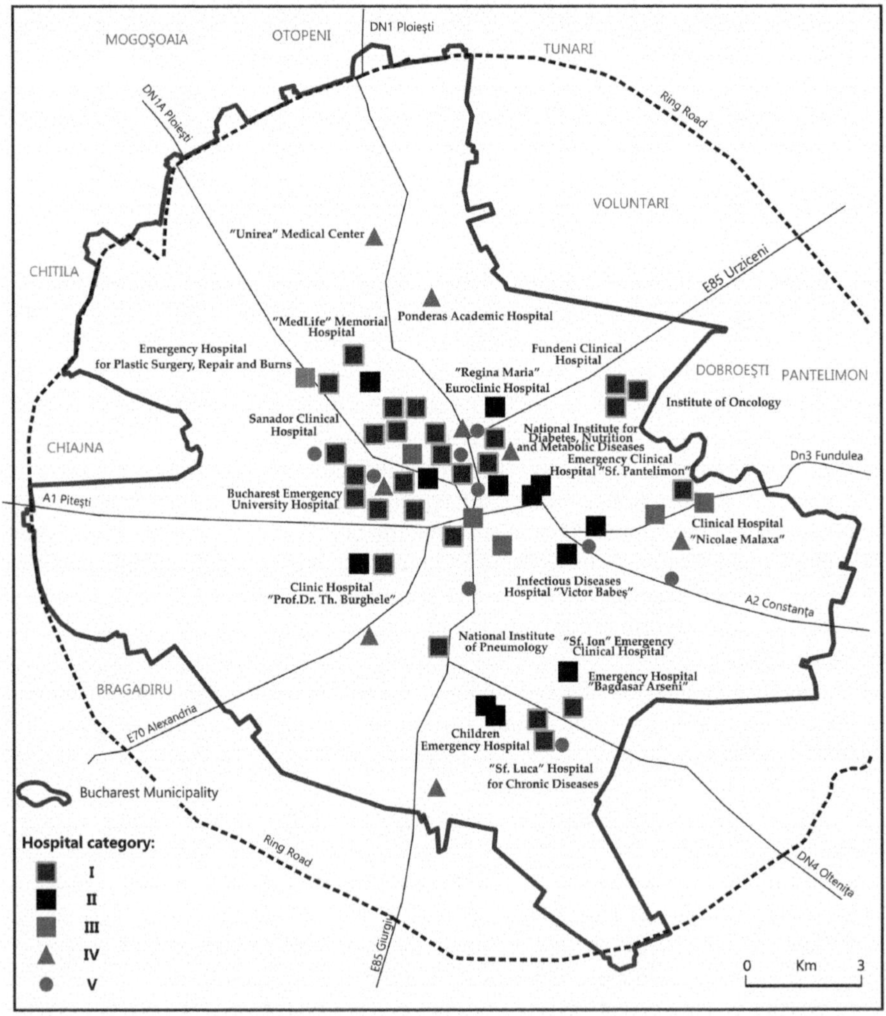

Fig. 24.2 Distribution of hospitals (public and private) by category

Although there have been many discussions and even projects to build new hospitals in Bucharest, after 1990, the public health sector has not been benefited from them.

Despite their large number, most of the public hospitals in Bucharest are overcrowded. This situation mostly results from a large number of patients from Bucharest or surrounding localities, who turn to hospital services even for simple investigations, and patients transferred from other hospitals in the country which, due to lack of equipment or specialised medical personnel, are unable to solve complex cases. These hospitals also face a lack of specialised personnel, especially after the 2008–2010 crisis that caused salaries cuts of 25%, and a hiring block in the public sector thus determining many health professionals to emigrate and practice abroad.

There were over 460 vacant positions in public hospitals in 2013 out of which 172 for physicians and over 230 for nurses; most of them were in large emergency or university hospitals, however, the reduced number of applications proved the lack of interest for medical practice in the public sector in Romania.

The main private hospitals in Bucharest are: Euroclinic (opened in 2005, and now owned by Regina Maria), Life Memorial (Medlife, opened in 2007), Spitalul de bstetrică Ginecologie Maternitatea Regina Maria (opened in 2008), West Eye Hospital (2010), Delta Hospital (2011); Paediatric Hospital (Medlife), Orthopaedics Hospital (Medlife) (2011) and Medicover Hospital (2012). They only constitute an alternative for a small population segment, usually the employees of multinationals companies and people on high incomes, which can afford full costs or copayments. So, in theory, the two healthcare systems coexist and local population is benefited from a variety of options and good accessibility to health care, in reality, the higher cost is limiting the addressability to private care, and pressure is higher on the public sector and public funds.

'The standard of living is most commonly assessed in terms of annual household level income or a way of life to which a group of people are accustomed, consciously or unconsciously (McGregor and Goldsmith 1998: 5)'. Higher rates of unemployment certainly have negative economic effects but can also represent a potential strain when the inhabitants' quality of life is subjectively evaluated (Dolan et al. 2008). Stress and coping theory is a potentially valuable model for understanding the association between family and economic stress. More than that, unemployment level, income level and purchasing power are important factors that can influence the negative perception towards personal life and quality of life in general. At European level, unemployment is one of the top three most important issues when ranking quality of life in 58 cities (EC 2013).

According to Eurostat data, the Bucharest-Ilfov Region registered an economic growth of more than 4.3% which would have meant a real increase in living standards for inhabitants. Transformation in PPS unit households' income presents significant differences. Berlin, for example registered an available household income of 18,000 PPS units while in Bucharest, it was only of 14,400 PPS units (Eurostat 2017). In general, higher income differentiation contributed to social polarisation among households.

Preserving the environmental conditions are undeniably connected to well-being and quality of life (Marans 2003; Streimikiene 2015; Orru et al. 2016) and the inhabitants' perception is rather different. Recent studies also observe these differences (Eurostat 2016). Air quality is the aspect on which views diverge; at least 50% are dissatisfied in 20 cities. Dissatisfaction with air quality is particularly high in Krakow (83%), Ostrava (76%) and Bucharest (75%). Central and local authorities are compelled to respect environmental standards, and they have to make it a priority in city management. In Europe, for example the standards for air quality are described in the 2008/50/EC Directive, which explains a limit of 40 $\mu g/m^3$ for the annual mean concentration of nitrogen dioxide and a limit of 200 $\mu g/m^3$ not to be exceeded for more than 18 h in a year. Unfortunately, Bucharest suffers from a high nitrogen dioxide concentrations. This high nitrogen dioxide concentration in Bucharest was recorded and found exceeding 200 $\mu g/m^3$ at the 19.00 h in 2013 (EC 2016a).

On 29 August 2014, Bucharest joined the WHO European Healthy Cities Network, thus showing the desire and commitment of local authorities to improve health and well-being for all. Moreover, although initiatives in this regard included investing in educational infrastructure, preserving and increasing green spaces, encouraging physical activity by developing a network of bicycle lanes, the major healthy city objectives are still far from being achieved.

24.5 Conclusions

The CEE cities have structurally changed from the point of view of land use, property rights, infrastructure, transport network and connectivity, commercial and residential developments. Also, cities gradually adapted to the principles of functional market economies to which the population-related social and economic pressures and strains concerning the quality of life and well-being (especially regarding low wages, unemployment, the housing crisis, social polarisation, increasing social vulnerability) were inevitably added.

In approximately three decades, since the fall of the socialist regime, in 1989, the demographic changes and urban sprawl played an essential role in the spatial reconfiguration of the city. Bucharest was spatially revitalised and reconstructed by different promoters and developers. Based on studies of Landsat TM imagery and statistical data, the built-up area of the city and its surroundings rose during 2003–2010 from 273.4 km^2 la 309.92 km^2. This phenomenon had a similar dynamic at the peak of the socialist era, translated into an increase in built-up area to the detriment of farming and forest areas (Mihai et al. 2015).

The uncontrolled urban sprawl phenomenon is currently in full progress, and it is generated mostly by private initiative, without public coordination (Suditu 2009), as well as by the real dysfunctions of urban planning legislation. Urban planning could play an essential role in reconsidering urban development strategies, increasing city sustainability and promoting a cleaner, greener, and healthier city. Therefore, a new consensus about planning goals and decisions need to be established; planners should consider the quality of life as a 'strategic resource for supporting continued development and achieving the future satisfaction of citizens' (Myers 1987: 356).

Reducing socio-spatial inequalities and increasing population accessibility to amenities are key ambitions. Socio-economic segregation as well the social division of urban space is slightly increasing (Marcińzak et al. 2014; Tammaru et al. 2016). The population may adapt or adjust to different circumstances, whether in relation to health, housing conditions, income level or other socio-economic factors when striving to achieve a better quality of life. An important mediator of this adaptation process is 'response shift', whereby internal standards and values are changed and hence the perception of quality of life (Sprangers and Schwartz 1999). Our results showed that the issue of dwellings and economic affordability could be a burden element that would lead to a negative perception about the quality of life.

Presently, there is no functional real estate market in which the public sector can actively get involved and directly support poor and vulnerable social groups. Following recommendations of the World Bank, implementing a National Real Estate Strategy would control and diminish these realities and create a functional real estate market, and would better value private investments towards the construction of affordable housing, knowing that the private sector adopted fully marketing-oriented strategies for middle and high-income social groups.

Public housing constitutes only 2% of the real estate stock and is insufficiently developed. The renting market is not well developed and is poorly regulated, and the 2008–2010 financial crisis affected the construction sector leading to a decrease in housing prices with more than half located in high-end areas; this led to the bankruptcy of many real estate developers and many households experienced loses in terms of quality of life. Multiple programmes funded by the state budget cover the expenditures for public housing, but the GDP percentages allocated to social housing is lower than the average level in other middle–income countries (MDRAP 2017).

Lastly, beyond the objective evaluation of the urban quality of life and sustainability, in general, the quality of life is inevitably subjective and depended upon individual perceptions. Qualitative assignment represents the result of value judgments built according to a reference system. This reference system is based on representations, experiences, feelings and affections of every citizen and there is no universal consensus value scale. Even more, linking the objective and subjective approach is extremely important for all actors involved; particularly, urban planners are managing the city, and they need to know how their decisions may affect resident's satisfaction with overall quality of life (McCrea et al. 2006).

Even if post-socialist transformations became less relevant during the last few years according to social scientists (Hirt 2013; Tuvikene 2016), we would consider the process through which political actors quantify and evaluate the outcomes of quality of life and urban sustainability as very important. The decision-making actors should further sustain and implement adequate policies and encourage participative planning. 'Genuine involvement of local people in local planning, urban design, and in implementation is far from having been achieved' (Chapman and Larkham 1999: 229). The role of the local public administration needs to be consolidated in order to implement reliable projects of urban revitalization by involving all the urban actors in order to increase resident's empowerment and urban quality of life.

References

Active Property Services. (2017). *Romania real estate market report March 2017, Bucharest.* Retrieved December 15, 2017, from https://www.activpropertyservices.ro/en/.

Brown, J., Bowling, A., & Flynn, T. (2004). Models of quality of life: A taxonomy, overview and systematic review of the literature. In *European Forum on Population Ageing Research.*

Castells, M. (1983). *The urban question: A marxist approach.* London: Edward.

Chapman, D. W., & Larkham, P. J. (1999). Urban design, urban quality and the quality of life: Reviewing the department of the environment's urban design campaign. *Journal of Urban Design, 4*(2), 211–232.

Codreanu, C. M. (2012). Source of variation in quality of life in Romania. *Procedia-Social and Behavioral Sciences, 58,* 645–654.

Conger, B. W. (2015). On livability, liveability and the limited utility of quality-of-life rankings. *The School of Public Policy, 7*(4), 1–8.

Cummins, R. A. (1997). Assessing quality of life. In R. I. Brown (Ed.), *Quality of life for people with disabilities: Models, research and practice* (2nd ed., pp. 116–150). Cheltenham: Stanley Thornes.

Cushman & Wakefield. (2010). *European city monitor 2010.* Retrieved February 20, 2018 from, http://81.47.175.201/ETMS/index.php/c-w-european-cities-monitor.

Dahlrup, B., Ekstrom, H., Nordell, E., & Elmstahl, S. (2015). Coping as a caregiver: A question of strain and its consequences on life satisfaction and health related quality of life. *Archives of Gerontology and Geriatrics, 61*(2), 261–270.

Das, D. (2007). Urban quality of life: A case study of Guwahati. *Social Indicators Research, 88,* 297–310.

Diener, E., Suh, E. M., Lucas, R. E., & Smith, H. L. (1999). Subjective well-being: Three decades of progress. *Psychological Bulletin, 125*(2), 276–302.

Dolan, P., Peasgood, T., & White, M. (2008). Do we really know what makes us happy? A review of the economic literature on the factors associated with subjective well-being. *Journal of Economic Psychology, 29,* 94–122.

Dumitrache, L. (2014). Défis, incohérences et échecs de la réforme sanitaire en Roumanie.In Anna Krasteva et Despina Vasilcu (eds.), *Migration en blanc. Medecins d'est en ouest* (pp. 21–40). Paris: L'Harmattan, coll. Global & Local.

Dumitrache, L., Zamfir, D., Nae, M., Simion, G., & Stoica, I.-V. (2016a). The urban nexus: Contradictions and dilemmas of (post) communist (sub) urbanization in Romania. *Human Geographies. Romanian Journal of Studies and Research in Human Geography, 10*(1), 39–58.

Dumitrache, L., Nae, M., Dumbrăveanu, D., Simion, G., & Suditu, B. (2016b). Contrasting clustering in health care provision in romania: Spatial and aspatial limits. *Procedia Environmental Sciences, ECOSMART—Environment at Crossroads: Smart Approaches for a Sustainable Development, 32,* 290–299.

European Commission. (2013). *Quality of life in cities. perception survey in 79 European cities, Luxembourg.* Publications Office of the European Union.

European Commission. (2016a). *Quality of life in European cities 2015.* Regional and Urban Policies, Luxembourg. Publications Office of the European Union. Retrieved December 19, 2017, from http://ec.europa.eu/regional_policy/sources/docgener/studies/pdf/urban/survey2015_en.pdf.

European Commission. (2016b). Directive of the European parliament and of the council amending directive 2010/31/EU on the energy performance of buildings. Retrieved February 23, 2018, from http://eur-lex.europa.eu/legal-content/EN/TXT/?qid=1490877208700&uri=CELEX:52016PC0765.

European Commission. (2017). *The cultural and creative cities monitor 2017.* Edition JRC. Retrieved February 20, 2018, from https://ec.europa.eu/jrc/en/publication/eur-scientific-and-technical-research-reports/cultural-and-creative-cities-monitor-2017-edition.

Eurostat. (2016). Housing statistics. https://ec.europa.eu/eurostat/statistics-explained/index.php/Housing_statistics
Eurostat. (2017). *Eurostat Newsrelease*. 2015 GDP per capita in 276 EU regions, 52/2017, 30 March 2017. Eurostat Press Office. Retrieved December 19, 2017, from http://ec.europa.eu/eurostat/documents/2995521/7962764/1-30032017-AP-EN.pdf/4e9c09e5-c743-41a5-afc8-eb4aa89913f6.
Field, A. (2009). *Discovering statistics using SPSS*. London: Sage.
Goode, W. (1960). A theory of role strain. *American Sociological Review, 25,* 483–496.
Hagerty, M., Cummins, R. A., Ferriss, A. B., Land, K., Michalos, A. C., Peterson, M., et al. (2001). Quality of life indexes for national policy: Review and agenda for research. *Social Indicators Research, 55,* 1–96.
Hamnett, C. (1994). Social polarisation in global cities: Theory and evidence. *Urban Studies, 31,* 401–424.
Hamnett, C. (1996). Social polarisation, economic restructuring and welfare state regimes. *Urban Studies, 33,* 1407–1430.
Hirt, S. (2013). Whatever happened to the (post) socialist city? *Cities, 32*, S29–S38.
Hofstede, G. (1984). The cultural relativity of the quality of life concept. *Academy of Management Review, 9*(3), 389–398.
Hosmer, D. W., Lemeshow, S., & Sturdivant, R.X. (2013). *Applied logistic regression*. New York: Wiley.
Ianoș, I., Sîrodoev, I., Pascariu, G., & Henebry, G. (2016). Divergent patterns of built-up urban space growth following post-socialist changes. *Urban Studies, 53*(15), 3172–3188.
IBM Corp. (2011). IBM SPSS Statistic for Window (version 17.0.), IBM Corp, Armonk, New York.
Iojă, C., Pătroescu, M., Niculiță, L., Pavelescu, G., Niță, M., & Iojă, A. (2008). Residential areas with deficient access to urban parks in Bucharest—priority areas for urban rehabilitation. *Environmental Problems and Development*, 71–74.
Kahneman, D., Deiner, D., & Schwarz, N. (Eds.). (1999). *Well-being: The foundations of hedonic psychology*. New York: Russell sage foundation.
Kaklauskas, A., Zavadskas, E. K., Radzeviciene, A., Ubarte, I., Podviezko, A., Podvezko, V., et al. (2018). Quality of city life multiple criteria analysis. *Cities, 72*(2018), 82–93.
Kane, R. A. (2001). Long-term care and a good quality of life: Bringing them closer together. *The Gerontologist, 41,* 293–304.
Lambiri, D., Biagi, B., & Royuela, V. (2007). Quality of life in the economic and urban economic literature. *Social Indicators Research, 2007*(84), 1–25.
Light, D., & Young, C. (2010). Reconfiguring socialist urban landscapes: The 'left-over' spaces of state-socialism in Bucharest. *Journal of Human Geography, 4*(1), 5–16.
Liu, B. C. (1976). *Quality of life indicators in U.S. metropolitan areas: A statistical analysis*. New York: Praeger Publishers.
Marans, R. W. (2003). Understanding environmental quality through quality of life studies: The 2001 DAS and its use of subjective and objective indicators. *Landscape and Urban Planning, 65,* 73–83.
Marcińczak, S., Gentile, M., Rufat, S., & Chelcea, L. (2014). Urban geographies of hesitant transition: Tracing socio-economic segregation in post-Ceausescu Bucharest. *International Journal of Urban and Regional Research, 38*(4), 1399–1417.
Marcuse, P., & van Kempen, R. (2000). *Globalising cities: A new spatial order?*. Oxford: Blackwell.
Marcuse, P., & van Kempen, R. (2002). *Of states and cities: The partitioning of urban space*. Oxford: Oxford University Press.
Mărginean, I. (2004). *Quality of life in Romania*. Bucharest: Expert Publishing.
Mărginean, I., & Bălașa, A. (Eds.). (2004). *Calitatea vieții în România*. București: Editura Expert.
Mărginean, I., & Precupețu, I. (Eds.). (2010). *Diagnoza anuală a calității vieții*. București: Editura Expert.
Massam, B. H. (2002). Quality of life: Public planning and private living. *Progress in Planning, 58,* 141–227.

McCrea, R., Tung-Kai Shyy, Stimson, R. (2006). What is the strength of the link between objective and subjective indicators of urban quality of life? *Applied Research in Quality of Life 1*, 79–96.
McGregor, L. T., & Goldsmith, E. (1998). Expanding our understanding of quality of life, standard of living, and well-being. *Journal of Family and Consumer Sciences, 1998*(90), 2–22.
Mihai, B., Nistor, C., & Simion, G. (2015). Post-socialist growth of Bucharest, Romania—a change detection analysis on Landsat imagery (1984–2010). *Acta Geographica Slovenica, 55*(2), 223–234.
Ministerul Dezvoltării Regionale și Administrației Publice/MDRAP. (2017). *Strategia națională a locuirii*. București. Retrieved October 30, 2017, from http://mdrap.ro/comunicare/presa/comunicate/mdrap-analizeaza-propunerile-primite-in-dezbaterea-publica-privind-strategia-locuirii.
Myers, D. (1987). Internal monitoring of quality of life for economic development. *Economic Development Quarterly, 1*, 268–278.
Myers, D. (1988). Building Knowledge about quality of life for urban planning. *American Planning Association Journal of the American Association, 54*(3), 347–358.
Myers, D. G., & Diener, E. (1995). Who is happy? *Psychological Science, 6* (1), 10–19.
Nae, M. (2006). *Geografia calităţii vieţii urbane*. Metode de analiză: Editura Universitară, Bucureşti.
Nae, M. (2009). *Municipiul București—dezvoltare urbană și calitatea vieții*. București: Editura Universitară. [in Romanian].
Nae, M. (2014). Le système de santé et sa réforme: représentations dans le cyberespace. In Anna Krasteva et Despina Vasilcu (Eds.), *Migration en blanc. Medecins d'est en ouest* (pp. 45–65). Paris L'Harmattan, coll. Global & Local.
Nae, M., & Erdeli, G. (2008). La ville de Bucarest, espace de (post)transition entre restructuration et étalement urbain, *Méditerranée, revue géographique des pays méditerranéens, Bulgarie - Roumanie – les nouveaux horizons de l'Union Européenne*, Editions de la Maison Méditerranéene des Sciences de l'Homme, Aix en Provence, 110/2008, 55–63.
Nae, M., & Turnock, D. (2011). The new Bucharest: Two decades of restructuring. *Cities. The International of Urban Planning, 28*(2), 206–219.
Nagelkerke N. J. D. (1991). A note on a general definition of the coefficient of determination. *Biometrika, 78*(3), 691–2.
National Institute of Statistics. (2014). Coordonate ale nivelului de trai în România. *Veniturile și consumul populației*. Retrieved December 3, 2017, from http://www.insse.ro/cms/en/content/household-income-and-expenditure.
National Institute of Statistics. (2018). *Tempo online statistics*. Retrieved December 28, 2017, from http://statistici.insse.ro/shop/?lang=en.
Numbeo. (2012). *Europe*: *Quality of life index 2012*. Retrieved September 3, 2017, from https://www.numbeo.com/qualityof-life/region_rankings.jsp?title=2012-Q1&region=150.
Numbeo. (2013). *Europe: Quality of life index 2013*. Retrieved September 3, 2017, from https://www.numbeo.com/qualityof-life/region_rankings.jsp?title=2013-Q1&region=150.
Numbeo. (2014). *Europe: Quality of life index 2014*. Retrieved September 3, 2017, from https://www.numbeo.com/qualityof-life/region_rankings.jsp?title=2014&region=150.
OECD. (2011). Compendium of OECD well-being indicators. *Technical report, OECD better life initiative*. www.oecdbetterlifeindex.org.
Orru, K., Orru, H., Maasikmets, M., Hendrikson, R., & Ainsaar, M. (2016). Well-being and environmental quality: Does pollution affect life satisfaction? *Quality Life Research, 25*(3), 699–705.
Pacione, M. (1982). The use of objective and subjective measures of life quality in human geography. *Progress in Human Geography, 6*(4), 495–514.
Pacione, M. (2003). Quality-of-life research in urban geography. *Urban Geography, 24*(4), 314–339.
Phillips, D. (2006). *Quality of life: Concept*. Routledge, USA: Policy and Practice.
Rapley, M. (2003). *Quality of life research. A critical introduction*. London: Sage Publications.
Romania Regional Development Programm and World Bank. (2015). *Către o strategie națională în domeniul locuirii*. Armonizarea investițiilor publice. Componenta 4. Raport Final.

Romice, O., Thwaites, K., Porta, S., Greaves, M., Barbour, G., & Pasino, P. (2017). Urban design and quality of life. In G. Fleury-Bahi, E. Pol, & O. Navarro (Eds.), *Handbook of environmental psychology and quality of life research. International handbooks of quality-of-life*. Cham: Springer.

Rosenberg, R. (1995). Health-related quality of life between naturalism and hermeneutics. *Social Science and Medicine, 41,* 1411–1415.

Rowley, A. (1998). Private—property decision makers and the quality of urban design. *Journal of Urban Design., 3*(2), 151–173.

Smith, T. J., & McKenna, C. M. (2013). A comparison of logistic regression pseudo R2 indices. *Multiple Linear Regression Viewpoints, 39*(2), 17–25.

Spicer, J. (ed.) (2005). *Logistic regression and discriminant analysis* (pp. 123–151). Sage: Making Sense of Multivariate Data.

Sprangers, M. A. G., & Schwartz, C. E. (1999). Integrating response shift into health-related quality of life research: A theoretical model. *Social Science and Medicine, 48,* 1507–1515.

Streimikiene, D. (2015). Environmental indicators for the assessment of quality of life. *Intellectual Economics, 9*(1), 67–79.

Siemens, A.G. (2012). European Green City Index. A summary of the Green City Index research series. http://www.siemens.com/press/pool/de/events/2012/corporate/2012-06-rio20/GCI-Report-e.pdf

Suditu, B. (2009). Urban sprawl and residential mobilities in the Bucharest area—reconfiguration of a new residential geography. *Human Geographies. Journal of Studies and Research in Human Geography, 3*(2), 79–93.

Suditu, B. (2011). *Mobilități și strategii rezidențiale urbane și periurbane. Studiu de caz - București.* București: Editura Universității din București.

Suditu, B., Nae, M., Neguţ, S., Dumitrache, L., & Gheorghilaş, A. (2014a). Suburban landscapes in Romania: From 'forting- up' to 'informal- up' and limits of public action. *European Journal of Science and Theology, 10*(5), 125–138.

Suditu, B., Dumitrache, L., Vârdol, D., & Vâlceanu, D-G. (2014b). New trajectories of post-socialist residential mobility in Bucharest. *Human Geographies. Journal of Studies and Research in Human Geography, 8*(1), 75–82.

Sudman, S., & Bradburn, N. (1982). *Asking questions: A practical guide to questionnaire design.* San Francisco, California: Jossey-Bass Inc.

Tammaru, T., Marcińczak, S., Van Ham, M., & Musterd, S. (2016). *Socio-economic segregation in European Capital Cities: East meets West.* London: Routledge.

Thorton, M., & Travis, S. S. (2003). Analysis of the reliability of the modified caregiver strain index. *Journal of Gerontology, 58B*(2), S127–S132; The Gerontological Society of America.

Tuvikene, T. (2016). Strategies for comparative urbanism: Post-socialism as a de-territorialized concept. *International Journal of Urban and Regional Research, 40,* 132–146.

Zamfir, C. (2014). Romania, quality of life. In A. C. Michalos (Ed.), *Encyclopedia of quality of life and well-being research* (pp. 243–311). Dordrecht: Springer.

Zamfir, D., Dumitrache, L., Stoica, I.-L., & Vîrdol, D. (2015). Spatial inequalities in health care provision in Romania: Milestones for territorial sustainable development. *Carpathian Journal of Earth and Environmental Sciences, 10*(3), 177–188.

Chapter 25
Transformation of Urban Land Use from Traditionality to Modernity—A Study of the Old Shanghai Town and Its Creek Landscape from Quality of Life Perspective

Jun-Fan Wu

Abstract Transformation or change in land use is directly or indirectly related to the sociocultural aspects of people and in turn affects the quality of life. Transformation of urban land use greatly affects land cover, agricultural land, demographic characteristics, environment, and urban landscape particularly in rural–urban fringe area. These play a significant role and assist the policy-makers, planners, and practitioners in improving the quality of life of people by making balance between urbanization and living environment in space and time. So far as the study of historical land use is concerned, much of the fruit produced by Chinese scholars concentrate on the rural style of land use, while the urban style is scarcely treated of; this has some relationship with the minor status of ancient Chinese cities in a powerful agricultural economy and life condition of people. This paper takes the Old Shanghai Town, a city located on the eastern edge of the Yangtze Delta, for a detailed case study. It deals with a transitional period between tradition and modernity, but other periods are also referred to when necessary from quality of life perspective. The author tries to explain the connection between the mode of urban land use and regional environment and also aims to find out the natural and social factors that affect urban land use and quality of life of the inhabitants. The conclusion is that while factors such as experiences, new concepts, and the regional environment all have an effect on urban land use, the basic and permanent one is the regional environment and its restricting power. Besides, to understand the "transformation" properly is also important to the studies in urban land use toward quality of life in modern China.

Keywords Change · Land use · Regional environment · Shanghai · Urban

J.-F. Wu (✉)
Shanghai Normal University, Shanghai, China
e-mail: 051039004@fudan.edu.cn

B. R. K. Sinha (ed.), *Multidimensional Approach to Quality of Life Issues*,
https://doi.org/10.1007/978-981-13-6958-2_25

25.1 Introduction

Land cover is considered to be a good interface between humans and nature, so its changing course and history can provide many illustrations for global environmental studies, and help to unfold the story of the evolution of human society and its driving forces. The International Social Science Council (ISSC) set up the Human Dimensions Programme (HDP) in 1990, in which the Land Use and Cover Change (LUCC) was the major concern. The plan of LUCC, aiming to discover some patterns of environmental change on a global scale and the relevant human-nature interactive system, soon became a hot subject in the academic circles. In 1996, the LUCC plan was again pinned down as the main task in both IGBP (International Geosphere Programme) and IHDP (International Human Dimensions Programme on Global Environmental Change). Nowadays, this topic is being attended by researchers from wider academic fields.

To approach the final aim of the LUCC plan, the study of different historical periods and geographic regions is urgently needed. This is the prerequisite for success and also the most difficult part of the whole program. Chinese scholars, utilizing the rich and well-preserved historical records, have already contributed much to the studies in the land use change in history. However, much fruit in this area concentrates on the rural style of land use, while the urban style is scarcely treated of, and that has some relationship with the minor status of ancient Chinese cities in a powerful agricultural economy. As to the previous defects, Professor Man Zhi-min, organized the research program on Chinese historical land use change in the Institute of Historical Geography Studies of Furman University, suggests that the urban style research can start from the cities with typical ecological characteristics. He believes that to choose the right urban objects is a vital step, and that to connect particular natural conditions with their social environment is equally important. Following Professor Man's idea, this paper takes the Old Shanghai Town, a city located on the eastern edge of the famous Yangtze Delta, for a detailed case study. It deals with a transitional period between tradition and modernity, but other periods are also referred to when necessary.

25.2 Problems to Be Solved

In this paper, "traditional age" is differentiated from "modern age" by the year of 1843, when Shanghai was opened to foreigners as a trading port, and this division is well received in the field of Shanghai studies.

"The Old Shanghai Town" in this paper refers to the usual title for the central town of Shanghai County since the late Qing Dynasty, as opposed to the new urban area built by the Foreign Settlement on the north. In 1927, Shanghai County was promoted to the status of city under the direct jurisdiction of the central government, while the original urban area was expanding, the name of the Old Shanghai Town continued to be used in memory of the original part of this city. The Town covered not only the administrative, business, residential districts surrounded by the rampart, but also the trade and port region outside the Eastern City Gate along the Huang-pu River. Located on the eastern edge of the Yangtze Delta, which is famous for the network of creeks and canals, the town of Shanghai was once called "a city of water." The interlaced creeks served as "the vital resources for living," with respect to transportation, drinking, cleaning, drainage, fire fighting, etc. Creeks, especially the tidal one, protect its adjacent lands from flooding and the scenic vistas and enhance property value and quality of life of people inhabiting the area. In fact, creeks are the sources of different types of resources which in turn help enhance quality of life of the inhabitants.

According to the gazettes of Shanghai County during the Ming and Qing Dynasties, the structure of the creek network in the Town remained stable after the year 1553, when the rampart was first built to protect citizens from Japanese invaders. Later, two changes occurred: (1) a new floodgate called Little Southern Gate, besides the old ones, was opened in 1598, so that the Xue-jia Creek within the city was connected with the Huang-pu River outside; (2) one more city gate was added to the northern part of the rampart to help resist Li Xiu-cheng's soldiers, a troop of the Heavenly Kingdom of Great Peace. These changes, however, had little effect on the whole creek system. In the city, numerous canals and bridges were still the most spectacular sight, "with the interlaced creeks leading to almost every house." Such urban sight remained until late Qing, as is shown in Fig. 25.1, which is based on a map in *The Official History of Shanghai County* (the 11th year of the Tong-zhi Period of the Qing Dynasty, i.e., 1872).

In the 1872 Issue of *Shanghai Gazette*, the layout of creeks in the city was described in detail:

The Zhao-jia Creek is the largest trunk canal in this city. It connects with the Huang-pu River beyond the Eastern Gate, where the tide enters and runs westward via many smaller canals in the city, and finally empties into the Pu-hui Creek. Under the Deng-yun Bridge near the center of the city ran another main branch called Core Creek, flowing south off the trunk canal via the Xi-cang Bridge and the Ning-he Bridge.

The Fang Creek is another Trunk River, which also connects with the Huang-pu River and takes in the tide from the west. Under the Xi-ma Bridge the trunk separates into two main branches: one goes northward and empties into the Lou-xiang Park Lake; the other runs southwest and joins the Zhao-jia Creek. The Hou-jia Creek is also a big branch of the trunk, and because it runs through the Hei-qiao Bridge, it is habitually called Hei-qiao Creek.

From the above citation, we know that the Zhao-jia Creek, the Fang Creek, the Core Creek, the Hou-jia Creek, and the Hei-qiao Creek were backbones of the canal network in the Town. However, toward the end of the Qing Dynasty (from 1905 onward), there came a sharp turn in the use of these creeks: they were filled up one after another and at the same time wide roads were built on them, which is considered to be a sign for the Town's modernization by later generations. By the year 1917, only a small number of creeks remained (see Fig. 25.2).

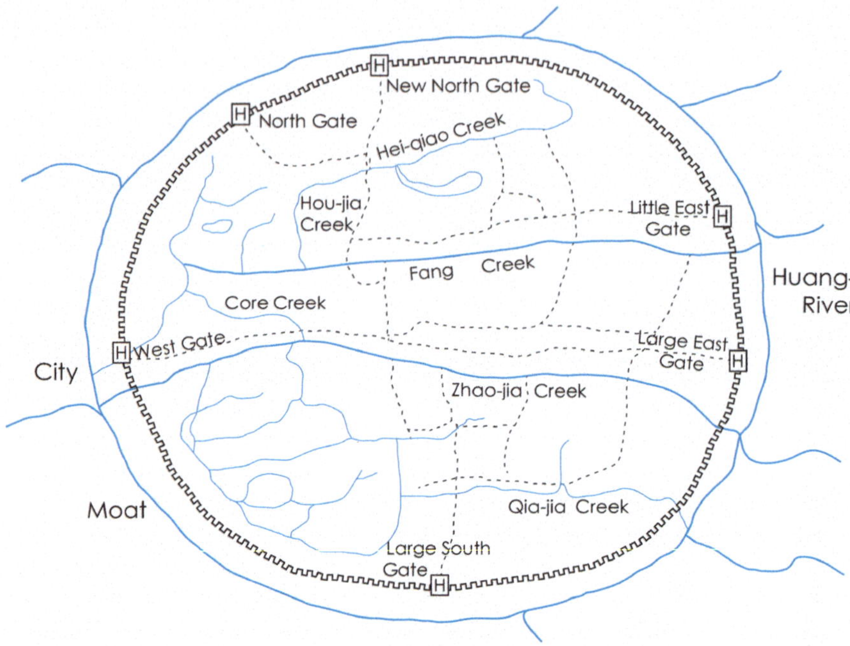

Fig. 25.1 The structure of the creek network (the blue lines) in the Old Town in the traditional period

There was so big a change in the landscape that it greatly influenced the town's history and attracted a great deal of attention then. The Town Planning Bureau, a semi-official institution at that time, announced that most creeks were filthy and dirty, just like open sewers, and that they should be filled up as soon as possible. Shortly the Chancellor of Shanghai County announced to the public on March 24th, 1906.

Most creeks in the Town have been too foul and dirty, and things are even worse when summer comes. Lots of diseases have been brought up by the creek water. This leads to depreciate health and health-related quality of life. In view of this, we have decided to fill up the Hei-qiao Creek now, which is the worst of all.

In fact, a review in *Shanghai City Paper* (the most famous newspaper in Shanghai at the time) on July 7th, 1905, had pleaded to the government urgently: "Since the creeks have become so odorous, all the citizens hope that the government will immediately take some measures."

It can easily be found that all the quotations cited above focus on the natural conditions of the creeks, which were thought to be harmful to the local people's health and well-being. Today, most scholars who are doing researches in the historical development of the city praise the filling of creeks and road building at the beginning of the twentieth century as the fruit of modernization. They believe that this greatly improved the economic environment of the Old Shanghai Town; but they have not made a more intensive investigation into the changes and effects this has caused to

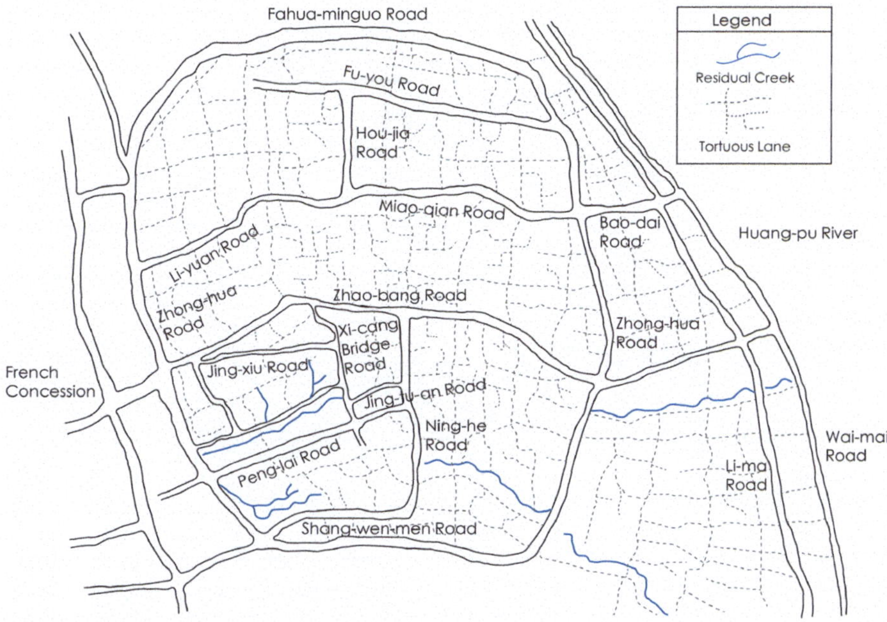

Fig. 25.2 The remaining creeks (the blue lines) and the newly built broad roads (the black double line) in the town. ("…" indicates the numerous walking lanes in the town.)

the natural environment. In fact, the filling of creeks indicates a turn in the land use typical of the areas south of the lower reaches of the Yangtze River, and thus calls for an elaborate study of the entire history of land use and the change-determining factors. This paper studies a typical case in the Old Shanghai Town and attempts to make some contributions to the LUCC program, which is now carried out in many parts of the world.

25.3 The Role of Human Factors in the Urban Landscape

In the landscape of the Old Shanghai Town before the end of the nineteenth century, two features were most noticeable: one was the interlaced creeks, which served for transportation, drainage, and other daily activities of the local people; the other one was the narrow walking lanes. The transportation of goods relied on larger creeks, but not the lanes, as was often the case with cities in the areas south of the lower reaches of the Yangtze River.

A map of the Old Shanghai Town in 1898 first attracted attention because the lanes in the map look so narrow and circuitous that they can hardly be distinguished from the creeks. So, we were inspired to investigate the history of the old lanes and creeks (Fig. 25.3).

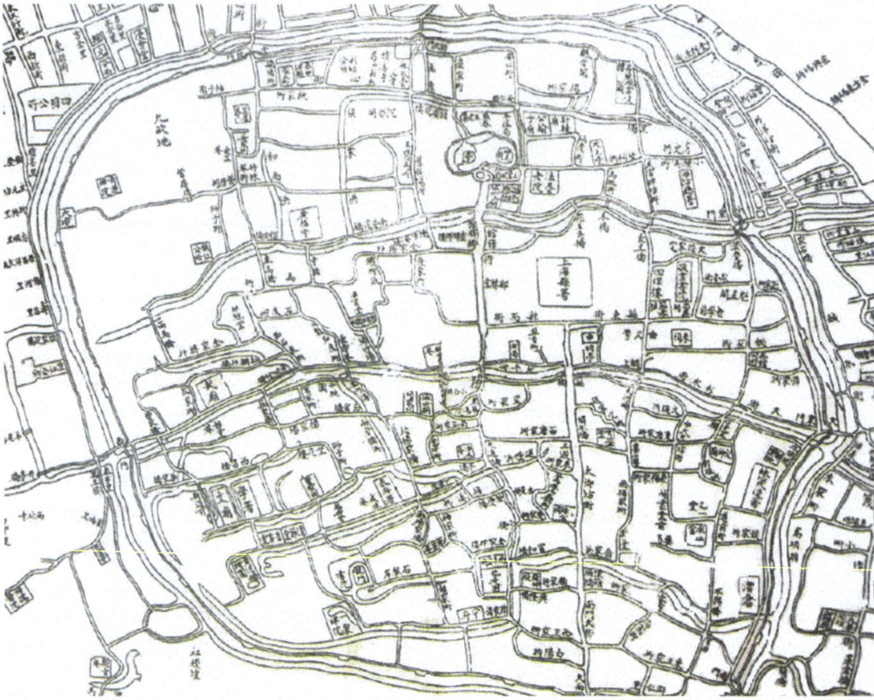

Fig. 25.3 The map of creeks and lanes of the Old Shanghai Town in 1898. (This map was taken from *Maps of Old Shanghai during the past 150 years*, Shanghai Pictorial Press, 2001, pp. 16–17.)

In order to explain this phenomenon, the following more maps were studied to make the following analysis.

According to Fig. 25.4a, b, the geographical transformation from creeks to lanes can be clearly seen, and this helps to explain why the lanes of this city looked so similar in shape to the creeks. But there is still a problem: the abovementioned case happened between 1910 and 1917, when the officially planned creek-filling movement since 1906 was proceeding, and so this transformation will possibly be understood as the fruit of modernization characterized by the flooding Western ideas in China after the mid-nineteenth century. Therefore, it is necessary to seek more evidence from the lanes in a longer period.

The old South Hong-qiao Lane and the Tai-ping Lane, built during the early Qing Dynasty with the age of nearly 200 years, lay in the downtown area. If we compare them with the creeks in Fig. 25.5b lying in the countryside, a big similarity in shape can be noticed. Although the area in Fig. 25.5b was part of the French Settlement in 1917, it remained rural because the foreigners did not develop it. So it is reasonable to conclude: the creek net in Fig. 25.5b can be seen as the reduction of the whole creek system of this area, which was created by local people for agriculture from the Northern Song Dynasty. The Old Shanghai Town, which had been serving as

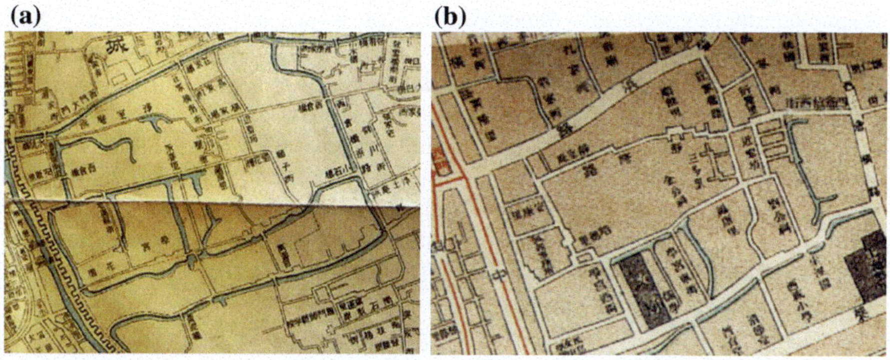

Fig. 25.4 **a** (left) The net of the creeks inside the Western City Gate of the Old Shanghai Town in 1910. (From *Maps of Old Shanghai during the past 150 years*, pp. 14–15.) **b** (right) the net of the lanes in the same area in 1917. (From *Maps of Old Shanghai during the past 150 years*, pp. 70–71.)

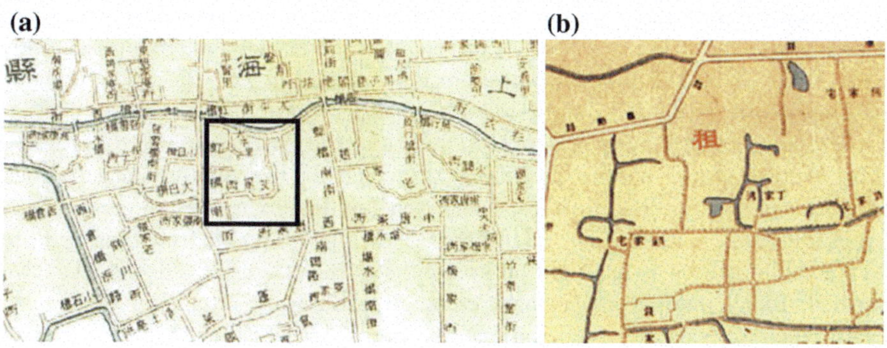

Fig. 25.5 **a** (left) The old South Hong-qiao Lane and the Tai-ping Lane. (From *Maps of Old Shanghai during the past 150 years*, pp. 14–15.) **b** (right) the creeks in the western suburb of the Old Shanghai Town in 1917. (From *Maps of Old Shanghai during the past 150 years*, pp. 44–45.)

the capital of Shanghai County since the early Yuan Dynasty, gradually expanded to such a rural land with interlaced creeks. Now the answer seems clear: the older lanes in downtown were also probably built on creeks, and that is why they looked so similar.

The preceding conclusions are mostly drawn from the maps, and then we will turn to another approach. It can be seen in Figs. 25.4a and 25.5b that most of the creeks ran alongside with the footpaths. Is there any relationship between these paths alongside the creeks and the lanes we have studied in the previous paragraphs? In order to find out the answer, we have to go on to research the earliest history of the paths. On such low and wet country land as the Yangtze Delta, farms, since the Tang Dynasty, had been developed after the *wei* pattern for the special geographical environment. *Wei* was a large piece of farmland encircled by canals used for drainage and irrigation, with a few smaller ditches dividing the farm into many parts inside.

The smaller ditches were all connected with the canals around and farther with natural creeks. Farmers built ditches for irrigation and banks along the canals for farm protection; they also made repairs to the banks from time to time. The banks served as the footpaths, the most convenient walking passage for the people there. The Old Shanghai Town was built on such rural land covered with canals and creeks, so the function of the rural paths began to change with the expansion of the city. The city people came, leveled the farmland, and widened the footpaths, changing the rural land into a commercial area. As to the canals or creeks along the footpaths, they widened and deepened the larger ones for transportation, and the smaller ones were used for urban drainage and everyday life. In this way, footpaths and creeks became a typical landscape of the Old Shanghai Town. Today in some towns in the Yangtze Delta, such a landscape is still very common. But now the problem is: how did the creeks beside the paths disappear whereas only the lanes remained?

The main reason lies in people's invading and occupying the creek land. With the population of the city growing, more commercial and residential space was needed. As a public resource, the creek land best satisfied individuals' needs for space. Since the creeks were not labeled anybody's private estate, everyone thought himself entitled to some of it. The following passage is quoted from *The Official History* of *Song-jiang Region* (the Jia-qing Period of the Qing Dynasty).

There are a great number of people in this city, who are accustomed to throwing rubbish into the creeks, because they think the creek bed is the cost-free and capacious space for holding rubbish. Besides, many rich families living on the creek banks always invade the river for more useful land. They first fill up the river little by little and then build houses on the filled-up part of the river. As a result, a few creeks have vanished. Today, many ill effects have come up. Little water remains in the creeks, because the riverbeds are blocked up and elevated by rubbish and people have not enough water for living. When the rainstorm comes, large quantities of rainwater cannot be drained away due to the shallowness of the riverbed, so the city often suffers from flood. In summer when it is so hot that the rubbish in the creek gives off very bad smells, people always get sick. When a fire breaks out, the creek cannot offer enough water for putting it out, so many houses will be reduced to smoking ashes. All these increase vulnerability of creeks which ultimately leads to potential property depreciation and lessens quality of life of communities. So, it is important for the local governments as well as local inhabitants and the whole communities to maintain and improve health of the existing creeks with a view to maintain health and overall quality of life people.

According to the writer, the quotation above refers to the condition of the creeks during the Wan-li Period of the Ming Dynasty (the period immediately before the founding of the Qing Dynasty), so it can be judged that invasion and occupation of the creeks had become a common illegal phenomenon when the Old Shanghai Town began its development and expansion. The main driving force is that the city, as a trading center in the eastern Yangtze Delta, was too crowded and people were always thirsty for more land because the leveled land was more precious for city people than for country people. In the countryside, creeks were as valuable as the farmland, because the agriculture of this area depended largely on these creeks; while in the city, smaller creeks, except for their function as drainage systems, did not seem that useful and naturally became people's objects of desire for private occupation. And only larger creeks were well kept both by the government and by citizens for the purposes of transportation, drinking, washing clothes, etc.

Now it is easy to understand the relationship between the paths along creeks and the lanes without creeks beside. If people valued both the creek and the path along it, this land use pattern, typical of this area, would be maintained; when people thought some smaller creeks to be less useful, they would gradually change them into urban constructive land and walking passages. The process of the disappearance of the creeks demonstrates the spatial growth of the Old Shanghai Town, and it can be called the typical pattern of urban land use in the areas south of the lower reaches of the Yangtze River.

But a problem still calls for explanation. That is, why did the government not stop the citizens from invading the creeks since it was public resources? Actually, according to various literature texts of Shanghai County, the government was all along strongly against the invasion of the creeks and had never ceased to afflict punishment on such behavior. However, the result was not that satisfactory. The main reason for that has been analyzed above, which is related to people's continuous needs for urban land. But if the government had taken measures severe enough, the citizens' invasion of creek land could have been brought under control. But why did creeks keep vanishing? Why were more and more lanes and houses built up? And why this urban land use pattern continued to the beginning of the twentieth century? In order to answer these questions, we have to turn to the natural features of the creeks in this area.

25.4 The Role of Natural Factors in Land Use Patterns

The historical records of Shanghai County often contain the following descriptions of the natural features of its creeks:

The lower reaches of the Wu-song River (one of the most important rivers in the Yangtze Delta) tend to become stagnant with the silt brought in by tides, because it is close to the mouth of the Yangtze River and the Yellow Sea. The land here is higher than the upper reaches (the area around the Tai-hu Lake), so it is hard for the silt to be rushed into the sea. As a result, all the branch creeks connected with the Wu-song River are also filled with tide silt, and soon they will become stagnant and need dredging. If these creeks cannot be dredged in time, the crops will be badly damaged by drought or flood sooner or later and successively this situation will harm the prosperity and quality of life.

Shanghai County just lies at the lower reaches of the Wu-song River; as its land is higher than that at the upper reaches, the silt brought in by tides blocked not only the creeks of the rural area, but also those in and around the city. Thus, the blocked riverbed will become shallow and narrow and unable to keep enough water. But these creeks depend much on tides for water renewal, with the freshwater from the mouth of the Yangtze River coming up and the dirty water from the city flushed away. If the creeks were seriously silted up and polluted, tides could not go up and down smoothly and the rubbish would not be easily carried away. A record about the Kang-xi Period of the Qing Dynasty (from *The Official History of Song-jiang Region*) describes the tidal effect upon the urban creeks in detail:

The creeks such as the Zhao-jia Creek, the moats, and many other smaller ditches are all vital resources for the people in the city, but now they are badly blocked with tide silt and rubbish. When the tide ebbs, there is no water but mud left in the riverbed. This reduction in the value of creeks encourages the citizens to illegally snatch more land by filling up parts of the creeks. Now it is much difficult to get the creeks back to its original condition. The Chancellor of Shanghai County is trying to have the creeks dredged, and he orders the houses built on the riverbed to be removed immediately. Besides, it is also suggested that all the creeks and ditches should be dredged and cleansed at the same time, because they are connected to each other and any one stagnant will affect the water running in others. For example, if the moat remains uncleansed, it will be no use cleansing the Zhao-jia Creek; and if the Zhao-jia Creek remains uncleansed, tide cannot reach any other smaller creeks or ditches.

The natural features of the creeks combined with the local people's illegal invasion and occupation made it very hard to do creek dredging and restoration. Every few years, the government would invest a great deal of money and labor in creek restoration, but could not achieve the desired effect. This was not only connected with the citizen's benefit-seeking actions, but also with the creeks' tendency to get stagnant and foul. If more people threw rubbish into the creeks, the whole creek system would soon become silted and filthy. When a creek's condition was too bad to maintain, even the government would agree to fill it up to increase the space for civil building. Compared to the reason given in the previous text, this is a better explanation to the history of winding lanes in the city, and it also better explains why the urban land use mode south of the Yangtze River can continue all through. It is known that Shanghai was opened as a trading port to foreigners in 1843, and since then Western ideas and new economic concepts have entered this traditional city and brought about great changes in many social fields. But as regards the traditional mode of creek use, did any obvious changes occur immediately? Did the double factors, i.e., the natural features of the creeks and people's illegal invasion still function? Especially how did the natural factors function? We will approach this problem by using the materials from William Lockhart's *The Medical Missionary in China: A Narrative of Twenty Years' Experience*. Lockhart was a missionary from England, and stayed in Shanghai for a long time; he later wrote down what he learnt about China and published this book in 1861. He wrote:

This city is scattered with numerous creeks, and people here use boats for travel and transportation. All the creeks depend much on tide, because tides raise the water level in the riverbed twice every day. But almost all the branch creeks have got somewhat silted because people always throw rubbish into them, as a result of this, tide cannot run smoothly, the creek water cannot be cleansed and is getting odorous. Last spring the Chancellor ordered all the creeks to be dredged completely in order to improve transportation and sanitation, and soon great deal of silt was taken out of the riverbed and then piled on the banks(Lockhart 38).

Obviously, both human factors and natural factors receive much attention from Lockhart. He points out that the worsening of the creek water was caused by the joint work of the two factors. In fact, Lockhart's description is not essentially different from the records in the past local newspapers. All this proves that the traditional problems with the creeks persisted even after the opening-up of Shanghai to foreigners.

However, with the population growing fast, the status of creeks changed soon. A piece of news from *Shanghai City Paper* on March 23, 1876 can serve as a telltale proof.

Since it was opened as a trading port, Shanghai has been a busier city, with crowds of people swarming into this small town every day. Those who come to Shanghai for business surely also like to do some sightseeing, and so all the main streets and famous sites such as the Hong-qiao Lane, the North Gate Lane, the Old Training Ground, Si-pai-lou, etc. are always full of people that the road stones have been trampled smooth. When it rains, people tend to fall over because of the wet and slippery ground. The condition of the creek water has declined much owing to the rubbish thrown into the creeks and the illegal occupation on the part of the citizens. Even if the tide comes every day, its cleansing power is getting weaker. Anyway the creek water has become too foul and odorous to serve as drinking water, and even not fit for other uses. So, there is need for paying attention to improve the overall health of the creeks from the point of view of social well-being.

This piece of news emphasizes the degeneration of the natural condition of the creek caused by the growing population and the excessive use. As a result, most creeks in the town were going from bad to worse. When people used creeks more powerfully, the natural condition of the creeks became worse. That is just how humans and natural power worked together on the creeks after this city's opening-up, which was somewhat the same as in earlier historical periods.

But it should be pointed out that the condition of the creek was going bad faster after Shanghai's opening-up, which brought about more inconveniences to citizens' daily life. According to another piece of news from *Shanghai City Paper* on May 19, 1876, every day when the tide came up, people had to walk a long distance to the Huang-pu River outside the Eastern Gate in order to get drinking water, because the water in the creeks within the city was not at all fit for drinking. There were so many people carrying water on the trunk roads that the road surface got too wet and muddy owing to the water spilt from buckets. The muddy road caused many people to fall over and some even got killed in such petty accidents. At that time, fires frequently broke out because most houses were made from wood, but people had no water to put out the fire if the tide could not bring enough water. The riverbed was shallow, and the creek water, dirty and stagnant, was in small quantity. Some people fell ill after drinking the creek water. Up to the beginning of the twentieth century, even the government considered some of the creeks to be "waste ditches," which were of little use to anyone.

With the human and natural factors working together, the problem of the stagnation and sanitation of the creeks had become very serious by the beginning of the twentieth century. The local government had no choice but to seek an effective way to ameliorate the present state. In the past, the usual measure was to dredge the trunk creeks as well as some branch ones to clear a smooth passage for the tide, for which the official did not hesitate to spend much money and labor. However, this time there came a sharp turn in dealing with the whole matter. With the local government's approval and the effort of the wealthy people in the town, within a period as short as a year, most of the trunk creeks were filled up and roads were built on them. The change of the urban landscape, slow for many years, was now being accelerated, and the previously forbidden action of filling up the creek was eventually approved by the government. The speed of the change in the urban landscape of the Old Shanghai Town in 1905 and the contributing factors should attract more attention from scholars. That is exactly why we will focus on the new concepts of social mechanism brought in by foreigners, and the resultant influence on the environment of the Old Shanghai Town in the following section. Obviously, the research only on the traditional factors is not enough.

25.5 The Influence of the Modern Concepts from the West

Such factors as people's illegal occupation of the creek land, a large population polluting the creek water, and the creeks' own natural features can all be regarded as the routine factors contributing to the change of the creek system in the Old Shanghai Town. They played their parts all through the traditional period of this city, and hence the formation of the traditional mode of creek use. But some new factors, rising with the transformation of society, can sometimes exceed all the usual factors. Therefore, Western concepts that came with the foreign settlement in the Old Shanghai Town after the opening-up of Shanghai should be duly noticed. There are two influential concepts of the creek land use: one is the building of roads under municipal management (in the past, lanes in the Old Shanghai Town mostly came into being naturally or built by some wealthy gentries, and there was no special municipal institution in charge of road building); the other is the modern concept of public health.

After the opening-up of Shanghai to foreigners, the idea of building wider roads just as those in the foreign settlement was soon appreciated by people of the Old Shanghai Town; but it was too difficult to carry out. The urban land was so precious, the houses were so crowded, and the lanes were so narrow that no space could be spared for wider roads. Although a semi-official municipal institution, modeled upon its Western counterpart, was set up in the 1890s, the only thing they could do was punish the lane and creek invaders. The few lanes that had been broadened were only three meters wide. In 1906, the government at last agreed to fill up waste creeks and build roads on them, and actually it was due to the influence of the Western concept of public health.

In the latter half of the nineteenth century, the West, with the series discoveries of pathogenic bacteria, was experiencing an era of bacteria in the field of public health. The westerners in the settlement of Shanghai believed that the polluted water in creeks or wells could cause cholera and other dangerous epidemics. In 1883, the foreigners in the settlement purified the river water and produced clean running water for drinking. Of course, the people in the Old Shanghai Town soon learnt about the new health concept, and then they began to doubt the cleanness of the creek water. Between the 1860s and the 1870s, even ordinary people would know that the dirty creek water could cause illness. Lots of the articles in *Shanghai City Paper* were about the sanitation of the creeks and expressed great concern about public health and public quality of life. For example, a report in the December of 1881 said appallingly: the water in the moat and other creeks was as dirty as that in a sewer, and so the government was under an obligation to widen and deepen the riverbed immediately as well as to punish the creek land invaders. Otherwise, more and more people would fall ill after drinking the creek water. The sanitation of the creeks was an old problem that the citizens of Shanghai had to face. And in the 1880s, the government began to seek other means to solve the problem other than the old ways of dredging and cleansing the creek. To imitate the practice of producing running water in the foreign settlement was the most important measure.

In fact, long before the running water program was completed in the settlement, the people of the Old Shanghai Town had planned to learn from the foreign practice. A proposal in *Shanghai City Paper* on December 5, 1873 says:

I know the foreign settlement is preparing for setting up a running water system, but I don't know why the plan ceased recently. If the running water plan cannot succeed in the settlement for certain reasons, it doesn't matter. After all, the roads there are broad enough for people carrying river water to walk on. But it's a great pity that the Old Shanghai Town has no running water, and the lanes here are too narrow. When people are carrying water from the river, the water spilt turns the lane wet and muddy, which is troublesome for walkers. If the running water system is set up in the Old Shanghai Town, people will get clean water easily and do not have to go outside the city in order to get purer water.

The government also made a good effort to carry out this program. In 1876, a man was sent to Hong Kong to learn the techniques. At last in 1902, the Old Shanghai Town built up its own running water system. Up to 1904, there had been 5700 families in the town depending on running water for living.

With the water system drawing plentiful clean water from the Huang-pu River, the traditional value of the creeks declined drastically, because people would no longer depend on creek water for drinking. At the same time, whenever a fire broke out, running water could be conveniently obtained to put it out, and was never restricted by the tide. So now the potential value of creek land began to be better recognized than that of creek water. There were two options. If people were willing to invest money in developing the land occupied by creeks, the reclaimed land could be used for urban construction immediately, for example, widening the narrow lanes and constructing wider roads. If people let them be, the dirty creeks would just lie there as a hotbed of diseases, and would get even dirtier because no more money would be invested in the dredging. It was under such a condition that in 1905 some local gentries held a meeting to discuss how to collect money from local businesses in order to fill up some odorous creeks and to improve the sanitation of the city. They hated dirty creeks and wanted to improve them for the public good; but they had no right to decide how to deal with the land occupied by the creeks, which had been regarded as official. In March 1906, the Chancellor of Shanghai County at last announced that the filled land from the waste creeks could be used for constructing wider roads and widening the old lanes. The document says:

Chancellor Wang has issued the following decree: because most of the creeks in the town have got foul and silted, in which the tide can not run smoothly, they are no longer useful and are a hotbed of diseases especially in hot weather. Now you are authorized to fill up the Hei-qiao Creek first, the most odorous one. But before filling up the creeks, you must cleanse the riverbed by using concrete pipes of one-meter diameter wide for drainage. And then you can fill up the creek and pave the surface. Besides, you will also have much difficulty in removing so many crowded houses built over the creek; so you can seek help from the chief administrative officer. The Chancellor hopes that this project can proceed successfully with broader roads and flourishing businesses.

The movement of creek-filling sanctioned by the local government at last started. In the past, the creek land had not been allowed for private occupation, but now the government took the initiative to turn it into urban construction land. It was really a remarkable transformation of the pattern in creek use in the Old Shanghai Town. It seemed that the Western concept of public health played a catalytic role. When people were seeking a solution to the sanitation problem of the creeks, the idea of public health met their requirements. Soon they solved the problem by creating clean running water, which diminished one of the most important values of the creeks. Then the creeks that were regarded as useless were filled up. This can be considered to be a special choice at the transitional period of society. But for the influence of the foreign concept, the original mode of creek use would have been continued. While on the other hand, the foreign concept would not have played its role without the long historical accumulation in nature and in human society. That is to say, the traditional factors would have kept their functions, whether or not the external factors had come in. When the new factor joined in, the speed of the creek system transformation got higher.

Through 1 year's worth of engineering work, the urban landscape was greatly changed. A few new roads were constructed on the former creek land such as Fu-you Road, Hou-jia Road, Peng-lai Road, Ning-he Road, etc., which were broader and tidier than so many other old lanes in the city.

25.6 New Environmental Problems After the Trunk Creeks Were Filled Up

The creek-filling and road-building, which were initiated by the Western concept of public health, actually satisfied people's needs for the improved sanitation of the creeks; but the citizens soon found that there seemed no end to the movement. Not only did the trunk creeks in the Town such as Hei-qiao Creek and Hou-jia Creek disappear as the first fruit of this new action, but also the rest creeks in or outside the Town got fouler and further silted owing to the worsening circulation capability of the tide in the whole creek system. Soon the local government had to fill up more creeks in the suburbs because people's life had been strongly affected by the odorous creeks. In the Town, after the trunk creeks were filled, many small branches and broken channels were left there; and they immediately caused great harm to people's health because the water in them could not flow any longer. The whole creek system was broken up quickly. Now the local government needed much more money to cure the environmental problem, but collecting money was always hard work for any official institution. So, there emerged a serious contradiction between the sour creeks everywhere and the embarrassed financial status. As a result, the problem with the creeks at the time was more serious than previously.

In fact, the abovementioned new problem should be explained separately on two levels. Concerning the rest small creeks inside the Town, at first the local government had planned to reserve them for the purpose of drainage. But the citizens could not wait because the creeks got fouler and fouler, and they urged the government to fill them up as soon as possible. The local government lacked financial ability and then tried to seek a way out by dredging. But who was willing to spend money on these half-waste channels? So the proposal of dredging the creeks was rejected. Under such a condition, the environmental problem with the creeks lasted until the 1940s, with its sanitary situation being bad all along. As to the creeks in the suburbs, affected by the anti-creek fervor both in the Old Shanghai Town and the foreign settlement, the tide could not flow smoothly as before, as the result of which they became silted too. Farms in the countryside still depend on them for irrigation, but the creeks could not afford adequate and qualified water for agriculture. So, conflicts between farmers and the municipal government often occurred. On the other hand, the merchants who had purchased land in the newly expended urban areas hoped that the dirty creeks could be filled up as soon as possible so that better commercial surroundings could be created. They urged the municipal government to fill up the dirty creeks. But they were so impatient that they often privately filled and invaded some of the creek land without any permission from the government. Faced with such a dilemma, the local government found it very hard to deal with the suburban creeks. They were always squeezed between the urban people and the farmers, but no solution seemed to be satisfactory to both sides. As a result, the government decided on filling up creeks and took a *laissez-fair* attitude toward the land usurpers, most of whom were wealthy enough to afford the big cost of filling up creeks and then building new passages. They often offered much money to the municipal institution and urged the officials to fill up any section of the creek they liked. Thus, the route changing of the suburban creek system was in the charge of the private land usurpers, and the environmental situation at last went chaotic. Under such a condition, to plan the creek use on the whole was not possible at all.

Another negative effect was that illegal occupation and invasion of the creeks became more and more serious. Since the government paid less and less attention to the ownership of creek land and ignored the maintenance work during this transformation period, the traditional public land could certainly boast as a better place for living. So the poor immigrants swarmed into the expanding city. These poor people could not afford to rent houses, and so they had no choice but to build huts over the creeks, with all the rubbish poured into the creeks. Soon the former canals became odorous sewers. The abovementioned phenomenon could be seen mostly at the gray zones between the city and the countryside, which accelerated the collapsing of the whole creek system.

Up to 1937, the City Hall of Shanghai (Shanghai County was promoted to Shanghai City in 1927) announced: "The citizens are permitted to be in possession of the waste creek land everywhere and exploit it as they like, provided they pay a sum of money to the city government." This was the most important turn of the government's attitude toward the land use of public creeks. Since ancient times, all the creeks had been protected carefully as public properties in the areas south of the Yangtze River and the private occupation had always been forbidden. But when history proceeded to modern times after the opening-up of the port of Shanghai and the introduction of Western concepts, great changes occurred to the mode of creek use. The abovementioned new laws also indicate the obvious changes in the regional environment such as the worsening of the creek system around the city with the urban expansion, which forced the government to change the rural land of many natural resources into a mere urban construction land. This new mode of using natural resources sheds some light on the relationship between humans and nature.

Today for visitors to Shanghai, the disappearance of natural creeks and the landscape typical of the areas in the lower reaches of the Yangtze River is always a pity. The picture of the harmonious coexistence of water and land is hard to see even in the suburbs of the city. Besides, there is another tough task for the city government to deal with. Now in the downtown area, more than 200 creeks still exist, which give off bad odors and in which the tide can hardly flow. Although every year the government will devote a great deal of money to improve them, yet the effect is not satisfactory enough. Recently, a new technique has been adopted to restore the natural environment of some big creeks, and some good effects have been obtained.

25.7 Conclusion

In this paper, a fairly thorough study on the creek use mode of the Old Shanghai Town has been made to trace the whole course of its history and transformation in modern times. It is believed that while such factors as historical accumulation in nature and humans (people's pursuit of economic profits), new concepts, and the regional environment all have exerted much influence upon the urban land use, the basic and permanent factor is the regional environment with its restricting power.

In this case, people's illegal occupation of the creek land was always changing the ecosystem of the creeks, and as a result small canals became constructive sites or lanes. But whenever the occupation became severe, the ecosystem of the creeks would be disturbed, and then the government would try to restore the ecology of the creeks. People lived partly on the creek resources and the creek system was restored slowly. This is the traditional mode of creek use, in which people's behavior was in fact restricted by the natural condition of the creeks. It also explains the relationship between humans and nature during the traditional period. After the opening-up of Shanghai, some new concepts came from the West, one of which affected the traditional mode of creek use, and it is none other than the concept of public health and quality of life. It met the need of the local environment and soon established itself. It played down the traditional factors and greatly changed the natural equilibrium of the creek system. So trunk creeks were filled up and broad roads were constructed, and the urban sanitation and landscape was temporarily promoted. However, all these new concepts and measures could not prevent the creek system from getting worse. The regional environment has never stopped showing its power. The negative effects of the creek-filling not only existed in the city, but also spread to the farther suburbs. This contemporary mode of creek use also indicates that the basic and permanent factor affecting the urban land use is the regional environment with its restricting power. The case of the Old Shanghai Town suggests that the characteristics of the regional environment should always receive enough attention during the urban land exploitation. It is very important to maintain the functioning mechanism of the main factors that act upon the urban land use and to understand the proper degree of man's use of natural resources.

Besides, there should be a moderate understanding about the "transformation" from traditionality to modernization for society. "Transformation" does not mean a sudden break, because it on the one hand is based on historical accumulation, and on the other will face many new problems. Therefore, the "transformation" of society should be examined within a long history and from various aspects. Since the year 1840, most of the Chinese cities have been receiving new concepts from the West, and their patterns of urban construction have changed a lot. Therefore, to properly understand the concept of "transformation" there is need for studying intensively the urban land use and existing creeks in modern China with a view to enhance the overall well-being and quality of life of the people of Old Shanghai Town.

References

(1) Archives and Historical Materials

Cai, Y.-T. (Ed.). (2005). *The history of title deeds in Shanghai*. Shanghai: Shanghai Press of Chinese Classics.

Gu, Y.-W. The advantages and disadvantages of Nations in the World.

Geng, J. (1980). *The technique of building Wei Field*. Beijing: Agricultural Press.

Zhang, C.-S. *On the irrigation system in the Southeast of China* (the 7th Year of the Guang Xu Period in the Qing Dynasty).

Zheng, J-Y. *Information on the Tai-hu Lake*.

Li, W.-Q. (1989). *The history of rural Shanghai*. Shanghai: Shanghai Press of Chinese Classics.
Xu, X.-Y. (Ed.), (1985). *A brief history of the social and economic development in modern Shanghai (1882–1931)*, Shanghai Social Sciences Institute Press.
The Official History of *Song-jiang Region* (the Jia-qing Period of the Qing Dynasty).
The Official History of Shanghai County (the 11th year of Tong-zhi Period of the Qing Dynasty).
Additional Information on the History of Shanghai Country (the 7th Year of the Republic of China).
Additional Information on the History of Jia-ding County (the Republic of China).
The History of Shanghai. (1993). Shanghai: Shanghai People's Press.
The History of Nan-shi District of Shanghai City. (1993). Shanghai: Shanghai Academy of Social Sciences Press.
Wang, T. (1989). *Sketches of oversea experiences*. Shanghai: Shanghai Press of Chinese Classics.
The Conference records of the Shanghai Municipal Council of the Shanghai English Settlement (1854–1943). (2001). (Vol. 1–28). Shanghai: Shanghai Press of Chinese Classics.
Library, S. (Ed.). (2001). *Maps of old Shanghai*. Shanghai: Shanghai Pictorial Press.
On Dredging the Creeks in the Old Shanghai Town and Throwing Mud into the Huang-pu River. (1873, May 23). *Shanghai City Paper*.
Suggestions to the Gentries of the Town on Producing the Running Water. (1873, December 5). *Shanghai City Paper*.
Creek Dredging within the Town. (1876, March 23). *Shanghai City Paper*.
On Fetching Water from beyond the Town. (1876, May 19). *Shanghai City Paper*.
Fire Broke Out in the Town. (1876, August 19). *Shanghai City Paper*.
Investigating the Quantity of Consumed Drinking Water. (1877, May 25). *Shanghai City Paper*.
Creek Dredging within the Town. (1881, December 18). *Shanghai City Paper*.
On the Price of the Running Water. (1899, July 14). *Shanghai City Paper*.
Announcement of the Creek Dredging in the Town. (1901, September 7). *Shanghai City Paper*.
The Chancellor Ordered the Canals in the Town to be Dredged. (1902, February 7). *Shanghai City Paper*.
Discussions on the Improvement of the Fire Fighting. (1903, March 24). *Shanghai City Paper*.
Widening the Roads. (1904, November 19). *Shanghai City Paper*.
The Advantages of Running Water. (1904, December 6). *Shanghai City Paper*.
Banning the Illegal Occupation of Creek Land. (1905, April 16). *Shanghai City Paper*.
The Chancellor Ordered the Illegal Occupation of Creek Land to Be Punished. (1905, April 27). *Shanghai City Paper*.
Meeting Held to Discuss the Roads Widening. (1905, May 1). *Shanghai City Paper*.
Meeting Held to Discuss the Creek-filling. (1905, July 7). *Shanghai City Paper*.
Asking for Instructions to Fill Up the Waste Creeks. (1906, March 1). *Shanghai City Paper*.
The Chancellor's Order to Fill Up the Hei-qiao Creek and Remove the Houses over the Creek. (1906, March 24). *Shanghai City Paper*.
The Chancellor Banned the Goods that Block the Roads. (1906, July 27). *Shanghai City Paper*.
Tax Paid for Reconstructing Houses. (1907, September 21). *Shanghai City Paper*.
Mr. Shen Xin-hai Submitted Proposals to the Director of the Public Benefit Association on Keeping the Public Sanitation of the Town. (1908, May 10). *Shanghai City Paper*.
The Town-planning bureau Asked the Chancellor for instructions to repair the roads and dredge the Canals of the Town. (1908, June 10). *Shanghai City Paper*.
Two Hundred and One Creeks in the Downtown Area Say Goodbye to Foul Odors. (2005, December 22). *Wen-hui News*.
The Archives of the Engineering Administrative Bureau in Southern Shanghai, Q205-1-92. Files on Filling Up the North Tang-jia-wan Creek and Building Road on it: In Response to Wang Cheng-yi's Request for the Ownership of the Filled Creek Land.
The Archives of the Engineering Administrative Bureau in Southern Shanghai, Q205-1-124. Files on Filling Up the Xue-jia Creek.
The Archives of the Engineering Administrative Bureau in Southern Shanghai, Q205-1-216. Files on the Cases of Illegal Occupation and Invasion of Public Creeks and Roads.

The Archives of the Engineering Administrative Bureau in Southern Shanghai, Q205-1-72. Files on Yu Mao-pei's Request for Instructions to Fill Up the Song-jia Creek.

Archives of the Shanghai Municipal Council of the English Settlement, U1-1-1072. Files on the Scheme of Drainage in the Settlement of 1870.

Archives of the Shanghai Municipal Council of the English Settlement, U1-2-1194. Files on the Land Use Regarding the Road Extension of the Year 1905.

Archives of the Shanghai Municipal Council of the English Settlement, U1-14-1261. Files on the Flood Prevention Program on Bubbling Well Road.

Archives of the Shanghai Municipal Council of the English Settlement, U1-16-4650. Files on the Annual Report of 1899 of the Public Health Department.

Archives of the Shanghai Municipal Council of the English Settlement, U1-14-5365A. Files on the Public Labor Department's Reply to the Appeals.

Archives of the Shanghai Municipal Council of the English Settlement, U1-16-4653, U1-14-4654, U1-14-4655, U1-14-4656.

Archives of the Municipal Bureau of the Shanghai City, Q215-1-6956. Files on the Bill of Citizens' Request for the Ownership of the Public Creek Land.

Archives of the Municipal Bureau of the Shanghai City, Q215-1-6956. Files on Cases of Citizens Asking for the Ownership of the Public Creek Land and Public Road Land.

(2) Books and Papers

Elvin, M. (2000). Towns and watercourse: the Shanghai County of 1480–1910. In W. Skinner (Ed.), *The cities during the late empire of China*. Beijing: China Book Company.

Fu, H. (2004). *Research on the history of land use in Henan Province*. Diss: Fudan University.

George, R. (1910). *A history of public health*. London: The Johns Hopkins University Press.

Lockhart, W. (1862). *The medical missionary in China: A narrative of twenty years' experience*. London: Hurst and Blackett Publishers.

Man, Z.-M. (2005). Report on the Change of the Urban Space, Settlements, and the Creek System after the Opening of Shanghai Port. *The Collected Papers of Research Programs of the Ministry of Education of Jan*. 2005 (unpublished).

Tan, Q.-X. (1962, July 21). Study on the Exact Beginning Time of the Name of Shanghai and the Township Establishment. *Wen-hui News*.

Wang, J.-G. (2006). Mill wheel and rice seedling: A scene of rice field draining and agricultural recovery in Jiang-nan in the Qing Dynasty. *Research on the History* of the *Qing Dynasty*, *2*, 1–11.

Wu, A.-N. (2005). The ecological reconstruction of the Urban creeks and the evaluating method. *Water Conservancy Transaction, 36*(9), 1088–1093.

Xiong, Y.-Z. (Ed.). (1999). *A general history of Shanghai*. Shanghai: Shanghai People's Press.

Zhang, X.-H., & Man, Z.-M. The driving forces of the land use in the South of Shaanxi province during the Qing Dynasty. *Issues on Chinese Historical Geography*, *17*(4), 114–125.

Zhao, Y. (2006). *The driving forces of the land use in the Jiang-su and An-hui area (1500–1937)*. Diss: Fudan University.

Zheng, Z.-A. (2001). The Rampart and City gates of the old Shanghai Town. In Z.-A. Zheng (Ed.), *Silhouette of Old Shanghai*. Shanghai: Shanghai Lexicographical Press.

Chapter 26
Adaptive Management of Green Spaces and Life Quality in Glasgow (Scotland) and Ottawa (Canada)

Michael O'Neal Campbell

Abstract Green spaces (greenbelts surrounding urban areas and greenhearts within urban areas) are increasingly recognised as vital for urban ecological health, this concept encompassing air quality, wildlife presence and habitat development, and with consequent contributions to human quality of life. Adaptive management (AM), a broadly sourced evaluative methodology for project appraisal, is eminently suitable for the analysis of the role of green spaces in human life quality. This chapter examines the utility of an adaptive management perspective applied to two established 'green' cities: Glasgow in Scotland (UK) and Ottawa, Canada. Background information was derived from interviews with personnel employed in relevant institutions, time series images and maps, and point count surveys of birds and mammals. Both cases examined the environmental histories and problems, relevant stakeholder roles, and the allocation of the AM framework as detailed by Nyberg (1998) (problem assessment, project design and implementation, monitoring and evaluation, and policy adjustment). Both cases showed use of the tenets of the AM framework especially at the project identification design and implementation phases, but with more issues at the monitoring and evaluation phases, and consequent possibilities for policy adjustment. These results inform general management theory and urban planning.

Keywords Greenbelt · Urban · Management · Project · Glasgow · Ottawa

26.1 Introduction

Urban vegetated areas, usually termed as green spaces, contribute strongly to the quality of human life in urban areas, due to the relaxing atmosphere, recreational possibilities, air quality regulation and exotic wildlife presence in such areas (Campbell 2002; Kuhn 2003; Chiari and Seeland 2004; Konijnendijk et al. 2006; Reith and Orova 2015; Martos et al. 2016; Ahmad et al. 2017; Konijnendijk 2017). Two common types of urban green areas are greenbelts that surround cities and

M. O. Campbell (✉)
Simon Fraser University, Burnaby, Canada
e-mail: ecol55@hotmail.com

B. R. K. Sinha (ed.), *Multidimensional Approach to Quality of Life Issues*,
https://doi.org/10.1007/978-981-13-6958-2_26

green hearts that are surrounded by urban areas. One method for assessing, developing and managing such developments is adaptive management (AM) . This was designed during the 1970s to assess such urban and ecological developments for possible improvement and environmental impacts (Lee 1999; Johnson 1999; Agrawal 2000). AM is described as 'an innovation that implements policies as experiments', 'mobilizes available information for objectives that are less susceptible to unexpected outcomes' (Agrawal 2000: 326) and 'probes the responses of ecosystems as people's behavior changes' (Lee 1999: 3). Basically, 'adaptive management tries to incorporate the views and knowledge of all interested parties' (Johnson 1999, 8) and incorporates process, learning participation and reappraisal into the management process (Wollenberg et al. 2000; Campbell 2017; Konijnendijk 2017).

Ministry of Forestry (2004: 1) considered 'active' adaptive management, 'experimentally compared selected policies, and alternative hypotheses about the system being managed' as the most effective form of AM. AM may comprise six steps or stages: (1) assessment of the problem; (2) design of the project; (3) project implementation; (4) monitoring; (5) evaluation; and (6) a response, usually adjustment (Nyberg 1998; Ministry of Forestry 2004). However, especially in the case of urban landscapes, insufficient attention has been paid to monitoring, evaluation and adjustment, especially in a comparative and historical mode (Reid and Mace 2003; Pretty and Smith 2004). Urban green spaces require adaptive management, due to their multifunctionality and multiple stakeholder interests (Konijnendijk 2017), strong 'recreational, aesthetic and emotional' values (Ong 2003: 197) and factors for enhanced quality of life (Kuhn 2003; Campbell 2017). Therefore, recent studies have examined the relations between ecology, urban planning, social action and participation within green space planning (Chiari and Seeland 2004; Konijnendijk et al. 2006; Konijnendijk 2017).

Glasgow (Scotland, UK) and Ottawa (Canada) (Figs. 26.1 and 26.2) are recognised as 'green' cities, in terms of green space area, recreation, life quality, wildlife and tourism. Glasgow (55° 52′ N, 4° 15′ W, population 629,501 General Register Office for Scotland 2012) is the economic capital and largest city of Scotland. It derives its name from the Gaelic word 'Ghlaschu', which in English translates to 'dear green place'. Glasgow is 'better endowed with green spaces than other European cities'; over 20% of its area is vegetated (Glasgow City Council GCC (2003a, b, c: 1, 2017). Ottawa (45° 19′ N, 75° 40′ W, population 883,391 Statistics Canada 2008), the political capital and fourth largest city in Canada, is 'one of the greenest metropolitan cities in North America' (City of Ottawa 2004a: 1). Although Ottawa is not 'well known for progressive, contemporary greenway planning efforts' (Erickson (2004: 0.199), it 'invests considerable money' in these green spaces (City of Ottawa 2004a: 1). Both Glasgow and Ottawa are surrounded by smaller satellite towns, and are near rivers and canals. These are the rivers Clyde and Kelvin, and the Forth and Clyde Canal for Glasgow; and the Ottawa and Rideau Rivers, and the Rideau Canal for Ottawa. These waterways form corridors, along which several green spaces are located, and there is a major human land use, especially recreation and tourism.

This chapter's hypotheses are that: (1) insufficient attention has been paid to the *monitoring, evaluation and adjustment* phase of AM (hereafter termed MEA), and

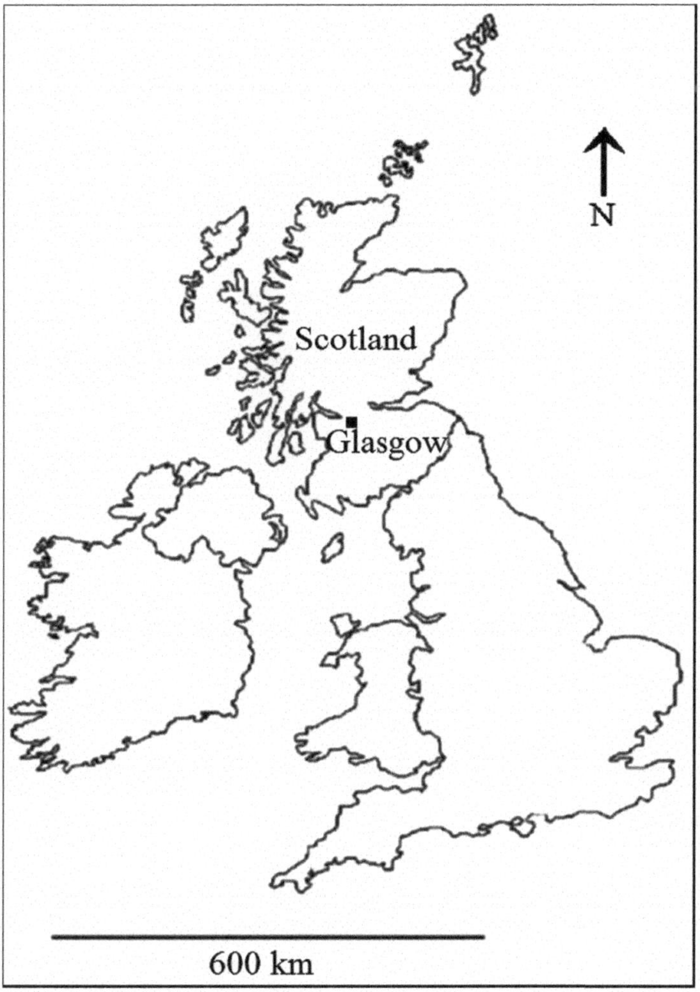

Fig. 26.1 Glasgow, Scotland

to the *project identification and project design and implementation* phase (hereafter termed PIDI); and (2) spatial and temporal comparative analysis, which has been relatively neglected in the AM literature, offers a strong method for the appraisal of such AM applications. The objectives of the chapter are to (1) devise and demonstrate a methodology sufficiently robust, to derive the information for these hypotheses; (2) investigate the historical and spatial issues of environmental management in these two cities; and (3) illustrate how PIDI and MEA were implemented and organised. The following sections examine the interdisciplinary methodology and discuss the importance of the results for AM applications and possibilities for extrapolation to other studies.

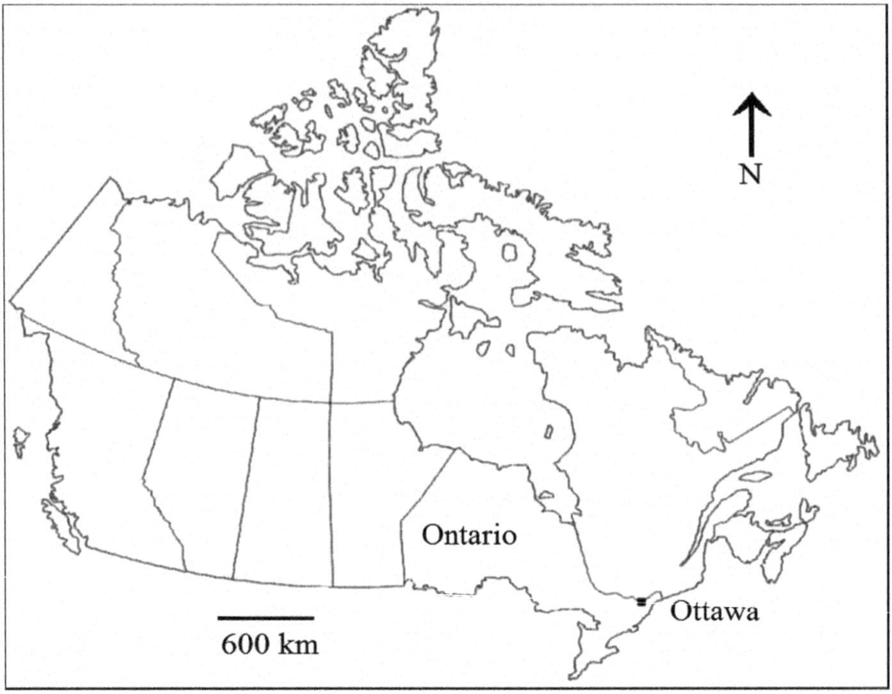

Fig. 26.2 Ottawa, Canada

26.2 Methodology

A qualitative research methodology, using interviews and documentary sources (Patton 2002; Erickson 2004), was integrated with a quantitative ecological analysis, as used in Bayne and Hobson (2000). For the Glasgow survey, interviews were also conducted with employees of Scottish Natural Heritage (SNH) (the Scottish government's statutory adviser on environmental issues), Glasgow City Council (GCC) and Scottish Wildlife Trust (SWT) (a leading voluntary charity, and member of the Scottish Urban Wildlife Partnership), concerning wildlife, air quality and land use. Other sources were the Glasgow City Archives, websites, old and current maps, aerial photographs and unpublished reports from the GCC, SNH, the Scottish Environment Protection Agency (the main government environment agency), Scottish Wildlife Trust and the Scottish Executive's Environment and Rural Affairs Department (SEERAD). To evaluate the ecological status of the green spaces, a sample of green spaces was also monitored for wildlife (diurnal birds and mammal species) using field appraisal and the point count method to determine the extent to which these multifaceted spaces served as habitats as well as places of human recreation. One hundred and seventy-nine points were used in green spaces, recording all signs of bird and mammal presence, between September 2003 and June 2004. The hypothesis for this survey was that smaller spaces support fewer species, as described by Fahrig (2001).

For the Ottawa survey, a similar methodology was employed. Interview sessions were conducted with employees of the National Capital Commission (NCC, the Federal Crown Corporation in change of the greenbelt) , the City of Ottawa, the Ontario Ministry of Natural Resources (OMNR), Geomatics Canada and the Map Library of Carleton University. Other sources were websites, old maps and aerial photographs and Landsat images, as well as unpublished reports of the NCC, City of Ottawa, Environment Canada, Geomatics Canada, the Regional Municipality of Ottawa Carleton (RMOC), the Greenbelt Master Plan (GBMP) , the OMNR and the Canada Parks and Wilderness Society. A sample of green spaces was also monitored for vegetation and wildlife (diurnal birds and mammal species) using field observation and the point count method. One hundred and sixty-two survey points were surveyed in the green spaces and the greenbelt, between October 2000 and August 2002.

The Glasgow and Ottawa surveys both cases examined: (1) the historical origins of environmental issues in the urban green spaces; (2) the stakeholders for environmental management; (3) the environmental problems; (4) the importance of environmental issues within the policy frameworks and in social assessments; (5) the extent to which the AM framework as detailed by Nyberg (1998) (problem assessment, project design and implementation, monitoring and evaluation, and policy adjustment) was followed; and (6) the methodological and management problems.

26.3 Results

26.3.1 Glasgow

Green spaces include 74 sites of importance for the conservation of nature (SINCS), 11 habitat corridors related to waterways and transport networks (GCC 2003a) and many treed avenues, river banks, kerb patches, isolated trees, gardens, gravesites and patches in derelict lots (GCC 2016, 2017). There is complex greenbelt around the city, comprising a mixed forest-farm mosaic, contiguous with numerous satellite towns such as Paisley, Motherwell, Coatbridge, Hamilton and East Kilbride. While PIDI was historically comprehensive, there was less evidence of a historically effective MEA, despite recent institutional and managerial developments (GCC 2016, 2017).

Historically, PIDI in park development was problem based, with social class engagement. Relevant stakeholders included the middle and upper classes of the West End and the working and industrial classes of the north and east, and tourists (Smith 1852; Carrick 1884; Mclellan 1894; Hart 1982; Conway 1991). Church involvement also lent symbolic and practical support (Whitton 1919; Maver 1998). Environmental factors for park development included industrial pollution, wildlife conservation and residential proximity.

The first park, the Glasgow Green (frequently termed the people's park, due to its mainly working-class clientele (Mclellan 1894)), was a public laundry and cattle herding area from the twelfth to 19th centuries and a public recreational forested park in the seventeenth century, after tree planting and landscaping by the Glasgow Town Council (GTO, the predecessor of the GCC). Subsequently, recreation was dominant, with landscaping to 'give the Green a more park-like appearance' and the cessation of cattle grazing and wildlife was documented (Mclellan 1894, pp. 18–25, 40).

The problem-based rationale for green space development was strongly manifested in the later park projects. Air pollution, perceived as serious and epidemic for industrial cities such as Glasgow, was considered ameliorated by green parks, which were also valued as symbols of 'regeneration' and 'evidence of the civic beneficence' (Maver 1998: 323). For example, Alexandra Park was developed in 1866 on land purchased from private ownership in northeast Glasgow (originally a 'cold bare bleak hill, with very few trees' (Mclellan 1894: 86)), and was founded partly to reduce the strong air pollution largely originating from the Blockchain iron works. Created in the popular (tree lot, grass and pond) model, it survived, despite the impact of pollution on trees. A swimming pond was created out of an old quarry, and large numbers of poplars and willows were planted.

Similarly, Victoria Park (1887) was developed principally to regenerate the industrial area of Partick. The landscaping project provided employment during a serious decline in the ship-building industries. This park too was designed in what had become a classic format: a tree belt along the park edges, with artificial ponds. Ruchill Park, developed by the GTO on purchased private land, was also founded to provide recreation for the large industrial classes of North Glasgow (Possil Park, Cowcaddens, Kelvinside and Maryhill) (Mclellan 1894). The recreation needs of the new middle class based in Western Glasgow, contributed to the foundation of Kelvingrove Park, near the river Kelvin, purchased from private land interests by the GTO (1883). The Botanical Gardens, located nearby (1887), had a similar function (Mclellan 1894).

Having established a basis for PIDI, the next issue is the translation of these into MEA. The historical literature documents park visitation and wildlife observations. For example, Mclellan (1894) numbers the Sunday visitors during August 1893, but there is little evidence that these surveys were analysed for adjustments in park management and/or urban policy concerning engagement of green spaces with nearby areas. More recent social and technical surveys, conducted by different agencies on different topics, provide a strong basis for MEA, if organised into an effective information base for decision-making. The Glasgow Panel Survey (GCC 2003b) used a park user survey to show strong social support for parks, with nearly 80% of respondents giving positive assessments and 50% making at least monthly park visits. Reasons for visiting park included 'peace and tranquillity' (32%) and wildlife sightings (24%). The Glasgow Green (28% of visitors) and the Botanic Gardens (24%) were the most popular, others being Alexandra Park, Queen's Park, Kelvingrove Park, Pollock County Park, Victoria Park, Tollcross Park, Bellahouston Park and Hogganfield Park. Problems noted included dog's excrement and behaviour, vandalism and graffiti, poor toilet facilities, crime and antisocial visitors. This survey served as a basis for future adjustments, and in association with historical documentation, verified the longstanding popularity of green spaces. Future plans envisaged further developments (GCC 2016, 2017).

In terms of pollution and waste management, the GCC (2003c) has also been monitoring air quality, although this is now related to transport (98%), rather than industry as noted by Mclellan (1894) in the nineteenth century. Air pollutant monitoring is, however, confined to the built-up areas, with no assessment of park impact on air pollution (GCC 2003c). The Scottish Environment Protection Agency SEPA (2001, 2003) concluded assessments of waste production and management in Glasgow, including parks, a relevant topic as the Glasgow Panel Survey (GCC 2003b) mentioned waste deposition as a problem. Five thousand, five hundred and twenty-one tonnes of waste were collected in parks from 2000 to 2001, and 5690 from 2001 to 2003. These figures have increased subsequently (Audit Scotland 2007 and remain a problem in green spaces (GCC 2016).

For ecological and zoogeographical assessments, McCall and Doar (1997) assessed Glasgow's parks among others. Bean (2001) and Zisman (2001) summarised the contribution of SNH and the Royal Society for the Protection of Birds (RSPB) in knowledge acquisition for the Clyde valley. The Scottish Ornithologists Club publishes the Clyde Bird Report, and the Glasgow Natural History Society publishes *The Glasgow Naturalist*, both of which document local species. The SWT (2003) also increased management of nature sites in Glasgow, produced the Greenspace Action Pack (Parker and Stewart 2000) targeting local communities, and after the publication of a green space strategy (2000) worked in collaboration with the SNH, the Scottish Executive and Scottish Local Authorities in green space developments from 2000 to 2004 (SWT 2004).

The SNH also awarded £1.6 million to the Glasgow and Clyde Valley Greenspace Trust for the creation and improvement of green spaces, working in some cases with the GCC (SNH 2003). The British Trust for Conservation Volunteers (BTCV) in collaboration with the Scottish Executive also ran a pilot scheme for biodiversity management in Glasgow and nearby areas (Scottish Executive 2002a). The GCC's Local Biodiversity Plan (2001) described conservation strategies for species and habitats. This initiative involved 20 partners including the SNH, SWT, Forestry Commission, SEPA, Kelvin Clyde Greenspace (a Glasgow and Clyde Valley Greenspace Trust project) and the RSPB, which also share the funding. The GCC also contacted groups, agencies and the public, through the publication of a questionnaire booklet by Parks Review, and GCC, a City Woodland Initiative, was developed, in response to the available information. Further plans were developed (GCC 2016, 2017).

Such activities have had policy impact. The Glasgow and Clyde Valley Structure Plan, which was approved by the Scottish parliament in 2002, looking at development over the period 2002–2022 is an example (Scottish Executive, 2002b). As noted in the Scottish Executive's (2004: 1) National Planning Framework (NPF) Environmental Assessment Report, the European Union Directive 2001/42 (or the Strategic Environmental Assessment (SEA) Directive) states: 'environmental assessment is an important tool for integrating environmental considerations into the preparation and adoption of plans and programmes which are likely to have significant effects on the environment… because it ensures that such effects of implementing plans and programmes are taken into account during their preparation and before adoption'.

Despite publications on parks and wildlife, the relationship between park size, location and wildlife presence was neglected (green space location in relation to social classes and air quality was by contrast well documented). On the topic of park size, location and wildlife presence, the field survey confirmed park design descriptions in the historical literature (Mclellan 1894; Sterry et al. 1998; Clyde Birds 2003; GCC 2003a) (at least 30% treed stands, mostly deciduous, with shrubs, grass and a few ponds covering the rest) and wildlife presence. In the field survey of the current study, mammal species recorded included the red deer *Cervus elaphus*, red fox *Vulpes vulpes*, grey squirrel *Sciurus carolinensis* and red squirrel *Sciurus vulgaris leucurus*. Birds included carrion crows *Corvus corone corone*, magpies *Pica pica*, great grey heron *Ardea cinerea*, lesser black backed gull *Larus fuscus*, black-headed gull *Larus ridibundus*, herring gull *Larus argentatus*, wood pigeon *Columba palumbus,* rock dove *Columba livia*, stock dove *Columba oenas,* common buzzard *Buteo buteo*, house sparrow *Passer domesticus*, black bird *Turdus merula*, song thrush *Turdus philomelos* and starling *Sturnus vulgaris*. The number of observed species increased with the area of the green spaces and the proximity of the green city edges ($r = 0.69$, $r^2 = 0.48$, $F = 98.33$, $p < 0.05$). There was also a high positive correlation between the number of animal species and water proximity ($r = 0.64$, $r^2 = 0.41$, $F = 87.46$, $p < 0.05$).

26.3.2 Ottawa

Polices for green space development in Ottawa were also problem based, with developed design and implementation, but less evidence of monitoring, evaluation and adjustment (NCC 2013). A much younger city than Glasgow, Ottawa developed from the old settlement of Bytown (Historical Atlas of Carleton County 1879; Ross 1927; Reid 1990; Larson et al. 1999), as a mill town, for lumber (Erickson 2004: 207) and farming (Nepean Museum 2004). Green spaces planning started with the Holt Report (1915) recommending in which 1214 ha of recreation parkland. Like Glasgow, a canal system was developed (Federal Plan Commission of Ottawa and Hull 1915: 105). From 1950, the greenbelt plan of Jacques Greber (Greber 1950) was implemented, one 'of the most far sighted plans of the 20th century' (NCC 1996: 15). The main implementing agency, the National Capital Commission NCC, founded in 1958, created greenbelt through the purchase of private lands, after the 1950s, with some landowner opposition. On completion, the greenbelt covered approximately 200 square kilometres of the National Capital Region (NCR) around Ottawa (Wickware and Rubec 1989), including forests, farms, meadows, rivers, lakes and wetlands (NCC 2013).

For the greenbelt, there were three problems: the control of urban sprawl, recreation and conservation (NCC 2013). Like Glasgow, urban congestion was identified as a problem, although pollution was less important, because of the lack of a heavy waste producing industry. Urban sprawl was serious, as in contrast to Glasgow's declining population, Ottawa has the third largest population growth rate among Canadian cities, especially in the satellite towns (Kanata, Orleans, Leitrim, South Gloucester (Riverside South), Stittsville and South Nepean). These were linked to Ottawa by urban corridors, especially Kanata and Nepean (Ottawa 20/20, 2002), by the Regional Official Plans (1969, 1988 and 1997) of the Regional Municipality of Ottawa Carleton RMOC (founded in 1969, which became the City of Ottawa in 2001). The urban area expanded and the population density decreased from 57 to 28 people per hectare between 1925 and 2001 (Ottawa 20/20, 2002). This resulted in the virtual encirclement of the greenbelt by satellite towns. The greenbelt acquired the appearance of a large green space within the city, what may be termed a greenheart.

In 1991, greenbelt ecology was studied (Hough Stanbury Woodland Limited 1991) and later there were studies for the creation of natural areas within the greenbelt (Brunton 1997; City of Ottawa 1991; Brownell and Larson 1995; Brownell and Blaney 1997; RMOC 1997; International Committee for Local Environmental Initiatives 2004). Vegetation (Spiwak 1996), ice storm impacts (Nielsen 2001) and mammal–human interactions (Brown 2000; City of Ottawa 2003) were also studied. Road kills, especially of white-tailed deer recorded by the police increased from 233 in 1994 to 685 in 2000 (Brown 2000). The number of visitors to the main conservation area in the greenbelt (Stony Swamp Conservation Area) was documented (NCC 1999). Campbell (2002) assessed this area using GIS, field surveys, aerial photographs, and aerial photographs covering the period 1955–1999 and concluded that there were important gaps in the short-term current knowledge of field dynamics, requiring more short-term assessments. Such studies were replicated through the years (NCC 2013). Like the Glasgow case, such studies tend to be isolated, rather than integrated into a coherent framework for policy adjustment.

The Green Belt Master Plan (GBMP) was developed to take stock of developments after the establishment of the greenbelt, and to involve stakeholders in the strategy for future enhancement. The GBMP involved intensive social participation in planned problem-solving. There was a 600-person public opinion survey in 1990, public open houses in 1991 and the use of studies by planning students as working documents (1992). Public consultation involved five main issues: (1) road impacts, (2) commercial restrictions recreation support, (3) the self-sustaining possibilities of conservation areas within the greenbelt, (4) removal of economic activity outside the greenbelt and (5) and the removal of urban land use from natural areas (NCC 1996). Increased policy flexibility was advocated. The City of Ottawa (2004b) also listed 301 smaller green spaces, many near the Rideau and Ottawa Rivers and the Rideau canal, and in built-up areas. Corridors were planned in 1991 (City of Ottawa Department of Engineering Works 1993), but these were only slowly implemented. One constraint was the lack of information on the environment, which was assessed for a solution by the Natural and Open Space Study (Erickson 2004).

The policy and institutional framework, which situated the NCC and the City of Ottawa as the prime movers for green space management, differed from the Glasgow case where a multi-private and public agency approach existed for information acquisition and policy support. However, in both cities, the monitoring and evaluation of the implemented projects was at least temporarily uncertain, weakening the possibilities for policy adjustment. Monitoring and evaluation of the greenbelt and its associated conservation areas and the green spaces in Ottawa were largely ad hoc. A reactive Municipal Evaluation Report was planned to help in the assessment, from which policy adjustments may be made (Erickson 2004: 216), along with envisaged adjustments (Ottawa 20/20 2002).

Like Glasgow, the field study of the current study was on the relationship between green space vegetation configuration, size and location and the presence of wildlife species. The results found the configuration of green spaces to be like those of Glasgow, but a few more evergreens were recorded (>10%, rather than <6%). Far more species (sightings, nests and road kills) were recorded within the contiguous greenbelt than the smaller green spaces, and the size of the green spaces was positively correlated with the number of species observed ($r = 0.63$, $r^2 = 39.7$, $F = 54.56$ $p < 0.05$) an issue largely ignored in the Canadian literature (Campbell 2002). Species numbers increased near water bodies ($r = 0.71$, $r^2 = 50$, F 76.43, $p < 0.05$). Commoner mammal species were white-tailed deer *Odocoileus virginianus*, black bears *Ursus americanus*, fishers *Martes pennanti* racoons *Procyon lotor lotor*, groundhogs *Marmota monax* black and grey *Sciurus carolinensis* and red squirrels *Tamiasciurus hudsonicus*, chipmunks *Tamias striatus*, and red foxes *Vulpes vulpes*. Birds recorded included red-tailed hawks *Buteo jamaicensis*, great blue herons *Ardea herodias*, starlings *Sturnus vulgaris*, blue jays *Cyanocitta cristata*, mallard ducks *Anas platyrhynchos*, Canada geese *Branta canadensis* and loons *Gavia immer.*

26.4 Discussion

26.4.1 Monitoring, Evaluation and Adjustment

The utilisation of an AM method for environmental management in Glasgow and Ottawa concerned the management of MEA phases: the available information, the utilisation of this for evaluation and the extent to which this resulted in policy adjustment. The historical assessments provided important information and evidence of the long-term sustainability of social interests in green spaces from recreational and conservation perspectives. The problem identification phase was extended in both cases, as important contextual hurdles concerning environmental assessment, land acquisition and in some cases social support and opposition was overcome. These developmental stages allowed involvement of both environmental and political interests, a key issue in such planning (Reid and Mace 2003). These narratives also provide evidence that, although occurring prior to the articulation of such issues as AM, PIDI was well organised.

A strong aspect of AM, participation, was developed in the early stages of the Glasgow case, and later consultation occurred in both cities. In both cases, despite limitations in the links between PIDI and MEA through much of the twentieth century, responses to MEA were demonstrated, and a strategy emerged based on increased information sources (e.g. SEPA 2001, 2003; GCC 2003a, b, c; Brunton 1997; RMOC 1997). Recognition of the importance of MEA has moved from planning to practice, hence the futuristic plans (e.g. Ottawa 20/20 2002; Scottish Executive 2004) based on such information sources.

Despite the difference between the multi-agency approach in Glasgow and the simpler structure in Ottawa, similar efforts were made by these stakeholders to link with both current MEA and futuristic plans. The success of such attempts at integrating a cohesive framework for MEA appeared moderately feasible, as in both cases future goals (summarised as effective MEA) represented objectives envisaged at the formative stages of green space development, and substantial supporting information existed. The pattern of incremental MEA development reflected the difficulty of bridging the gap between MEA and PIDI. Experimentation with both research and broad consultative and socio-environmental methods were identified in both cases.

26.4.2 The Comparative and Integrated Methodology

A comparative methodology emphasises the strengths of respective cases. The results show (1) how public and private cooperations may contribute in different settings (land purchases, agency cooperation and public involvement); (2) recreation may be integrated into conservation, where there are both declining (Glasgow) and increasing populations (Ottawa) ; and (3) different time frames (>100 years for Glasgow, <70 for Ottawa) may not necessarily affect the sustainability of green space interest provided the base is broad and deep.

However, some studies which employ a comparative methodology neglect monitoring and evaluation as a tool for policy adjustment and future directives Kuhn (2003). Those studies that examine broader methodologies (e.g. Salafsky and Wollenberg 2000; Wollenberg et al. 2000) are generally not comparative or historical works; hence, the derivation of generic principles is difficult. This also applies to issues within green spaces. For example, Yamsaki et al. (2001) distinguish between the links of socio-economic indicators and ecological indicators, and those between ecological indicators. These differences were neglected (e.g. the relationship between animal species and green space area). While acknowledging contextual differences (cited as important by Salafsky and Wollenberg 2000), it is apparent in the current paper that the strengths and core issues are more readily tested in such works, if an element of comparison is used for illustration.

Both policy environments favoured an adaptive management approach and were striving for full implementation, although this was not explicitly stated in the policy directives and plans of either case study. Consequently, it is argued that an effective version of adaptive management would fill the gaps needed for more comprehensive green space . This requires an investigation of (1) the strengths and weaknesses of the existing systems; (2) availability of relevant social and environmental studies;

(3) futuristic policies and programmes, which indicate an awareness of the need for improvement; and (4) institutions geared towards the strengthening of socio-environmental policies.

26.5 Conclusions

The hypothesis of the paper was that for an effective assessment of the AM implementation, there must be an assessment of the MEA phases, within an incorporation of both spatial and temporal comparative analyses. The results support this position. The existence of strong historical and contemporary problem identification and project design and implementation systems does not guarantee an effective monitoring, evaluation and adjustment process. It requires a critical assessment of linked processes and strategic planning. Also, a comprehensive synthesis for effective holistic planning must not be taken for granted. A critical comparative method, from spatial and temporal positions, informs on the possibilities for the implementation of AM. The weakness of the study was the small number of case studies. Further studies must include more detailed experimentation with AM methods, across several contextually variable cases and a comparison with other methods. This will require a more comprehensive methodology, possibly involving GIS-based databases. This will provide the information for competent decision-making, the establishment of cross-referencing frameworks between case studies and a willingness to undertake policy adjustments in response to the findings of such AM methods.

References

Agrawal, A. (2000). Adaptive management in transboundary protected areas: The Bialowieza National Park and Biosphere Reserve as a case study. *Environmental Conservation, 27*(4), 326–333.

Ahmad, P., Misni, A., Kamaruddin, S. M., & Daud, N. (2017). Green neighborhood adaptive model for urban living: A conceptual review. *Environment-Behavior Proceedings Journal, 2*(5), 55–63.

Audit Scotland (2007). *Sustainable waste management*. Edinburgh: Audit Scotland.

Bayne, E., & Hobson, K. (2000). Relative use of contiguous and fragmented boreal forest by red squirrels *Tamiasciurus Hudsonicus*. *Canadian Journal of Zoology, 78*, 359–365.

Bean, C. (2001). Nature conservation and the River Clyde. In *Conference on the Ecology and Management of the Firth of Clyde* (pp. 5–13). Clydebank: Firth of Clyde Forum.

Brown, C. (2000). *Deer Collisions*. Ottawa: City of Ottawa.

Brownell, V. R., & Blaney, C. S. (1997). *Planning our region: Summary natural area reports for natural areas east of Rideau River*. Ottawa: Regional Municipality of Ottawa-Carleton.

Brownell, V. R. & Larson, M. H. B. (1995). *Planning our region: An evaluation framework for natural areas in the Regional Municipality of Ottawa-Carleton* (Vol. 1). Regional Municipality of Ottawa-Carleton, Ottawa.

Brunton, D.F. (1997). *Planning our region: Summary natural area reports for Natural Areas West of the Rideau River 500 Series*. Regional Municipality of Ottawa-Carleton, Ottawa.

Campbell, M. (2002). *The assessment of biogeographical change in the western Greenbelt of Ottawa using Geomatics Unpublished MA Thesis*. Ottawa: Carleton University.
Campbell, M. (Ed.). (2017). *Biological conservation in the 21st century: A conservation biology of large Wildlife*. New York: Nova Science Publishers.
Carrick, J. (1884). The progress of Glasgow. In Reid, S. (Ed.), *Glasgow Past and Present* 1 (p. xxxv). Glasgow.
Chiari, C. G., & Seeland, K. (2004). Are urban green spaces optimally distributed to act as places for social integration? *Results of a Geographical Information System GIS Approach for Urban Forestry Research Forest Policy and Economics, 6,* 3–13.
City of Ottawa. (1991). *Vegetation cover classification*. Ottawa: City of Ottawa.
City of Ottawa Department of Engineering Works. (1993). *Land and water background report state of the environment reporting programme*. Ottawa: City of Ottawa.
City of Ottawa. (2003). *Report on Ottawa road safety*. Ottawa: City of Ottawa.
City of Ottawa. (2004a). *Parks and Recreation*. Retrieved from https://www.ottawaca/city_services/recreation/index_enshtml.
City of Ottawa. (2004b). *Parks and recreation—park locations*. Retrieved from https://www.ottawaca/city_services/recreation/parks/locations.
Clyde Birds. (2003). Retrieved from https://www.clydebirdscom/.
Conway, H. (1991). *People's parks: The design and development of victorian parks in Britain*. Cambridge: Cambridge University Press.
Erickson, D. L. (2004). The relationship of historic city form and contemporary greenway implementation: A comparison of Milwaukie Wisconsin USA and Ottawa Ontario Canada. *Landscape and Urban Planning, 68,* 199–221.
Fahrig, L. (2001). How much habitat is enough? *Biological Conservation, 100,* 65–74.
Federal Plan Commission of Ottawa and Hull. (1915). *Report of the Federal Plan Commission on a General Plan for the Cities of Ottawa and Hull*. Ottawa: FPCOH.
General Register Office for Scotland. (2012). *Glasgow city council area: Demographic factsheet*. Retrieved from May 31, 2012.
Glasgow City Council. (2001). *Local biodiversity action plan* GCC, Glasgow. Retrieved from https://www.ukbaporguk/lbapaspx?ID=414.
Glasgow City Council. (2003a). *Glasgow's wildlife*. Retrieved from https://www.wildlifeglasgowgovuk/.
Glasgow City Council. (2003a). *Local air quality management: Update and screening assessment 2003*. Glasgow: GCC.
Glasgow City Council. (2003b). *Glasgow panel survey*. Glasgow: GCC.
Glasgow City Council. (2016). *Glasgow green management plan 2016–2019*. Glasgow: GCC.
Glasgow City Council. (2017). *City development plan 2017. sg6: Green belt & green network supplementary guidance*. Glasgow: GCC.
Greber, J. (1950). *Plan for the national capital general report submitted to the National Capital Planning Committee*. National Capital Planning Service Ottawa.
Hart, T. (1982). Urban growth and municipal government: Glasgow in a comparative context 1846–1914. In A. Slaven & D. Aldcroft (Eds.), *Business banking and urban history: essay in honour of sg checkland* (pp. 193–219). Edinburgh: John Donald Publishers.
Historical Atlas of Carleton County (1879). *H Belden and Co*, Ottawa.
Limited, Hough Stanbury Woodland. (1991). *Ecological analysis of the greenbelt*. Ottawa: National Capital Commission.
International Committee for Local Environmental Initiatives. (2004). *The environmental conservation and management strategy of the city of Ottawa*. Toronto: ICLEI.
Johnson, B.L. (1999). The role of adaptive management as an operational approach for resource management agencies. *Conservation Ecology* 3(2), 8. Retrieved from https://www.consecol.org/vol3/iss2/art8.

Konijnendijk, C. C. (2017). Cities and nature: Urban forestry for greater biocultural diversity. In Biological Conservation. In Campbell, M. (Ed.), *Biological Conservation in the 21st Century: A Conservation Biology of Large Wildlife* (pp. 15–30). New York: Nova Science Publishers.
Konijnendijk, C. C., Ricard, R. M., Kenney, A. & Randrup, T. B. (2006). Defining urban forestry—A comparative perspective of North America and Europe. *Urban Forestry & Urban Greening 4*(3–4), 93–103.
Kuhn, M. (2003). Greenbelt and green heart: separating and integrating landscapes in European city regions. *Landscape and Urban Planning, 64,* 19–27.
Larson, B. M., Riley, J. L., Snell, E. A., & Godschalk, H. G. (1999). *The woodland Heritage of South Ontario: A study of the ecological change, Distribution and Significance*. Ottawa: Don Mills Federation of Ontario Naturalists.
Lee, K. N. (1999). Appraising adaptive management. *Conservation Ecology, 3*(2), 3. Retrieved from https://www.consecol.org/vol3/iss2/art3.
Martos, A., Pacheco-Torres, R., Ordonez, J. & Jadraque-Gago, E. (2016). Towards successful environmental performance of sustainable cities: Intervening sectors. *Department of engineering construction and project management*. Spain: University of Granada.
Maver, L. (1998). Glasgow's public parks and the community 1850–1914: A case study in Scottish civic interventionism. *Urban History, 25*(3), 323–347.
Mccall, A., & Doar, N. (1997). *The state of Scottish greenspace SNH review report 88*. Perth: SNH.
Mclellan, D. (1894). *Glasgow public parks*. Glasgow: John Smith and Son.
Ministry of Forestry Government of British Columbia. (2004). *Definitions of adaptive management.* Victoria: Government of British Columbia.
National Capital Commission. (1996). *Greenbelt master plan*. Ottawa: NCC.
National Capital Commission. (1999). *Project of research on gatineau and greenbelt: Study on traffic in stony swamp-summer season*. Ottawa: NCC.
National Capital Commission. (2013). *Canada's capitalgreenbelt master plan*. Ottawa: NCC.
Nepean Museum. (2004). *History Sheet*, Nepean Museum, Nepean.
Nielsen, C. (2001). Ice storm 1998-forest research conference. *The Forestry Chronicle, 77*(1), 16–18.
Nyberg, J. B. (1998). Statistics and the practice of adaptive management In Sit V. & Taylor B. (Eds) *Statistical methods for adaptive management studies.* Ministry of Forestry Government of British Columbia, Victoria.
Ong, B. L. (2003). Green plot ratio: an ecological measure for architecture and urban planning. *Landscape and Urban Planning, 63,* 197–211.
Ottawa 20/20. (2002). *Background—Development in Ottawa: A history.* Ottawa city of Ottawa.
Parker, D., & Stewart, F. (2000). *Greenspace action pack.* Edinburgh: SWT.
Patton, M. Q. (2002). *Qualitative research and evaluation methods*. Beverly Hills: Sage Publications.
Pretty, J., & Smith, D. (2004). Social capital in biodiversity conservation and management. *Conservation Biology, 18*(3), 631–638.
Regional Municipality of Ottawa—Carleton. (1997). *Candidate natural area evaluation.* Ottawa: RMOC.
Regional Municipality of Ottawa—Carleton. (1969). *Official Plan.* Ottawa: RMOC.
Regional Municipality of Ottawa—Carleton. (1988). *Official plan.* Ottawa: RMOC.
Regional Municipality of Ottawa—Carleton. (1997). *Official plan.* Ottawa: RMOC.
Reid, R. M. (1990). *The Upper Ottawa valley to 1855.* Ottawa: Carleton University Press.
Reid, W. V., & Mace, G. M. (2003). Taking conservation biology to new levels in environment decision-making. *Conservation Biology, 17*(4), 943–945.
Reith, A. &Orova, M. (2015). *Ecological indicators: Do green neighbourhood ratings cover sustainability*? (Vol. 48, pp. 660–672). Budapest: ABUD Engineering Ltd.
Ross, A. H. D. (1927). *Ottawa past and present.* Toronto: The Masson Book Company Limited.
Salafsky, N., & Wollenberg, E. (2000). Linking livelihoods and conservation: a conceptual framework and scale for assessing the integration of human needs and biodiversity. *World Development, 28*(8), 1421–1438.

Scottish Environment Protection Agency. (2001). *Local authority waste arisings survey: Results for Glasgow city council*. Stirling: SEPA.
Scottish Executive (2002a). *BTCV Scotland—Linking Biodiversity Edinburgh Scottish Executive*.
Scottish Executive. (2002b). *Plan to boost Glasgow and Clyde Valley Approved*. Retrieved from https://www.scotlandgovuk/pages/news/2002/05/SEsj008aspx.
Scottish Executive (2004). *National planning framework: environmental assessment report*. Edinburgh: Scottish Executive.
Scottish Natural Heritage. (2003). *Biggest ever grant Greens Glasgow and the ClydeValley*. https://www.greenspaceorguk/data/greenspace/GreenspaceTrustmediainviteandmediareleasepdf.
Scottish Wildlife Trust. (2003). *Annual review 2003*. Edinburgh: Scottish Wildlife Trust.
Scottish Wildlife Trust. (2004). *Our priorities for 2000—2004 Scottish Wildlife Trust Edinburgh*. Retrieved from http://www.swtorguk.
Smith. C. (1852). *Parks and pleasure grounds: Or practical notes on Country residences, villas, public parks and gardens*. London: Reeve and Company.
Spiwak, A. (1996). *Changes through time: Variations in spatial patterns of land cover with the stony swamp region of the Ottawa Greenbelt*. Unpublished MA thesis. Carleton University, Ottawa.
Statistics Canada (2008). *Census Statistics Canada* Ottawa: Statistics Canada.
Sterry, P., Cleave, A., Goodfellow, P. & Clements, A. (1998). *Field guide to the birds of Britain and Europe*. Windsor: Automobile Association Developments.
Whitton, J. (1919). *The public parks of Glasgow*. Glasgow: John Smith and Son.
Wickware, G. M., & Rubec, C. D. A. (1989). *Ecoregions of Ontario: Ecological land classification series 26*. Ottawa: Environment Canada Sustainable Development Branch.
Wollenberg, E., Edmunds, D., & Buck, L. (2000). Use scenarios to make decisions about the future: Anticipatory learning for the adaptive co-management of community forests. *Landscape and Urban Planning, 47*, 65–77.
Zisman, S. (2001). The RSPB and its perspective on the management of the Firth of Clyde. In *Conference on the Ecology and Management of the Firth of Clyde* (pp. 14—15). Clydebank: Firth of Clyde Forum.

Chapter 27
Household-Level Quality of Life of People in Bolpur Town of Birbhum District, W.B.

Mahuya Sen and Braj Raj Kumar Sinha

Abstract A household is the most micro level important spatial unit of study. The size, number of persons, physical and socio-economic characteristics of this spatial unit has a great bearing on the quality of life. Different socio-cultural and economic components determine the quality of a person's life. If one member of the family has achieved a high quality of life, this will have a positive impact on the other members of the family and on the rest of the household. The household is often taken as the basic unit of analysis in many social, microeconomic and government studies. In this paper, attempt has been made to study variation in the quality of life of urban inhabitants at the household level. To accomplish the work, Bolpur town from Birbhum District of West Bengal was chosen. Bolpur town lies in a socio-economically backward region. The study involves primary data obtained from 350 households. The quality of life at the household level was found varying across households of different social groups, different categories of educational achievement, income and occupation. The majority of households belonged to the lower income category. Only a small number belonged to the category of higher educational achievement but these enjoyed a better quality of life as did the families whose earning member was in the service sector.

Keywords Society · Development · Social group · Quality of life · Household · Achievement

27.1 Introduction

Analysing the quality of life of people at household level is a matter of great concern to geographers. The study of quality of life at any spatial unit is rather different from

M. Sen (✉)
Birbhum Mahavidyalaya, Suri, Birbhum, West Bengal, India
e-mail: mahuyasen74@gmail.com

B. R. K. Sinha
Department of Geography, Institute of Science, Banaras Hindu University, Varanasi, UP, India
e-mail: sinha_brk@yahoo.co.in

B. R. K. Sinha (ed.), *Multidimensional Approach to Quality of Life Issues*,
https://doi.org/10.1007/978-981-13-6958-2_27

the study of standard of living. In fact, the study of quality of life is very important from the point of view of the development of an area. In this sense, quality of life is one of the major aspects of developmental studies. Wealth, material possessions, access to health care, etc. can all be measured but this only reveals the standard of living. Thus, anyone who lacks the basic human needs of food, water, shelter, freedom and access to education has necessarily a poor standard of living. 'Quality of Life' is much more than this and aims to assess a person's overall happiness and is, therefore, an extremely complex phenomenon. Standard indicators include not only wealth and employment but also the environment, physical and mental health, recreation, leisure time and social belonging. The World Health Organization (WHO) defines the term 'quality of life' as a perception about the status of one's life with regard to the prevailing cultural systems in which he/she lives and in relation to their goals, expectations, standards and concerns. In the opinion of Diener and Suh (1997) feelings are also indicative of the quality of life as feelings are for the most part a reaction to the effect of external forces. Normally, the word well-being is also used while explaining the quality of life. This involves several emotional aspects that happened in the life of someone. Thus, in evaluating a person's life one should include how frequently and intensely the person experiences pleasure, unhappiness or despair, resentment, anxiety or tension and how much affection he/she receives from family, friends and society. All these are factors of a person's emotional well-being. Diener and Suh evaluated a respondent's replies about his/her emotional experiences against a scale which they had devised. Ferrans and Powers (1985) (https://qli.org.uic.edu/overview/overviewhome.htm) devised quality of life index (QOLI) for computing the level of satisfaction with life. This index provides an idea about the satisfaction and importance concerning different dimensions of life. According to Ferrans (1990, p. 15) quality of life is 'a person's sense of well-being that stems from satisfaction or dissatisfaction with the areas of life that are important to him/her'. They pointed out that the quality of life index is generally the result of health and its functioning, psychological and spiritual aspect, socio-economic aspect and aspects related to family.

Man is a social animal and a society is formed by a large combination of households and its people. A household may be defined as a house or home and all its members who share meals cooked in one pot. It is a self-contained unit and supports itself financially and provides sustenance to nurture its members with physical and emotional care. It relies on the infrastructure of the State to provide education, medical care, drinking water, roads, public transport, police protection, etc. All these internal and external factors have a bearing on the lives of the household members. Different socio-cultural and economic components determine qualitatively the life of a person. If the quality of life of a person is high, this, in turn, has a positive impact on other family members as well as on the household.

27.2 Objective

This study aims at analysing variation in the level of quality of life of the surveyed persons at household level across different social groups, family size, educational achievement category, income and occupational category and to put forth some appropriate suggestions for the enhancement and maintenance of quality of life.

27.3 Approach of the Study

This paper is based exclusively on the primary data collected from personal field survey. For this the study area 'Bolpur Town' of Birbhum District, West Bengal was selected. This area is divided into 18 wards (Fig. 27.2). From each ward, the number of households selected was purposely fixed in the range of 15–20. The households in this range from each ward were randomly selected. While conducting the household survey it was kept in mind that the numbers of household in each ward from each social group namely General Caste (G.C.), Other Backward Caste (O.B.C.), Muslim, Scheduled Caste (S.C.) and Scheduled Tribe (S.T.) should be almost equal. However, most of the wards have very few numbers of Muslim and S.T. households as the majority of households in almost all wards in Bolpur town are from G.C., O.B.C. and S.C. In this way, the total number of households from all 18 wards became 350. At least one respondent from each household was selected to fill up a questionnaire. Thus, the total number of households and respondents became 350 who furnished the information of about 1,748 persons. Quality of life index was calculated after giving weightage to all the determinants. Individual's weightage of all the determinants of a household are summed up to get household-level weightage (Fig. 27.1).

27.4 Location of the Study Area

The study area is situated in the south-eastern portion of Birbhum District, West Bengal. Bolpur town is situated in Bolpur subdivision under Bolpur Police Station. The geographical location of Bolpur town is 23° 39′ 46.01″ N and 87° 41′ 49.02″ E. The town is almost in the central part of the jurisdiction of Bolpur Police station and also in between Kopai River in the north and Ajoy River in the south. It is situated on the Burdwan–Sahebganj loop line of Eastern Railway which has immense importance in the development of this town.

27.5 Demographic Attribute of the Study Area

Demographic attributes of an area play a significant role in the life condition. Such attributes are also known as population characteristics and have some direct or indirect effect on quality of life. Demographic attributes may include size, distribution, density, growth and population change over time, age and sex, literacy/education,

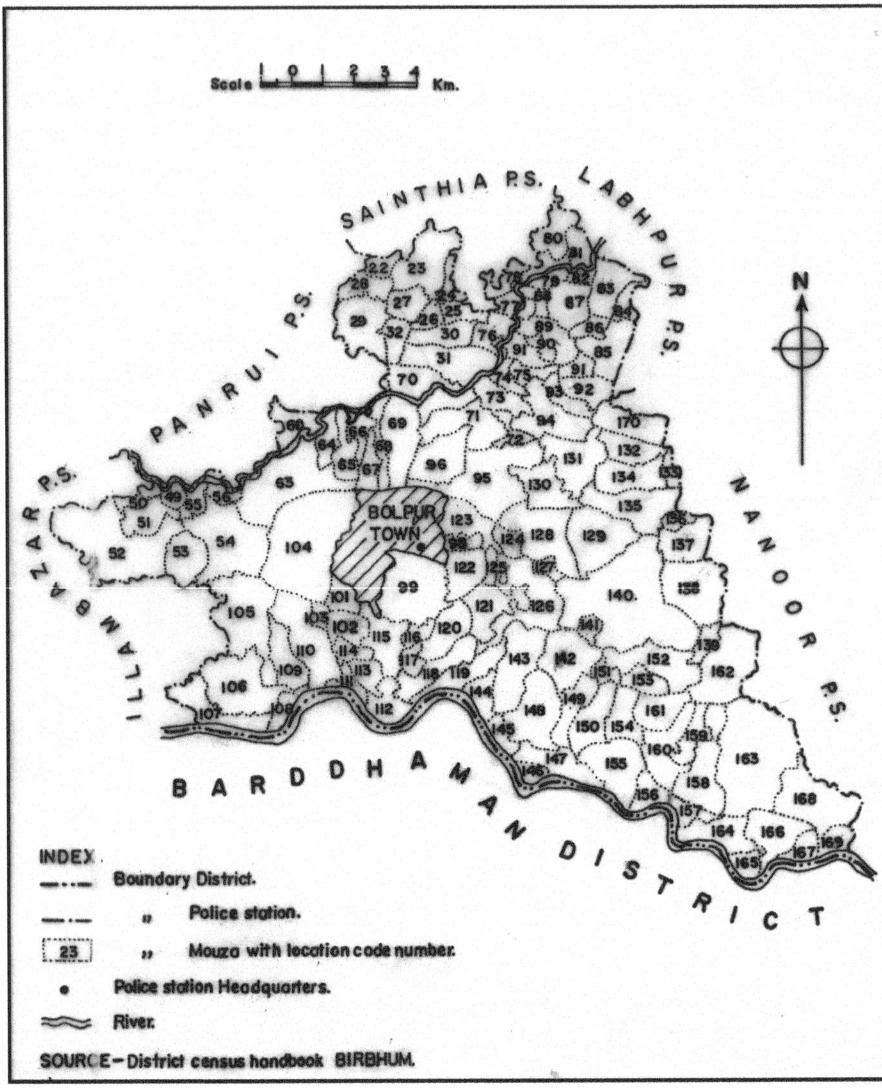

Fig. 27.1 Reference map: Location Code Number of Mauza in Bolpur Police Station of Birbhum District, West Bengal

health, social structure, income, occupation in a defined area and in a given time. Population characteristics may be grouped into quantitative and qualitative aspects of the human population. The population can be analysed from a demographic point of view from the moment it is subject to a continuous process of change as time goes on. Age–sex composition is one of the important aspects of population study. It has profound effects on the socio-cultural and economic conditions under which a population lives.

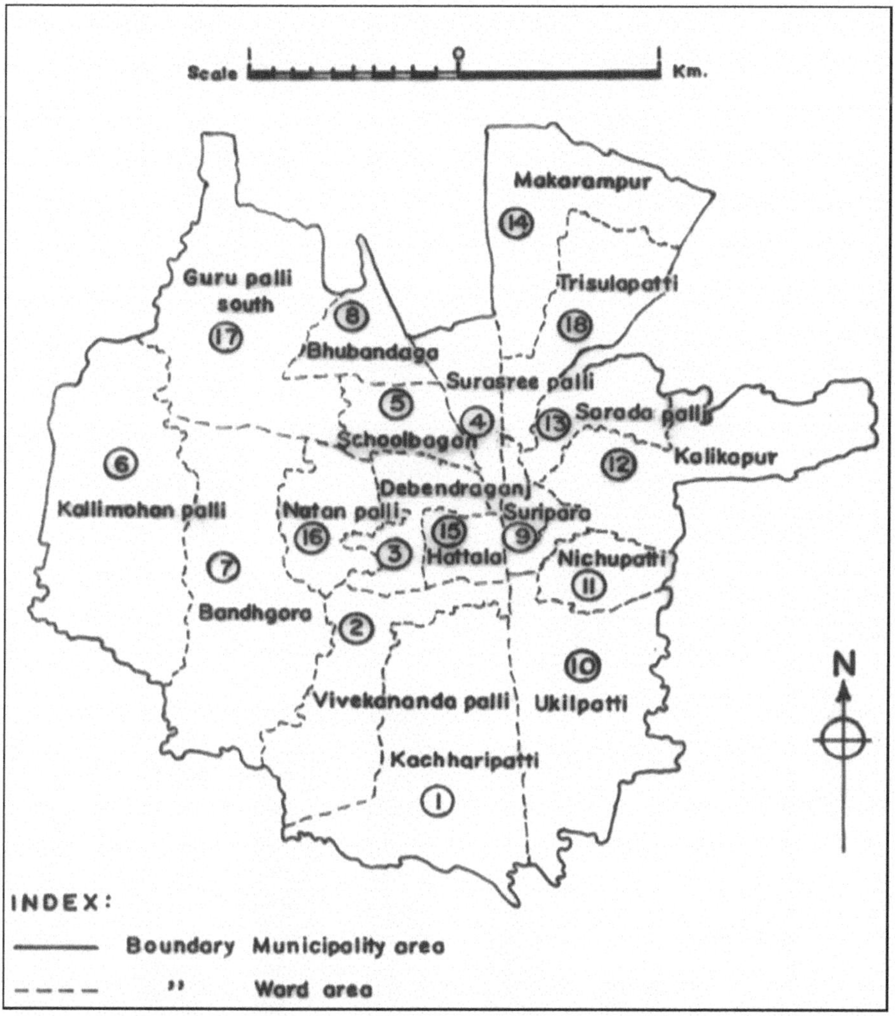

Fig. 27.2 Reference map: Ward Map of Bolpur Municipality

Table 27.1 and Fig. 27.3 clearly show the distribution of households. It is evident that the maximum percentage of urban males and females are found in the 15–34 year age group and next is in 35–59 year age group. The percentage of respondents is comparatively much lower than the independents. Thus, the total dependency ratio is calculated as 41.08%.

Table 27.2 and Fig. 27.4 exhibit that the largest number of households belongs to Scheduled Caste (29.43%) of the surveyed urban households, 92 (26.29%) households were from Higher Caste, 82 (23.43%) were from Other Backward Caste, 41 (11.71%) were from Muslim families and Scheduled Tribe households were only (9.14%).

Table 27.1 Pattern of the surveyed population by age group and sex in Bolpur town

Age group	Gender		Total population
	M	F	
0–4	46 5.26[a]	50 5.72	96 (5.49)[b]
5–14	121 13.84	136 15.56	257 (14.70)
15–34	346 39.59	326 37.30	672 (38.44)
35–59	278 31.81	289 33.07	567 (32.44)
60+	83 9.50	73 8.35	156 (8.92)
Grand total	874 (50.00)	874 (50.00)	1748 (100.00)

Source Investigator's Household Survey (Bolpur town) 2005

[a]Unbracketed lower figures in the cells are the percentages to total male or female population of all age groups

[b]Bracketed lower figures are the percentages to the grand total population

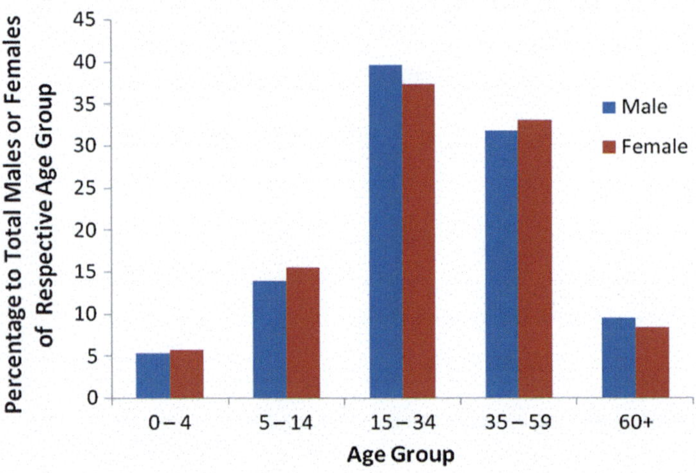

Fig. 27.3 Age and sex wise pattern of surveyed population in Bolpur town

Table 27.2 Pattern of households by social group in Bolpur town

Number and % of households	Social group					Total surveyed households
	H.C.	O.B.C.	S.C.	S.T.	Muslim	
Number of households	92	82	103	32	41	350
% to total households	26.29	23.43	29.43	9.14	11.71	100.00

Source Investigator's Household Survey (Bolpur town) 2005

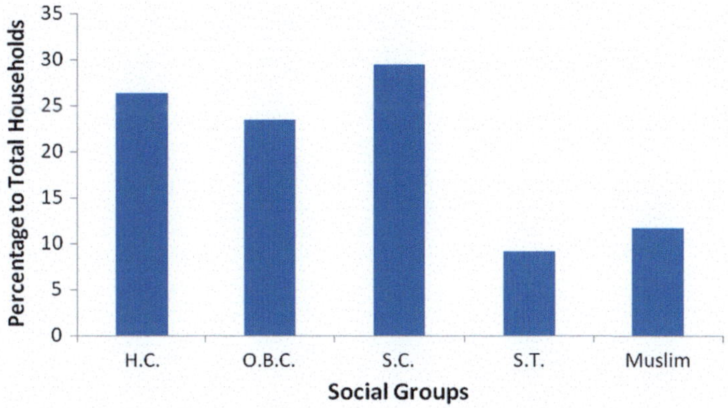

Fig. 27.4 Social group wise pattern of surveyed population in Bolpur town

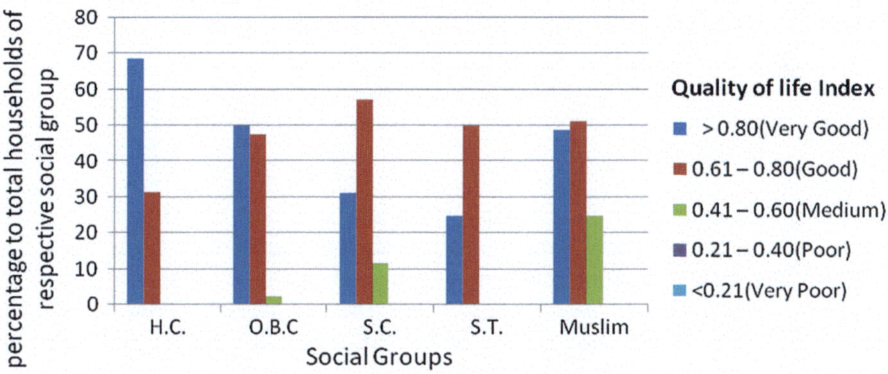

Fig. 27.5 Quality of life index and surveyed households of different social group in Bolpur town

27.6 Households Level Quality of Life

Quality of life varies with different components like social groups, educational achievement category, family size, occupational category, gross income, per capita income, etc. at household level. The spread of value and attitude can be achieved through education and one of the important needs of life is education.

Quality of life of the families varies across different social groups as mentioned above. This is because of variation in the social–cultural, economic and environmental conditions of the concerned area. From Table 27.3 and Fig. 27.5 it is found that 63 (68.48%) houses of Higher Caste enjoyed very good quality of life and 29 (31.52%) a good quality of life. In the same way 41 (50%) Other Backward Caste houses were found in very good quality of life category, 39 (47.56) in good quality of life category and rest 2 (2.44%) houses were found enjoying medium category of quality of life.

Out of the total Scheduled Caste households 59 (57.28%) were in good quality of life category that is between 0.61 and 0.80 quality of life index. 32 (31.07%)

Table 27.3 Pattern of surveyed households of different social groups by quality of life index in Bolpur town

Quality of life index and level	Social group wise households					Total households
	H.C.	O.B.C.	S.C.	S.T.	Muslim	
>0.80 (very good)	63 68.48	41 50.00	32 31.07	8 25.00	20 48.78[a]	164 (46.86)[b]
0.61–0.80 (Good)	29 31.52	39 47.56	59 57.28	16 50.00	21 51.22	164 (46.86)
0.41–0.60 (medium)	–	2 2.44	12 11.65		8 25.00	22 (6.29)
0.21–0.40 (poor)	–	–	–		–	–
<0.21 (very poor)	–	–	–		–	–
Grand total	92 (26.29)	82 (23.43)	103 (29.43)		32 (9.14)	350 (100.00)

Source Investigator's Household Survey (Bolpur P.S.) 2005
[a]Unbracketed lower figures are the percentages to total households of respective social group
[b]Bracketed lower figures are the percentages to grand total surveyed households

households belong to very good quality of life category and 12 (11.65%) were in the medium category that is between 0.41 and 0.60 on the quality of life index. 21 (51.22%) Muslim houses were found enjoying a good quality of life and 20 (68.48%) found to be enjoying a very good quality of life, whereas 16 (50%) of the Scheduled Tribe houses were in the good quality of life category and 8 (25%) each were in medium and very good quality of life categories.

The detailed picture of the distribution of urban households across different social groups shows that the majority of families from Higher Caste and Other Backward

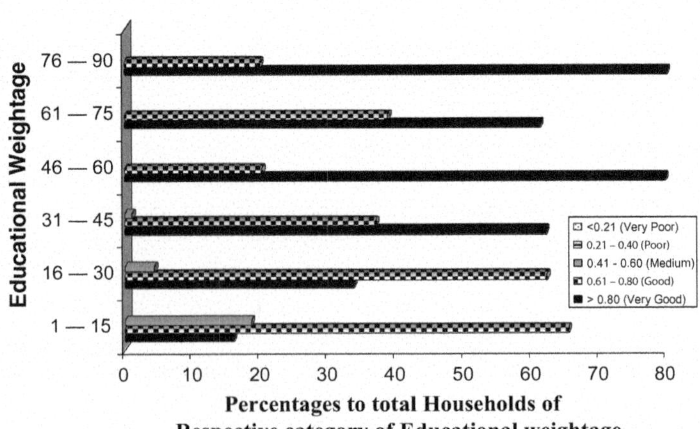

Fig. 27.6 Quality of life index and surveyed households by educational weightage in Bolpur town

Caste houses enjoy a very good quality of life, whereas the majority of families from Muslim, Scheduled Caste and Scheduled Tribe enjoy good quality of life. However, most families from Scheduled Caste, Scheduled Tribe and a few from Other Backward Caste houses were found enjoying medium category of quality of life too. This indicates that in general, the quality of life of the H.C. and Other Backward Caste families is relatively better than that of the families of other social groups. This is a result of differential socio-economic conditions of the houses.

Quality of life of the families of urban houses also varies from one category of educational weightage to another as shown in Table 27.4 and Fig. 27.6. Out of 350 urban households 344 belonged to different levels of educational achievement. Only 6 urban households were from the totally illiterate category. From Table 27.4 and Fig. 27.6, it is evident that the majority of urban houses belonged to very good quality of life index and have the highest educational weightage, i.e. 76–90, whereas the households having a lower educational weightage were in the medium quality of life index. Therefore, it can be said that education is one of the determinants of quality of life.

Out of the total 350 urban households, 16 (4.57%) belong to the family size of <3 persons. 223 (63.71%) and 94 (26.86%) belong to the medium family size between

Table 27.4 Households level scores of educational weightage by quality of life index in Bolpur town

Quality of life index and level	Category of household level scores of educational weightage						Total households
	1–15	16–30	31–45	46–60	61–75	76–90	
>0.80 (very good)	12 16.00[a]	32 33.68	57 61.96	47 79.66	11 61.11	4 80.00	163 (47.38)[b]
0.61–0.80 (good)	49 65.33	59 62.11	34 36.96	12 20.34	7 38.89	1 20.00	162 (47.09)
0.41–0.60 (medium)	14 18.67	4 4.21	1 1.09	–	–	–	19 (5.52)
0.21–0.40 (poor)	–	–	–	–	–	–	–
<0.21 (very poor)	–	–	–	–	–	–	–
Grand total	75 (21.80)	95 (27.62)	92 (26.74)	59 (17.15)	18 (5.23)	5 (1.45)	344 (100.00)

Source Investigator's Household Survey (Bolpur town) 2005

[a]Unbracketed lower figures are the percentages to total households of respective category of educational scores

[b]Bracketed lower figures are the percentages to grand total households

Table 27.5 Surveyed households by family size and quality of life index in Bolpur town

Quality of life index and level	Family size (in terms of number of persons)				Total households
	0–2	3–5	6–8	9–11	
>0.80 (very good)	6 37.5[a]	108 48.43	47 50	3 (17.65)	164 (46.86)[b]
0.61–0.80 (good)	7 43.75	103 46.19	40 42.55	14 (82.35)	164 (46.86)
0.41–0.60 (medium)	3 18.75	12 5.38	7 7.45	–	22 (6.29)
0.21–0.40 (poor)	–	–	–	–	–
<0.21 (very poor)	–	–	–	–	–
Grand total	16 (4.57)	223 (63.71)	94 (26.86)	17 (4.86)	350 (100.00)

Source Investigator's Household Survey (Bolpur P.S.) 2005
[a]Unbracketed lower figures are the percentages to total households of respective category of family size
[b]Bracketed lower figures are the percentages to grand total households

3–5 and 6–8 persons, respectively. 17 households constituting 4.86% belonged to the larger family size of 9–11 persons. When one looks at the quality of life index, it is found that 108 (48.43%) households having family size of 3–5 persons were in the very good and good quality of life categories and only 22 (6.29%) households having a family size of 3–5 and 6–8 persons were in the medium category of quality of life. In this study area, medium size families (3–5 and 6–8 persons) dominate the study area. The above pictures are clearly exhibited in Table 27.5 and Fig. 27.7.

Household level quality of life varies at income level too. From Table 27.6 and Fig. 27.8, it is evident that out of the total (350) urban households the highest number of households, i.e. 94 (26.86%) were found in the income category of Rs. 1000–3001 and very few households were in the income category of Rs. 30,001–40,000 and only 10 (2.86%) households were in the income category of Rs. <1000. Thus, the majority of urban households of the study area were in lower and middle-income categories. The number of households was found decreasing towards the higher income category. This pattern indicates that the urban houses enjoying a very good quality of life have a high level of income and the urban houses enjoying very poor quality of life have lower income.

Table 27.7 and Fig. 27.9 evidently show variation in the pattern of household level quality of life across per capita income category. The highest number of households was found in the lowest per capita income category, i.e. in Rs. <500 and a very small number of households were found towards higher per capita income category. Urban households having a high per capita income were found enjoying a very good quality of life whereas, households having medium and low per capita income were found in the good and medium category of quality of life index.

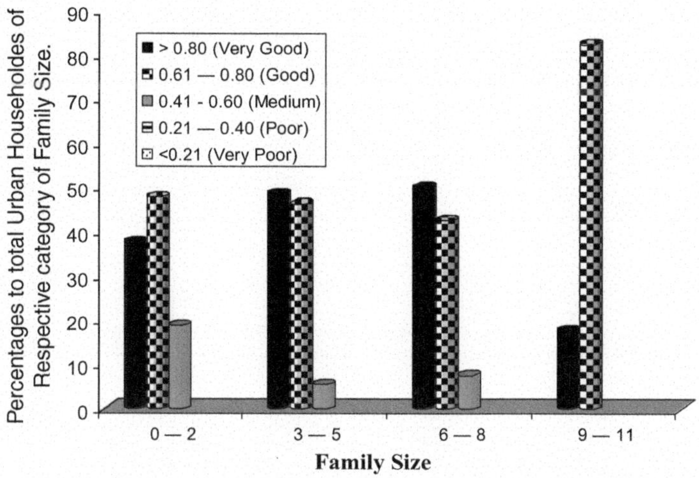

Fig. 27.7 Quality of life index and surveyed households by family size in Bolpur town

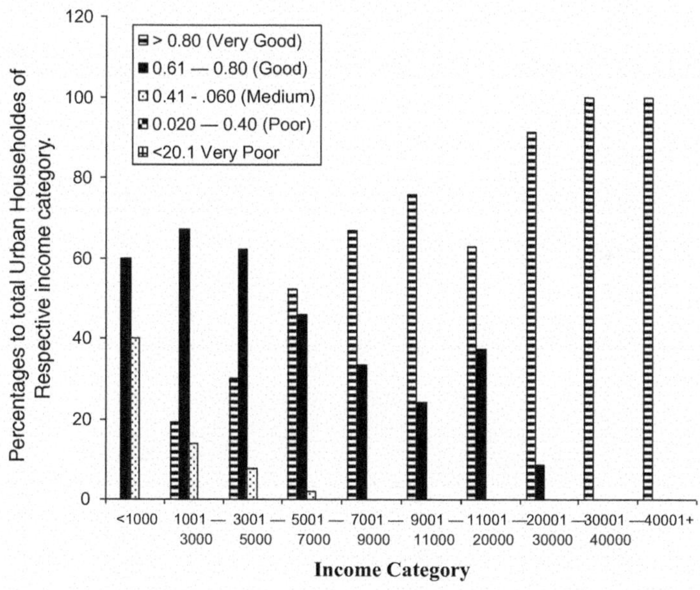

Fig. 27.8 Quality of life index and surveyed households by income category in Bolpur town

Table 27.6 Quality of life index and surveyed households by household income category in Bolpur town

Quality of life index and level	Household level income category										Total house-holds
	<1000	1001–3000	3001–5000	5001–7000	7001–9000	9001–11,000	11,001–20,000	20,001–30,000	30,001–40,000	40,001+	
>0.80 (very good)	–	18 19.15[a]	16 30.19	25 52.08	18 66.66	22 75.86	37 62.71	21 91.30	6 100.00	1 100.00	164 (46.86)[b]
0.61–0.80 (good)	6 60.00	63 67.02	33 62.26	22 45.83	9 33.33	7 24.14	22 37.29	2 8.70	–	–	164 (46.86)
0.41–0.60 (medium)	4 40.00	13 13.83	4 7.55	1 2.08	–	–	–	–	–	–	22 (6.29)
0.21–0.40 (poor)	–	–	–	–	–	–	–	–	–	–	–
<0.21 (very poor)	–	–	–	–	–	–	–	–	–	–	–
Grand total	10 (2.86)	94 (26.86)	53 (15.14)	48 (13.71)	27 (7.71)	29 (8.29)	59 (16.86)	23 (6.57)	6 (1.71)	1 (0.29)	350 (100.00)

Source Investigator's Household Survey (Bolpur P.S.) 2005

[a]Unbracketed lower figures are the percentages to total households of respective income category

[b]Bracketed lower figures are the percentages to total households

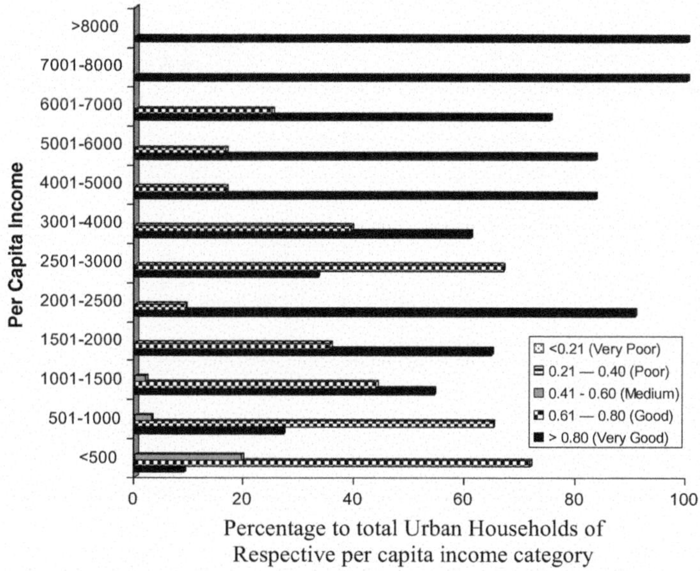

Fig. 27.9 Quality of life index and surveyed households by per capita income category in Bolpur town

From Table 27.8 and Fig. 27.10, it is found that out of the total 350 urban households 343 households were found with certain types of economic activities but 7 households were such which did not report any type of occupation because such houses belonged to retired persons and other types of persons were found depending on the income and occupation of other family members. The maximum households were in trade and commerce and in other services. Since the study area is urban, very few households were found in primary activity. Only a few households were in the secondary sector of the economy due to lack of industries. Those families whose major occupations were other services and trade and commerce enjoy a better quality of life.

27.7 Conclusion

The study area 'Bolpur town' is a town for national importance and derives its meaning and significance from Santiniketan, the traditionally rich centre of Indian culture and a site of education. Quality of life of urban households varies across different social groups, income categories, educational levels, per capita income and occupational categories. Houses belonging to higher caste were found enjoying a better quality of life. Out of the total 350 households, 344 households belonged to different levels of educational achievement. Only 6 urban households were from the

Table 27.7 Quality of life index and surveyed households by per capita income category in Bolpur town

Quality of life index and level	Per capita income category												Total households
	<500	501–1000	1001–1500	1501–2000	2001–2500	2501–3000	3001–4000	4001–5000	5001–6000	6001–7000	7001–8000	>8000	
>0.80 (very good)	7 9.09[a]	20 27.03	26 54.17	31 64.58	29 90.63	2 33.33	17 60.71	10 83.33	10 83.33	3 75.00	2 100.00	7 100.00	164 (46.86)[b]
0.61–0.80 (good)	55 71.43	48 64.86	21 43.75	17 35.42	3 9.38	4 66.67	11 39.29	2 16.67	2 16.67	1 25.00	–	–	164 (46.86)
0.41–0.60 (medium)	15 19.48	6 8.10	1 2.08	–	–	–	–	–	–	–	–	–	22 (6.29)
0.21–0.40 (poor)	–	–	–	–	–	–	–	–	–	–	–	–	–
<0.21 (very poor)	–	–	–	–	–	–	–	–	–	–	–	–	–
Grand total	77 (22.00)	74 (21.14)	48 (13.71)	48 (13.71)	32 (9.14)	6 (1.71)	28 (8.00)	12 (3.43)	12 (3.43)	4 (1.14)	2 (0.57)	7 (2.00)	350 (100.00)

Source Investigator's Household Survey (Bolpur P.S.) 2005

[a]Unbracketed lower figures are the percentages to total households of respective per capita income category

[b]Bracketed lower figures are the percentages to total households

Table 27.8 Surveyed urban households by different occupations and quality of life index in Bolpur town

Quality of life index and level	Occupational status								Total households
	Cultivators	Agricultural labourers	Livestock farmers	Construction works	Industrial works	Trade and commerce	Transport and communication	Other services	
>0.80 (very good)	3 50.00[a]	–	–	1 3.26	3 13.64	61 44.85	9 31.03	85 66.41	162 (47.23)[b]
0.61–0.80 (good)	3 50.00	–	–	16 84.21	13 59.09	70 51.47	14 48.28	43 33.59	159 (46.35)
0.41–0.60 (medium)	–	–	3 100	2 10.52	6 27.27	5 3.68	6 20.69		22 (6.41)
0.21–0.40 (poor)	–	–	–	–	–	–	–	–	–
<0.21 (very poor)	–	–	–	–	–	–	–	–	–
Grand total	6 (1.75)	–	3 (0.87)	19 (5.54)	22 (6.41)	136 (39.65)	29 (8.45)	128 (37.32)	343 (100.00)

Source Investigator's Household Survey (Bolpur P.S.) 2005
[a]Unbracketed lower figures are the percentages to total households of respective occupational category
[b]Bracketed lower figures are the percentages to total households

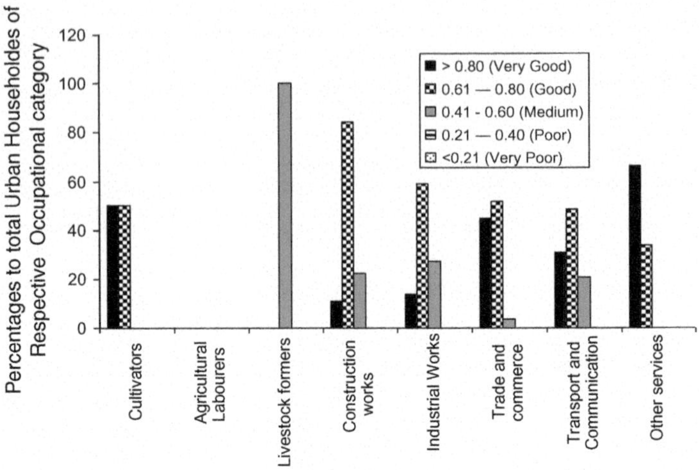

Fig. 27.10 Quality of life index of surveyed households by different occupations in Bolpur town

totally illiterate category. Even despite a close connection of the study area with the milieu of the educational hub of Visva-Bharati, Santiniketan (a central university), the majority of households were in the medium level category of educational achievement. Households having high educational weightage enjoy very good quality of life. Majority of the houses belonged to the category of lower family size and shows a trend of increasing nuclear family. Small family sized households were found enjoying a very good quality of life. The study area is not sound from the point of view of economic development because most of the houses showed medium level household and per capita income. People of such houses had medium and poor category of quality of life. Very few households had a high household income and high per capita income. Such households normally enjoy better quality of life. Therefore, there is a need for formulating appropriate plans and policies with a view to increase education and income. Diversification of occupations would be an alternative mechanism for creating jobs for educated youths.

The households having a predominance of trade and commerce and other services enjoy comparatively better quality of life say, very good quality of life. Such occupations generally generate a better income which in turn helps increase the educational level. To sum up, more emphasis needs to be given on developing the economy of the study area as well as on improving the level of education with a view to increase the quality of life of common people in the study area.

References

Diener, E., & Suh, E. (1997). Measuring quality of life: Economic, social and subjective indicators. *Social Indicators Research, 40,* 189–216.

Ferrans, C. E. (1990). Development of a quality of life index for patients with cancer. *Oncology Nursing Forum, 17*(3), 15–19. Retrieved from https://qli.org.uic.edu/overview/overviewhome.htm.

Ferrans, C. E., & Powers, M. (1985). Quality of life index: Development and psychometric properties. *Advances in Nursing Science, 8,* 15–24.

The World Health Organization (WHO). Retrieved from http://www.who.int/healthinfo/survey/whoqol-qualityoflife/en/.

Index

B. R. K. Sinha (ed.), *Multidimensional Approach to Quality of Life Issues*,
https://doi.org/10.1007/978-981-13-6958-2

O

P

Q

R

The manufacturer's authorised representative in the EU is Springer Nature Customer Service Centre GmbH, Europaplatz 3, 69115 Heidelberg, Germany. If you have any concerns regarding our products, please contact ProductSafety@springernature.com

Printed and bound by CPI Group (UK) Ltd, Croydon, CR0 4YY

30/09/2026

02225304-0018